Essentials of Surgical Specialties

THIRD EDITION

Essentials of Surgical Specialties

THIRD EDITION

SENIOR EDITOR

PETER F. LAWRENCE, MD
Bergman Professor and Chief of Vascular Surgery
Department of Surgery
David Geffen School of Medicine at UCLA
Los Angeles, California

EDITORS

RICHARD M. BELL, MD
Professor and Chairman
Department of Surgery
University of South Carolina School of Medicine
Columbia, South Carolina

MERRIL T. DAYTON, MD
Professor and Chairman
Department of Surgery
State University of New York at Buffalo
Buffalo, New York

TEXTBOOK CONTENT EDITOR

MOHAMMED I. AHMED, MBBS, MS (SURGERY)
Clinical Instructor
Department of Surgery
Affiliated Institute for Medical Education
Chicago, Illinois

QUESTION BANK EDITOR

JAMES C. HEBERT, MD
Professor
Department of Surgery
The University of Vermont College of Medicine
Burlington, Vermont

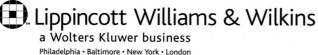 Lippincott Williams & Wilkins
a Wolters Kluwer business
Philadelphia • Baltimore • New York • London
Buenos Aires • Hong Kong • Sydney • Tokyo

Acquisitions Editor: Nancy Anastasi Duffy
Developmental Editor: Catherine C. Council and Kathleen H. Scogna
Marketing Manager: Jennifer Kuklinski
Associate Production Manager: Kevin P. Johnson
Designer: Holly Reid McLaughlin
Compositor: Maryland Composition
Printer: Courier

Printed in the United States of America

First Edition, 1993
Second Edition, 2000

Library of Congress Cataloging-in-Publication Data

Essentials of surgical specialties / senior editor, Peter F. Lawrence ; editors, Richard M. Bell,
Merril T. Dayton ; textbook content editor, Mohammed I. Ahmed ; question bank editor,
James C. Hebert. — 3rd ed.
    p. ; cm.
Includes bibliographical references and index.
ISBN 0-7817-5004-0
1. Surgery. I. Lawrence, Peter F. II. Bell, Richard M. III. Dayton, Merril T. IV. Title.
[DNLM: 1. Surgical Procedures, Operative. 2. Specialties, Surgical — methods. WO 500
E783 2007]
RD31.E875 2007
617 — dc22

                    2006011197

---

06 07 08 09 10
1 2 3 4 5 6 7 8 9 10

Contents

Preface

Approximately half of all medical students enter such primary care fields as family practice, general internal medicine, and obstetrics and gynecology. The clinical problems that they will address in daily practice should be the basis for their clinical training in undergraduate medical education. Previous studies have shown that more than 50% of primary care practice involves surgical problems. Other studies indicate that more than 60% of emergency room visits are surgically related. Because the types of clinical problems faced by primary care and emergency room physicians often require knowledge of surgery, surgical principles are best taught by surgeons, whether from orthopedics, otolaryngology, ophthalmology, or urology. For example, the otolaryngologist, who sees the anatomy and pathology of the ear daily, is best equipped to teach the approach to diseases of the ears, including common problems such as otitis media in children.

We believe that this textbook, *Essentials of Surgical Specialties*, should be of great value to all medical students, particularly those who are not entering a surgical field. The surgical specialists contributing to this book have been asked to address only the most important principles and the common diseases pertaining to their specialty. Uncommon diseases are not discussed. Consequently, if you, the student, master the material in this textbook for each of these surgical specialties, you will have a solid foundation and understanding of most of the surgically related problems you will see in your everyday practice, whether you enter a primary care field, a nonsurgical specialty, or a surgical specialty.

We have included diagrams and instructions to assist you in learning the most common technical procedures that all physicians need to master in each specialty. An example is bladder catheterization, an extremely common procedure used to diagnose genitourinary problems and monitor urine output in many clinical situations. Knowledge of the anatomy of the bladder and the urethra as well as familiarity with the proper technique for catheter insertion will reduce the likelihood of unsuccessful bladder catheterization. Additionally, knowledge of the common causes of urethral stricture, which may preclude catheter placement, should help you understand the potential complications or causes of failure of catheterization.

This textbook is designed to be used in conjunction with our textbook in general surgery, *Essentials of General Surgery*. Like the general surgery textbook, the specialties book has multiple-choice questions accessible on the Lippincott Williams and Wilkins CONNECTION web site (http://connection.lww.com/lawrence). Students can use these USMLE-type questions to review and test themselves on material contained in the chapter. Important terms appear in boldface in the text and are defined in the glossary.

We hope that this volume of our surgical educational program will prepare you to care for patients with clinical problems in the specialty fields of surgery and anesthesia. Best wishes for your career in medicine, whether it is in a surgical or a nonsurgical field.

Acknowledgments

This project was nurtured by many members of the Association for Surgical Education (ASE), whose advice and expertise I would like to acknowledge. At its annual meetings, the ASE provides an excellent forum to discuss and test ideas about the content of the surgical curriculum and methods to teach and evaluate what has been learned.

Dr. Mohammed Ahmed, MBBS, MS (Surgery), has recently joined our team of editors and has added greatly to the textbook quality by carefully reading and editing the content of every section and chapter. My thanks go as well to Cathy Council, our editor in Salt Lake City, who has spent two years editing, revising, and coordinating all components of this project. I also thank my editors at Lippincott Williams & Wilkins, Donna Balado and Kathleen Scogna.

Contributors

Gerald Berke, MD
Professor of Surgery
Chief, Division of Head and Neck Surgery
David Geffen School of Medicine at UCLA
Los Angeles, California

Andrew Celmer, MD
Clinical Instructor
Division of Head and Neck Surgery
David Geffen School of Medicine at UCLA
Los Angeles, California

Alan S. Crandall, Jr., MD
Professor and Senior Vice Chair
Ophthalmology and Visual Sciences
John A. Moran Eye Center
University of Utah
Salt Lake City, Utah

Barry P. Duel, MD
Assistant Clinical Professor
Division of Urology
School of Medicine
University of California, Irvine
Irvine, California

Gregory R.D. Evans, MD
Professor of Surgery and Biomedical Engineering
Chief, Aesthetic and Plastic Surgery Institute
University of California, Irvine
Irvine, California

Toni M. Ganzel, MD
Professor of Surgery
Division of Otolaryngology
Department of Surgery
University of Louisville
Louisville, Kentucky

Joel Gelman, MD
Assistant Clinical Professor
Division of Urology
School of Medicine
University of California, Irvine
Irvine, California

Richard C. Haydon, MD
Professor of Surgery
Division of Otolaryngology
Department of Surgery
University of Kentucky
Lexington, Kentucky

Constance H. Hill, MD
Clinical Professor of Anesthesia
State University of New York at Brooklyn
Brooklyn, New York

Marshall L. Jacobs, MD
Professor of Cardiac Medicine and Surgery
Drexel University College of Medicine
Chief of Cardiothoracic Surgery
St. Christopher's Hospital for Children
Philadelphia, Pennsylvania

Isaac Yi Kim, MD, PhD
Assistant Professor
Division of Urology
The Cancer Institute of New Jersey
Robert Wood Johnson Medical School
New Brunswick, New Jersey

Mark E. Linskey, MD
Associate Professor and Chairman
Department of Neurological Surgery
University of California, Irvine
Irvine, California

John J.A. Marota, MD, PhD
Assistant Professor of Anesthesia
Harvard Medical School
Cambridge, Massachusetts

John J. Murnaghan, MD
Assistant Professor of Orthopaedic Surgery
Division of Orthopaedic Surgery
Faculty of Medicine, University of Toronto
Toronto, Ontario, Canada

Barbara Pettitt, MD
Assistant Professor of Surgery
Emory University School of Medicine
Chief of Pediatric Surgery
Grady Health System/Hughes Spalding Children's
   Hospital
Atlanta, Georgia

Dan Poenaru, MD
Adjunct Professor of Surgery and Paediatrics
Queen's University
Kingston, Ontario
Hon. Professor of Surgery
Aga Khan University
Nairobi, Kenya

Susan L. Polk, MD, MSEd
Professor of Clinical Anesthesia and Critical Care
University of Chicago
Chicago, Illinois

Irving Raber, MD
Clinical Assistant Professor of Ophthalmology
Wills Eye Hospital
Jefferson Medical College
Philadelphia, Pennsylvania

David Rogers, MD
Professor of Surgery and Pediatrics
Southern Illinois University School of Medicine
Springfield, Illinois

Arthur J.L. Schneider, MD
Professor of Anesthesiology
Medical College of the Pennsylvania State University
Hershey, Pennsylvania

Manisha R. Shende, MD
Assistant Professor
Department of Surgery
Division of Cardiothoracic Surgery
Robert Wood Johnson Medical School
New Brunswick, New Jersey

Alan Spotnitz, MD
Professor of Surgery
Surgical Director, Heart Center of New Jersey
Robert Wood Johnson Medical School
New Brunswick, New Jersey

Michael P. Teske, MD
Associate Professor of Ophthalmology and Visual
   Sciences
John A. Moran Eye Center
University of Utah
Salt Lake City, Utah

Joseph Valentino, MD
Associate Professor of Surgery
Division of Otolaryngology
Department of Surgery
University of Kentucky
Lexington, Kentucky

George L. White, Jr., PhD, MSPH
Professor and Director of Public Health Programs
Department of Family and Preventive Medicine
University of Utah
Salt Lake City, Utah

Garrett A. Wirth, MD
Assistant Clinical Professor of Surgery
Aesthetic and Plastic Surgery Institute
University of California, Irvine
Irvine, California

Philip J. Wolfson, MD
Professor of Surgery
Thomas Jefferson University
Chief, General Pediatric Surgery
Alfred I. duPont Hospital for Children
Wilmington, Delaware

SUSAN L. POLK ■ CONSTANCE H. HILL
JOHN J. A. MAROTA ■ ARTHUR J. L. SCHNEIDER

Anesthesiology

OBJECTIVES

1 Describe the information that the anesthesiologist should obtain from the patient during the preanesthetic visit.
2 Differentiate among the types of anesthesia, and give the indications for selection of type, based on the various surgical procedures.
3 Distinguish between general and regional anesthetics in terms of time course, general pharmacology, and toxicology.
4 Describe the pharmacologic and physiologic properties of commonly used sedative and local anesthetic agents.

5 Discuss the basic principles of airway management.
6 Describe the methods and devices used in anesthesiology to monitor the patient's oxygenation, circulation, respiration, and temperature.
7 Describe the immediate complications of anesthesia that occur in the postanesthesia care unit and discuss their management.
8 Discuss the management of postoperative pain.
9 Discuss the ways in which chronic medical conditions affect the patient in the perioperative period, and describe any special preoperative testing and preparation that is required.

Anesthesiologists render patients insensitive to surgery, manage their medical problems, and maintain their physiology at near normal during and immediately after the operative period. They are also involved in caring for patients in critical care units, managing the pain of labor and delivery, treating acute pain in the postoperative or postinjury period, and managing chronic pain syndromes. Basic knowledge in anesthesiology is derived from the fields of pharmacology and physiology and is helpful to physicians who manage patients who require surgery. This chapter discusses the role of the anesthesiologist in perioperative care, specific intraoperative drugs and anesthesia techniques, monitoring in the operative period, management of acute postoperative pain, and implications of concurrent medical conditions in the perioperative period. This chapter will familiarize students with the risks and hazards of anesthesia so that they can learn to prepare a patient, both physically and psychologically, for anesthesia and surgery. Students will also become acquainted with problems that are specific to anesthesia so that they can consult with the anesthesiologist about medical problems that may affect the patient's response to anesthesia and

surgery. Because many types of physicians supervise sedation for minor procedures, a brief discussion of local anesthetic and sedation drugs will provide basic knowledge necessary to ensure patient safety during those procedures.

PREOPERATIVE EVALUATION

Except in an emergency, no patient should undergo surgery until he or she is in optimal medical condition. Before surgery, the anesthesiologist must evaluate the patient's risk for the anesthetic and facilitate plans for anesthetic technique, monitoring, and postoperative care. During the preoperative evaluation, the anesthesiologist must prepare the patient and family psychologically for the upcoming procedure and must also establish physician–patient rapport. The anesthesiologist should discuss the planned anesthetic technique with the patient and document that the risks and benefits have been reviewed. The anesthesiologist should tell the patient when to stop eating and drinking before surgery, indicate the projected time of surgery, discuss the planned premedication, and explain what monitors will be used in the operating room. The patient should be prepared for the recovery room and recognize the possible need for ventilatory assistance, prolonged endotracheal intubation, or invasive monitoring. The patient should be told to expect some discomfort, be aware of postanesthesia procedures, and understand how he or she can contribute to restoring normal function (e.g., by coughing and deep breathing). Finally, the patient is asked to give informed consent for the anesthetic and monitoring interventions.

Traditionally, the preoperative evaluation for anesthesia was performed in the hospital on the day before surgery. Early preoperative evaluation allows the anesthesiologist and surgeon time for appropriate laboratory tests and consultations. Today, many patients arrive at the hospital on the day of surgery and must be evaluated either as outpatients or immediately before surgery. Test results or consultations may be difficult to obtain on short notice, so a clinic visit a few days before surgery is often arranged for any patient who is suspected of having a medical condition that might affect the choice of anesthetic technique. Some practices use telephone or computer-assisted screening to determine which patients should come to the preanesthesia clinic. In emergency procedures, the preoperative visit is made just before surgery because little time is available to test or adjust the patient's condition.

On completion of the preoperative visit, a summary of pertinent findings is written in the patient's record. Included in the summary are details of the patient's medical and anesthesia history, the patient's medication history, pertinent family history, physical examination findings, and laboratory data. Healthy, asymptomatic women who are younger than 40 years of age and have normal findings on physical examination need few laboratory tests (e.g., complete blood count [CBC] or just a hematocrit), although many experts think even these are not productive. Men with a similar profile often require no tests. The laboratory data that are traditionally requested for healthy patients who are older than 40 years of age include CBC, urinalysis, serum electrolytes, renal function tests, electrocardiogram, and chest x-ray, if indicated. Recent recommendations for patients who are 40 to 49 years old do not include a chest x-ray (unless there is a history of cardiac or pulmonary disease) or CBC, unless major blood loss is anticipated. Pregnancy tests are often ordered for women of childbearing age, but the American College of Obstetricians and Gynecologists recently issued a consensus report indicating that the routine use of such a test for anesthesia purposes is not cost-effective because little information indicates that anesthesia presents a risk to the fetus. Further tests are requested based on history, symptoms, or surgical procedure. Finally, a physical status classification is assigned based on criteria established by the American Society of Anesthesiologists (ASA). The ASA classification is not a prediction of anesthetic risk (of death) per se, but rather a description of the overall condition of the patient for purposes of comparison with other patients

Table 1-1	American Society of Anesthesiologists (ASA) Physical Status Classification
ASA I	Healthy patient
ASA II	Patient with mild systemic disease
ASA III	Patient with severe systemic disease that limits activity, but is not incapacitating
ASA IV	Patient with incapacitating systemic disease that is a constant threat to life
ASA V	Moribund patient who is not expected to survive 24 hours with or without surgery
ASA VI	Organ donor for harvest already declared brain dead
E	Notation added to the classification if the procedure is performed as an emergency

(Table 1-1). In cases of elective surgery where the patient is not in optimal medical condition, the anesthesiologist should discuss with the patient's primary physician or surgeon the possibility of postponing surgery.

History

The preanesthetic history should include a review of the following systems: cardiovascular, pulmonary, renal, hepatic, endocrine, metabolic, hematologic, and central nervous. For a thorough discussion of the interaction between disease and anesthesia, see the section on patient factors that influence anesthesia. A brief dental history should also be obtained, and the presence of dentures, loose teeth, and chipped, missing, or capped teeth noted. The time, composition, and amount of the last oral intake should be determined. In women, an obstetric and gynecologic history that includes the date of the last menstrual period should be obtained. A social history should include drug, alcohol, and tobacco use. A history of previous surgical and anesthetic procedures is important, including type of anesthesia and complications. A family history of anesthetic problems should also be obtained to rule out inherited conditions (e.g., cholinesterase abnormalities, malignant hyperthermia, porphyria). The medication history should include the names of drugs, their dosage and schedule, and allergies or unusual reactions. The time of the last dose is also noted. Dietary supplements and other herbal or nontraditional medicines are investigated because of the actions many have on sedative pharmacodynamics and coagulation function. Most medications are continued until the time of surgery. The exceptions are anticoagulants, herbal medicines that cause anticoagulation effects, and aspirin. If anticoagulant therapy is needed, warfarin should be withdrawn and heparin substituted for titration through the perioperative procedure.

Physical Examination

The physical examination is usually confined to the upper airway, the lungs, and the cardiovascular system. To assess possible difficulties in airway management, evaluation of the head and neck should include the size of the mouth and tongue, the condition of dentition, and the range of motion of the temporomandibular joint and cervical spine. Obesity, short neck, and tracheal deviation signal potential difficulties. The lungs are auscultated for the presence of abnormal breath sounds, rales, and wheezing. The cardiovascular examination consists of measurements of blood pressure, skin turgor, heart rate and rhythm; auscultation for cardiac murmurs and carotid bruits; and, in appropriate situations, assessment of intravascular volume status. If nasotracheal intubation is anticipated, the patency of both nasal passages should be assessed. Sites for intravenous access, invasive monitoring, and regional anesthesia should be examined for infection and anatomic abnormalities.

Psychological Preparation and Preoperative Medication

The goals of premedication are sedation, anxiolysis, and pain relief. In the immediate preoperative period, the patient should be calm and pain-free, but cooperative and easy to arouse. There is no recipe for this mental state, and drugs and doses must be tailored to the individual patient. Some anesthesiologists believe that the psychological preparation provided by the preoperative visit should address the patient's fear, thereby precluding the need for pharmacologic premedication. Elderly and debilitated patients usually require reduced or no premedication. Patients with increased intracranial pressure (ICP), chronic or acute lung disease, blood volume depletion, or altered levels of consciousness should not be premedicated until they are under the constant observation of the anesthesiologist, if at all. Premedication is often avoided in outpatients because it may prolong recovery time. Premedicants are classified as sedatives, narcotics, and anticholinergics. Other drugs administered before anesthesia might include those designed to reduce the possibility of regurgitation and aspiration of gastric contents or to prevent an allergic reaction to intravenous dyes and other drugs administered intraoperatively (most notably vancomycin). Table 1-2 lists commonly used premedication drugs with their doses and timing of administration.

Sedatives

Benzodiazepines and antihistamines are commonly used as preanesthetic sedatives. Benzodiazepines are tranquilizers that produce minimal cardiorespiratory depression when used in appropriate doses. They usually produce anterograde amnesia and may cause prolonged sedation. However, they are well known to ameliorate postanesthesia delirium, especially in children. Antihistamines have both sedative and antiemetic properties. They potentiate the sedative and analgesic properties of narcotics.

Table 1-2	Preoperative Medications		
Classification	**Medication**	**Dosage**	**When Administered**
Benzodiazepines	Diazepam (Valium)	5 mg PO	About 1 hour preop
	Lorazepam (Ativan)	0.5–2 mg PO	About 1 hour preop
	Midazolam (Versed)	1–2 mg IV	Immediately preop
Antihistamines	Promethazine (Phenegran)	25 mg IM	1 hour preop
	Hydroxazine (Vistaril)	25–50 mg IM	1 hour preop
Narcotics	Morphine	5–10 mg IM	1 hour preop
		2–5 mg IV	Immediately preop
	Demerol	25–50 mg IM	1 hour preop
		12.5–25 mg IV	Immediately preop
	Fentanyl	50–100 μg	Immediately preop
Anticholinergics	Atropine	0.02 mg/kg, up to 0.6 mg	Immediately preop
	Scopolamine	0.02 mg/kg, up to 0.4 mg	
	Glycopyrrolate (Robinol)	0.01 mg/kg, up to 0.2 mg	
Antacids	Cimetidine (Tagamet)	300 mg PO	The night before and the morning of surgery
	Ranitidine (Zantac)	50 mg IV	Immediately preop
	Famotidine (Pepcid)	20 mg IV	Immediately preop
		20 mg PO	Immediately preop
	Sodium citrate (Bicitra)	20 mL PO	Immediately preop
Gastric volume reduction	Metoclopramide (Reglan)	10 mg IV	Immediately preop
Allergy prophylaxis	Cimetidine	As above	As above
	Ranitidine	As above	As above
	Famotidine	As above	As above
	Benadryl	25–50 mg IV	Immediately predrug
	Hydrocortisone	100 mg IV	

Narcotics

Narcotics produce analgesia in patients with preoperative pain. They are also used to reduce discomfort in patients who are undergoing insertion of invasive monitoring lines or regional anesthesia. Because narcotics produce respiratory depression, they are best avoided in patients with decreased pulmonary reserve and in those in whom respiratory depression may be harmful (e.g., patients with increased ICP). Side effects include nausea, vomiting, orthostatic hypotension, and smooth muscle contraction. Narcotic premedication should be administered intravenously only when the patient can be monitored full time until induction of anesthesia.

Anticholinergics

Anticholinergic drugs are administered for their antisialagogue (salivation-reducing) effect, for prevention of reflex bradycardia (especially in children), and for their sedative and amnesic effects. Their intramuscular administration 1 hour before surgery has fallen into disfavor with many anesthesiologists because all of these agents are as effective and much more comfortable for the patient when given intravenously immediately before the induction of anesthesia. An antisialagogue effect is useful for intraoral surgery, when intraoral or nasal topical anesthesia is used, when intubation is planned with a fiberoptic bronchoscope, or when the use of a laryngeal mask airway is anticipated. Scopolamine and, to a lesser degree, atropine cross the blood–brain barrier and produce sedation and amnesic effects.

Side effects of anticholinergic drugs include central nervous system (CNS) toxicity (delirium or prolonged somnolence after anesthesia), tachycardia, elevation of body temperature, relaxation of the lower esophageal sphincter that results in passive gastric reflux, mydriasis, and cycloplegia. If the drugs are in effect while patients are conscious, patients usually complain of a dry mouth.

Prophylaxis for Pulmonary Aspiration

Sedation or anesthesia decreases both gastroesophageal sphincter integrity and airway protective reflexes, increasing the risk of aspiration. Although there is still some controversy about this, normal patients are usually assumed to have an empty stomach if they have refrained from solid food for 6 hours and from clear liquids (anything that can be seen through well enough to read) for at least 2 hours before induction. Infants may have milk up to 4 hours before anesthesia. Characteristics of patients who are at high risk for aspiration pneumonitis are listed in Table 1-3. Gastric contents flow into the pharynx either actively or passively and then are inhaled into the trachea during spontaneous or controlled respiration. An endotracheal tube with the cuff inflated is not a reliable seal of the trachea. The adverse effect of aspiration pneumonitis is markedly reduced by decreasing the acidity and volume of gastric contents.

Table 1-3	When to Assume a Full Stomach

Solid food intake within 6–8 hours in a normal adult
Pregnancy, regardless of last oral intake
Trauma victim, regardless of last oral intake
Bowel obstruction
Peritonitis
Ascites
Septic shock
Morbid obesity
Elderly patient with autonomic dysfunction
Diabetic patient with autonomic dysfunction
Parkinson's disease
Hiatal hernia, GERD
Esophageal abnormalities (achalasia, diverticula)
Hypothyroidism
Addison's disease
Chronic neuromuscular disorder

Acid Reduction

The H_2 antagonists cimetidine (Tagamet), ranitidine (Zantac), and famotidine (Pepcid) increase gastric fluid pH by inhibiting the ability of histamine to induce the secretion of gastric acid. Cimetidine prolongs the elimination of many drugs, including diazepam, lidocaine, theophylline, and propranolol. Proton pump inhibitors are effective for at least a day after regular use is discontinued and effectively prevent acid reflux. They include omeprazole (Prilosec), esomeprazole (Nexium), rabeprazole (Acidophex), lansoprazole (Prevacid), and pantoprazole (Protonix). Because particulate antacids (e.g., Maalox) can produce serious pneumonitis if aspirated, they are not used in this setting. Sodium citrate (Bicitra) orally on call to the operating room or immediately preinduction, is a safe, effective means of increasing the pH of gastric contents when a full stomach is anticipated. Although this agent increases the volume of gastric contents slightly, its ingestion does not increase the incidence of regurgitation or vomiting on induction of anesthesia.

Volume Reduction

Metoclopramide (Reglan) is a cholinergic stimulant that speeds gastric emptying by increasing the motility of the upper gastrointestinal tract and decreasing pyloric sphincter tone. It decreases intragastric volume, but has no effect on gastric fluid pH. It should be included in the preoperative preparation of patients who are suspected of having a significant volume of gastric contents.

OPERATIVE ANESTHETIC TECHNIQUES

Anesthetic techniques fall into one of three categories: general, regional, or local. These may be used either alone or in combination. General anesthesia is maintained by the use of gas, volatile anesthetics, intravenous drugs (narcotics, sedatives), and often muscle relaxants. Regional anesthesia is achieved by central or regional techniques. Central techniques include spinal, epidural, and caudal anesthesia. Peripheral techniques include nerve, plexus, and intravenous (Bier) blocks. The surgeon usually performs local anesthesia (infiltration of the tissues at the surgical site), although the anesthesiologist may stand by to monitor and sedate the patient, thus managing the patient's ongoing medical condition during surgery. The choice of anesthetic technique is the combined responsibility of the anesthesiologist, surgeon, and patient; often, there are several comparable options. After the alternatives, risks, and benefits of each are explained, the patient should be allowed to choose a technique. When deciding on anesthetic technique, several factors are taken into consideration. Most important is whether a local or regional technique will provide adequate analgesia given the site of surgery. The duration of the procedure and the position of the patient during the procedure must also be considered. Patient factors that influence the choice of anesthetic include the presence and type of coexisting diseases, bleeding tendencies, infection, patient age, and the possibility of a full stomach. Finally, the surgeon's and anesthesiologist's personalities and skill are important to consider when suggesting that a patient be conscious during surgery.

General Anesthesia

General anesthesia should provide analgesia, unconsciousness, muscle relaxation, and autonomic control. It is used whenever complete insensitivity is required, when the surgery involves a part of the body that is not amenable to regional or local anesthesia, when mechanical ventilation is necessary, or when the position required for the procedure does not allow the patient to be comfortable when awake. General anesthesia is achieved with a combination of inhalational anesthetics and other drugs (e.g., narcotics, sedatives, muscle relaxants).

Induction

Before induction, the patient is preoxygenated to minimize hypoxemia on induction. Induction begins with the intravenous injection of an ultra–short-acting drug, usually a barbiturate or propofol. Table 1-4 lists other drugs

that cause rapid loss of consciousness and may be used. When intubation of the trachea is planned, a **depolarizing** (succinylcholine) or **nondepolarizing** (pancuronium, atracurium, vecuronium, mivacurium, cisatracurium, rocuronium) **neuromuscular-blocking agent** (muscle relaxant) is given to facilitate the process. An alternative to intravenous induction is inhalation induction, which is more gradual and may not be as pleasant for the patient. For inhalation induction, the patient breathes oxygen with or without nitrous oxide and a gradually increasing concentration of volatile anesthetic agent, usually sevoflurane or halothane. Enflurane, isoflurane, and desflurane are usually considered too pungent for a smooth mask induction.

Intravenous Induction Agents

Intravenous induction agents cause rapid loss of consciousness because their early peak plasma levels are delivered directly to the brain. Consciousness returns when the drug is redistributed to other tissues. Differences in their elimination half-lives cause lingering mild sedation after one dose with some agents and, in most cases, prolonged effects with continuous infusion or repeated doses. Specific agents and their characteristics are listed in Table 1-4. The barbiturate thiopental is most commonly used because it is inexpensive. Pharmacologic differences among the induction agents are summarized in Table 1-5.

The choice of an induction agent depends on the patient's preexisting medical condition, the length of the surgery, the anticipated length of hospital stay, and the particular needs of the anesthetic. Rectal or intramuscular induction is used in children who will not allow an intravenous catheter; it also avoids mask induction with inhalation agents. Either route allows a young patient to fall asleep outside the operating room while held by the parents. The child is then transported to the operating room. Monitors and an intravenous catheter are placed, and anesthesia is begun without frightening the child. Induction by these alternative routes has the disadvantage of prolonging the recovery period. Ketamine is different from the other induction agents, whether used intramuscularly or intravenously, because of its unique CNS actions. The drug is a hallucinogen in adults and causes signs of excitement in children. Anesthetic depth is difficult to assess because there are often neuromuscular excitatory signs

Table 1-4	Characteristics of Induction Anesthetics				
Drug	**Route**	**Dose (mg/kg)**	**Onset of Sleep**	**Duration of Sleep (min)**	**Elimination Half-Life (hr)**
Thiopental (Pentothal)	Intravenous	3–5	1 circulation time	5–10	5–12
Etomidate	Intravenous	0.3	1 circulation time	3–5	1.2–4.5
Ketamine	Intravenous	1–2	1 circulation time	10–15	2–3
	Intramuscular	4–6	5–15 min	20–30	2–3
Propofol (Diprivan)	Intravenous	2–2.5	1 circulation time	3–5	0.9
Diazepam (Valium)	Intravenous	0.3–0.6	2–3 min	6–15	20–40
Midazolam (Versed)	Intravenous	0.15–0.4	3 min	6–15	2–4

Table 1-5	Advantages and Disadvantages of Intravenous Induction Agent	
Agent	**Advantages**	**Disadvantages**
Thiopental	Inexpensive Rapid acting May be given rectally in children Decreases ICP profoundly Brain protection Onset in 1 circulation time Excellent anticonvulsant No muscle relaxation	Long elimination half-life; postoperative sedation Myocardial depression Hypotension No analgesic effect Difficult to use as sedative Causes apnea and hypotension at sedative and anticonvulsant doses Contraindicated in porphyria
Diazepam	Less myocardial and respiratory depression than barbiturates Amnesia Muscle relaxant Excellent sedative in low doses Excellent anticonvulsant	Pain on injection Phlebitis Prolonged sedation Longer time to onset of sleep; difficult to use alone as induction agent
Midazolam	Less myocardial and respiratory depression than barbiturates No pain on injection or phlebitis Retrograde and antegrade amnesia Excellent sedative in low doses Excellent anticonvulsant	Questionably safe in porphyria More myocardial depression than diazepam Prolonged sedation Prolongs opioid action, apnea Slow onset time
Etomidate	Little effect on cardiovascular system Safe in porphyria Onset in 1 circulation time Less respiratory depression than barbiturates Less postoperative sedation than barbiturates or benzodiazepines Decreases ICP Decreases cerebral O_2 consumption	Questionably safe in porphyria Postoperative nausea and vomiting No analgesia Pain on injection Depresses adrenal steroid production May cause myoclonus on induction No evidence of analgesic effect Probably safe in porphyria
Propofol	Shortest duration of sedation of any intravenous agent Onset in 1 circulation time Safe in porphyria Rarely causes nausea and vomiting Allows early airway manipulation	Pain on injection Involuntary muscle action Most cardiovascular depression on any intravenous induction agent No analgesia
Ketamine	Excellent analgesic Increases blood pressure and pulse rate in intact patient Little if any respiratory depression Maintains protective airway reflexes No muscle relaxation Probably safe in porphyria Rarely causes nausea and vomiting	Causes hallucinations in adults May cause myocardial ischemia in susceptible patients Causes increased secretions Difficult to assess level of anesthesia Increases intracranial pressure Causes myocardial depression when sympathetic nervous system is depressed

such as nystagmus, purposeful and nonpurposeful movements, and myoclonus. During the recovery period, auditory stimulation causes excitement in children that may be secondary to nightmares. Although ketamine induces signs of CNS stimulation, paradoxically, it suppresses seizure activity. When administered in very small doses, ketamine is an excellent sedative for use with local or regional anesthesia. Its profound analgesic effect is not seen in any other nonnarcotic intravenous anesthetic, so it is often used for short, painful procedures (e.g., dressing changes, suture removal or insertion, fracture reductions in children).

Barbiturates remain the most popular induction agents. Porphyrias and allergy are the only contraindications. Although etomidate, the benzodiazepines, and ket-

amine support blood pressure in normal patients, this effect does not extend to patients with hypovolemia or little cardiac reserve. The search for new induction agents results from a desire to identify one that has a very short elimination period, a good analgesic effect, and no undesirable emergence effects. Propofol is especially popular in the ambulatory setting because it approaches the ideal in its characteristics, although it is the most expensive agent.

Maintenance

Inhalation agents, intravenous agents (discussed earlier), or a combination of both are used to maintain anesthesia. These agents may be supplemented with a muscle relax-

Table 1-6	Physical Characteristics of Inhaled Anesthetics			
Agent	Minimum Alveolar Concentration (%)	Vapor Pressure (mm Hg at 20°C)	Blood/Gas Solubility	Lipid/Gas Solubility
Nitrous oxide	104.00	—	0.47	1.40
Halothane	0.74	243	2.30	224.00
Enflurane	1.68	175	1.80	96.50
Isoflurane	1.15	239	1.40	90.80
Desflurane	7.3	699	0.42	18.7
Seroflurane	1.7	157	0.63	47.5

ant, depending on the need for operative exposure and controlled ventilation. All drugs used for anesthesia are selected according to their pharmacologic effects on the patient's physiologic function, keeping in mind the patient's medical condition and the surgical requirements. The anesthesiologist's goal is to minimize the stress response to surgery while maintaining the patient's cardiovascular system as close to the preoperative state as possible.

Inhalation Agents

Inhalation agents have the most profound effects on the physiology of the patient, adding to or even potentiating the effects of other drugs. The five agents commonly used are nitrous oxide, halothane, isoflurane, desflurane, and sevoflurane. Enflurane is still available but is used less commonly in the United States. The physical characteristics of these agents are compared in four areas: the minimum alveolar concentration (MAC), vapor pressure, blood–gas solubility, and lipid–gas solubility. MAC is the alveolar concentration of gas at 1 atmosphere that prevents movement in response to a surgical stimulus (e.g., skin incision) in 50% of patients. It is the standard by which the potency of anesthetics is compared and is roughly proportional to the lipid solubility. The vapor pressure determines the concentration of agent in the

carrying gas. Blood–gas solubility is a measure of how much of the agent remains dissolved in the blood as it is carried to the brain and other tissues. Lipid–gas solubility determines how easily the agent enters brain and neural tissue to exert its anesthetic effect and is roughly proportional to its potency. Table 1-6 summarizes the important physical characteristics of inhaled agents currently in use and gives the MAC of each. Table 1-7 summarizes the physiologic effects of the commonly used inhalation agents. All of the agents depress respiration (N_2O less so than the volatile agents) and the cardiovascular system, although these effects are moderated by varying degrees of autonomic reflex depression.

Nitrous oxide is different from the other inhaled agents (see Tables 1-6 and 1-7). First, it is a gas, whereas the others are volatile agents: they are supplied as liquids and are vaporized in a carrier gas. In most hospitals, N_2O is piped in through a central system. Otherwise, it is supplied in blue cylinders that attach to the anesthesia machine. Its MAC of 104%, determined under hyperbaric conditions (greater than atmospheric pressure), indicates its relative impotency. Because anesthetic gas mixtures should deliver at least 30% oxygen to ensure adequate tissue oxygenation, it is possible to administer safely a maximum of only 70% N_2O at sea level, and less at high altitudes. It is evident,

Table 1-7	Physiologic Effects of Inhaled Anesthetics					
	Cardiac Effects		Vascular Effects		Nervous System Effects	
Agent	Contractility	Rate	Arteriolar	Venous	Sympathetic	Neuromuscular
N_2O	Decrease or no change	No change or increase	No change or constrict	No change	Stimulate	No effect or increased tone
Halothane	Decrease	Decrease or no change	Dilate	Dilate	Abolish reflexes	Relax
Enflurane	Decrease	Increase	Dilate	Dilate	Decrease reflexes	Relax
Isoflurane	Decrease	No change or increase	Dilate	Dilate	Slight decrease of reflexes	Relax
Desflurane	Decrease	No change or increase	Dilate	Dilate	Slight decrease of reflexes	Relax
Sevoflurane	Decrease	No change or increase	Dilate	Dilate	Slight decrease of reflexes	Relax

then, that N_2O cannot be used as the sole anesthetic in most patients. It must be supplemented with narcotics, intravenous induction agents (e.g., propofol) in a continuous infusion, or a volatile agent to cause unconsciousness and analgesia. Because it has few effects on the cardiovascular system and is an excellent analgesic, it is often used to potentiate the effects of other anesthetic agents. Its principal drawback is that it diffuses into closed air spaces much faster than nitrogen can diffuse out, and so causes a rapid increase in the volume of entrapped air. Thus, it is not indicated for use in surgery for an obstructed bowel or for any other abdominal surgery where an increased volume of bowel gas would interfere with the surgical procedure, increase trauma, or make closure difficult. Nitrous oxide is contraindicated in patients with pneumothorax, large alveolar bullae, and pneumocephalus. It must be used with caution in patients who need a high inspired oxygen concentration for any reason. It is also the only inhaled anesthetic that has toxic effects with prolonged exposure. Bone marrow depression, chronic neuropathy, and possible teratogenicity are also reported. It inactivates methionine synthetase, which in turn inhibits vitamin B_{12} for up to 4 days after exposure. This inhibition is postulated to be the reason for its toxicity. It must be emphasized, however, that N_2O is still used in many general anesthetics, and it is often the analgesic of choice for dental and other procedures. When patient outcomes are compared, it is the safest of all anesthetics. The advantages of N_2O are that it is not metabolized, is rapidly taken up and exhaled, is easy to administer, and causes minimal cardiovascular and respiratory depression at clinical concentrations.

The hepatic microsomal enzymatic system metabolizes all of the volatile agents to varying degrees. The kidneys excrete most of the metabolites (Table 1-8). The lungs excrete unmetabolized drug. In hepatic hypoxia, a reductive pathway may metabolize halothane. It is postulated that the metabolites from this reductive metabolism cause hepatocyte toxicity. Thus, halothane has the undeserved reputation of being a liver toxin. In the national halothane study of the 1960s, halothane hepatitis, or massive hepatic necrosis, occurred in 1 of 35,000 administrations. Besides the direct toxicity, in some patients there appears to be an immune component to halothane-related liver dysfunction. Current recommendations are that halothane not be

administered to any patient who has a history of unexplained liver dysfunction after a previous halothane anesthetic or to one who has altered liver perfusion for any reason. Hepatic dysfunction after the administration of the other inhaled anesthetics is believed to be related to global or surgical effects on liver perfusion rather than to the agent itself.

The metabolites of all volatile agents include small amounts of inorganic fluoride ion, but in concentrations that are too low to cause renal toxicity. Halothane metabolism may also cause a measurable blood level of bromine, which may have some sedative effects of its own. Halothane is measurable in exhaled air many hours after the anesthesia is discontinued. Its metabolites are measurable in urine up to several days postoperatively.

In summary, with the exception of halothane, the inhaled anesthetics are remarkably inert metabolically. They rarely cause toxicity. Although they cause profound cardiovascular, respiratory, and neurologic system depression, they are safe when used under controlled conditions. Combining volatile agents with N_2O, and all inhaled agents with the adjunctive drugs discussed below, produces profound general anesthesia with little interference with tissue perfusion and oxygenation.

Muscle Relaxants

Muscle relaxants allow a much lighter plane of anesthesia to provide conditions required for surgery. They facilitate such procedures as endotracheal intubation and abdominal surgery, which require a degree of muscle relaxation that often cannot be safely achieved by inhalation agents alone. Controlled ventilation is also facilitated by muscle relaxants, extending their use beyond the operating room and into intensive care units.

The normal reflex response to a noxious stimulus is withdrawal. Movement of a patient during anesthesia indicates that the depth of anesthesia is not sufficient to prevent this motor response. Because muscle relaxants might mask a sign of inadequate anesthesia, the anesthesiologist relies on autonomic rather than motor reflexes as a sign of depth of anesthesia. These reflexes include increases in heart rate or blood pressure, attempts at spontaneous respiration, sweating, increased respiratory tract secretions, and bronchoconstriction. Thus, the use of muscle relaxants is a safe method to reduce inhalational anesthetic requirements to a level that does not cause dangerous cardiovascular depression and other ill effects.

Two classes of muscle relaxants are in use today. The depolarizing relaxants activate the postsynaptic cholinergic receptor of the neuromuscular junction, then dissociate slowly from that receptor, binding it so that it will not fire again until it is free. The nondepolarizing relaxants prevent muscle contraction by competitively blocking the postsynaptic receptor from binding with acetylcholine, but do not activate the receptor. Monitoring the response to single and repeated supramaximal twitch stimuli and tetanic stimulation differentiates the two types (Table 1-9) and determines the percentage of receptors blocked at any

Table 1-8	Metabolism of Volatile Anesthetics
Agent	**Percentage Metabolized**
Halothane	25
Enflurane	3
Isoflurane	0.20
Desflurane	0.02
Sevoflurane	5

| Table 1-9 | Monitoring Neuromuscular Blockade with a Peripheral Nerve Stimulator |

Type of Relaxant	Single Twitch	Train-of-Four[a]	Tetanic (50 Hz) Stimulation	Posttetanic Twitch
Depolarizing	Decreased height in proportion to dose	No fade; all four equally decreased	No fade; tetany depressed in proportion to dose	No facilitation; twitch same as pretetany
Electromyogram	Drug injection			Posttetanic facilitation; first twitches greater in height than pretetanic twitch
Nondepolarizing	Decreased height in proportion to dose	Fade in proportion to dose	Rapid fade	
Electromyogram	Drug injection			

[a]Train-of-four is four twitches delivered at a rate of one every 0.5 second.

one time. A simple nerve stimulator applied over the ulnar nerve at the elbow or wrist or the ophthalmic branch of the trigeminal nerve that is just anterior to the ear is used to monitor twitch response. A single stimulus applied at a rate of 1 per second, a train-of-four stimulation applied at a rate of 2 per second, or a tetanic stimulation applied at 50 or 100 cycles per second may be used to determine the percentage of muscle receptors blocked by the muscle relaxant. As shown in Table 1-9, 75% to 80% of receptors must be blocked before the twitch response is depressed, whereas 90% to 95% of receptors must be blocked before there is no response to a single twitch. Fade (a progressive decrease in the height of successive twitches) is seen in the train-of-four stimulation sequence when 70% to 75% of receptors are blocked. A train-of-four sequence consists of four supramaximal stimuli delivered at a rate of 2 cycles per second (2 Hz). Tetanic stimulation at 50 Hz leads to appreciable fade when 75% to 80% of receptors are blocked. At 100 Hz, fade is seen when 50% of receptors are blocked.

Succinylcholine, the only depolarizing agent currently in use, consists of two acetylcholine molecules joined together. It produces relaxation of short duration after initial generalized contraction, which is clinically visible as fasciculations. Succinylcholine is not metabolized at the neuromuscular junction by acetylcholinesterase. Instead, it diffuses into the blood, where it is rapidly hydrolyzed by **plasma cholinesterase** (pseudocholinesterase). Its onset of action is almost immediate, and a single dose of 1 mg/kg has a duration of approximately 10 minutes. Despite its side effects (Table 1-10), it is the choice of many anesthesiologists for endotracheal intubation because of its rapid onset. It is the relaxant most used for emergency intubations. Many of these side effects can be ameliorated by

preceding the injection with a small, defasciculating dose of a nondepolarizing relaxant (d-tubocurarine 3 mg). However, this action also increases the time to onset, the duration, and the dose of succinylcholine required to suppress neuromuscular transmission. Nondepolarizing relaxants do not have these side effects.

Hyperkalemia after succinylcholine injection occurs as a consequence of depolarization. It can be clinically significant in patients with massive soft tissue injury, including burns (at least 48 hours old), acute and chronic denervation injuries, renal failure, or preexisting hyperkalemia. In these situations, cardiac arrest is not uncommon and is not effectively prevented by pretreatment with nondepolarizing agents. Increases in intracranial and intraocular pressure occur with succinylcholine, even in the absence of both fasciculations and increased venous pressure. The reason for the increase in ICP is not known, but the rise in intraocular pressure is initiated by contracture of extra-

| Table 1-10 | Side Effects of Succinylcholine |

Vagal stimulation (common in children)
  Bradycardia (especially with repeat injections)
Sympathetic stimulation
  Tachycardia and hypertension in adults
Increased intracranial pressure
Increased intraocular pressure
Fasciculations
  Hyperkalemia
  Increased intra-abdominal pressure
  Further increase in intracranial pressure
  Further increase in intraocular pressure
  Postoperative myalgia

ocular muscles and may be enhanced by transient dilation of choroidal blood vessels. Therefore, extrusion of vitreous may occur in patients with an open globe injury. The increase in intra-abdominal pressure is caused by contractions of the abdominal muscles and may be significant enough to cause regurgitation of stomach contents and aspiration into the lungs if protective measures are not taken. Nonetheless, succinylcholine is the favorite relaxant of many anesthesiologists for rapid endotracheal intubation, especially in patients with a full stomach, because of its rapid, reliable onset of action.

Succinylcholine triggers the onset of malignant hyperpyrexia (MH) in susceptible individuals. MH is a rare, inherited myopathy in which muscles undergo sustained contracture when triggered by depolarizing relaxants, inhaled anesthetics, or other physiologic stressors. A hypermetabolic state ensues that is characterized by hypertension, tachycardia, hyperkalemia, hypercapnia, and hyperthermia. MH is often associated with chronic neuromuscular diseases. Because these diseases may be subclinical in small children at the time of surgery, some anesthesiologists believe that the drug should be used only when indicated in children.

The action of succinylcholine is prolonged in patients with abnormal or deficient plasma cholinesterase and in those with chronic neuromuscular disease. Severe liver failure results in low levels of plasma cholinesterase. Succinylcholine may be safely used as a continuous-infusion relaxant for short procedures, with constant assessment of its effect with a twitch monitor. Large doses of the drug cause a phase II (or desensitization) block, a prolongation of effect that cannot reliably be reversed pharmacologically and must be allowed to wear off gradually. Monitoring the twitch shows the onset of signs of a nondepolarizing blockade (fade on tetanic stimulation and posttetanic facilitation) when this phase II block develops.

Nondepolarizing agents are used for prolonged relaxation during the surgical procedure. They can be used for endotracheal intubation, but they take longer than succinylcholine to complete relaxation of the jaw (approximately 2 minutes) when twice the ED_{95} (dose required to block 95% of receptors) is administered. The nondepolarizing agents that are currently in use and their doses, durations, and side effects are listed in Table 1-11.

The cardiovascular effects of nondepolarizing relaxants are the result of ganglionic blockade, vagal stimulation, and histamine release. Ganglionic blockade and histamine release result in hypotension, whereas vagal blockade results in tachycardia. The way in which drugs are metabolized and eliminated determines which drugs are used for patients with hepatic, renal, or some metabolic dysfunctions (Table 1-12). Most nondepolarizing relaxants are partially metabolized in the liver. The rest are excreted unchanged in urine or bile.

Most anesthesiologists monitor the twitch response when using neuromuscular-blocking agents because the concurrent administration of inhalational agents potentiates their effect, and many physiologic factors may affect

their excretion and metabolism. Although relaxation may be antagonized by the administration of neostigmine, pyridostigmine, or edrophonium, this effect is not reliable when doses of nondepolarizing relaxants that are sufficient to block all twitch responses at the time of administration are used.

Airway Maintenance

The patient's airway must be maintained when a general anesthetic is being administered. As soon as the patient loses consciousness, the upper airway structures relax and the tongue falls backward, obstructing the glottis. This obstruction is corrected by pulling the lower jaw upward and forward, hyperextending the neck, and inserting an oropharyngeal airway. However, if an oropharyngeal airway is inserted before the pharyngeal and laryngeal reflexes are obtunded, laryngospasm may occur. Obese patients and those with a short, muscular neck tend to obstruct easier and earlier during induction. If the patient is not anesthetized deeply enough for the mouth to be opened, a nasopharyngeal airway may be inserted.

It is critical to select the right size of oropharyngeal and nasopharyngeal airways. One may estimate the correct-sized oropharyngeal airway by placing it against the side of the face, the flange (wide opening) at the lips. The tip of the airway should reach the angle of the jaw. If the airway is too large, it will not fit. If it is too small, it will cause obstruction by delivering the gas mixture to the soft tissue of the tongue. The proper length of the nasopharyngeal airway is from the nares to the tragus of the ear. If it is too long, it may damage pharyngeal structures or cause vagal stimulation resulting in bradycardia.

If the patient's airway cannot be maintained with a mask, or if a long period of airway control is anticipated, a laryngeal mask airway or endotracheal intubation becomes necessary. The laryngeal mask airway is a recent innovation and provides a conduit for inspired gas directly to the supraglottic area (Fig. 1-1). However, it does not provide a reliable seal to protect from aspiration of saliva or gastric contents. It also does not provide a tight seal for controlled ventilation, because it is not in the trachea. The great benefit of this device is that it does provide an open airway in the vast majority of cases without requiring perfect positioning, and it may also be used as a conduit for endotracheal intubation in most patients if other methods have not been successful. Generally, if the patient requires help with ventilation, an endotracheal tube is required. Muscle relaxants facilitate intubation. However, because they inhibit spontaneous ventilation, they should not be given until the anesthesiologist can manually ventilate the patient through a mask. If mask ventilation is impossible, the depth of anesthesia must be decreased and the endotracheal tube must be inserted with the patient awake and breathing spontaneously. Intubation is facilitated by the use of a laryngoscope. Figure 1-2 shows a laryngoscope with a curved, Macintosh-3 blade. Batteries in the handle of the laryngoscope power a small light bulb on the side

Table 1-11	Characteristics of Nondepolarizing Relaxants			
Relaxant	ED$_{95}$ (mg/kg)	Intubating Dose (mg/kg)	Time to 5% Recovery (min)[a]	Side Effects
d-Tubocurarine	0.51	0.6	30–45	+ + + Histamine release Blocks ganglionic transmission No effect on vagus
Metocurine	0.28	0.4	30–45	+ + Histamine release Blocks ganglionic transmission less than curare No effect on vagus
Pancuronium	0.07	0.1 0.2	45 129	+ + Vagal blockade (tachycardia) No histamine release No ganglionic effect
Vecuronium	0.05	0.1	20–30	No effect on vagus No ganglionic effect No histamine release
Atracurium	2.8	3.5	20–30	No effect on vagus No ganglionic effect + Histamine release
Cisatracurium	0.05	0.2	40	No effect on vagus No ganglionic effect No histamine release
Gallamine	2.8	3.5	30–45	+ + + Vagal blockade (tachycardia) No ganglionic effect No histamine release
Mivacurium	0.08	0.2–0.4	16–19	+ Histamine release No effect on vagus
Rocuronium	0.3	0.6	18	No histamine release No effect on vagus No ganglionic effect
Pipecuronium	0.05–0.06	0.1	80–120	No histamine release No vagal effect
Doxacurium	0.025	0.06	80–120	No histamine release No vagal effect No ganglionic effect

[a]After intubating dose.
ED, dose required to block 95% of receptors.

Table 1-12	Metabolism and Excretion of Nondepolarizing Neuromuscular Blocking Drugs		
Drug	Renal Elimination (%)	Hepatic Metabolism (%)	Other
Gallamine	100	0	0
Metocurine	60–90	10–40	0
Pancuronium	30–80	15–40	≤10% biliary excretion
d-Tubocurarine	40–60	0	40%–60% biliary excretion
Pipecuronium	38	60	2% biliary excretion
Doxacurium	25–60	15–40	
Vecuronium	15–25	50–60	≤50% biliary excretion
Rocuronium	9–33		54% biliary excretion
Atracurium	<10	0	>90% Hoffman elimination
Cisatracurium	<5	0	>90% Hoffman elimination
Mivacurium	<10	0	Metabolized by plasma cholinesterase

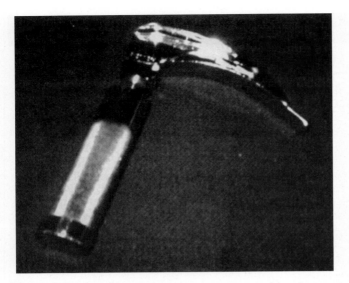

Figure 1-1   A battery-operated laryngoscope with a 3-Macintosh blade.

of the blade. The operator holds the handle in the left hand and opens the patient's mouth with the right hand. The blade is inserted from the right side of the mouth and slides back along the right margin of the tongue to the vallecula (the area between the base of the tongue and the epiglottis). With the blade in the proper position and the patient's neck slightly extended in the sniffing position, lifting the handle raises the epiglottis and brings the vocal cords into direct vision (Fig. 1-3). Figure 1-4 shows the difference between the curved and the straight blades in

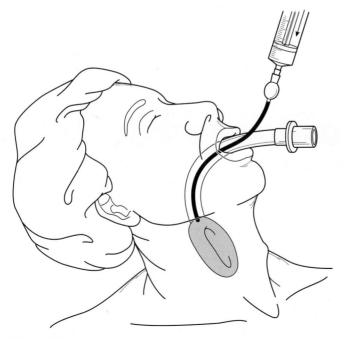

Figure 1-2   A laryngeal mask airway in place.

various sizes. In all patients except newborns, the straight blade is placed over the epiglottis to lift it, along with the base of the tongue, to expose the larynx. Another device being used with increasing frequency, especially in the case of difficulty visualizing the glottis with the laryngoscope, is the fiberoptic laryngoscope. This device is similar to the fiberoptic bronchoscope but is smaller in diameter to allow the endotracheal tube to be inserted over it. The tube is placed over the bronchoscope and held at its top while the glottis is visualized and the scope is advanced into the trachea. The tube is then advanced over the bronchoscope while the operator continues to visualize the carina. This intubation method obviously requires considerable practice, but saves many patients from undergoing an emergency surgical airway (tracheostomy) when difficulty is encountered with routine airway management.

In general, endotracheal intubation is required whenever the anesthesiologist does not have immediate access to the airway, when mechanical ventilation is required because of muscle relaxation or physical characteristics of the patient, or when there is risk of aspiration. Intubation of the trachea in a poorly anesthetized patient results in massive autonomic stimulation, which is seen as hypertension, tachycardia or bradycardia, arrhythmias, and bronchoconstriction. Endotracheal intubation never guarantees an adequate airway. Secretions may obstruct the tube, it may kink, it may become displaced either out of the trachea or down into a bronchus, or the patient may aspirate pharyngeal contents despite the presence of an inflated cuff. To minimize the risk of aspiration of gastric contents, patients who are suspected of having a full stomach can be intubated either awake under topical anesthesia or after being anesthetized with a rapid sequence (or crash) induction. In a rapid sequence induction, the patient is preoxygenated until the expired oxygen concentration approaches 100%. Then anesthesia is rapidly induced with the induction agent and muscle relaxant while an assistant provides downward pressure on the cricoid cartilage of the neck. This pressure is applied to compress the lumen of the esophagus between the posterior ring of the cartilage and the vertebral body. It prevents passive regurgitation of gastric contents through the esophagus. To avoid pushing air into the stomach and increasing gastric pressure, the anesthesiologist intubates the trachea without ventilating the patient with the mask. When the position of the tube in the trachea is verified and the cuff is inflated, the assistant releases the cricoid pressure. Indications and complications of endotracheal intubation for general anesthesia are listed in Table 1-13.

If the uvula and tonsillar pillars are easily visible when the patient opens the mouth and sticks out the tongue, then the anesthesiologist can safely assume that intubation will be possible with direct laryngoscopy. A difficult intubation may be anticipated in patients who have a short, muscular "bull" neck, a receding chin, protruding upper incisors, or a high-arched palate in a narrow mouth. Inability to open the mouth wide or to extend the neck also predicts difficult laryngoscopy. Finally, any space-occupy-

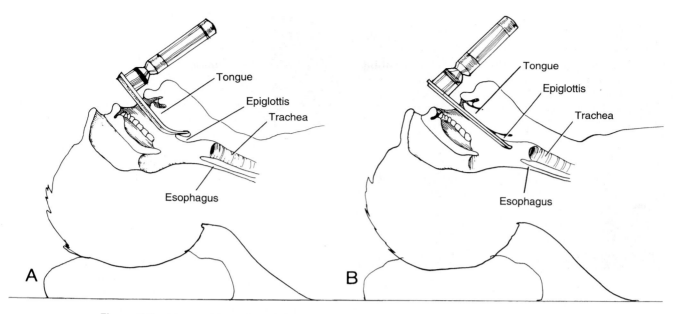

Figure 1-3 The position of the **(A)** curved blade and **(B)** straight blade in exposing the larynx.

ing lesion of the mouth, pharynx, larynx, or neck makes direct laryngoscopy difficult. In these cases, conventional induction and intubation may not be appropriate. Alternative methods include awake intubation under direct vision with topical anesthesia, awake blind nasal intubation, intubation over a fiberoptic bronchoscope inserted into the trachea with the patient either awake or asleep, and tracheotomy under local anesthesia.

Emergence

A patient who is not critically ill should be returning to a normal state when leaving the operating room. In this

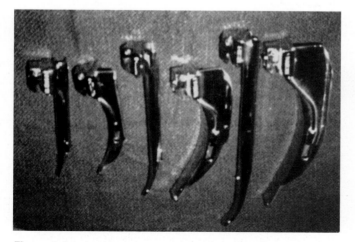

Figure 1-4 Curved and straight laryngoscope blades of various sizes. *Left to right:* 1-1/2-Wis-Hipple and 1-Macintosh blades for small children; 3-Miller and 3-Macintosh blades for most intubations; 4-Miller and 4-Macintosh blades for very large adults.

condition, respiratory obstruction, pulmonary aspiration, and cardiovascular instability are unlikely. Recovery from anesthesia begins when anesthetic drugs are discontinued. Oxygen at 100% is administered while the anesthetic gases are being excreted through the lungs. The patient's alveolar ventilation, the lipid solubility of the agent, and the duration of the anesthetic determine how quickly gases are eliminated. An agent that is highly lipid-soluble tends to remain sequestered in body fat, dissolving slowly and providing a long period of low blood concentration as it dissolves. The recovery rate from intravenous anesthetics depends on the amount administered, time of last injection, lipid solubility, hepatic metabolism, and renal excretion. If muscle relaxants are used, the degree of remaining blockade is monitored with a nerve stimulator. If neces-

Table 1-13	Endotracheal Intubation During Anesthesia
Indications	**Complications**
Inability to maintain airway	Trauma to teeth or oropharyngeal soft
Requirement by surgeon for	tissue
muscle relaxation	Aspiration
Inaccessibility of the airway or	Hypoxemia
shared airway with surgeon	Obstruction by secretions
Patient with a full stomach or at	Endobronchial intubation
risk for aspiration	Accidental extubation
Need for tracheal toilet	Autonomic response
Patients who require positive	Hypertension, tachycardia,
pressure ventilation	bradycardia, arrhythmias
Massive upper airway secretions	Bronchospasm
or bleeding	Endotracheal tube obstruction

sary, blockade effects are neutralized by neuromuscular antagonists. All monitoring continues until the patient leaves the operating room; it begins again in the recovery room. In unstable patients, monitoring continues during transportation. Because hypoxemia is documented consistently in the immediate postanesthesia period, oxygen is administered as the patient is transported to the recovery room.

Extubation of the Trachea

Patients are safely extubated when the criteria in Table 1-14 are met. Before extubation, the patient breathes 100% oxygen until the expired oxygen concentration is nearly 100% and the oropharynx is suctioned. The endotracheal tube may be suctioned if necessary. The cuff is deflated to allow easy removal of the endotracheal tube. Complications that may follow extubation postanesthesia include laryngospasm, aspiration, pharyngitis or laryngitis, and vocal cord dysfunction. The most common and most serious is laryngospasm, which occurs when the vocal cords are irritated. Laryngospasm is treated by administering positive pressure oxygen by mask and by maintaining an unobstructed airway. Occasionally, a small amount of muscle relaxant is necessary to relax the vocal cords sufficiently to allow air to enter. The patient's respirations must be controlled until the relaxant wears off.

Regional Anesthesia

Regional anesthesia provides loss of pain perception in the area of surgical intervention. The patient usually remains awake and can breathe adequately. Monitoring and observation in the operating room and recovery room are identical to those for general anesthesia. The most common regional anesthetics are those of the lower spinal nerve roots (spinal, epidural, and caudal blocks) and the brachial plexus.

Table 1-14	Criteria for Postanesthesia Extubation

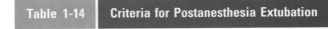

Adequate spontaneous respiration
  Normal respiratory rate
  Adequate tidal volume
  Vital capacity >15 mL/kg
  Expired CO_2 <45–50 mm Hg
Return of protective reflexes (gag and cough)
Responsive to verbal commands
Cardiovascular stability
Metabolic stability (temperature >35°C)
No residual neuromuscular blockade
  By nerve stimulator
  Sustains head lift for 5 seconds
  Good muscle tone
  Negative inspiratory force > −20 cm H_2O

Figure 1-5 shows the lower spinal canal and the different needle placements for subarachnoid (spinal), epidural, and caudal blocks. Each approach provides adequate anesthesia and operating conditions for surgical procedures below the waist. If the procedure will be performed on the upper abdomen, or if extensive manipulation of the viscera is required, adequate analgesia may be achieved only with the addition of a celiac plexus block (to denervate the viscera). Combined techniques with regional and general anesthesia recently became popular, especially in small children. The regional block is designed to provide analgesia into the postoperative period.

Spinal Anesthesia

Spinal anesthesia is an ideal technique for surgery on the lower part of the body. When a small amount of local anesthetic is injected into the subarachnoid space at a level below L2, it diffuses through the cerebrospinal fluid (CSF) to a height determined by the specific gravity and concentration of the anesthetic solution and the position of the patient. After the drug is injected, an almost immediate sympathetic blockade occurs, which results in vasodilation, pooling of blood in dependent areas, and decreased cardiac output. This sympathetic effect is best treated by administering fluids and raising the patient's legs to increase venous return. The Trendelenburg position is contraindicated soon after a spinal injection. It elevates the level of block to higher than desired in the case of a hyperbaric (specific gravity greater than that of CSF) anesthetic solution and to lower than expected in the case of a hypobaric (specific gravity less than that of CSF) solution. If the level of sympathetic blockade is higher than T1 to T4, the cardioaccelerator sympathetic nerves are blocked and bradycardia ensues.

During a spinal anesthetic, the sympathetic blockade is several levels higher than the sensory blockade, and the motor blockade is several levels lower than the sensory level. If the level of motor blockade is higher than C3, the diaphragm and intercostal muscles are paralyzed, and the patient cannot breathe adequately. Apnea may also occur secondary to ischemia of the medullary centers as a result of profound hypotension induced by the anesthesia. If respiration is compromised, the patient is intubated and ventilated until the level recedes enough for spontaneous respiration to resume. The anesthesiologist must ensure that the patient who is receiving a spinal anesthetic is fully monitored during and after the block. A reliable intravenous line must be running, oxygen must be available, and all anesthetic drugs and equipment must be within arm's reach as the block is being performed. Patient preparation should be as complete for a regional technique as for a general anesthetic (i.e., the patient should be in optimal medical condition, have an empty stomach, and be psychologically prepared).

Headache, the most common complication of a spinal anesthetic, once occurred in approximately 25% of cases, mostly among younger patients. It is more common when

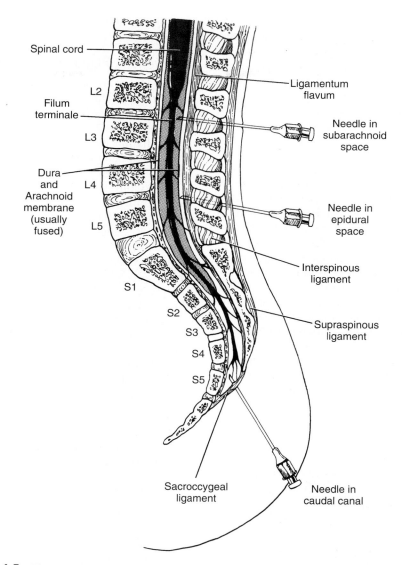

Spinal cord

L2

Filum terminale

L3

Dura and Arachnoid membrane (usually fused)

L4

L5

S1

S2

S3

S4

S5

Ligamentum flavum

Needle in subarachnoid space

Needle in epidural space

Interspinous ligament

Supraspinous ligament

Sacroccygeal ligament

Needle in caudal canal

Figure 1-5 The lumbosacral spinal canal showing needle placement for subarachnoid, epidural, and caudal blocks. The spinal cord terminates at approximately L2, and the dural sac terminates at approximately S2. Below S2, the sacral canal contains only the dura-enclosed sacral nerve roots.

anesthetic is continuously administered, a technique involving insertion of a small catheter into the subarachnoid space for repeated injections. Headache usually begins the day after the spinal and is related to posture, occurring when the patient is upright and disappearing when the patient lies down. The headache is caused by leakage of CSF through the dural puncture. Using a 25- or 27-gauge needle for the puncture reduces the probability of **spinal headache** to 5% to 10% in the most susceptible population. Use of a "pencil point" needle further reduces the incidence to 2%. Hydration and bed rest are usually adequate treatment, but if the headache is prolonged (1–2 days), it is treated by injecting 5 to 10 mL of the patient's own blood into the epidural space at the level of the previous spinal injection (epidural blood patch).

Epidural Anesthesia

When anesthesia is needed in the lower half of the body, epidural anesthesia is another option. The epidural space is the area within the spinal canal outside the dura and arachnoid. In the area below L2, it contains fat, an extensive venous plexus, and the dura-enclosed cauda equina. A large volume of local anesthetic is injected into the space. The level of the block depends on the actual volume injected. Continuous analgesia is obtained by giving additional doses of the anesthetic through a catheter inserted through the needle at the time the epidural space is identified. The concentration of anesthetic determines whether the block is sympathetic, sensory, or complete (i.e., including motor fibers).

The onset of epidural anesthesia is slower than that of spinal anesthesia. However, the level and characteristics of the block are much more controllable because anesthetic can be added in small increments through the indwelling catheter placed in the epidural space. Because of anatomic abnormalities that may be present in the space, a "patchy" block is much more likely to result from an epidural than from a spinal block. Hypotension and respiratory insufficiency may develop, but less frequently than with a spinal anesthetic because of the more gradual onset of blockade. The needle used in an epidural block is larger than that used in a spinal block. For this reason, if the dura is accidentally punctured during its insertion, a spinal headache is more likely to ensue. Backache also is more likely after an epidural block because tissues are more likely to be injured when the larger, blunter needle is inserted through the ligaments that support the spinal column. Anesthetic unknowingly injected into the subarachnoid space because of unrecognized dural puncture results in a total spinal, with total blockade of all of the spinal nerves. If the anesthetic reaches the level of the brain stem, unconsciousness and apnea occur. If the anesthetic is injected into one of the numerous epidural veins, systemic toxicity occurs. These complications are rare and epidural anesthesia is the gold standard for many lower extremity, pelvic, and lower abdominal surgeries, as well as for analgesia during labor and delivery.

Caudal Anesthesia

The caudal block is a variation of the epidural block, in which the needle is inserted through the sacral hiatus at the bottom of the sacrum and anesthetic is injected into the epidural space. Larger volumes of anesthetic are required to achieve the same level of analgesia with this route, but there is virtually no possibility of an unrecognized subarachnoid injection. Because of anatomic variations that are present in a large percentage of the population, however, reliable anesthesia is often difficult to achieve with this technique. For this reason, it is used less often than the epidural block, except in small children, in whom the anatomy is less variable.

Brachial Plexus Blocks

The brachial plexus may be blocked in the interscalene area, supraclavicular area, or axilla. Any of these approaches results in reliable anesthesia of the forearm and hand. Anesthesia of the upper arm with a brachial plexus block is less reliable. The plexus is identified with a needle by eliciting paresthesia or by motor response to stimulation by a nerve stimulator attached to the needle. A relatively large volume (35–50 mL) of local anesthetic, usually 1.5% to 2% lidocaine, 0.5% bupivacaine, 1.5% mepivacaine, or 2% chloroprocaine, is injected when the plexus is located. Anesthesia of all of the nerves in the plexus depends on the volume and concentration injected. Complications of brachial plexus blocks are related to the volume of anesthetic or the proximity of the injection site to the carotid or axillary artery, the dome of the pleura, and the spinal canal.

Intravenous Regional Block (Bier Block)

When the surgical procedure can be performed with a tourniquet on the extremity, a Bier block provides reliable anesthesia of an arm or leg. The block is achieved by exsanguinating the extremity with an elastic compression bandage, inflating a proximal tourniquet above arterial pressure, and replacing the blood volume of the extremity with a dilute solution of local anesthetic (usually 0.5% lidocaine). Complete blockade occurs almost immediately and continues until the tourniquet is released. If a second tourniquet is placed just distal to the first and inflated after the block is effective, the proximal tourniquet may be deflated and tourniquet pain (ischemic pain under the tourniquet) is avoided. If the tourniquet is not inflated to a sufficiently high pressure, or if it is released or leaks during the procedure, the block fades as anesthetic escapes into the circulation. If this escape occurs within half an hour of the injection, systemic toxicity may occur because of the large load of anesthetic that may be released. At the end of the procedure, the tourniquet is released and the block diminishes rapidly. If the procedure lasted less than half an hour, the tourniquet is released slowly and intermittently to minimize systemic blood levels of local anesthetic.

Nerve Blocks and Local Infiltration Anesthesia

Nerve Blocks

Injections of local anesthetic are used to provide adequate analgesia for limited surgery. The following peripheral nerves are easily blocked: digital for finger or toe surgery; intercostal for thoracic or abdominal wall procedures; sciatic, obturator, and femoral for lower leg procedures; mandibular for lower jaw procedures; retrobulbar for eye procedures; penile for circumcisions; and ankle for foot procedures. Nerve blocks are effective for distal procedures that include skin, subcutaneous tissue, muscle, fascia, bone, joints, and periosteum. Peritoneum, pleura, and pericardium cannot be rendered insensitive by peripheral nerve block because they have both autonomic and somatic innervation. An epinephrine local anesthetic solution should not be used for nerve blocks on the digits or penis because epinephrine can cause local vasoconstriction that leads to peripheral ischemia. The only contraindications to nerve blocks for appropriate procedures are unacceptability to the patient, local infection at the injection site, coagulopathy, and allergy to both kinds of local anesthetic.

Local Anesthesia

Local anesthesia is achieved by infiltrating a local anesthetic into the skin and underlying tissue around the operative site. Local infiltration of anesthetic is sufficient for limited superficial procedures that involve skin, subcutaneous tissue, muscle, and fascia. It is difficult to desensitize bone and periosteum with local infiltration. Preemptive analgesia by presurgical infiltration of the incision area reduces postoperative pain and suffering. The same contraindications as for nerve blocks apply.

Local anesthetics may be administered by several routes: topically (directly on the skin, cornea, or mucous membrane), by infiltration around a peripheral nerve or plexus, in the subarachnoid space, in the epidural space, or even intravenously. To provide a drier surgical field and to prolong the block, epinephrine is added to the local anesthetic. Because virtually every practitioner uses local anesthetics to some extent, a working knowledge of their pharmacology and toxicity is important. All local anesthetics except cocaine consist of a tertiary amine and an unsaturated aromatic ring separated by either an ester or an amide link. The benzene ring imparts lipid solubility that is necessary to permeate nerve sheaths and coverings. The amine imparts water solubility that is necessary to diffuse and bind to the axonal site of action. The amide

or ester link determines the route and speed of drug metabolism: those with an ester linkage are metabolized rapidly by serum cholinesterase and acetylcholinesterase; those with an amide linkage are metabolized more slowly by the hepatic microsomal system. Table 1-15 lists local anesthetics that are currently in use, the ways in which they are used, and their important characteristics.

Local anesthetics are classified according to their duration of action. The drugs in each category have similar toxicities and potencies. Adding epinephrine or another vasoconstrictor to the injected solution usually prolongs the duration of action by one third to one half and reduces the toxicity of the drug secondary to retarding its rapid vascular uptake. Because epinephrine causes vasoconstriction, it is not used in areas that are prone to ischemia (e.g., nostril, external ear, digits, penis).

True allergic reactions to local anesthetic agents, especially those with an amide linkage, are rare but life threatening. A patient who has a history of allergy to local anesthesia should undergo skin testing with several agents to determine whether they are truly contraindicated. Although it is not 100% reliable, skin testing, which involves

Table 1-15	Characteristics of Local Anesthetic Agents					
Agent	**Linkage**	**Uses**	**Concentration Used and Dose**	**Onset[a] (min)**	**Duration[a] (min)**	
Benzocaine	Ester	Topical	20% ointment	Immediate	30	
			20% aerosol	Immediate	30	
Chloroprocaine	Ester	Infiltration	1%–2%, up to 1 g	5	30	
		Epidural/caudal	2%, 5–10 mL increments, up to 25 mL	15	30–90	
Cocaine	Ester	Topical	4%, up to 4 mL	Immediate	60	
Dibucaine	Ester	Spinal	0.07%–0.5%, 1–2 mL	Immediate	30	
Procaine	Ester	Infiltration	1%, 2%, up to 1 g	Immediate	20	
		Spinal	10%, 1–2 mL	5	30	
Tetracaine	Ester	Spinal	1%, 1–2 mL	5–10	60–140	
Bupivacaine	Amide	Infiltration	0.25%–0.5%, up to 200 mg	15	200 ± 33	
		Spinal	0.5%–0.75, up to 1 mL	10	120–240	
		Epidural/caudal	0.25%–0.5%, 5–10 mL increments up to 25 mL	17	195 ± 30	
Etidocaine	Amide	Infiltration	0.25%–1%, up to 300 mg	4–5	300	
		Epidural/caudal	0.5%–1%, 5–10 mL increments up to 25 mL	11	170 ± 57	
Lidocaine	Amide	Topical	1%–5%, up to 500 mg	3	30	
		Infiltration	0.5%–2%, up to 500 mg	Immediate	75–127	
		Spinal	5%, up to 1 mL	3–6	30–45	
		Epidural/caudal	0.5%–2%, 5–10 mL increments up to 25 mL	15	100 ± 20	
Mepivacaine	Amide	Infiltration	1%–2%, up to 500 mg	30–60	60–180	
		Epidural/caudal	2%, 5–10 mL increments up to 25 mL	15	115 ± 15	
Prilocaine	Amide	Infiltration	1%–3%, up to 900 mg	10	100–150	
Ropivacaine	Amide	Infiltration	0.5%–1%, up to 2.5 mg/kg	15	200	
		Epidural	0.5%–1%, up to 2.5 mg/kg	17	200	

[a]Onset and duration of surgical analgesia when anesthetic was used without vasoconstrictors.

applying an intradermal patch and looking for wheal and flare, is accepted as adequate screening for local anesthetic allergy. True allergy to lidocaine and other amides has been reported only a few times in millions of administrations. Distinguishing an allergic reaction from systemic toxicity is difficult because most reactions to local anesthetics are the result of accidental intravascular injections or overdoses rather than true allergies. The maximum recommended doses of commonly used local anesthetic agents are shown in Table 1-15. Systemic toxicity is the greatest potential risk associated with their use. Symptoms include ringing in the ears, perioral numbness, and a metallic taste in the mouth. These symptoms signal the onset of CNS excitation that may then progress to jitteriness, shivering, convulsions, and coma. Treatment of local anesthetic toxicity consists of oxygenation and injection of anticonvulsants, preferably short-acting intravenous agents (e.g., thiopental, diazepam, midazolam). Prevention is easily accomplished by calculating the dose to be administered, ensuring that the agent is not injected into a vessel by aspirating frequently during injection, and premedicating with a benzodiazepine to reduce CNS toxicity whenever it is anticipated that large doses of local anesthetics will be used.

All local anesthetics (with the exception of cocaine) cause myocardial depression, peripheral vasodilation, and depression of autonomic responses in a dose-related fashion. Lidocaine is associated with a short-lived blockade of the myocardial conduction system. Bupivacaine causes a more prolonged blockade associated with malignant reentrant dysrhythmia, which is difficult to reverse and occurs at blood levels only slightly above those that cause CNS excitation. Emergency lifesaving support may be necessary, including prolonged cardiopulmonary resuscitation, bretylium rather than lidocaine for ventricular ectopy, and, often, large doses of epinephrine. If convulsions also occur after bupivacaine injection, they are controlled with a short-acting muscle relaxant (e.g., succinylcholine). Anti-

convulsants are contraindicated because they may cause further cardiac depression.

Cocaine is different from the other local anesthetics because it blocks the presynaptic uptake of norepinephrine into sympathetic nerve terminals. For this reason, it has local vasoconstrictive effects that make it useful as topical anesthesia for surgery of the nose and throat. Cocaine also has profound CNS effects, similar to those of antidepressants or amphetamines, accompanied by cardiovascular stimulation. It is associated with coronary arterial vasospasm. The drug fell out of favor with many anesthesiologists because of the difficulty in keeping it "off the street," and because the same effects can be achieved with a combination of other topical anesthetics and vasoconstrictors (e.g., phenylephrine).

Anesthetic Supplements

Opioids

Opioids are used to supplement local or regional anesthesia, to supplement inhalational anesthetics so that lower concentrations may be used, and with other drugs as a part of total intravenous anesthesia. Fentanyl, sufentanil, and alfentanil are often given as a continuous intravenous infusion or in small, frequent doses after an initial bolus dose. Remifentanil is usually given as a continuous infusion. The longer-acting opioids are given as incremental small doses during the anesthetic to establish a baseline narcosis that continues through the immediate postoperative period. With the exception of remifentanil, which is metabolized in plasma by esterases, opioids are all metabolized by the liver and the metabolites are excreted through the kidneys. Table 1-16 characterizes the opioid receptors and identifies their commonly used agonists and antagonists. Table 1-17 shows the opioids that are used intravenously in the operating room and their relative potencies, onset times, and elimination half-lives.

Table 1-16	Opioid Receptors, Agonists, and Antagonists				
Receptor	**Actions**	**Agonists**		**Partial Agonist/Antagonist**	**Antagonists**
μ	Supraspinal analgesia Respiratory depression Euphoria Physical dependence	All morphine-like drugs	3/1 2–3/2 1/3	Buprenorphine (Buprenex) Butorphanol (Stadol) Pentazocine (Talwin) Nalbuphine (Nubain) Levallorphan (Lorphan) Nalorphine (Nalline)	Nalorphine Naloxone
κ	Spinal analgesia Respiratory depression	All morphine-like drugs Nalorphine (partial) Butorphanol Nalbuphine Pentazocine			Naloxone
Σ	Dysphoria Hallucinations Vasomotor stimulation	Nalorphine Butorphanol Nalbuphine			Naloxone

Table 1-17	Opioids Used Intravenously During Anesthesia			
Drug	**Relative Potency**	**Time to Peak Effect[a] (min)**	**Duration of Action**	**Elimination Half-Life (hr)**
Morphine	1	10	Long	2.9
Meperidine	0.1	10	Intermediate	4.2
Methadone	1	30	Long	35
Fentanyl	100	5	Intermediate	3.7
Sufentanil	500–1,000	2–5	Intermediate	2.7
Alfentanil	25	1–2	Short	1.5
Remifentanil	100	Immediate	Short	0.15

[a]When given intravenously.

The CNS effects of opioids include analgesia, euphoria, drowsiness, miosis, depression of the cough reflex, nausea, and vomiting. Analgesia is caused by a reduction in the transmission of noxious stimuli at the peripheral, spinal, and central levels. Nausea and vomiting are caused by stimulation of both the vestibular system and the central chemoreceptor trigger zone in the medulla. High doses of opioids cause drowsiness and sedation, but do not reliably cause unconsciousness, so anesthesia must include other agents.

Cardiovascular effects include bradycardia that is caused by stimulation of vagal nuclei in the medulla and is easily treated with atropine. Meperidine may cause tachycardia in large intravenous doses, presumably because its chemical structure is similar to that of atropine. Only meperidine causes myocardial depression in clinically useful doses, which can be as low as 2 to 2.5 mg/kg. Morphine and meperidine stimulate the release of histamine in clinical doses, resulting in arteriolar and venous dilation and hypotension. Because fentanyl, sufentanil, alfentanil, and remifentanil do not show this effect, these narcotics are most often used in high doses during anesthesia.

All opioid agonists produce a dose-dependent respiratory depression that causes an equivalent right shift of the CO_2 response curve, but does not alter its slope (Fig. 1-6). The effect is equal for all drugs at equianalgesic doses. Lower doses decrease the respiratory rate without changing the tidal volume, but at higher doses, the tidal volume is also smaller. Pontine and medullary centers are depressed at still higher doses and breathing becomes irregular, with eventual apnea ensuing in the unstimulated patient.

Contrary to previous belief, opioids alone do not affect renal function or antidiuretic hormone secretion. Their effects on the liver are limited to contraction of the sphincter of Oddi and an increase in pressure in the biliary tree. Opioids decrease the motility of the gastrointestinal tract, causing ileus, delayed gastric emptying, and constipation.

All agonists can cause skeletal muscle rigidity when given in high intravenous doses, but only fentanyl, sufentanil, and alfentanil are given in sufficiently large boluses for this effect to be clinically significant. Large individual variation in this effect is seen; it can occur with doses as small as 1 mg/kg fentanyl. Rigidity is not caused by an action at the neuromuscular junction, but rather by a central effect. Nonetheless, sometimes a patient who has truncal rigidity after receiving intravenous narcotics cannot be ventilated until a muscle relaxant is administered. Muscle rigidity rarely occurs when opioids are given after an inhalation anesthetic is started.

In general, the narcotics used in the perioperative period are safe. The most common problems are respiratory depression and resultant hypoxemia. Hypotension is seen mainly with morphine because of its histamine-releasing effects or in severely hypovolemic patients. There is no evidence of teratogenicity, organ toxicity, or other delayed effects. Overdose is easily reversed with antagonists, although these drugs have serious side effects of their own (see later). Allergic reactions are rare, and they usually cause urticaria rather than anaphylaxis. Because they stimulate histamine release, morphine and meperidine may cause local wheal and flare formation at and near the site of injection. Meperidine is contraindicated in patients who are taking monoamine oxidase (MAO) inhibitors;

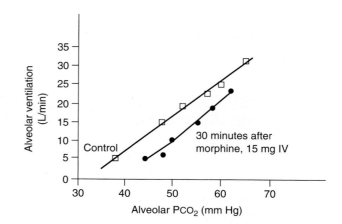

Figure 1-6 The CO_2 response curve is shifted to the right after opioid administration. (Modified from Bailey PR, Stanley TH. Narcotic intravenous anesthetics. In Miller RD, ed. *Anesthesia.* 3rd ed. New York: Churchill Livingstone; 1990.)

tachycardia and hypertension can lead to death with this combination of agents.

Opioid Antagonists

Naloxone and naltrexone are competitive antagonists at the m, k, and S receptors for all opioid effects, including analgesia. Naltrexone, a long-acting antagonist used only in an oral preparation, has no use in the perioperative period. Naloxone is used to reverse narcotic-induced ventilatory depression and sedation in the immediate postoperative period and to treat unwanted side effects of epidural, subarachnoid, or continuous-infusion narcotics. Unfortunately, doses that rapidly reverse ventilatory depression may lead to such rapid onset of pain that the accompanying sympathetic stimulation causes tachycardia, hypertension, and CNS excitement. Doses of 0.1 to 0.4 mg naloxone are associated with atrial and ventricular dysrhythmia, pulmonary edema, cardiac arrest, and convulsions. To balance the desired effect of analgesia with the undesirable effect of respiratory depression, ventilation is supported while reversal is titrated with small, incremental doses of naloxone. In this way, a balance can be achieved between analgesia and acceptable respiration. The effect of naloxone lasts only approximately 30 minutes, so repeated doses or continuous infusion may be necessary. The best course is to tailor narcotic administration to avoid respiratory depression.

Sedation

Sedation is used in the operating room as well as in special procedure areas, radiology, computed tomography scanning, magnetic resonance imaging, dental and other offices, and elsewhere. Anesthesiologists may or may not be involved in administering the sedation and monitoring the patient. The term "Monitored Anesthesia Care" (MAC) is used to describe anesthesiologist-provided sedation, medical management, and patient monitoring during surgery or other procedures. The Joint Commission on Accreditation of Health Care Organizations and other agencies have issued regulations governing patient sedation for procedures outside the operating room. Minimum monitoring standards include the presence of a qualified professional dedicated to caring for the patient. Within the hospital setting, the same standards for monitoring apply as when the patient is anesthetized. The term "conscious sedation" is often used to differentiate sedation provided outside the operating room from the sedation provided within the operating room. The definition of conscious sedation includes the presence of response to verbal and physical stimuli, maintenance of airway protective reflexes, and stable cardiovascular parameters. However, sedation is a continuum from the state of being awake to that of being unconscious (Table 1-18). Patients may slide along that continuum to the point of losing protective reflexes or respiratory drive and become endangered at any time. Therefore, the setting must provide sources of oxygen and suction, equipment for airway management, drugs for resuscitation, and personnel qualified to administer resuscitation. Sedatives are given according to carefully designed algorithms that consider the times to peak drug effects and individual patient differences. Intravenous sedation should be given only with a functioning infusion.

Monitoring the Anesthetized Patient

Continuous assessment of physiologic function is essential to maintain homeostasis and return the patient to the preanesthetic state. The anesthesiologist monitors the patient's oxygenation, level of consciousness, ventilation, circulation, and body temperature. Other monitors may also be necessary, depending on the patient and the surgical procedure. Table 1-19 summarizes monitors used in the operating room.

Basic Intraoperative Monitoring

Basic intraoperative monitoring for patients under the care of the anesthesiologist is described in standards published by the ASA (Table 1-20). Some states and malpractice insurance carriers also require basic monitoring.

Oxygenation

To prevent the administration of a hypoxic gas mixture, the concentration of oxygen in the inspired or expired gas

Table 1-18	Continuum of Sedation			
	Minimal Sedation (Anxiolysis)	**Moderate Sedation/ Analgesia (Conscious Sedation)**	**Deep Sedation/ Analgesia**	**General Anesthesia**
Responsiveness	Normal response to verbal stimulation	Purposeful[a] response to verbal or tactile stimulation	Purposeful[a] response following repeated or painful stimulation	Unarousable even with painful stimulus
Airway	Unaffected	No intervention required	Intervention may be required	Intervention often required
Spontaneous ventilation	Unaffected	Adequate	May be inadequate	Frequently inadequate
Cardiovascular function	Unaffected	Usually maintained	Usually maintained	May be impaired

[a]Reflex withdrawal from a painful stimulus is *not* considered a purposeful response.

Table 1-19	Intraoperative Monitors of the Body Systems

Cardiovascular system	Blood pressure
	    Pulse palpation
	    Auscultation
	    Oscillometry
	    Doppler
	    Automated sphygmomanometers
	    Intra-arterial measurement
	Cardiac rhythm and rate
	    Auscultation
	    Lead II electrocardiogram
	    Pulse palpation
	    Pulse oximetry
	Myocardial perfusion
	    Lead V electrocardiogram
	    Pressure wave form
	    ST segment trending
	    Transesophageal echocardiography
	Peripheral perfusion
	    Pulse palpation
	    Pulse oximetry
	    Arterial blood gases

Respiratory system	Observation and auscultation
	Inspired pressure gauge
	Spirometry
	Pneumotachograph
	Oxygenation
	    Observation
	    Pulse oximetry
	    Transcutaneous oxygen analysis
	    Mass spectrometry
	    Arterial blood gases
	Carbon dioxide excretion
	    Capnography
	    Mass spectrometry
	    Transcutaneous CO_2 analyzers
	    Arterial blood gases

Central nervous system	Observation
	    Eye signs
	    Respiration and heart rate
	Intracranial pressure monitoring
	Electroencephalogram, evoked potentials

Renal function	Urine output Electrolytes
Metabolic system	Body temperature Blood glucose Electrolytes Arterial blood gases
Circulating volume	Blood pressure Pulse characteristics Right and left ventricular filling pressures Urine output Arterial blood gases Electrolytes and hematocrit
Coagulation	Observation Laboratory tests
Integumentary and neuromuscular system	Direct observation of position and padding Nerve stimulator

Table 1-20	Standards for Basic Intraoperative Monitoring
Qualified anesthesia personnel present at all times	
Continual evaluation of the patient's oxygenation, ventilation, circulation, and temperature	
Oxygenation	Inspired oxygen concentration Pulse oximetry Skin color
Ventilation	Observation, auscultation Capnography (CO_2 content of expired air) to verify endotracheal tube placement throughout the anesthetic procedure unless the nature of the patient or procedure makes it impossible Spirometry Alarm disconnected when ventilator is used
Circulation	Electrocardiogram Blood pressure Heart rate Peripheral perfusion: palpation of pulse, heart auscultation, pulse oximetry, plethysmography, or intra-arterial pressure tracing
Temperature	Temperature monitoring in every patient receiving anesthesia when clinically significant changes in body temperature are intended, anticipated, or suspected

is measured with an oxygen analyzer. Several devices are available; most measure oxygen content by an electrochemical process (a current is produced that is proportional to the partial pressure of oxygen). These sensors require frequent calibration. They are attached to the anesthesia machine directly in line with the patient's inspired or expired gases in the breathing circuit, which connects the anesthesia machine to the patient. Among the sensors is an audible alarm that is set to the desired minimum concentration, usually 30%, before anesthetic delivery begins.

Adequate oxygen content in the patient's blood is a major concern during administration of an anesthetic. Several methods are available to evaluate oxygenation. The color of the patient's skin and of blood in the surgical field are the simplest, most direct monitors. Although these are the least quantitative measures, they should be evaluated continuously. Cyanosis usually is apparent when the concentration of deoxygenated hemoglobin reaches 5 g/dL. This assessment of color requires that the operating room be adequately illuminated and that a portion of the patient be exposed and available for observation. Observation of skin color may be unreliable in dark-skinned or anemic patients, but blood can usually be evaluated in the surgical field.

The development of the **pulse oximeter** greatly improved the adequacy and accuracy of patient monitoring. Pulse oximeters measure changes in the ratio of bright red, oxygenated hemoglobin to darker, deoxygenated hemoglobin. They display this ratio as percentage of oxygen saturation. Two different waveforms of light are projected through a translucent portion of tissue (e.g., fingertip, earlobe) to a detection cell on the other side. One frequency of light is absorbed by oxygenated hemoglobin; the other is absorbed by both oxygenated and deoxygenated hemoglobin. As hemoglobin enters the tissue with arterial pulsation, more light is absorbed. Microelectronics interpret the change in light absorption as a pulse and use the ratio of absorption of the two light waves to calculate the percentage of oxygen saturation in hemoglobin entering the tissue. In this way, the anesthesiologist is given a pulse-to-pulse update of the adequacy of oxygenation, as well as a monitor of tissue perfusion.

Arterial blood may also be sampled for blood gas analysis. This invasive technique is made easier by inserting an indwelling arterial cannula. Blood gas analysis is often used to check the accuracy of other monitors and to assess acid–base and electrolyte status and hematocrit. Catheters that have oxygen sensors at the tip to allow continuous monitoring of Pao_2 are being perfected.

Ventilation

The adequacy of ventilation must be monitored continually throughout an anesthetic administration. Several direct methods are used; the most direct is observation of chest excursion and change in volume in the reservoir bag of the breathing circuit during respiration. There is no substitute for auscultation of breath sounds, however, in evaluating respiratory status. A precordial stethoscope is a heavily weighted bell that is placed over the precordium, or sternal notch, during anesthesia. When the trachea is intubated, an esophageal stethoscope can be substituted. This instrument, which is a plastic tube with a soft balloon at the end, is placed directly into the esophagus. The anesthesiologist usually listens through a monaural earpiece that allows simultaneous monitoring of ventilation and communication with operating room personnel.

More quantitative monitors of ventilation are also used. The best monitor of ventilatory adequacy is arterial blood gas analysis. This technique is often used to assess the accuracy of the other monitors. Many operating room electrocardiogram (ECG) monitors provide a **pneumotachogram,** which is a respiratory trace of both chest motion and respiratory rate. Expansion of the chest may not indicate effective air movement if the upper airway or endotracheal tube is obstructed, however. A spirometer attached to the expiratory limb of the breathing circuit gives a breath-to-breath record of expired volume. The best constant monitor of adequate ventilation is the expired CO pressure ($Peco_2$), which is determined by a capnograph or respiratory gas analyzer. Unless there is a large ventilation–perfusion abnormality, the end expired CO_2, which reflects the alveolar CO_2 concentration, is very close to the arterial CO_2 concentration. Expired gas is monitored at the patient's endotracheal tube with a small infrared device or at the monitoring unit after a small quantity of expired gas is aspirated through a small catheter in the breathing circuit. Usually the monitor provides a plot of CO_2 partial pressure against time, displayed as a capnogram, and allows the anesthesiologist to assess the pattern of respiration. A slow rise in exhaled CO_2 pressure indicates obstructive airway dysfunction that may be caused by chronic disease, acute bronchospasm, or tube kinking. If the curve does not return to zero during inspiration, there is CO_2 in the inspired gas. A sudden drop in expired CO_2 may be caused by acute pulmonary embolism with air, blood clot, or another substance or by an acute drop in cardiac output that leads to failure of pulmonary perfusion and CO_2 excretion.

Correct placement of the endotracheal tube must be verified after every intubation. Undetected esophageal placement results in hypoxemia in apneic patients and is rapidly fatal. The first steps in confirmation are visualizing chest expansion and water vapor in the tube during expiration and hearing bilateral equal breath sounds over both sides of the chest. The sounds over the stomach should be distant if present. However, evaluation of chest excursion and breath sounds may be misleading. A decrease in oxygen saturation is a late indication of esophageal intubation and a sign that the patient is already in danger. A normal capnogram that is sustained over several breaths is the strongest evidence that the tube is in the trachea. Small disposable CO_2 detectors are now available to confirm tracheal placement outside of monitored areas. Endobronchial placement can be reliably detected by noting a large, otherwise unexplained difference in the partial pressure of oxygen between alveolar (inspired) and arterial measurements ($Pao_2 - Pao_2$) or by noting diminished breath sounds in one hemithorax compared with the other while auscultating the lateral chest walls. If only one lung is being oxygenated by fresh gas flow, a large portion of the cardiac output is not receiving oxygen. Direct observation of the carina through a fiberoptic bronchoscope inserted through the endotracheal tube past the tip or a chest x-ray are the only foolproof methods to confirm proper endotracheal tube placement.

During general anesthesia, a mechanical ventilator often controls the patient's breathing. Disconnection of the ventilator from the breathing circuit is fatal if the patient is paralyzed, hypocapnic, or apneic because of the respiratory depressant effects of the anesthetic. The anesthesia machine must be equipped with a low-pressure alarm in the breathing circuit that activates if positive pressure is not sensed within a certain period. Many machines also have a high pressure sensing system that sounds or automatically relieves pressure if a preset pressure is exceeded during the ventilatory cycle (e.g., the endotracheal tube becomes obstructed by kinking or a mucus plug or the patient's lung compliance suddenly decreases markedly because of tension pneumothorax).

Circulation

Without instrumentation, circulation can be measured continuously by listening to the heart and palpating a peripheral pulse. The speed of pulse upstroke provides a qualitative assessment of the force of myocardial contraction and cardiac output. The volume of heart sounds provides the same information. These methods also show changes in rhythm.

The ECG, a required operating room monitor, evaluates heart rate and rhythm and indicates myocardial oxygenation. Modern ECG monitors use a four- or five-lead system, with one or two standard leads continuously monitored on a cathode ray tube. Most have extensive filtering systems to reduce interference by other electrical equipment in the operating room. Many also store tracings so that comparisons can be made when change occurs or a hard copy is needed for later analysis. An audible beep is provided and QRS complexes are counted to provide an averaged heart rate, which is displayed on the screen. Lead II is most often used for rhythm analysis because the P wave is most evident in that lead. If ischemic episodes are of concern, lead V5 is preferred because it monitors the anterolateral wall of the left ventricle, where most ischemic episodes occur. If the area of the ventricle at risk is known preoperatively, a five-lead system allows the anesthesiologist to choose which area to monitor for S-T segment changes. Continuous simultaneous monitoring of leads II and V5 detects approximately 75% of intraoperative myocardial ischemic events. Many ECG monitors analyze S-T segment depression or elevation and are more accurate than the anesthesiologist's observational skills in detecting incipient events.

Various instruments are used to monitor peripheral circulation continuously. The most commonly used is the pulse oximeter (discussed previously). Doppler pulse monitors placed directly over a peripheral pulse detect changes in sound wave transmission of arterial pulsation and are monitored by an audible sound. Pulse plethysmography measures changes in light absorption in the tissue as blood volume changes with arterial pulsation. This method is similar to pulse oximetry, but lacks the second light wave needed to calculate oxygen saturation.

Systemic blood pressure must be assessed at least every 5 minutes and, along with the heart rate, recorded on the anesthesia record graphically. The 5-minute standard is generally accepted as the minimum interval to permit detection of trends early enough to allow successful intervention. The standard method of determining blood pressure uses a cuff over the brachial artery (although other peripheral arteries are occasionally used), an aneroid (non–fluid-containing) manometer, and a stethoscope affixed over the artery. Oscillometry can produce reliable measurements, but errors in diastolic pressure are more likely. A finger on the pulse, a Doppler probe, or a plethysmograph can be placed distal to the cuff to detect systolic blood pressure, but again, determining diastolic pressure is difficult without a stethoscope. Whatever the detection technique, for a sphygmomanometer to function accurately and reliably, the full cuff pressure must be transmitted to the artery. Ideally, the cuff should be 20% wider than the diameter of the limb on which it is positioned. If it is too narrow, an artificially high pressure will be obtained; if it is too wide, the pressure will be underestimated. The inflatable

rubber bladder within the cuff should just encircle the limb without overlapping and should be no shorter than half the limb circumference.

Several automated noninvasive blood pressure monitors are available and have almost replaced the manual devices in the operating and recovery rooms. These devices use either a Doppler or an oscillometric technique and display the systolic, diastolic, and mean pressures. They can also display the heart rate at an interval set by the user, which can be as frequent as 1 minute. Most are equipped with audible alarms for high or low values and for changes from previously determined values. These automated monitors are more accurate than manual techniques, and they function reliably even when the patient is profoundly hypotensive. They are valuable also because they free the anesthesiologist to perform other functions while they perform blood pressure determinations during busy or critical times.

Temperature

During surgery and anesthesia, a patient can lose a significant amount of body heat and become hypothermic. Severe hypothermia results in hemodynamic compromise, cardiac irritability, metabolic change, decreased coagulation, and postoperative shivering, with a corresponding increase in oxygen consumption. Almost all patients lose some body heat, but infants and geriatric patients are particularly at risk. An intraoperative increase in temperature is much less common, but must be detected early and treated because of the metabolic consequences (e.g., marked increase in oxygen consumption and carbon dioxide production). Malignant hyperthermia is a rare hypermetabolic response to anesthesia and surgery that causes profound morbidity and frequent death. Temperature rise is usually only a late manifestation of the syndrome. It occurs after earlier signs of tachycardia, hypertension, and increased CO_2 production (see Chapter 2, Perioperative Management of Surgical Patients, Lawrence et al., *Essentials of General Surgery*, 4th ed.).

Because these conditions must be treated early, continuous temperature monitoring in the operating room is desirable. The most common method in the intubated patient is the esophageal temperature probe, which may be incorporated into the esophageal stethoscope. Temperature probes can also be inserted in the rectum, nasopharynx, axilla, or external auditory canal near the tympanic membrane. Skin patches, usually placed on the forehead, provide a continuous digital display that uses liquid crystal thermography. They are useful for determining trends, but are not as accurate as probes placed nearer to the core.

The Anesthesiologist

Despite sophisticated technology, the anesthesiologist remains the principal monitor and should be present and alert at all times. The anesthesiologist should also keep an accurate, timely, and inclusive record of all events that occur in the operating room. This record, which should become a part of the patient's permanent medical record, should include information about positioning and padding; anesthetic technique; monitors used and information gathered from them; drugs and doses; fluids administered, including blood products; airway maintenance techniques; and all events related to the surgery. Vital signs and other physiologic data should be recorded graphically at 5-minute intervals. This record is useful in determining trends during the course of the anesthetic. It also provides valuable information for postoperative care.

Additional and Optional Monitors

Neuromuscular Blockade
Neuromuscular-blocking drugs are often administered during general anesthesia to provide relaxation that is essential for the surgery, to facilitate controlled ventilation, or to provide optimal conditions without the cardiovascular depression that is associated with deep anesthesia. Monitoring the extent of the blockade helps to determine subsequent doses, adequacy of reversal, and criteria for extubation at the end of the procedure. The extent of blockade can be estimated without instrumentation. Observation of the surgical field gives an indication of how well the muscles are relaxed. During abdominal surgery, the contents of the peritoneal cavity are extruded through the incision when abdominal wall tone is high and the surgeon has difficulty approximating the wound edges at closure. Increased abdominal and respiratory muscle tone is evident as decreased compliance (increased inspiratory pressure) during controlled ventilation. The recovery from blockade can be estimated by measuring respiratory tidal volume, vital capacity, and negative inspiratory force. In the conscious patient, adequate return of muscle function is indicated by the strength of the handgrip and the ability to hold the head off the table for at least 5 seconds.

The extent of neuromuscular function can be measured with a nerve stimulator. This instrument delivers a small electrical stimulus to skin electrodes that are placed over a motor nerve (usually ulnar). The response (flexion of the fourth and fifth digits) is observed. If the arm is not accessible, the forehead or foot can be used. The train-of-four stimulus pattern is usually chosen because it is the most sensitive to varying levels of blockade with a nondepolarizing relaxant (see Table 1-9). Other parameters monitored include the single-twitch response at a rate of one per 1, 5, or 10 seconds and the response to tetanic stimulation at a rate of 50 to 200 Hz.

Respiratory Gases
In addition to capnography and an oxygen analyzer in the circuit, other methods are used to monitor respiratory gases. The respiratory gas analyzer is used to sample and analyze both inspired and expired gases and to measure the content of oxygen, carbon dioxide, and each of the inhaled anesthetics. A small sample of the respiratory gas is withdrawn into a vacuum chamber through a catheter placed at the junction of the patient's endotracheal tube and the breathing circuit. The sample is then analyzed by ion or infrared detection. Most instruments provide a numeric display of inspired partial pressure or percent concentration and a continuous capnogram or graphic display of other gas concentrations.

Urine Output
To avoid overdistention of the bladder during long surgeries and to provide a monitor of renal function, Foley catheters are often positioned in the bladder before surgery. Frequently measured urine output is a good indicator of blood volume, renal function, and visceral perfusion. Intraoperative oliguria may be the result of decreased renal perfusion because of blood volume depletion, circulatory failure, the antidiuretic effects of anesthetics or other drugs, or the hormonal response to stress. It can also be caused by mechanical obstruction of the ureters or the catheter.

The quality of the urine is also a good monitor of physiologic status. The specific gravity can often be easily estimated from changes in urine color, giving a good indication of renal perfusion. If the urine becomes reddish, a microscopic examination and quick dipstick test will tell whether it contains blood, hemoglobin, or myoglobin. Blood indicates trauma to the kidneys, ureters, or bladder. Hemoglobin or myoglobin indicates a serious systemic problem that may easily result in renal or other end-organ damage. The cause should be found and treatment instituted immediately. Electrolyte and glucose content of the urine provides valuable information about the volume status and renal concentrating ability. The benefits of continuous urine output monitoring must be weighed against the risks. Catheterization has the potential for trauma to the bladder and urethra and introduces another source of infection.

Specialized and Intensive Monitoring

Invasive Hemodynamic Pressure Monitoring
Occasionally, a preexisting medical condition or the nature of the surgery necessitates highly specialized and invasive monitoring. Because of their potential complications, invasive monitors are reserved for situations in which conventional monitors do not provide adequate information. They are used for moment-to-moment assessment of patients who are at high risk for cardiovascular decompensation; in open-heart, major vascular, or intracranial surgery; and when high-volume or rapid blood loss is anticipated.

Intra-arterial blood pressure monitoring provides beat-to-beat analysis of blood pressure and pulse characteristics. The tracing gives a good indication of the volume of each pulse and may help the observer to draw conclusions about cardiac output and circulating volume, as well as the effect of dysrhythmias. This monitoring is particularly useful when rapid pressure changes are expected and measurement must be taken more often than once a minute (the fastest cycle of the automated, noninvasive monitors). An indwelling cannula is inserted into a peripheral artery (usually radial) and connected to a pressure transducer with noncompliant, small-bore tubing. The tubing is filled with heparinized saline and connected to a continual flushing system that provides a slow infusion of the heparinized solution to prevent clotting of the catheter or artery. Because the fluid in the tubing is noncompressible and the tubing is noncompliant, the pressure exerted on the fluid column at the tip of the cannula is accurately transmitted to the transducer. A wave form is generated by each arterial pulsation, and the systolic (peak), diastolic (nadir), and mean pressures are digitally displayed. The cannula also provides ready access for blood sampling, thereby making intraoperative determinations of arterial gases, pH, glucose, electrolytes, hematocrit, and other blood tests more convenient.

Transducers require special care, calibration, and "zeroing" to provide a valid pressure measurement. After the stopcock at the top of the transducer is opened to air, the transducer is positioned at the level of the patient's heart and the electronic components are adjusted to read zero. All pressure measurements must be made with the transducer at this reference level. Air bubbles in the tubing or transducer "damp" the tracing and provide inaccurate readings.

Intra-arterial monitoring may have complications. Clots can accumulate on the cannula tip, leading to thrombosis of the vessel, embolization, and even gangrene of the extremity. The use of heparin flush, small cannulas, and limited duration of cannulation can minimize the frequency of this complication. When cannulation of the radial artery is anticipated, the patency of cross-circulation from the ulnar artery is often assessed with a modified Allen test. After both the radial and ulnar arteries are occluded with the thumbs, the patient opens and closes the fist several times to blanch the hand. The hand is observed for flushing after the ulnar artery is released but the radial artery is still occluded. If the entire hand does not flush, the palmar arch is not completely patent. The radial artery should not be cannulated because its potential obstruction might cause hand ischemia. Recent literature questions the efficacy of the Allen test in predicting whether distal ischemia may follow radial artery cannulation, but it is still frequently performed.

When large changes in intravascular fluid volume are expected, fluid replacement is more easily managed by monitoring the central venous pressure (CVP). CVP is the hydrostatic pressure exerted by the blood in the right atrium. It is an indirect measure of the amount of blood filling the right ventricle. In the normally functioning heart, the pressure required to fill the left ventricle is 4 to 5 mm Hg higher than that for the right ventricle. Although lower than the left ventricle filling pressure, the CVP still varies directly with that pressure. When blood volume is diminished or venous capacitance is increased, less blood returns to the heart from the periphery, the ventricle is less well filled, and the CVP is correspondingly low. Increased circulating blood volume or peripheral vasoconstriction increases CVP. However, poor ventricular contraction or an impedance to ventricular outflow because of lung pathology elevates CVP, even with normal or diminished blood circulating volume.

Measuring CVP requires insertion (through the internal or external jugular, subclavian, or cephalic vein) of a fluid-filled cannula into the right atrium or superior vena cava, just above the atrium. The cannula may be connected to a water manometer or pressure transducer in a manner similar to that of an indwelling arterial cannula. Because intrathoracic pressures that result from respiration are transmitted to the heart, measurements are taken at the end of expiration. The wave form generated with a transducer monitoring system also provides information about atrial contraction and intracardiac valve function.

When left-sided heart failure or valvular dysfunction occurs, CVP is not an adequate measure of circulating blood volume. In this situation, a **pulmonary artery catheter,** the Swan-Ganz, provides more accurate determinations of left ventricle filling pressure. The Swan-Ganz catheter is a long, multilumen catheter with an inflatable balloon on the tip. The catheter is inserted through an access sheath placed in the external or internal jugular or subclavian vein. After it is threaded into the superior vena cava, the balloon is inflated with a small amount of air, and the catheter is advanced through the right side of the heart and into the pulmonary artery. The pressure wave from the distal port of the catheter is monitored while the catheter is being threaded into the pulmonary artery (Fig. 1-7). The balloon allows the catheter to flow more easily through the heart along with the flow of blood. As the catheter is advanced within the pulmonary artery, the diameter of the vessels decreases and the balloon eventually becomes "wedged." In this position, if there is no abnormality in the pulmonary vasculature distal to the balloon, the pressure sensed at the tip of the catheter reflects that of the left atrium. This pressure is called the pulmonary capillary occlusion pressure, pulmonary artery occlusion pressure, or more commonly (but inaccurately), wedge pressure. During surgery and anesthesia, the changes in pulmonary artery pressure, wedge pressure, and cardiac output provide the best information, allowing the anesthesiologist to optimize the patient's circulation with a combination of fluid administration, inotropic agents, and manipulation of peripheral resistance. Using right atrial pressure as a monitor of circulating volume is perfectly adequate in patients whose myocardial and valvular function is good because differences in right and left heart outputs are not usually seen. The pressure tracings displayed on the monitor are characteristic for each step of insertion. The tracings indicate exactly when the catheter tip enters the right atrium, right ventricle, pulmonary artery, and wedged position. When the catheter is correctly placed, deflating the balloon results in a normal pulmonary arterial pressure tracing. Reinflating it restores the tracing to the wedge configuration. Wedge pressures are obtained only intermittently. The balloon remains deflated at all other times to prevent ischemia of the distal lung or trauma to the vessel wall.

In the absence of pulmonary arterial disease or pulmonary hypertension, pulmonary arterial diastolic pressure

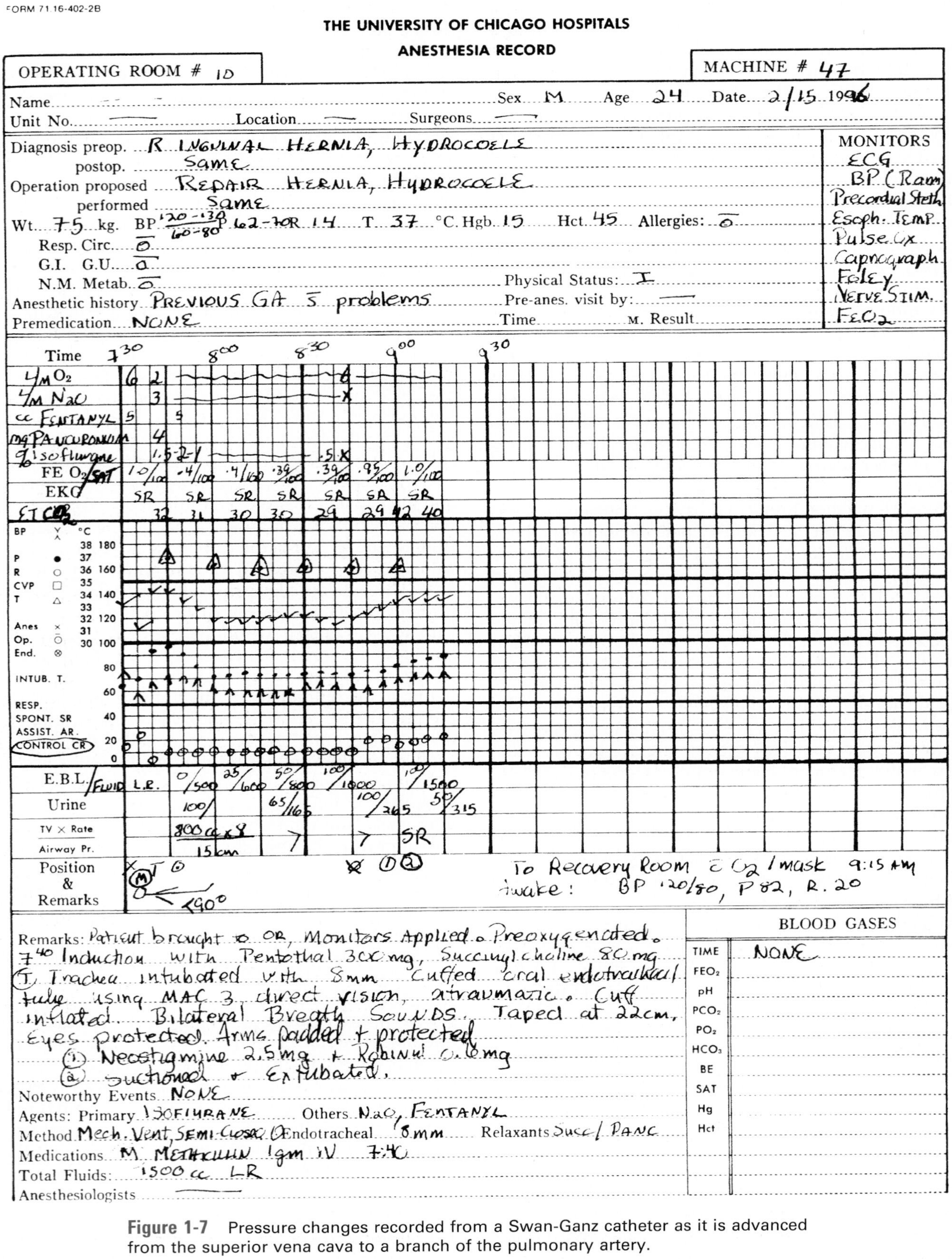
FORM 71.16-402-2B

THE UNIVERSITY OF CHICAGO HOSPITALS

ANESTHESIA RECORD

OPERATING ROOM # 1D

MACHINE # 47

Name ——— Sex M Age 24 Date 2/15 1996

Unit No. ——— Location ——— Surgeons ———

Diagnosis preop. R INGUINAL HERNIA, HYDROCOELE

postop. Same

Operation proposed REPAIR HERNIA, HYDROCOELE

performed Same

Wt. 75 kg. BP 120-130/60-80 P. 62-70 R. 14 T. 37 °C. Hgb. 15 Hct. 45 Allergies: ō

Resp. Circ. ō

G.I. G.U. ō

N.M. Metab. ō Physical Status: I

Anesthetic history PREVIOUS GA s̄ problems Pre-anes. visit by: ———

Premedication NONE Time M. Result

MONITORS: ECG, BP (Ram), Precordial Steth, Esoph. Temp, Pulse Ox, Capnograph, Foley, Nerve Stim., FeO2

Time	7:30	8:00	8:30	9:00	9:30
L/M O2	6 2 ——— 6				
L/M N2O	3 ——— X				
cc Fentanyl	5 5				
mg Pancuronium	4				
% Isoflurane	1.5-2-1 ——— .5 X				
FE O2/SAT	1.0/100 .4/100 .4/100 .39/100 .39/100 .95/100 1.0/100				
EKG	SR SR SR SR SR SR SR				
ET CO2	32 31 30 30 29 29 42 40				

BP ˅ ˄ °C; P ●; R ○; CVP □; T △; Anes ×; Op. ⊙; End. ⊗; INTUB. T.; RESP.; SPONT. SR; ASSIST. AR; CONTROL CR

E.B.L./Fluid	L.R.	0/500	25/600	50/800	100/1000	10/1500
Urine		100/	65/165	100/265	50/315	
TV × Rate		800 cc × 8	→	→	SR	
Airway Pr.		15 cm				

Position & Remarks: X T ⊙ Ⓜ ⊗ ① ② ← 90° To Recovery Room c̄ O2 / mask 9:15 AM Awake: BP 120/80, P 82, R. 20

Remarks: Patient brought to OR, Monitors Applied. Preoxygenated. 7:40 Induction with Pentothal 300 mg, Succinylcholine 80 mg Ⓣ Trachea intubated with 8mm cuffed oral endotracheal tube using MAC 3, direct vision, atraumatic. Cuff inflated. Bilateral Breath Sounds. Taped at 22cm. Eyes protected. Arms padded + protected.
① Neostigmine 2.5mg + Robinul 0.6mg
② Suctioned + Extubated.

Noteworthy Events NONE

Agents: Primary ISOFLURANE Others N2O, FENTANYL

Method Mech. Vent, Semi-Closed Endotracheal 8mm Relaxants Succ / Panc

Medications M. Methicillin 1gm IV 7:40

Total Fluids: 1500 cc LR

Anesthesiologists ———

BLOOD GASES	
TIME	NONE
FEO2	
pH	
PCO2	
PO2	
HCO3	
BE	
SAT	
Hg	
Hct	

Figure 1-7 Pressure changes recorded from a Swan-Ganz catheter as it is advanced from the superior vena cava to a branch of the pulmonary artery.

reflects the wedge pressure and, thus, the left atrial pressure. It can be used as a continuous monitor of left ventricular filling. The Swan-Ganz catheter also has a proximal port in the right atrium that allows the right atrial pressure to be monitored continuously and its pressure wave displayed. This catheter also allows the user to measure cardiac output by the thermodilution technique. A measured amount of iced or room temperature saline is injected through the right ventricular port while a thermistor sensor tip senses changes in blood temperature. A portable computer connected to the catheter calculates the cardiac output as the integrated time versus temperature change curve and displays this curve digitally.

The pulmonary artery catheter can also provide continuous monitoring of blood temperature by the thermistor. In addition, a pacing port can be used to allow a paced cardiac rhythm, and samples can be drawn to measure mixed **venous oxygen saturation** (SvO_2). This measurement provides the best available monitor of tissue perfusion and oxygen availability.

Pulmonary artery and right atrial pressure monitors are indispensable to anesthesiologists in many situations, but are not without risks and complications. Insertion sites are another source of infection. Arrhythmias commonly occur when catheters or guide wires irritate the conduction system. They are especially common when pulmonary artery catheters are inserted. The risk of air embolism is always present when central catheters are in place, and thrombus formation is not uncommon. Pulmonary artery catheters may knot in the ventricle, even around chordae, and damage heart valves. Rupture of the pulmonary vessels is reported, especially if the Swan-Ganz catheter is advanced too far or the balloon is not deflated. Finally, pneumothorax, hemothorax, or accidental carotid puncture occasionally occurs.

Transesophageal echocardiography (TEE) may be used intraoperatively for detailed monitoring of volume status, valvular function, and myocardial contractility, and for early detection of myocardial ischemia. The probe is located at the tip of a modified gastroscope that is inserted through the esophagus and positioned behind the heart to provide a continuous picture of the heart displayed on a television monitor. Early ischemic events are often diagnosed by decreased contraction of affected segments of the left ventricular wall before ECG evidence is apparent (regional wall motion abnormality). Volume status is easily assessed by the end-systolic diameter of the ventricle. With experience, the anesthesiologist can assess valvular efficiency and inotropy. TEE is especially useful in diagnosing air or particulate matter entering the circulation.

Complications of TEE in the anesthetized patient are limited to trauma to the mouth or esophagus caused by insertion of the gastroscope. The technology is expensive, but appears to be durable and reliable in providing an accurate, comprehensive monitor of cardiac status.

Central Nervous System Monitoring

In patients who have decreased intracranial compliance, further increases in ICP can rapidly cause brain stem deformation and death. Because anesthetics and small changes in hemodynamic and ventilatory parameters can profoundly affect ICP, monitoring this pressure is often useful during anesthesia. This monitoring is accomplished by the neurosurgeon, who drills a small hole in the skull and inserts a cannula connected to a pressure transducer into one of the ventricles of the brain. Alternatively, a subdural or extradural transducer is implanted. A pressure tracing is displayed, and the mean pressure is calculated and exhibited. The ventricular catheter also allows withdrawal of CSF, if necessary, to reduce the pressure. All of these methods are invasive and introduce the potential for infection.

Recently, the ability to monitor cerebral function by the EEG and its variations was introduced into the operating room. The EEG is a complex wave generated by the electrical activity of the brain. The electrical potential is measured between small electrodes, either adhesive patches or needles applied to the scalp. The resulting voltage differences are displayed so that the user can compare the activities of the two hemispheres. Several devices are available to process the EEG in various ways. The most common is currently bispectral analysis (BIS). BIS separates the EEG into component waveforms and analyzes the levels of synchronization, frequency, and amplitude. EEG and processed EEG monitoring are most useful when a compromise of the cerebral circulation is anticipated (e.g., during cranial vascular surgery, carotid artery surgery, or cardiopulmonary bypass). BIS is heavily marketed as a monitor of depth of anesthesia that allows more rapid emergence and prevents intraoperative awareness.

A more refined method of EEG monitoring, evoked potential response, measures the cortical response to sensory stimulation of a peripheral nerve. This measure is obtained by applying repeated stimuli to a sensory nerve. The resulting cortical activity is averaged and displayed in a waveform that allows comparison of the latency and amplitude of the response over time. Alternatively, sections of the motor cortex may be stimulated and the peripheral motor response evaluated with a twitch recorder. A normal sensory or motor-evoked potential response is a good indication of normal transmission from peripheral nerve to brain. These monitors are most useful during spinal cord or vertebral column surgery, but they are also used to monitor cranial nerve and brain stem integrity when surgery places those structures at risk.

Transcranial Doppler ultrasonography was recently introduced into the operating room for monitoring cerebral circulation, usually during carotid endarterectomy or cardiopulmonary bypass. Its usefulness is limited because it provides information only about the large arteries and not about tissue perfusion of the brain.

Intraoperative Fluid, Electrolyte, Blood, and Component Therapy

Venous Access

Intravenous catheters are usually placed before the patient enters the operating room. Injection of a small dermal wheal of local anesthetic immediately before the procedure or application of lidocaine and prilocaine cream (EMLA) and an occlusive dressing an hour before the procedure minimizes pain. Cannulation sites depend on the location of the surgical procedure and the patient's preexisting medical conditions. Most anesthesiologists cannulate large veins on the dorsum of the nondominant hand or in the lower forearm with a 14- to 18-gauge plastic cannula. If significant blood loss is anticipated, several sites are cannulated with large-gauge catheters. Alternative sites include the cephalic or brachial veins, the external or internal jugular veins, the foot veins, or the subclavian veins. Cannulation of lower extremity veins in adults should be performed only as a last resort because of the possibility of superficial phlebitis. Femoral veins are rarely used, but few complications are reported if steps are taken to avoid infection. In infants, scalp veins are often used, but these may be more fragile than those of the extremities. The only contraindication to any site is an infection in the area. Veins distal to an infected area should not be used, nor should any veins distal to an arteriovenous fistula that has been established for hemodialysis, because the patency of the proximal veins may be compromised. A distal intravenous infusion should not be started in patients who have had a lymph node dissection or surgery on vessels in the axilla or groin. These patients may not have normal venous drainage from that extremity. Before inducing anesthesia, the anesthesiologist must confirm that vascular access is adequate for rapid infusion of fluid, the cannula is firmly secured, and all connections are tight.

Fluid and Electrolyte Therapy

Intraoperative fluid therapy begins with an assessment of volume status when the patient comes to the operating room. Despite recent evidence that a prolonged period of fasting is probably not necessary, most patients who come to surgery have had no fluid intake for the previous 8 to 12 hours. Infants and small children often have been administered clear liquids up to 2 hours before surgery. In both cases, at least part of that deficit is replaced with maintenance fluids. Preoperative "bowel prep," vomiting or nasogastric suction, fever, chronic or acute diuretic therapy, and chronic hypertension all contribute to the preoperative volume deficit. In most cases, some attempt at volume repletion should be made with a balanced isotonic solution (lactated Ringer's solution, normal saline, or Plasma-Lyte) before anesthesia is induced. Patients who are severely hypovolemic because of blood loss or bowel pathology have postural hypotension, even if they have been able to compensate by vasoconstriction. Generally, a normal heart rate and blood pressure indicate that the circulating volume is adequate and that induction can proceed without undue concern about the vasodilation that follows administration of anesthetics. (For a detailed discussion of fluid and electrolyte therapy, see Chapter 3 in Lawrence et al, *Essentials of General Surgery*, 4th ed.) In normal adults, administration of glucose is not necessary

and may even be detrimental. Whether infants need glucose is controversial, but the availability of rapid glucose determinations should allow the anesthesiologist to monitor glucose levels and plan fluid administration appropriately. Even moderate hyperglycemia increases the damage that results from hypoxic brain injury.

In replacing lost fluid and electrolytes, preexisting conditions and insensible, or unmeasurable, losses must be taken into account. Preexisting conditions (e.g., inflammation, ascites, pleural effusions) continue intraoperatively. Insensible loss occurs through the respiratory tract, exposed surfaces (e.g., muscle, peritoneum, pleura), perspiration, and the bowel. Several liters can be sequestered in the bowel if it is traumatized or if it becomes ischemic. Respiratory insensible losses can be decreased by humidifying inspired gases and by using a low flow of gases so that they are rebreathed after they pass through the carbon dioxide absorber (a closed or semiclosed breathing circuit). Losses through perspiration can be minimized by maintaining a normal body temperature in the patient and anesthesia deep enough to prevent sympathetic stimulation. Evaporation from exposed surfaces can be decreased somewhat by maintaining a lowered ambient temperature with high humidity.

Third-space loss is the volume of fluid that enters the extravascular, extracellular space in response to the disease and the trauma of the surgical procedure. Formulas for fluid replacement during surgery take into account the site and nature of the procedure. For moderately traumatic surgery (e.g., procedures on the extremities or superficial structures), 2 to 5 mL/kg/hr is infused. For more extensive surgery that requires prolonged dissection and trauma to major organs, 5 to 10 mL/kg/hr is recommended. A balanced isotonic crystalloid solution most closely resembles the characteristics of fluid lost. Third-space loss continues postoperatively, often for 2 to 3 days, and must be considered when calculating fluid requirements during this period. Unreplaced third-space loss should be suspected when urine output or central pressure falls despite seemingly adequate volume infusion.

Colloid solutions (e.g., albumin, hetastarch [Hespan], plasma) may also be used to replace insensible and third-space losses, but considerable controversy surrounds their use. They are expensive and expose the patient to the risk of infection if they are prepared from donated blood. If crystalloid alone is used, the total volume infused can be three to five times greater than that of colloid. Most patients would not be harmed by a large, rapid fluid infusion, but some may have cardiovascular, brain, or pulmonary consequences. Current recommendations are that colloid be considered to replace large, rapid fluid losses in the following situations: (a) if there is difficulty maintaining hemodynamic stability with crystalloid despite minimal external losses; (b) if the risk of fluid deficit is high because of concomitant vasodilator therapy, preexisting cardiac or pulmonary pathology, or cerebral edema; (c) if hemodynamic status cannot be monitored invasively; or (d) if the colloid oncotic pressure is lower than 15 mm Hg. (See the National Institutes of Health Consensus Conference cited at the end of this chapter.)

Blood and Component Therapy

Surgical teams, including anesthesiologists, administer more than half the blood given to patients in the United States. Blood transfusions are given to maintain oxygen-carrying capacity when blood loss occurs. Unless blood loss is extensive, volume repletion is not an indication for transfusion because it is adequately achieved with crystalloid or colloid solutions. Blood is usually replaced by component therapy: packed red blood cells are given to provide oxygen-carrying capacity; fresh frozen plasma is given to correct decreased levels of coagulation factors; and platelets are administered to correct low platelet concentrations or dysfunctioning platelets. Decisions about which components to transfuse would be much simpler if fresh whole blood were readily available because it would replace exactly what is lost. Unfortunately, the tremendous cost and administrative difficulties associated with maintaining an adequate supply of such blood make the practice prohibitive. If packed cells are used to replace blood loss, they must be accompanied by crystalloid in a 3:1 ratio or by colloid in a 1:1 ratio to replenish the volume lost.

In determining when to transfuse, the major factor to consider is the lowest hemoglobin concentration, or hematocrit, that will maintain adequate tissue oxygenation. A 1988 National Institutes of Health consensus conference recommended that blood not be transfused when the hematocrit is 30% or higher, noting that patients with chronic anemia tolerate much lower levels without ill effect. In 1989, the Food and Drug Administration recommended that patients with adequate circulating blood volume not undergo transfusion until the hemoglobin falls below 7 g/dL. Patients with ischemic cardiovascular disease or pulmonary pathology that precludes normal oxygen uptake need higher hemoglobin concentrations. The ASA published a practice guideline for perioperative transfusion in 1996 (see Suggested Readings). This guideline summarized previously issued guidelines and revised them based on evidence in the literature that suggests that patients differ in their need for hemoglobin to carry oxygen.

Despite the common practice of transfusing fresh frozen plasma and platelets when 5 to 10 units of blood are given, these components should not be given unless there is demonstrated clinical coagulopathy in the surgical field or unless laboratory tests prove a deficiency in coagulation factors of less than 50,000 platelets per high-power field. It is evident from this brief discussion that the responsible practice of transfusion therapy requires a method of rapid assessment of hemoglobin, hematocrit, and coagulation function. Many operating rooms are equipped to provide these tests, and the recent appearance of small, handheld prothrombin time and activated partial thromboplastin time analyzers has made the anesthesiologist's job much easier.

Complications

The major complications of blood or component administration are transfusion reactions, allergic reactions, electrolyte and acid–base abnormalities, dilutional coagulopathy, and infection. Major transfusion reactions are rare and are usually caused by errors in identifying patients. Approximately 1 in 100 patients has an irregular antibody that should be detected in crossmatching. The risk of an incompatible transfusion is 0.2% when ABO–Rh type-specific blood is administered. The risk decreases to 0.06% with an antibody screen and to 0.05% with a full crossmatch. A major hemolytic transfusion reaction (incidence of 1:4,000–1:6,000) is diagnosed under anesthesia by sudden hypotension, hemoglobin in the urine, and severe coagulopathy (i.e., uncontrollable bleeding in the surgical field and at sites of vascular cannulation). Treatment includes immediate discontinuation of the transfusion, hemodynamic support, maintenance of urine output by fluid administration and diuretic therapy, and administration of sodium bicarbonate to alkalinize the urine and prevent precipitation of acid hematin in the distal tubules of the kidney. Coagulopathy must be diagnosed accurately and treated appropriately, perhaps with the help of a hematologist.

Nonhemolytic transfusion reactions are febrile or allergic and are caused by the presence of allergens or pyrogens in the transfused blood. Allergic reactions occur in approximately 3% of transfusions. They rarely involve anaphylaxis. They are treated by antihistamines and fluid administration as needed. Anaphylactic shock requires intensive monitoring, hemodynamic support, epinephrine and steroid administration, and fluid replacement that may approach tens of liters in volume because of profound vasodilation and capillary leakage.

Banked blood that is preserved with citrate phosphate dextrose undergoes significant chemical and hematologic changes that increase with the length of storage. Table 1-21 summarizes those changes, indicating the scope of electrolyte and acid–base abnormalities that must be compensated for when transfusing massive amounts. Most patients do not have biochemical effects from transfusion of up to 10 units of packed cells. Rapid electrolyte and blood gas determinations are available to detect any such effects. Table 1-21 shows that there is a rapid decrease of platelet concentration and coagulation factors over time, increasing the risk of dilutional coagulopathy.

Infections that are currently attributed to the transfusion of blood components include hepatitis, cytomegalovirus (CMV), and human immunodeficiency virus. Screening of donor blood eliminates most, but not all, of these infections. Some viruses have a long incubation period during which antigens or antibodies are not evident, and some hepatitis viruses cannot be characterized as B or C. The risk of transfusion-associated viral infection is currently estimated at 1:83,000 units transfused. Table 1-22 lists the viral infections and their associated risks. Hepatitis was estimated at 1:100 transfusions before the availability of a screening test for hepatitis C in 1990. CMV is almost nor-

Table 1-21	Changes in CPD-Preserved Blood with Storage			
	Day of Storage			
Test	**1**	**7**	**14**	**21**
pH	7.1	7.0	7.0	6.9
Pco$_2$ (mm Hg)	48.0	80.0	110.0	140.0
Lactate (mEq/L)	41.0	101.1	145.0	179.0
Plasma bicarbonate (mEq/L)	18.0	15.0	12.0	11.0
Plasma potassium (mEq/L)	3.9	12.0	17.0	21.0
Plasma glucose (mg/100 mL)	345.0	312.0	181.0	231.0
Plasma hemoglobin (mg/100 mL)	1.7	7.8	13.0	19.0
Platelets (%)	10.0	0	0	0
Factors V and VII (%)	70.0	50.0	40.0	20.0

CPD, citrate phosphate dextrose.

mal in adults, causing no disease or symptoms. If transmitted to infants or immunocompromised patients, however, it can cause severe illness. Components transfused to this population are tested for CMV antibodies, thus eliminating most of the risk. The risk of infection is not reduced when directed donor blood is used. This startling finding is explained by the fact that persons asked to donate blood for a friend or family member are not as likely to disclose important information as a routine volunteer donor.

Retransfusion

The previous discussion shows that exposure of the patient to transfusion of blood or blood products from other people must be minimized. The amount of donor blood transfused during most surgery can be markedly diminished by preoperative donation by the patient and by intraoperative and postoperative salvage and retransfusion of shed blood. Additionally, most healthy patients can safely tolerate acute intraoperative hemodilution, which is accomplished by withdrawing 1 or 2 units of blood and replacing it with crystalloid or colloid solutions. At the end of the procedure, the patient's blood is retransfused to restore normal hemoglobin levels. Infusion of predonated blood is directed by the same criteria used for blood from another donor because errors of identification and infection may still occur.

Blood is salvaged intraoperatively and postoperatively with a suctioning apparatus. This device channels shed blood to a reservoir, where it is filtered and kept with heparinized saline until enough is collected to warrant retransfusion. The blood is centrifuged, washed with saline, concentrated, and emptied into a transfusion bag. The resulting solution resembles packed red blood cells, but has a hematocrit in the high 20s. Retransfusion of this blood does not cause major complications as long as it is filtered on transfusion. However, platelet counts may fall to less than 100,000 in the 2 to 3 days after surgery because of mechanical damage. Enough heparin is removed from the solution to prevent coagulopathy. Contraindications to intraoperative salvage include malignancy and infection in the surgical field.

Patients who adamantly refuse transfusions may safely undergo surgery if they are adequately prepared with iron or the red cell–stimulating drug epoetin alfa (Epogen). Some may consent to a closed-circuit hemodilution technique or a salvaging procedure. Otherwise, blood loss is replaced by crystalloid and hetastarch. With careful intraoperative and postoperative attention to volume, perfusion, and oxygenation, very low hematocrits may be tolerated. Infusions of non–red cell oxygen-carrying substances are expected to be available soon.

POSTOPERATIVE RECOVERY

Recovery from most anesthetics occurs in the postanesthesia care unit (PACU) or recovery room under the supervision of specially trained nurses. An anesthesiologist and the surgeon are available to manage any complications. Patients who receive brief general anesthetics, some regional anesthetics, and most local anesthetics with sedation may recover in a phase 2 area. Patients in this area are less intensively monitored and are prepared rapidly for discharge. Immediate postoperative anesthetic problems include pulmonary and circulatory complications, renal dysfunction, bleeding abnormalities, hypothermia, pain, nausea, and vomiting.

Table 1-22	Risk of Transfusion-Related Viral Infections
Virus	**Risk of Infection**
HIV	1:1.4 to 2.4 million units transfused
HTLV I and 2	1:250,000 to 2,000,000 units transfused
Hepatitis B	1:58,000 to 149,000 units transfused
Hepatitis C	1:872,000 to 1,700,000 units transfused

Pulmonary Complications

Postoperative pulmonary problems are usually caused by the respiratory depressant effects of the inhaled or intravenous agents or a residual neuromuscular blockade. Upper airway obstruction results from occlusion of the pharynx by the tongue or other soft tissue. Laryngeal obstruction occurs as a result of laryngospasm or injury. Laryngospasm is caused by irritation of the larynx and pharynx by secretions or upper airway manipulation. Signs of upper airway obstruction include flaring of the nares and suprasternal and intercostal retractions. The obstruction is usually easily treated by neck extension and anterior displacement of the mandible. If these maneuvers are not successful, a nasopharyngeal or oropharyngeal airway is inserted. If the obstruction persists, positive pressure ventilation by mask or insertion of an endotracheal tube may be necessary to prevent hypoventilation and hypoxemia.

Because cyanosis is a late symptom of decreasing oxygenation, most PACUs use pulse oximetry to detect early arterial desaturation. In addition to airway obstruction and hypoventilation, reasons for hypoxemia in the recovery period include ventilation–perfusion abnormalities (e.g., atelectasis, remaining anesthetic effects), pulmonary vascular congestion and edema, and aspiration of gastric contents. Most patients show some degree of postoperative hypoxemia and benefit from supplemental oxygen therapy. To counteract the irritation caused by airway manipulation, the oxygen is usually heated and humidified. If the patient will be discharged from the PACU without supplemental oxygen, pulse oximetry is continued for at least 15 minutes while the patient is breathing room air.

Circulatory Complications

The most common circulatory complications in the immediate postanesthesia period include hypotension, hypertension, and cardiac arrhythmias. Hypovolemia is the most common cause of hypotension, usually because of inadequate replacement of blood or because of third-space loss as a result of surgery. Unrecognized postoperative hemorrhage is a serious complication that must remain foremost in the differential diagnosis of hypotension. If hypovolemia is the cause of hypotension, the treatment is fluid or blood resuscitation. Until the hypovolemia is corrected, elevation of the legs is helpful and pharmacologic support with a pressor may become necessary. Monitoring of volume status is the same in the recovery period as intraoperatively. Other complications include residual effects of anesthetics, acute myocardial ischemia or infarction, preexisting ventricular dysfunction, pulmonary embolus, and pneumothorax. If the hypotension is caused by myocardial dysfunction, it is helpful to follow pulmonary arterial and wedge pressures while treating it.

Postoperative hypertension is often caused by pain, excitement, or delirium on emergence from anesthesia. If antihypertensive therapy is withdrawn preoperatively, postoperative hypertension may be magnified. Volume over-load, arterial hypoxemia, hypercarbia, acidosis, and hypothermia should also be suspected in the hypertensive patient. Treatment is based on the etiology of the hypertension. When pain or excitement is the cause, hypertension is treated only if it persists after adequate pain control is achieved. If hypoxemia or hypercarbia is the cause, appropriate measures to restore adequate respiration and oxygenation are instituted immediately. Volume, temperature, or acid–base status should be corrected as rapidly as possible. If pharmacologic therapy is instituted, its effects must be monitored adequately.

Cardiac arrhythmias can be caused by hypoxemia, hypercarbia, electrolyte abnormalities, pain, excitement, or myocardial ischemia. The underlying cause should be determined before antiarrhythmic drugs are administered.

Virtually every patient in the PACU should be monitored with an ECG, frequent blood pressure determinations, a pulse oximeter, and observation of respiration. Patients who have had or are expected to have large volume changes should have their status assessed by urine output and, if indicated, CVP. If these parameters are followed, sudden circulatory changes are evident and easily correctable.

Renal Dysfunction

Oliguria is the result of either hemodynamic or mechanical compromise. Postoperative renal insufficiency is common in patients who have preexisting renal disease, sepsis, massive trauma, major vascular or cardiac surgery, or pelvic pathology with intraoperative trauma to either the ureter or renal vessels. Because of the effects of aging on renal circulation and tubular function, geriatric patients are more likely to have postoperative renal dysfunction. Patients who have prolonged hypotension during surgery or who require massive blood transfusion often have intraoperative renal insufficiency continuing into the postoperative period. Patients who are at risk for postoperative renal dysfunction should be monitored with Foley catheter drainage of urine throughout the perioperative period. In patients who have no predisposing factors, oliguria might be caused by an obstructed catheter or by residual anesthetic or surgical effects (e.g., edema causing obstruction of a ureter). After mechanical obstruction is ruled out, the first step in the treatment of developing oliguria in the PACU is to optimize the patient's volume status and cardiac output. Only then should diuretics be administered because they further deplete the patient's intravascular volume and prevent the use of urine output as a monitor of volume status.

Other Complications

Postoperative bleeding is usually caused by inadequate hemostasis during surgery. It may occur because blood pressure is higher in the PACU than it is under anesthesia. Coagulopathy may have been present preoperatively or may develop because of a massive transfusion of banked blood, the intraoperative administration of anticoagulants, a transfusion reaction, or the release of tissue substances that interfere with normal coagulation. After surgical hemostasis is ruled out, laboratory tests are performed to indicate which specific factor deficiencies must be corrected.

Hypothermia occurs because operating rooms are cold and the patient's temperature-regulating mechanism is compromised during anesthesia. The anesthesiologist counters these effects by providing warm gases, warming intravenous fluids, using a heating blanket, and covering nonsterile parts of the body. Nonetheless, postoperative hypothermia is not uncommon. It causes shivering, continued somnolence, and prolonged action of muscle relaxants. Shivering causes hypertension, pain, and a marked increase in oxygen consumption. It is treated aggressively by warming the patient and providing supplemental oxygen. In addition, small intravenous injections of benzodiazepines, thonzylamine (Thorazine), or meperidine (Demerol) may be required.

Pain, the most common postoperative complication, is discussed in the next section. The most painful surgical procedures are upper abdominal, thoracic, and orthopedic. After pain, nausea and vomiting are the most common postoperative complications. They are often the result of treatment of pain with narcotics. Prolonged nausea and vomiting are the most common causes of unplanned admissions of patients scheduled for ambulatory surgery. These complications are more common in patients who have abdominal or ophthalmologic surgery and in those who have abdominal distention. Almost all anesthetic agents are implicated. Agents used to treat nausea and vomiting may contribute to prolonged somnolence and cardiovascular instability. The drugs of choice include prochlorperazine 10 mg and metoclopramide 10 mg. If they are ineffective, ondansetron 4 mg or dolasetron 12.5 mg is usually administered. Ondansetron and dolasetron are not the first drugs of choice because they are much more expensive than the others.

Discharge Home

Currently, more than half of all surgical procedures are performed on patients who will be discharged home after recovery from anesthesia. The patient must be accompanied by a responsible adult who will drive the patient home and be available to provide assistance. To qualify for discharge, the patient should be awake and alert, ambulate without exhibiting weakness or postural hypotension, drink fluids without vomiting, and (most anesthesiologists agree) be able to urinate. In addition, the surgical site should be dry and dressed to ensure sterility. The patient should be instructed not to drive or operate machinery and not to drink alcohol or take any medication not prescribed by the surgeon or anesthesiologist.

Approximately 5% of surgical outpatients are admitted postoperatively, usually because of intractable vomiting or for pain requiring narcotic injections. Far less common causes are urinary retention, surgical or anesthetic compli-

cations, or the need for intensive treatment of concurrent medical conditions (e.g., diabetes, hypertension).

MANAGEMENT OF POSTOPERATIVE PAIN

Why Treat Postoperative Pain?

By blunting the reflexes that cause undesirable metabolic and motor responses, postoperative pain control may lead to improved patient outcome. Unlike patients who are in pain, patients who are comfortable can readily breathe deeply, cough, ambulate, and cooperate with physical and respiratory therapy. The metabolic responses to surgery are mediated by the autonomic nervous system. They include increased production of adrenocorticotropic hormone (ACTH), cortisol, catecholamines, renin, angiotensin II, and glucagon and decreased production of insulin. These metabolic responses produce such physiologic responses as tachycardia, hypertension, hyperglycemia, sodium and water retention, increased systemic vascular resistance, increased cardiac work, and increased myocardial oxygen consumption. The motor response to injury is characterized by splinting (involuntary local muscle contracture) and resistance to movement of the injured area. This resistance can result in the inability to take a deep breath (leading to atelectasis, hypoxemia, and pneumonia), or it can result in the inability to move about (increasing the risk of deep vein thrombosis). Thus, good postoperative pain control can prevent complications, facilitate therapy, and hasten recovery and discharge.

The most common method of providing postoperative analgesia is the systemic administration of opioid analgesics. **Patient-controlled analgesia** (PCA) allows the patient to control opioid administration. Nociceptive (pain-transmitting) impulses can be blocked by the administration of local anesthetics or occasionally by neurodestructive techniques (e.g., cryoprobe). Subarachnoid or epidural administration of local anesthetics or opioids allows profound analgesia. However, all of these modalities are associated with risks and side effects. The ability of the medical and nursing staff to recognize and treat these problems, the limitations of the particular hospital situation, and the needs of the local patient population must be considered when instituting any program to treat postoperative pain. Nonsteroidal anti-inflammatory agents are successful in treating the postoperative pain caused by most minor procedures.

Psychological Interventions

People differ in their reactions to pain. The suffering associated with pain may be reduced if an individual knows what to expect, is taught how to exercise some control over pain, and is reassured that help will be available. All patients deserve, consistent with their age and mental status, a description of what will take place on the day of surgery, a description of the sensations that they will experience, and an explanation of the analgesic plan. The patient should be encouraged to ask for analgesia when needed and taught how to minimize pain (e.g., how to cough or move in bed). Finally, the patient should be reassured that personnel will be available to treat postoperative pain.

Systemic Opioids

Postoperative pain is most commonly treated by the intermittent administration of opioid analgesics. The goal is to achieve an opioid blood level that provides analgesia without excessive sedation or respiratory depression. A number of opioid analgesics are used in the immediate postoperative period. Table 1-23 summarizes commonly used opioids, doses by various routes, and the timing of administration. Systemic opioids have various side effects. All opioid agonists depress respiration. Significant respiratory depression is treated by the administration of naloxone 0.04 to 0.4 mg intravenously. Life-threatening respiratory depression may necessitate endotracheal intubation and mechanical ventilation until the effect of the drug subsides. Nausea and vomiting, which result from opioid stimulation of the chemoreceptor trigger zone, can be treated with transdermal scopolamine, with prochlorperazine 5 to 10 mg intramuscularly, or by changing to a different opioid. Opioids cause constipation by delaying intestinal transit, depressing small intestinal propulsive contractions, and decreasing colonic peristalsis, resulting in increased water absorption and desiccation of feces. Biliary tract pressure is increased and may cause biliary colic that is manifested by epigastric or chest pain. The biliary spasm may be reversed by naloxone or glucagon.

Patient-Controlled Analgesia

Systemic administration of opioids by the oral, intramuscular, or subcutaneous route has one disadvantage: the analgesia produced is often inadequate because of patient differences in rates of drug absorption and metabolism. For example, after intramuscular meperidine, peak blood levels between individuals can vary threefold to fivefold, and the time to reach peak blood level can vary threefold to sevenfold. The blood level necessary to achieve analgesia is also variable; the variation for meperidine is approximately fourfold. Further, the therapeutic window is very small. A change in meperidine concentration of as little as 0.05 mg/mL may be the difference between complete pain relief and no pain relief. The combination of unreliable drug delivery methods and variable therapeutic blood levels makes adequate opioid analgesia with traditional delivery methods very difficult. Added to these problems are the widespread misunderstanding of opioid pharmacology and an excessive concern about side effects. The result is poor postoperative analgesia for many patients.

In the 1970s, the first PCA devices became available. The device is programmed to deliver, on demand by the patient, a very small dose of drug through an intravenous cannula. For pain control, the patient pushes a button connected to the PCA device, which then delivers the drug. At that point, a lockout interval begins, during which time any demands by the patient are not honored. After the lockout interval is completed, the patient may demand another dose. The lockout interval ensures that the patient waits for the peak analgesic effect of one dose before receiving another dose. Most PCA devices allow for a slow continuous infusion of drug in addition to intermittent doses.

Most PCA devices have numerous safety mechanisms. One is an antisiphoning valve to prevent drugs from leaking out of a broken or improperly loaded syringe. One-way valves on Y-connectors in the tubing prevent the drug from traveling into secondary intravenous lines instead of into the patient. PCA tubing connected directly to the intravenous cannula also minimizes the amount of drug in the dead space of intravenous tubing. Locks on access doors and programming panels prevent tampering. Microprocessor software is designed to eliminate many common programming errors by requiring such precautions as min-

Table 1-23	Systemic Opioids for Postoperative Pain: Suggested Adult Dose			
Drug	**Oral Dose (mg)**	**Intramuscular Dose**	**Intravenous Dose**	**Duration (hr)**
Buprenorphine (Buprenex)		0.3–0.4	0.3–0.4	6
Butorphanol (Stadol)		1–4	0.5–2	3
Codeine	15–60	15–60	15–60	4
Hydrocodone (Vicodin)	5–10			6
Hydromorphone (Dilaudid)	3 (rectal) 2 (oral)	1–2	1–2	4
Levorphanol (Levo-Dromoran)	2	2 (subcutaneous)		6
Meperidine (Demerol)	100–200	75–100	25–50	3
Methadone	20	10	10	24 (oral) 4 (intramuscular, intravenous, or subcutaneous)
Morphine	10–30	10	10	4
Oxycodone (Numorphan)	5			6

imum lockout intervals or by limiting maximum PCA or continuous infusion doses. Alarms for line occlusion, low battery, empty syringe, and other malfunctions are often included. A running total of the amount of drug administered is constantly updated, allowing the physician to determine the pattern and intensity of drug usage and, hence, the rate of decrease in postoperative pain.

To provide satisfactory postoperative analgesia with PCA therapy, the physician, nursing staff, and patient must be educated. The physician and nursing staff must understand the proper assembly and use of the PCA device, the pharmacology of the drug chosen, and the signs and treatment of side effects. The patient must understand that the device must be used properly and that complete pain relief may not be achieved (although distressing pain can be avoided). Further, the patient should understand that the device can be used to minimize the pain associated with ambulation, dressing changes, and physical therapy, if used before these maneuvers.

The ideal opioid for PCA has a rapid onset and an intermediate duration of action. Drugs with a long duration of action (e.g., methadone, buprenorphine) are difficult to control. Drugs with a short duration of action (e.g., fentanyl, sufentanil) require the patient to administer doses frequently, which may interfere with sleep. The maximum analgesic effect of mixed agonist–antagonist drugs is often inadequate for postoperative pain, and increasing doses beyond those that achieve the ceiling effect only produce more side effects. In practice, the most commonly used drugs for PCA are morphine, hydromorphone, and meperidine.

A typical protocol for initiating PCA therapy is as follows. Before leaving the operating room or on arriving in the PACU, the patient receives a loading dose of opioid. The amount depends on such factors as the characteristics of the individual patient, the type of anesthetic given, and the amount of narcotic given intraoperatively. A typical loading dose for morphine is 0.1 mg/kg. For meperidine, it is 1 mg/kg, given over 15 to 30 minutes until adequate analgesia is achieved. The loading dose of hydromorphone is 0.2 mg. The patient assumes control of the PCA device after he or she sufficiently recovers from anesthesia. If the dose is inadequate, as evidenced by inadequate analgesia after frequent administration, it is increased by approximately 50%. If the dose is excessive, as evidenced by sedation or dizziness, it is decreased by approximately 50%. A continuous infusion of morphine 1 mg/hr or meperidine 10 mg/hr is sometimes used to decrease the frequency with which the patient needs to demand doses, thereby improving sleep. However, continuous infusion should be used with caution in the elderly and in patients who have renal or hepatic insufficiency or cardiac failure. Typical morphine consumption on PCA is 1 to 2 mg/hr; for meperidine, it is 10 to 20 mg/hr. Therapy is continued until the patient can tolerate opioids orally or until analgesia is not needed. For orthopedic patients, PCA therapy is often con-

Table 1-24	Patient-Controlled Analgesia for Postoperative Pain: Suggested Drugs, Adult Doses, and Lockout Intervals		
Drug	Dose (mg)	Lockout (min)	Continuous Infusion Dose (mg/hr)
Morphine	0.5–3	5–20	1–2
Meperidine	5.0–30	5–15	5–25
Hydromorphone	0.1–0.6	5–15	5–15

tinued until physical therapy begins. Table 1-24 shows suggested doses and lockout intervals for three narcotics commonly used for PCA therapy.

Whenever opioids are given, resuscitation equipment and naloxone should be readily available. In addition, the side effects of pruritus, constipation, nausea, vomiting, and urinary retention should be expected and treated. Pruritus is best treated with diphenhydramine, 25 to 30 mg intramuscularly or intravenously. Nausea and vomiting are treated with prochlorperazine 10 mg intramuscularly or metoclopramide 10 mg intravenously or intramuscularly. Urinary retention is treated with a single straight bladder catheterization. If the patient still has retention after straight catheterization, a Foley catheter may be used for 12 to 24 hours. The use of a standard set of orders simplifies the process because this makes it easier to remember to order treatment for side effects. Excessive sedation is treated by decreasing the dose and discontinuing any continuous infusion of narcotics. Respiratory depression may be treated with naloxone 0.1 to 0.4 mg intravenously or with intubation and ventilatory support. For patients who are receiving PCA therapy, all orders for narcotics, sleeping pills, and other sedatives should be written by the same individual or service to minimize unnecessary and potentially hazardous duplication of orders.

Complications related to PCA therapy are rare. They are minimized by training the medical and nursing staff, understanding the pharmacology of the opioid used, educating the patient, selecting the patient carefully, and using a dilute opioid solution (e.g., morphine 1 mg/mL or meperidine 10 mg/mL). However, a more concentrated opioid solution may be needed because of tolerance or other factors. Only the patient should push the button. Parents, nurses, physicians, or visitors should not be allowed to control analgesic delivery.

Epidural and Spinal Analgesia

The widespread use of epidural and spinal analgesia for postoperative pain control is a recent development. Epidural or subarachnoid infusion of local anesthetics produces profound analgesia at the price of variable degrees of sensory, motor, and sympathetic blockade, depending on the drug and technique used. The discovery of spinal opioid receptors in the late 1970s led to the use of subarachnoid opioids for postoperative analgesia. Subarachnoid opioids produce reliable analgesia without sensory, motor, or sympathetic blockade. However, profound respiratory depression may occur as late as 24 hours after injection. Various combinations of local anesthetics and opioids are used to minimize the side effects associated with each agent, but the ideal agent or technique has yet to be found.

Epidural Analgesia

Epidural analgesic agents are administered by intermittent techniques, patient-controlled epidural analgesia (PCEA), or by continuous infusion. Regardless of the method used, the best results are obtained when the agent is deposited at the vertebral level that approximates the middle of the spinal segments affected by the surgery. The epidural catheter is inserted with normal sterile technique and securely fixed with tape. An occlusive dressing is used when contamination by fluid or incontinence is a problem. Depending on the site of surgery, the catheter is then draped across the back toward the neck or brought along the flank to the lateral position. Often the anesthesiologist inserts the catheter before surgery; uses it to inject opioids or local anesthetics during surgery, with or without general anesthesia; and then leaves it in for postoperative analgesia.

To minimize the frequency of redosing and tachyphylaxis, long-acting local anesthetics (e.g., bupivacaine 0.125%–0.25%) are most commonly used for continuous infusion in the postoperative period or during labor. The concentration of 0.125% to 0.25% bupivacaine provides sensory analgesia with a minimum of motor blockade. Shorter acting local anesthetics may be used for PCEA. Sympathetic blockade may occur with epidural administration of local anesthetics and could be dangerous in a patient with cardiac disease or hypovolemia. On the other hand, sympathetic blockade causes vasodilation and improved tissue blood flow, which is advantageous in vascular surgery or in patients who are at risk for thromboembolism.

Opioids are also used for epidural analgesia. Usually a loading dose is given (morphine 2–3 mg or fentanyl 0.05–0.1 mg). Analgesia is maintained with intermittent reinjection of the same dose when the patient becomes aware of pain or with continuous infusion of 0.5 mg/hr morphine or 0.075 mg/hr fentanyl, usually with 0.125% bupivacaine. The greatest risk associated with epidural opioids is respiratory depression, which may occur early (within 1 hour) because of vascular uptake of drug or late (up to 24 hours) because of diffusion of opioid from the spinal cord to the brain. Highly lipid-soluble opioids (e.g., fentanyl, sufentanil) are associated with early respiratory depression. Less lipid-soluble agents (e.g., morphine) are associated with late respiratory depression.

Side effects that occur with epidural opioids include pruritus, nausea and vomiting, and urinary retention. Pruritus is highly variable, nonsegmental, and most commonly seen with morphine. The mechanism is unknown.

Benadryl 25 mg intramuscularly or naloxone 0.04 to 0.1 mg intravenously usually helps. Naloxone can be titrated to minimize side effects while retaining analgesia. Nausea and vomiting are less common and are probably related to stimulation of the chemoreceptor trigger zone in the medulla. They are successfully treated with prochlorperazine 5 to 10 mg intramuscularly, metoclopramide 5 to 10 mg intravenously, or transdermal scopolamine patches. Urinary retention occasionally occurs. The cause is poorly understood, but may be related to inhibition of the micturition reflex. Usually intermittent bladder catheterization is sufficient, but an indwelling catheter may be used as well.

Combinations of local anesthetics and opioids are being used epidurally more often because low concentrations of both agents provide analgesia with minimum side effects. In a healthy adult patient, a combination of 0.1% bupivacaine with 0.05 mg/mL morphine or 0.005 mg/mL fentanyl is infused at a rate of 5 to 7 mL/hr through a thoracic epidural catheter. If a lumbar epidural catheter is used, the rate is 5 to 12 mL/hr.

Spinal Analgesia

Both opioids and local anesthetics may be given intrathecally, but this technique has several drawbacks. Headache occasionally occurs after lumbar puncture. In addition, pruritus, nausea and vomiting, urinary retention, and respiratory depression are more common when opioids are given intrathecally rather than epidurally. When local anesthetics are used, motor blockade may limit postoperative ambulation as well as physical and respiratory therapy. As with epidural analgesia, a catheter may be placed in the subarachnoid space before surgery and used to supplement the anesthetic in the operating room as well as to provide postoperative analgesia.

Monitoring

Patients who receive local anesthetics intraspinally must be monitored for side effects of sympathetic blockade, hypotension, systemic toxicity, seizures, cardiac arrhythmia, motor blockade, and urinary retention. Patients who receive opioids intraspinally must be monitored for side effects of nausea and vomiting, pruritus, urinary retention, respiratory depression, and sedation. Various protocols and devices are used to monitor these side effects. Patients are monitored in intensive care settings and general units with such devices as motion sensors, strain gauges, impedance monitors, pulse oximeters, and expired CO_2 monitors. However, no monitoring technique or protocol is clearly superior. The safe, effective use of these analgesic techniques requires that the patient be monitored regularly by trained personnel who can recognize and treat complications. In addition, physicians must be available on a 24-hour basis to respond to problems.

Other Techniques

Nonsteroidal Anti-inflammatory Drugs

Although the use of nonsteroidal anti-inflammatory drugs (NSAIDs) for pain control is increasing, their exact role has not been defined. NSAIDs appear to produce analgesia during tissue injury by inhibiting the release of prostaglandins, which sensitize peripheral nociceptors. When the nociceptive impulse delivered to the CNS is increased, the perception of pain is increased. Prostaglandins may also exert hyperalgesic effects in the CNS. Although the use of NSAIDs before surgery appears worthwhile, several side effects may limit their usefulness. NSAIDs inhibit platelet function, which may interfere with hemostasis. In addition, prostaglandins may be necessary for wound healing. The antipyretic activity of NSAIDs may mask the febrile response to infection and thus delay its treatment. Renal insufficiency and failure are also associated with the use of these compounds. Ketorolac is most commonly given intravenously at the end of surgery to provide immediate postoperative analgesia, but most NSAIDs are administered only orally or rectally, limiting their immediate postoperative use.

Peripheral Neural Blockade

Regional anesthetic techniques to control postoperative pain involve the use of local anesthetic agents to interrupt the transmission of nociceptive impulses to the CNS. In addition to analgesia, most neural blockade techniques produce complete sensory and motor blockade. If analgesia is desired for more than a few hours, a repeat block or an infusion technique is used. Patients who receive neural blockades are monitored for side effects (e.g., toxicity of the local anesthetic agent from either peripheral absorption or intravascular injection, unexpected spinal or epidural blockade, circulatory depression because of sympathectomy). The patient may not adequately protect an anesthetized area of the body; therefore, all anesthetized areas must be shielded from injury. If a lower extremity is anesthetized, ambulation is delayed. Pneumothorax may occur with intercostal blocks, with interpleural blocks, and occasionally with brachial plexus blocks. Neural blockade for postoperative pain control requires an increased level of nursing surveillance, care, and perhaps help with ambulation. The availability of such care, often in a special "step-down" unit, should be determined preoperatively.

A variety of techniques are used to provide peripheral blockade of postoperative pain. The surgical wound may be infiltrated or simply washed with local anesthetics before incision or suturing. Brachial plexus blockade is used for upper extremity surgery. Lumbar plexus or femoral, obturator, and sciatic nerve blocks are used for lower extremity procedures. Intercostal nerve blocks are used for chest wall and abdominal wall pain. Interpleural blockade is used to control pain in a variety of abdominal surgical procedures and in painful conditions of the chest wall (e.g., rib fractures, mastectomy). It is not as useful for control of pain after thoracotomy. In small children, caudal or spinal blocks are administered after induction of anesthesia for postoperative analgesia when immediate ambulation is not anticipated. These techniques may be performed intermittently or continuously. A catheter is used to infuse local anesthetic.

Some blocks require specialized techniques or personnel that may not be available at many medical centers. However, many single-injection regional blocks can be performed by the surgeon at the time of surgery. These blocks are often effective and have an acceptably low incidence of complications, but unfortunately, they are underused. Inguinal, iliohypogastric, and dorsal penile nerve blocks are used successfully for a variety of surgical procedures in the inguinal and genital regions. Direct infiltration and topical application of local anesthetics to a surgical wound are used to control pain in many cases. Preemptive analgesia, initiated preoperatively, may decrease the requirements for postoperative pain control.

Cryoanalgesia

Cryoanalgesia is used most often to control chest wall pain after thoracotomy. The technique involves placing a cryoprobe, either percutaneously or under direct vision, at surgery on the nerve to be disrupted. The tip of the probe is cooled to approximately $-60°C$ with nitrous oxide or liquid nitrogen. Applying the probe to the nerve causes an ice ball to form around the nerve. Consequently, axonal degeneration occurs, but the nerve sheath architecture is spared. The nerve grows back at a rate of 1 to 3 mm/day without the scarring, neuritis, or neuroma occasionally seen with surgical sectioning of the nerve or with chemical neurolysis. The analgesia usually lasts a few weeks to a few months. This technique has several disadvantages. Analgesia is often incomplete, with residual pain in areas that are not affected by the blocks (e.g., shoulder, midback, chest tube sites). Cryogenic lesions of surrounding tissue or full-thickness skin destruction may occur. In addition, the necessary equipment is expensive. The usefulness of this technique must be considered before this investment is undertaken.

Transcutaneous Electrical Nerve Stimulation

In transcutaneous electrical nerve stimulation (TENS), analgesia is provided with a weak electrical current transmitted through the skin surface to a painful area. The mechanism of analgesia is not fully explained, but this technique probably inhibits pain transmission at the spinal or central level by the barrage of impulses generated by nonnociceptive receptor stimulation. TENS successfully controls pain after knee, hip, and lower back operations. It is not as effective after herniorrhaphy and thoracic procedures.

Various nonnarcotic, nonlocal anesthetic techniques are under investigation. These include intrathecal and epidural administration of such drugs as ketamine, clonidine, and calcitonin, as well as systemic administration of tricyclic antidepressants. The safety and efficacy of these techniques are not established, but this field has grown so rapidly in the last decade that new treatments are expected to be available soon.

PATIENT FACTORS THAT INFLUENCE ANESTHESIA

To maintain homeostasis during surgery, the anesthesiologist supports respiration and circulation and also interferes with the patient's stress response by blocking pain. In addition, the anesthesiologist manages endocrine responses with anesthetics and other drugs and oversees the patient's medical conditions. Even healthy patients have a complex physiologic response to stress, although the stress may not be consciously perceived. Preexisting medical conditions alter this response to the extent that it may become life threatening. Each patient responds uniquely to the drugs administered and to attempts to control the physiologic state during and after surgery. This section describes the effects of common medical conditions on surgical patients, describes what the anesthesiologist needs to know, and explains the importance of this information in clinical decision-making and patient outcome.

Cardiovascular System

Anesthesia almost always depresses normal cardiovascular function. The effects of surgery and resulting pain and inflammation cause a considerable insult to homeostasis. Consequently, when cardiovascular disease is present, the anesthesiologist must have a thorough knowledge of the patient's degree of dysfunction and the probable effects of surgery and anesthesia. Guidelines for perioperative cardiovascular evaluation for noncardiac surgery have been formulated and recently updated by a task force convened by the American College of Cardiology/American Heart Association and have been cited at the end of this chapter (see Suggested Readings). Clinical predictors of increased perioperative risk of myocardial infarction, congestive heart failure, and death are enumerated within the document, as are recommended workups and treatment options.

Hypertension

Preexisting hypertension makes intraoperative blood pressure control difficult. In normal patients, intraoperative hypertension is a sign of sympathetic stimulation because of inadequate analgesia or anesthesia. It is most effectively treated by increasing the depth of anesthesia with volatile agents, narcotics, or intravenous anesthetics. The patient who has preexisting hypertension that is not controlled with a stable medication regimen may have wide swings in blood pressure as a result of varying levels of stimulation, anesthetic administered, or attempts to control hemodynamic status with volume restriction or infusion. A patient who has controlled hypertension responds much like a

normal patient as long as medication is continued throughout the perioperative period.

The techniques used to control intraoperative hypertension are determined by the cause. If "light" anesthesia or pain is considered the cause, anesthesia is the treatment. Only when the level of anesthesia is appropriate, in the best judgment of the anesthesiologist, should β blockers or vasodilators be used. If fluid overload is strongly suspected as a contributing cause, then intravenous diuretic therapy may be indicated, provided that the continuing surgical procedure will not cause significant fluid loss.

A rare, but dangerous, cause of intraoperative hypertension is the interaction of monoamine oxidase (MAO) inhibitors or tricyclic antidepressants with catecholamines or catecholamine-like drugs (e.g., ephedrine). MAO inhibitors and tricyclics interfere with the metabolism of catechols and may allow dangerously high concentrations at the sympathetic nerve ending. The popular herbal supplement St. John's wort is a mild MAO inhibitor. Despite this potential danger, the most recent recommendation is to continue the drugs throughout the perioperative period to prevent dangerous withdrawal phenomena and to make every effort to avoid sympathetic stimulation or exogenous catechol administration intraoperatively.

Table 1-25 lists potential perioperative complications in the patient who is following an antihypertensive medication regimen. Despite these potential drug interactions, most data indicate that all antihypertensive medications, with the possible exception of diuretics, should be continued through the immediate preoperative period. When propranolol and clonidine first became commonly used to control hypertension, there was concern that their depressive effects on the cardiovascular system would preclude safe administration of anesthetics. However, it soon became evident that there was greater danger of rebound hypertension and tachycardia on their abrupt withdrawal.

The anesthesiologist should formulate a plan to deal with hypertension and hypotension intraoperatively long before intervention is required. The anesthetic and monitoring techniques should be carefully chosen, taking into consideration any possible interactions. A patient with chronic hypertension, even one who is on a medication regimen, has end-organ manifestations of the disease. Cardiovascular manifestations include ischemic disease, left ventricular dysfunction, aortic stenosis, and central and peripheral vascular insufficiency. Renal vascular disease leads to chronic renal insufficiency. Carotid and cerebrovascular disease leads to focal cerebral ischemia, altered autoregulation, and stroke. Therefore, for appropriate evaluation, each hypertensive patient needs a preoperative ECG; a chest x-ray; a determination of serum electrolytes, blood urea nitrogen (BUN), and creatinine; a CBC; and an assessment of neurologic function. Preoperatively, a careful history and physical examination should help determine the presence of angina, the degree of dyspnea on exertion, and the degree of congestive failure. If the ECG is abnormal, as it often is, further evaluation is needed to

Table 1-25	Effect of Antihypertensive Drugs on the Perioperative Period
Class of Drug (Examples)	**Potential Problems**
Diuretics	Hypovolemia Vasodilation Decreased urine output if omitted Electrolyte abnormalities (usually K^+) Denervation sensitivity to direct-acting pressors
Drugs that deplete neurotransmitters (reserpine, guanethidine)	Abnormal response to indirect-acting pressors Reserpine decreases MAC[a] by 20%–30% Bradycardia Orthostatic hypotension Decrease in MAC if centrally acting
False neurotransmitters (methyldopa)	Abnormal response to indirect-acting pressors Bradycardia Orthostatic hypotension
β-receptor-blocking agents	Additive hypotension and bradycardia with anesthetics Possible bronchiolar constriction Rebound hypertension and tachycardia on withdrawal
α_1-receptor-blocking agents (prazosin)	Additive hypotension with anesthetics Decreased MAC
α_2-receptor agonists (clonidine)	Rebound hypertension and tachycardia on withdrawal Additive hypotension with anesthetics
Arteriolar vasodilators (hydralazine)	Postural hypotension Decreased response to pressors
Calcium channel blocking agents	Hypotension, decreased contractility, and conduction delays additive to anesthetics Decrease in MAC of approximately 25% Potentiation of neuromuscular-blocking agents
Angiotensin-converting enzyme inhibitors	Hypotension with many anesthetics Hyponatremia

[a]MAC, a measure of anesthetic potency, is discussed in the section on pharmacology of inhalation agents. If MAC is decreased by another drug, that drug has an additive, or potentiating, effect on anesthesia.

determine the contractile state of the myocardium and the myocardial oxygen supply–demand status. Sometimes a dipyridamole–thallium scan or angiography is indicated, but the ready availability of echocardiography has replaced these more invasive procedures in many patients, especially when used with a dobutamine infusion as a stress test.

The anesthesiologist should determine the range of blood pressures and heart rates at which the hypertensive patient is asymptomatic and then set limits (usually within 10%–20% of this range) at which intervention during surgery becomes necessary. Finally, early planning of monitoring in consultation with the surgeon facilitates mainte-

nance of blood volume and myocardial and tissue oxygenation throughout surgery.

Ischemic Heart Disease

Myocardial infarction (MI) is the leading cause of death in elderly patients who undergo surgery. The anesthesiologist must administer just enough anesthetic to achieve anesthesia without causing undue cardiovascular depression or allowing a significant stress response. Either response can upset the myocardial oxygen supply–demand ratio and cause ischemic damage. Until proven otherwise, the patient who has any of the symptoms listed in Table 1-26 is considered to have ischemic heart disease, even if the ECG is normal. The anesthesiologist takes a preoperative history and conducts a physical examination. Tests should include an ECG, a chest x-ray, and other measures of myocardial oxygenation as indicated. Echocardiography is helpful in evaluating regional myocardial function. If emergency surgery precludes further evaluation, the patient is treated as though ischemic heart disease is present.

Surgery in the face of a recent MI or acute coronary vascular insufficiency carries a mortality rate of 1.7% to 27%, depending on the nature of the surgery, the time from infarction, and the perioperative management. Preoperative optimization of myocardial oxygenation with medication, angioplasty, or even coronary artery bypass graft (CABG) surgery reduces morbidity and mortality significantly. If possible, surgery should be delayed a few weeks after angioplasty or coronary stent placement because of the associated endothelial damage caused by these procedures. Patients who undergo successful CABG have a much reduced incidence and severity of perioperative morbidity from subsequent surgery. Delaying subsequent

Table 1-26	Clues to Ischemic Heart Disease
History	Chest pain with arm or neck radiation, especially if relieved by nitroglycerin Dyspnea on exertion, exposure to cold, straining, or after eating Orthopnea Paroxysmal nocturnal dyspnea Nocturnal coughing Peripheral or pulmonary edema History or electrocardiographic evidence of myocardial infarction Cardiomegaly Family history of coronary artery disease at patient's age
Concurrent disease	Carotid bruit Unexplained tachycardia Diabetes Hyperlipidemia Hypertension Left ventricular hypertrophy on electrocardiogram Peripheral vascular disease Aortic disease

surgery for 6 months after an MI greatly reduces surgical mortality. Perioperative beta blockade has been shown to reduce the incidence and severity of perioperative ischemia in patients at risk.

Patients who are at risk for ischemic episodes during anesthesia are carefully monitored with some combination of ECG, S-T segment trending, pulmonary artery and wedge pressures, cardiac output, and transesophageal echocardiography. Careful management is needed to maintain the correct myocardial oxygen supply–demand ratio for tissue oxygenation. Because myocardial perfusion occurs mainly during diastole, maintaining a slow heart rate is paramount. Patients who have a history of myocardial ischemia are usually treated with agents to lower the heart rate and contractility. They are also given drugs to reduce peripheral and coronary vascular resistance. These drugs are continued throughout the perioperative period. Intraoperatively, nitroglycerin is given as a continuous infusion (0.1–1 mg/kg/min) rather than as a dermal patch because skin perfusion is not predictable under anesthesia. As with hypertensive patients, a range of acceptable values for the patient is determined preoperatively, and a plan is formulated to maintain those values intraoperatively. Because the most likely time for reinfarction is 48 to 72 hours postoperatively, monitoring for ischemia with some or all of these methods is begun before anesthesia is induced. This monitoring continues long into the postoperative period.

Congestive Heart Failure

The failing heart causes various problems at surgery. It cannot easily maintain adequate output during surgery and anesthesia. However, pharmacologic agents that are used to treat congestive heart failure (CHF) affect anesthetics and other drugs used during surgery. Pulmonary hypertension and pulmonary edema seriously interfere with both oxygenation and uptake of inhaled anesthetic agents. Because the pharmacokinetics are usually abnormal, the dosage and timing of drug administration are carefully titrated.

In patients with CHF, the goal of preoperative preparation is to maximize cardiac output without compromising myocardial oxygenation so that vital organ perfusion continues despite reduced blood circulation. As with any other chronic medical problem, a stable therapeutic regimen should be in effect before elective surgery. In addition, medications should be continued throughout the perioperative period, although dosages may need to be modified. The patient's optimal ranges of blood pressure, heart rate, cardiac output, and peripheral resistance should be determined before surgery, along with the means that will be used to maintain them. Patients with severe CHF may be admitted to the intensive care unit the day before surgery so that a pulmonary arterial catheter can be inserted and a Starling curve calculated. The calculation correlates the effect on cardiac output of changes in pulmonary artery,

wedge, and right ventricular pressures and systemic vascular resistance.

In addition, patients with CHF often take digoxin, a drug that has a very narrow therapeutic window. Too little drug produces a less than optimal therapeutic effect; too much causes toxicity. Most patients with CHF also take diuretics to control their blood volume. For this reason, they are at risk for both hypovolemia (relative and absolute) and electrolyte imbalance. It is recommended that digitalized patients not be anesthetized for elective surgery if their serum potassium falls below 3.5 mg/dL. Instead, total body K^+ is returned to normal with therapy over 48 to 72 hours while the hazards of hyperkalemia are not overlooked. Table 1-27 lists the arrhythmias that are often associated with digoxin and hypokalemia, which are also indicators of digoxin toxicity.

The choice of anesthetic technique and agents depends on the patient's blood volume, pulmonary vascular resistance, optimal filling pressures, the state of myocardial oxygenation, and the ability of the heart to increase output on demand. Most anesthetics and sedatives, including local anesthetic agents, vasodilate or depress myocardial contractility. Patients who receive long-term diuretic therapy compensate for depleted blood volume by peripheral vasoconstriction. These patients become hypotensive when anesthetized and vasodilated. Therefore, these patients should receive carefully monitored prophylactic fluid before they receive any vasodilating drugs. The circulation should be monitored before the first drug is administered. If surgery can be performed with a regional anesthetic, the myocardial depression caused by most anesthetics and adjuncts may be avoided. However, in patients with CHF, clearance of local anesthetics is reduced. Therefore, blood levels are higher and the risk of toxicity is increased. For this reason, the original dose and the timing of repeat injections are altered. Hypotension that results from the sympathectomy that accompanies spinal or epidural anesthesia cannot be treated with volume infusion, as in normal patients. As the sympathectomy wears off, patients with CHF may not be able to excrete the excess fluids rapidly enough to prevent decompensation. Often a carefully titrated infusion of a vasoconstrictor (e.g., phenylephrine) is given to support the blood

Table 1-27	Arrhythmias Associated with Digitalization and Hypokalemia
Atrial	Sinus bradycardia
	Rapid atrial rate with 2:1 or 3:1 block
	Atrial premature contractions
	Sinoatrial block
Junctional	Atrioventricular node block, often with atrial tachycardia
	Junctional tachycardia
Ventricular	Ventricular premature contractions
	Ventricular tachycardia
	Ventricular fibrillation

pressure. Some patients with severe CHF cannot maintain adequate ventilation when lying supine on the operating table unless their respiration is assisted or controlled. For this reason, these patients are not candidates for major regional anesthesia unless it is used in combination with general anesthesia and mechanical ventilation.

To support cardiac output intraoperatively, either dopamine, dobutamine, inamrinone, or milrinone in continuous infusion is administered. Tachycardia is not tolerated in these patients, and heart rate cannot easily be controlled with β blockers or Ca^{++} channel entry blockers because they may cause myocardial depression. Increased peripheral vascular resistance must also be avoided because the failing heart cannot contract against an increased load.

Valvular Heart Disease

Every patient who has valvular disease must be carefully evaluated preoperatively to determine the status of the heart, lungs, and peripheral perfusion. Valvular disease can cause profound disruption of rate and rhythm, contractility, pulmonary and peripheral vascular resistance, and preload and myocardial oxygenation. The prevalence of rheumatic valve disease is declining, but the rates of congenital bicuspid aortic stenosis, mitral valve prolapse, hypertrophic cardiomyopathy (idiopathic hypertrophic subaortic stenosis), and calcific mitral insufficiency are all increasing. Endocarditis or MI can cause acute valvular insufficiency. A diseased valve is an ideal colonizing spot for circulating bacteria. Therefore, regardless of the lesion, antibiotic prophylaxis for *Staphylococcus* with ampicillin, erythromycin, or vancomycin is initiated before surgery and continued through the first postoperative day. Despite the potential for intraoperative and postoperative bleeding, anticoagulation is considered essential to prevent a fatal embolism. In this situation, regional anesthesia is contraindicated, as are blind needle sticks (e.g., for central venous access in the internal jugular or subclavian veins).

Stenosis
Stenotic lesions require maintenance of preload, contractility, rate, and rhythm within a narrow range. Atrial contraction is helpful in preserving cardiac output in mitral stenosis, so maintenance of sinus rhythm is desirable. Coronary vessel perfusion in patients who have aortic stenosis requires maintaining peripheral resistance (especially diastolic blood pressure) within a narrow range to allow flow across the stenosis into the coronary circulation.

Insufficiency
Patients with valvular insufficiency often benefit from reduced pulmonary or peripheral vascular resistance. The easier the forward flow, the less blood regurgitates across an incompetent valve. When valves are both stenotic and insufficient, the anesthesiologist must treat what appears to be the most hemodynamically significant lesion, yet be ready to alter the strategy if that choice is incorrect. Monitoring flow across the valves with the Doppler flow modality of a TEE is especially helpful.

Mitral Valve Prolapse
Mitral valve prolapse (MVP) is the most common valve lesion, occurring in approximately 6% of otherwise normal people. It is more prevalent in females and often occurs in association with other chest skeletal anomalies, von Willebrand's syndrome, autonomic dysfunction, and migraine anxiety syndrome. Signs and symptoms include palpitations, dyspnea, atypical chest pain, dizziness, and syncope. Episodes of supraventricular or ventricular tachycardia occur in as many as 50% of patients with MVP; 25% have episodes of bradycardia. Sudden death occurs in approximately 1% to 2% of patients with MVP, probably because of ventricular fibrillation. The presence of an unexplained murmur with any one of the listed symptoms signals the possibility of MVP and requires further investigation. Patients with MVP are at increased risk for morbidity from intraoperative and postoperative dysrhythmias and probably benefit from prophylactic antibiotics.

Idiopathic Hypertrophic Subaortic Stenosis
Idiopathic hypertrophic subaortic stenosis is an obstruction of the left ventricular outflow tract by hypertrophied septum muscle. Stenosis occurs when contraction of the ventricle approaches its maximum in mid to late systole. Mitral regurgitation may also occur. As the disease progresses, the left ventricle hypertrophies because of the pressure gradient across the stenosis. Arrhythmia is common because the conduction system is involved in the septal hypertrophy. Obstruction to the forward flow of blood is minimized by maintaining approximately the same peripheral blood pressure and ventricular volume that the patient typically functions with and by preventing an increased left ventricular contractile force. Patients who have idiopathic hypertrophic subaortic stenosis are usually treated with β-adrenergic blocking agents or Ca^{++} channel blockers. This therapy is continued throughout the perioperative period. Inhalation anesthetics reduce myocardial contractility and help maintain cardiac output during surgery.

Intravenous Drug Abuse
The chronic intravenous drug abuser who undergoes surgery may have bacterial endocarditis with resultant valvular lesions. Preoperative anticoagulation and antibiotic prophylaxis are used. Other common medical problems in intravenous drug abusers are pulmonary fibrosis and hypertension, renal and hepatic insufficiency, hepatitis, and acquired immunodeficiency syndrome (AIDS). Virtually every drug abuser, whether addicted or not, exhibits tolerance to sedatives, narcotics, and anesthetics. Patients who are under the influence of cocaine or other "uppers" may have increased sensitivity to adrenergic agonists and vasoconstrictors.

Disorders of Rhythm

Dysrhythmia in surgical patients may be benign, an indication of a more serious disorder, or life threatening.

Because pharmacologic intervention requires drugs with serious side effects, physicians must distinguish between dysrhythmias that require intervention and those that do not.

Tachycardia

Sinus tachycardia is associated with several conditions, most of which can be corrected or stabilized before surgery. Tachyarrhythmia in an otherwise normal patient is rare and is usually related to stress. A patient with sinus tachycardia should be evaluated for hypervolemia, hypovolemia, hypoxemia, hypercarbia, hyperthermia, drug toxicity, catecholamine-secreting tumors, thyrotoxicosis, and autonomic dysfunction. Atrial fibrillation or flutter with a rapid ventricular rate is usually a sign of serious cardiac dysfunction (e.g., ischemia, CHF). The patient will benefit from stabilization before anything but the most emergent surgery is considered.

Bradycardia

Except in aerobically fit sports enthusiasts, bradycardia usually implies a profound conduction system disorder. A patient who has unexplained dizziness or syncope should have a cardiac evaluation. Patients with a temporary or permanent complete atrioventricular (AV) block benefit from preoperative placement of a pacemaker. An incomplete AV block rarely progresses to a complete heart block. As a precaution, however, many anesthesiologists place an intravenous access sheath in a central vein preoperatively in case a temporary pacemaker is needed.

Pacemakers

Surgical patients who have a functioning pacemaker usually present little problem to the anesthesiologist. However, it is important to be aware of the original rhythm problem, the patient's current condition and drug therapy, and the exact type of pacemaker in place (i.e., the chamber sensed, the chamber paced, the sensing pattern, and the default rhythm). It is also important to know what to do if the pacemaker malfunctions because of radio frequency. The default rhythm is the rhythm to which the pacemaker resorts when a problem occurs with its normal function. Radio frequency from cautery or other instruments can inhibit firing, especially of demand pacemakers. In this situation, the pacemaker is immediately reprogrammed or converted to a fixed-rate pacer. Neither maneuver is difficult to accomplish if the necessary equipment (e.g., programmer) is available. To avoid this problem, bipolar (current passes only between the two prongs of the instrument) rather than unipolar (current passes from the unit to the grounding pad) cautery is used. To prevent cautery current from traversing the pacemaker wires, the grounding pad is placed so that the pacemaker wires are not located between the cautery and the operative site.

Ventricular Ectopy

Ventricular ectopy on the preoperative ECG presents a difficult problem. Certain patterns of premature ventricular contractions (PVCs) are associated with increased perioperative risk. The current recommendation is for further assessment if the PVCs occur more frequently than 3/min, if they occur in couplets or runs of more than two, or if they are multifocal. They may be a symptom of drug toxicity, electrolyte abnormality, or ischemia, all of which should be stabilized preoperatively. The next step in assessment is usually a 24-hour monitoring sequence for better diagnosis. Many drugs are currently used to treat PVCs (e.g., quinidine, procainamide, propranolol). The medication is begun preoperatively and generally continued during the perioperative period. The greatest risk associated with PVCs is the potential for tachyarrhythmia and decreased cardiac output.

Respiratory System

The preoperative preparation should identify the characteristics and consequences of pulmonary disease. Taking the patient's history and performing a physical examination are adequate in most patients, but further investigation is often needed to determine the degree of alteration in volume, flow pattern, oxygenation, and CO_2 excretion. Table 1-28 lists important features of the preoperative evaluation of the respiratory system that could indicate the need for further workup and formulation of a plan for perioperative therapy. If pathology is suspected, a chest x-ray film is obtained to determine the baseline state of the patient's lungs and heart and to establish that the patient has no reversible condition that requires treatment before surgery and anesthesia. In all patients who have preexisting pulmonary disease, the goals of preoperative testing and therapy should include those listed in Table 1-29.

Infectious Diseases

Most infectious diseases of the lungs are reversible to some extent. Chronic bronchitis and bronchiectasis can be im-

Table 1-28	Preoperative Evaluation of the Respiratory System
History	Dyspnea (with what degree of exertion?)
	Coughing (sputum production)
	Recent respiratory infection
	Hemoptysis
	Wheezing use of drugs for asthma
	Pulmonary complications from previous surgery
	Neuromuscular disease
	Smoking
	Age
Examination	Breathing frequency and pattern
	Body habitus (chest wall anatomy, obesity)
	Upper-airway evaluation
	Auscultation of lungs
Laboratory	Electrolytes
	Chest x-ray
	Arterial blood gases
	Pulmonary function tests

Table 1-29	Preparing the Patient Who Has Pulmonary Disease for Surgery and Anesthesia

Control infections
    Eradicate acute infections
    Suppress chronic infections with antibiotic treatment
Treat bronchospasm
    Institute treatment with bronchodilating drugs
    Document optimal treatment
        Obtain blood levels of drug
        Document relief with pulmonary function testing
Improve sputum clearance
    Institute pharmacologic therapy
    Treat with incentive spirometry, postural drainage, or other therapy
    Prepare patient for postoperative therapy
Optimize right ventricular performance
    Treat congestive heart failure
Institute measure to prevent pulmonary embolism
    Administer anticoagulants
    Institute sequential compression of lower extremities
    Arrange for early mobility
Encourage reduction or cessation of smoking

proved with antibiotics and measures to increase sputum clearance. Elective surgery is not undertaken in a patient with an acute lower respiratory infection, even if only a local anesthetic is planned. General anesthetics and surgery itself cause a temporary interruption of normal immune responses, decreased ciliary clearance of secretions and debris in the respiratory tract, and increased tenacity of secretions. Patients who have pneumonia or acute bronchitis are at risk for a worsening of their condition, a reactive airway with bronchospasm and laryngospasm, thick sputum obstructing the airways, and prolonged hypoxemia. They often require mechanical ventilation in the recovery period. Uncomplicated viral upper respiratory infections probably do not markedly increase the risk for surgery and anesthesia if they are not accompanied by bacterial infection and fever. However, many physicians postpone the procedure until the acute phase of the infection passes because manipulation of the airway and generalized immunosuppression can worsen the infection or bacterial **superinfection.**

Smoking

Approximately one fourth of American adults smoke cigarettes. Smoking increases airway irritability, sputum production, and obstructive airway disease and decreases oxygen-carrying capacity. Cessation 2 to 3 months before surgery permits maximal reversal of these effects. Sputum production and airway hyperreactivity do not diminish appreciably unless the patient quits smoking more than a few weeks before surgery. However, carboxyhemoglobin levels return to normal within a day or so, and oxygen delivery to tissues improves correspondingly.

Chronic Obstructive Pulmonary Diseases

Chronic obstructive pulmonary diseases increase the patient's susceptibility to bronchospasm and laryngospasm with airway manipulation. In addition to preoperative control of chronic infection and sputum mobilization, preparation of the patient who has severe symptoms includes an assessment of expiratory flow patterns with pulmonary function testing, a chest x-ray to determine the extent of bullae formation, and testing of blood gases on room air to determine the patient's baseline levels.

For these patients, the course of surgery is usually uneventful because most anesthetic agents relax bronchiolar smooth muscle. However, these patients must be monitored postoperatively as they assume spontaneous respiration and manage their secretions in the presence of continued sedation, narcotic suppression of respiratory drive, and pain-induced immobility. Although regional anesthesia may seem preferable to general anesthesia with intubation and prolonged sedation, often it is not. The supine (or any other) position decreases chest compliance, and a high level of motor blockade decreases the contribution of intercostal and abdominal muscles to expiration. In addition, during regional anesthesia, the patient might cough. The anesthesiologist could do nothing to control the cough, short of inducing complete muscle relaxation, which would require intubation and ventilation.

Asthma

Patients who have asthma should be in remission at the time of surgery and anesthesia. Even so, they have an increased risk of bronchospasm when the airway is manipulated, when intubation is performed, and whenever surgical stimulation causes an autonomic response. Asthma is controlled perioperatively by maintaining a therapeutic level of the patient's usual medication, by avoiding drugs with histamine-releasing or bronchoconstricting effects (e.g., certain muscle relaxants, β_2 antagonists, irritating inhalation anesthetics), and by using a stress-free anesthetic. Many patients use inhalers to control their attacks. Inhalers can be used just before induction, on emergence, and during anesthesia. The patient's preoperative history should include information about current or recent use of oral or inhaled steroid preparations, both perioperatively and postoperatively, so that steroid coverage can be maintained (see the section on adrenal insufficiency).

Nervous System

Patients with preexisting neurologic conditions have varied problems during surgery. Most of these problems can be anticipated with complete assessment and preparation. Increased ICP and cerebrovascular insufficiency may be the most difficult to manage, and acute or chronic spinal cord disorders present many dilemmas. Chronic neurologic conditions cause less of a management problem, but they usually coexist with other factors associated with debilitation. The anesthesiologist must consider these factors preoperatively.

Increased Intracranial Pressure

The most common conditions associated with increased ICP are tumor, trauma, hydrocephalus, and intracranial bleeding. Increased ICP usually accompanies hepatic failure; severe hyperglycemia, with or without ketoacidosis; acute hyponatremia or water intoxication; myxedema coma; and eclampsia. Preoperative management is the same, regardless of whether the surgical procedure is designed to relieve the intracranial hypertension. The most common methods used to reduce ICP are diuresis to decrease cellular water content, steroids to decrease cellular water and stabilize the blood–brain barrier, and acute hyperventilation to decrease intracranial volume by cerebral vasoconstriction. Diuresis and steroids provide long-term treatment. Hyperventilation is effective only for 24 to 36 hours.

Hyperventilation is used only in extreme cases because it requires endotracheal intubation and mechanical ventilation in the intensive care unit. Patients with increasing ICP are at risk for profound brain stem damage and death because of herniation of the cerebellar tonsils through the foramen magnum. Most anesthetic drugs, as well as glucose, fluid, and blood pressure alterations, exacerbate the condition. Spinal fluid drainage, intentional or not, may also cause herniation if an acute loss of CSF pressure occurs. Preoperative signs and symptoms of increased ICP are listed in Table 1-30.

When a patient who has increased ICP undergoes anesthesia, management consists of reducing the effect of surgical stimulation that further increases intracranial hypertension. A responsive patient is asked to hyperventilate voluntarily before the induction of anesthesia. Because all intravenous induction agents, except ketamine, profoundly decrease cerebral blood flow and metabolism, they are particularly useful in this setting. Intravenous lidocaine (1–1.5 mg/kg) is effective 1 to 2 minutes before intubation to prevent the increased cerebral blood flow associated with this stimulating event.

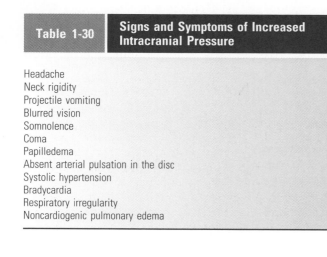

Table 1-30	Signs and Symptoms of Increased Intracranial Pressure

Headache
Neck rigidity
Projectile vomiting
Blurred vision
Somnolence
Coma
Papilledema
Absent arterial pulsation in the disc
Systolic hypertension
Bradycardia
Respiratory irregularity
Noncardiogenic pulmonary edema

Anesthesia is tailored to prevent sympathetic response to surgical stimulation, hypercarbia, and increased venous pressure that may be associated with coughing on the endotracheal tube or "fighting" the ventilator. When used in conjunction with hyperventilation, inhalation agents in moderate concentrations do not cause further intracranial hypertension ($PaCO_2 \leq 25$).

Cerebrovascular Insufficiency

Cerebrovascular insufficiency may be acute, chronic, or intermittent. Elderly patients with carotid artery disease and flow impairment often seek treatment for unrelated surgical procedures. The only finding in these patients is an asymptomatic carotid bruit. Carotid disease that is neither symptomatic nor marked by ulcerated plaques does not require correction before elective surgery. However, even if carotid disease is corrected, it is safe to assume that significant intracerebral vascular disease remains.

If a patient has suspected cerebrovascular insufficiency, measures are taken to prevent an ischemic episode intraoperatively. These measures include administering anticoagulants and cerebral vasodilators (e.g., nifedipine, nitroprusside, nitroglycerin); manipulating cerebral perfusion pressure; avoiding cerebral vasoconstriction by maintaining $PaCO_2$ in the normal range; and using anesthetics that decrease the cerebral metabolic rate (e.g., intravenous agents, isoflurane). As with cardiovascular disorders, in cerebrovascular disorders, the acceptable range of intraoperative values is chosen preoperatively, when the patient is awake and asymptomatic.

Surgical patients who have had a cerebrovascular accident may have a variety of related problems that require special attention. Bedridden patients are often cachectic and hypovolemic. They have skin breakdown, bony demineralization, and autonomic dysfunction. Cachexia leads to poor wound healing, infection, and hypoproteinemia-induced edema. It can be corrected by a period of preoperative nutritional support. Skin and bony abnormalities increase the risk of pressure sores and fractures during and after surgery. Hypovolemia and autonomic dysfunction make it difficult to manage intraoperative and postoperative blood volume changes without further risk to the CNS. Because of a proliferation of receptors in skeletal muscle, chronic denervation leads to life-threatening hyperkalemia in response to depolarizing muscle relaxants. Renal function is often compromised, leading to altered pharmacokinetics of anesthetic drugs and adjuncts. Bedridden patients often have postoperative respiratory and thromboembolic complications. Methods such as incentive spirometry and chest physical therapy are used to prevent atelectasis and congestion. Thromboembolism is prevented with physical therapy, anticoagulation, pneumatic stockings, and frequent position changes. Finally, the conscious stroke victim may have debilitating depression that can impede recovery and threaten survival.

Chronic Neuromuscular Disease

Patients who have chronic demyelinating diseases, whether bedridden or not, have many of the same problems as stroke patients. Many receive steroids or adrenocorticotropic hormone (ACTH) and require perioperative dosages that are large enough to cover possible acute stress-induced adrenal insufficiency (see the section on adrenal insufficiency). The anesthesiologist should prepare the patient to expect a postoperative relapse or worsening of neurologic symptoms because they often occur despite the best medical management.

Spinal Cord Injury

Acute cord injury, whether caused by compression, trauma, or vascular insufficiency, may leave the patient without sympathetic, motor, or sensory function below the level of the lesion. Usually the patient seeks treatment to relieve compression, hoping to reverse the injury, but more often to prevent further injury. The patient is often maximally vasodilated and cannot compensate for changes in position or blood volume. The patient is at great risk for further cord injury and loss of function while being positioned and during episodes of intraoperative hypotension. Thus, assessment and management of blood volume status is an important part of anesthetic management.

The patient with chronic paraplegia or quadriplegia may have any or all of the conditions previously discussed for debilitated patients. Additionally, patients with high cord lesions (T6 or above) are at risk for sudden, severe hypertension and tachycardia with ventricular ectopy caused by autonomic hyperreflexia. This reaction occurs with almost any stimulus below the level of intact cord, including a distended bladder. The frequency and severity of these episodes can be reduced during surgery by complete sensory deafferentation of the surgical site and the viscera with local, regional, or general anesthesia. Renal, cardiovascular, and psychological dysfunction often occurs in the cord-injured patient. It should be assessed carefully and optimized before surgery.

Epilepsy

The patient with chronic epilepsy is of concern because of drug therapy. Most anticonvulsants interact with anesthetics because of their effect on the CNS and because of the activity they induce in the hepatic microsomal enzyme system. This system also metabolizes most anesthetic drugs. If acute onset of seizures occurs during surgery, the cause must be found and treated (Table 1-31). Acute or chronic seizures should be controlled as well as possible before surgery, and the medication regimen should be continued throughout surgery.

Endocrine Disorders

Virtually every endocrine disorder can affect the patient during the perioperative period, but the three most common are diabetes mellitus, adrenal disease, and thyroid disorders.

Table 1-31	Causes of Acute Onset of Seizures

Drug intoxication (alcohol, cocaine, amphetamines)
Drug withdrawal (alcohol, narcotics, sedatives, hypnotics, tranquilizers)
Acute hypoxia
Hyponatremia
Hypocalcemia
Neoplasm
Infection
Fever
Uremia
Trauma
Cerebrovascular insufficiency
Cerebrovascular accidents
Eclampsia of pregnancy

Diabetes Mellitus

The two types of diabetes mellitus, insulin-dependent (type I) and noninsulin-dependent (type II), have different consequences and treatments. With either type, long-term tight control of blood glucose levels delays the onset of complications. Hypertension, myocardial ischemia and dysfunction, renal insufficiency, cerebrovascular insufficiency, peripheral vascular insufficiency, and peripheral neuropathy are often associated with diabetes in adults and occasionally in children. These conditions are of concern in the perioperative period (Table 1-32). Tight control of blood glucose during surgery may increase wound healing and decrease the infection rate in patients with type I diabetes. There is no evidence that it confers any benefit to patients with type II diabetes except during pregnancy and possibly during cerebral ischemic episodes. Extreme hyperglycemia should be avoided because it can cause cerebral edema, osmotic diuresis, and ketoacidosis in type I diabetes and hyperosmolar nonketotic coma in type II diabetes. On the other hand, hypoglycemia can cause hypotension and seizures in either type of diabetes.

To control intraoperative glucose levels, it is necessary

Table 1-32	Medical Conditions Commonly Associated with Diabetes Mellitus

Atherosclerotic disease	Autonomic dysfunction
Aortic	Gastroparesis
Carotid	Hypovolemia, hypervolemia
Cerebrovascular	Inadequate sweating
Peripheral	Sexual dysfunction
Myocardial ischemia	Altered response to infection
Silent	
Angina	Altered wound healing
Myocardial infarction	
Microvascular disease	
Neurovascular	
Renal	
Coronary	
Retinal	

to have a means of measuring blood glucose. A recommended regimen is to begin with half the usual morning dose of subcutaneous insulin, run a drip of dextrose 5% in water (D_5W) at approximately 125 mL/hr/70 kg, and use a sliding scale of regular insulin injections during and after surgery. Blood glucose is monitored hourly. An alternative plan is to administer a continuous intravenous drip of insulin (at a rate in units/hr equal to plasma glucose in mg/dL/150) and a separate drip of 5% glucose, regulated according to hourly blood glucose determinations. A safe blood glucose range is 80 to 200 mg/dL, but the closer it is to 100, the better. Patients with type II diabetes usually tolerate a much higher level without side effects, but they are at risk for hyperosmolarity as the glucose level approaches 600 mg/dL. In the hyperglycemic patient, urine output may not be a reliable monitor of blood volume status. In all patients, hyperglycemia increases the damage caused by cerebral ischemic episodes.

Adrenal Disease

Cushing's Syndrome

The most common cause of Cushing's syndrome is exogenous administration of steroids. Consequently, the adrenal glands atrophy because they are not called on to function. Other causes include increased production of ACTH secondary to pituitary microadenoma and ectopic production of ACTH by tumors of the lung, pancreas, or thymus. Adrenal adenoma or carcinoma accounts for fewer than 10% to 20% of cases of noniatrogenic Cushing's disease. Preoperative preparation of these patients includes evaluation and control of fluid status, hypertension, and hyperglycemia. If removal of the adrenal glands or the ACTH-secreting tumor is planned, mineralocorticoid and glucocorticoid replacement is commonly begun at the time of surgery and continued until the patient is weaned postoperatively. If surgery is performed for other reasons, a bolus dose of steroid is given on the day of surgery to prevent stress-induced adrenal insufficiency with cardiovascular collapse caused by hypovolemia or inadequate response of blood vessels to vasoconstrictive stimuli (see later).

Adrenal Insufficiency

Primary adrenal insufficiency, or Addison's disease, is usually caused by an autoimmune process that results in destruction of adrenocortical cells. Secondary adrenal insufficiency can be caused by tumor, hemorrhage into the gland, or withdrawal of steroid or ACTH therapy. In addition to a deficiency in steroid hormones, mineralocorticoid deficiency results in electrolyte abnormalities. These patients usually have hypovolemia, hyponatremia, and hyperkalemia, but do not have severe difficulties unless they are stressed by infection, injury, or surgery. Addisonian crisis can be prevented or treated by prompt administration of steroids at a dose equal to 300 mg hydrocortisone in a 24-hour period. This dose is given on the day of surgery. This dosage is believed to approximate the maximum output of the adrenal glands during a 24-hour period. Recently, however, doses of 100 mg/day hydrocortisone hemisuccinate or hydrocortisone phosphate also prevented addisonian crisis. The steroids can be tapered starting the next day. Patients with mineralocorticoid deficiency are likely to have hyperkalemic alkalosis, hyponatremia, and hypovolemia. In the untreated patient, dysrhythmia is caused by hyperkalemia.

Pheochromocytoma

Pheochromocytoma is a rare cause of hypertension, but 60% of patients with pheochromocytoma who die in the hospital are previously undiagnosed and die during surgery unrelated to their tumor. Inducing anesthesia in the undiagnosed patient can lead to severe hypertension and death. Occasionally, the only clue to pheochromocytoma is a history of unexplained severe hypertension or tachycardia during a previous anesthetic. The signs and symptoms of pheochromocytoma include unexplained episodic hypertension, tachycardia, flushing, sweating, and headache. Recognizing this disorder can be lifesaving. The patient who has a known pheochromocytoma can be well prepared preoperatively with α and occasionally β blockade. The goal of preoperative preparation is to control intermittent hypertension and tachycardia and to normalize the circulating blood volume and red cell mass. Electrolyte, BUN, and creatinine levels should be normal before surgery proceeds.

The perioperative mortality rate for resection of pheochromocytoma decreased from between 40% and 60% to between 0% and 3% with the introduction of preoperative α-adrenergic blockade. Prazosin or phenoxybenzamine counteracts the vasoconstriction induced by surges of catecholamines. These agents restore normal blood volume, control blood pressure, and reduce symptoms. Patients with tachycardia or dysrhythmia also benefit from β blockade, but only after α receptors are blocked, so that the vasoconstrictor effects of β blockade will not worsen the hypertension. α-Methylparatyrosine may be added to the regimen if needed. Most patients require a stabilization period of at least 2 weeks before surgery. Surgery can proceed when they no longer experience episodic symptoms. No particular anesthetic technique results in a better patient outcome than any other. A smooth perioperative course depends first on preparation and then on monitoring and immediate correction of intraoperative blood volume, blood pressure, and rhythm changes.

Thyroid Disorders

Hyperthyroidism

Hyperthyroidism in surgical patients is usually caused by diffuse multinodular enlargement of the gland (Graves' disease). It can also be caused by pregnancy, thyroiditis, choriocarcinoma, or a pituitary adenoma that secretes thyroid-stimulating hormone. In all but the most urgent cases, these patients are treated to reduce all symptoms, especially cardiac symptoms, before surgery. Treatment with propylthiouracil or methimazole for 6 weeks may be required before symptoms resolve. The current trend is to treat hyperthyroidism only with iodine and propranolol. Symptoms usually resolve in 7 to 14 days. However, this therapy may not normalize cardiac function. All medications are continued throughout the perioperative period. Table 1-33 contrasts the signs and symptoms of hyperthyroidism and hypothyroidism, and should alert students to suggested routes for preoperative investigation.

If surgery is urgent in the patient with hyperthyroidism, cardiac symptoms can be stabilized by administering β blockers to control heart rate and hypertension or by monitoring pulmonary artery and wedge pressure. There is risk, however, of further reducing ventricular function. Attention to intravascular volume status is necessary throughout the perioperative period, especially because most anesthetics cause vasodilation. A "thyroid storm," evidenced by the sudden onset of fever, severe hypertension, tachycardia, and disorders of consciousness, is treated immediately with β blockers and iodine to block the peripheral actions of thyroid hormone. At the same time, a search for precipitating stress (e.g., infection) should begin because successful treatment depends on controlling both the cause and effects of thyroid storm.

No one anesthetic technique is superior for avoiding intraoperative problems in patients with pheochromocytoma or hyperthyroidism. Important factors include preoperative preparation, continuation of therapy throughout the operative period, and anticipation of possible problems caused by hypovolemia or electrolyte, rhythm, or blood pressure abnormalities.

Hypothyroidism

Most patients with hypothyroidism who come to surgery have been treated with thyroid hormone replacement and have stable cardiovascular systems. Occasionally, patients with untreated myxedema require emergent procedures and acute management. T_3 hormone can be given intravenously, but must be carefully titrated to avoid myocardial ischemia. Volume and electrolyte status is carefully monitored, and special measures are taken to keep the patient warm. These patients have excessive responses to anesthetics, sedatives, narcotics, and muscle relaxants. Because postoperative ventilatory depression is common, the patient and family should be prepared for the possibility of prolonged sleepiness, intubation, and mechanical ventilation after anesthesia.

Renal Disease

As renal tubular function diminishes, patients become uremic and may come to surgery with varying degrees of renal failure. Long-term hemodialysis reverses many of the effects of uremia. Diabetes and chronic hypertension, the two most common causes of chronic renal failure, must be managed concurrently. Table 1-34 lists alterations that are expected in patients with renal failure, suggesting areas of particular concern in preoperative evaluation and preparation.

Cardiovascular stability is difficult to achieve in patients with renal disease because of anesthetic-induced depression, surgical stress–induced catecholamine activity, and the large shifts in blood volume that occur during surgery. Remaining renal function is preserved only by maintaining renal perfusion near baseline. Because renal excretion is so important in eliminating intravenous agents and muscle relaxants, doses of anesthetics are carefully tailored based on remaining renal function to avoid prolonged postoperative depression. Urine output is carefully monitored in patients with partial renal function. However, if diuretics are used or if the patient is hyperglycemic, urine output does not reflect volume status and invasive monitoring becomes necessary.

Table 1-33	Signs and Symptoms of Thyroid Dysfunction
Hyperthyroid	**Hypothyroid**
Weight loss	Weight gain
Diarrhea	Slow gastric emptying
Warm, moist skin	Dry, thick skin
Muscle weakness, wasting	Fatigue, weakness
Menstrual abnormalities	Slow mentation
Nervousness	Slow movement
Jitteriness, tremor	Cold intolerance
Heat intolerance	Bradycardia
Tachycardia	Cardiomegaly
Cardiomegaly	Dyspnea, orthopnea
Atrial fibrillation	Congestive failure
Mitral valve prolapse	Impaired free water clearance
Papillary muscle dysfunction	Pericardial and pleural effusions
Dyspnea, orthopnea	Decreased MAC[a] for anesthetics
Congestive failure	
Anemia, thrombocytopenia	
Increased alkaline phosphatase	
Hypercalcemia	
Bone loss	

[a]MAC, a measure of anesthetic potency, is discussed in the section on pharmacology of inhalation agents.

Table 1-34	Manifestations of Renal Failure
Decreased excretion of water and electrolytes	
Edema, pleural and pericardial effusions	
Hyperkalemia	
Anemia	
Coagulopathy	
Neuropathies	
Peripheral	
Autonomic	
Hypertension	
Atherosclerosis with vascular disease	
Pericarditis	
Congestive heart failure	

Patients with chronic renal failure who come to surgery immediately after dialysis have a low circulating blood volume. The anesthesiologist is concerned both with maintaining the patency of the vascular access site for hemodialysis and with protecting other organ systems. Immediate postoperative dialysis is often required because of the blood or fluid needed to maintain intraoperative homeostasis or to correct electrolyte abnormalities. This dialysis may be provided in the PACU.

Gastrointestinal System

This section discusses the patient who comes to surgery with a full stomach, bowel obstruction, morbid obesity, or hepatic failure.

Full Stomach

Patients with more than 25 mL of gastric content with a pH of less than 2.5 are at increased risk for pulmonary aspiration syndrome. Preoperative treatment and special induction techniques can reduce this risk to near zero. A high level of suspicion at the preoperative evaluation is often lifesaving. Table 1-2 summarizes the conditions that suggest a full stomach.

The preoperative preparation of the patient with a full stomach, designed to reduce the volume and increase the pH of the gastric contents, is discussed in the section on preoperative medication. Induction of anesthesia must proceed with extreme caution, even after pharmacologic preparation, because once the protective airway reflexes are abolished, aspiration cannot be prevented if regurgitation occurs. The risk of aspiration is not eliminated by inserting a nasogastric tube to suction the stomach or by using local or regional anesthesia. It is always possible for the patient to lose consciousness or control of the airway if the procedure does not go as planned.

Bowel Obstruction

Patients who undergo surgery for bowel obstruction are often critically ill, and little time can be spared for preoperative preparation. Bowel obstruction rapidly leads to perforation, peritonitis, and septic shock, especially in elderly or chronically ill patients. These patients are assumed to be hypovolemic, to have electrolyte abnormalities, and to have full stomachs not completely drained by nasogastric suction. If the obstruction has been protracted, abdominal distention and pain will interfere with lung expansion. In addition, accompanying atelectasis and pleural effusion can interfere with efficient oxygenation. The profound hypovolemia that usually accompanies this condition must be reversed before anesthesia can be induced safely. Even in the elderly patient with cardiovascular disease, several liters of crystalloid solution can be infused rapidly if filling pressures are monitored. Preoperative monitoring of urinary output is a useful guide to the adequacy of volume replacement.

The most life-threatening manifestation of bowel obstruction is septic shock, which may occur when the integrity of the bowel mucosa is lost and Gram-negative bacteremia ensues. Septic shock may cause a hyperdynamic state that includes hypotension, tachycardia, increased cardiac output, and high fever. When the patient is hypovolemic, as is usually the case with bowel obstruction or perforation, the hyperdynamic state may not be evident until fluid resuscitation occurs. Gram-negative bacteremia has a 47% mortality rate.

Early in septic shock, bacterial endotoxin activates mediators that act on smooth muscle and cause vasodilation and myocardial depression. Because these effects are impossible to reverse, the management of septic shock is particularly difficult. The heart attempts to compensate by increasing both rate and contractility, but if blood volume is low, this compensation is not adequate and blood pressure falls. Because of inadequate tissue perfusion, the patient becomes acidotic and cannot respond to catecholamines or other agents used to support the cardiovascular system.

Initial treatment consists of antibiotics and volume expansion. Fluid is infused rapidly, guided by careful hemodynamic and urine output monitoring and frequent determinations of pH, blood lactate, and mixed venous O_2 saturations to assess tissue perfusion. Antibodies to bind endotoxin are used experimentally. Vasoconstrictors are used only when volume is restored and systemic vascular resistance remains low. Myocardial contractility is improved with low-dose dopamine, dobutamine, inamrinone, milrinone, or epinephrine, which may be added to the volume restoration to increase cardiac output. High-dose corticosteroid therapy is ineffective. Patients in septic shock often have coagulopathy that must be treated throughout the perioperative period.

Controversy exists as to whether fluid resuscitation should be carried out with crystalloid or colloid solutions. Colloid solutions include albumin, plasma, and hetastarch. Proponents of crystalloid therapy cite the lower cost, decreased exposure to blood donors, and reduced lung water accumulation. In addition, there is no difference in outcome between the two techniques. Resuscitation with crystalloid solution requires three to four times as much volume, resulting in postresuscitation edema that may require a longer period of intensive care. Patients with bowel obstruction and septic shock require a period of postoperative ventilation, regardless of the resuscitation fluid therapy. As in any critical illness, red cell transfusions are used to maintain adequate oxygen-carrying capacity. There is controversy about the optimal hematocrit, but most critical care specialists agree that a hemoglobin level of more than 10 g/dL blood is usually necessary.

Morbid Obesity

Morbid obesity, defined as being twice the ideal body weight, increases the risk of anesthesia and surgery two to three times. Many pulmonary and cardiovascular problems stem from the fact that pulmonary compliance is mechanically reduced by the mass of fat on the chest wall and in the abdomen. Functional residual capacity is also diminished in these patients. The increased work of breathing results in an increased oxygen cost at the same time that oxygenation is reduced because of ventilation–perfusion abnormalities caused by incomplete expansion. These problems are magnified when the patient lies down. The high circulating blood volume and cardiac output are secondary to the large tissue mass that must be perfused. Pulmonary and systemic hypertension are caused in part by the high blood volume and relative hypoxemia, as well as by hyperlipidemia and other risk factors for cardiovascular disease. Polycythemia results from chronic hypoxemia. Sleep apnea (see Otolaryngology, Chapter 5), which initially occurs because of mechanical obstruction of the upper airway, may become central over time, increasing the respiratory depressant effects of anesthetics, sedatives, and narcotics. Table 1-35 lists common medical problems in morbidly obese patients; the preoperative evaluation should search for possible sources of increased risk.

These cardiovascular and respiratory abnormalities may eventually result in the Pickwickian syndrome (i.e., chronic alveolar hypoventilation, hypoxemia, hypercarbia, congestive heart failure, daytime somnolence). These patients, who represent 5% to 10% of all morbidly obese patients, may have acute pulmonary edema and die of dysrhythmia when they lie down. Thus, they are at great risk of death during surgery. Even the most normal morbidly obese patient needs supplemental oxygen from the time he or she lies down on the operating table until sev-

eral days postoperatively. These patients also should be considered to have a full stomach, no matter how long they have fasted, because of high intra-abdominal pressure. As in all patients, diabetes and hypertension should be treated carefully. The status of myocardial oxygenation should be assessed before surgery, and perioperative management should proceed as though the patient were at risk because of CHF and myocardial ischemia. Because the most prevalent cause of perioperative morbidity in this population is thromboembolic, the patient must be encouraged to resume activity early in the postoperative period. Low-dose anticoagulation regimens are also commonly used. Postoperative ventilatory support can be avoided with appropriate preparation and attentive nursing care. Because morbidly obese patients often have depression and a poor self-image, their psychological state also requires attention during this time. Their contribution to their own recovery is essential.

Liver Failure

Preoperative evaluation begins with an examination of hepatic function that includes bilirubin, enzymes, and a coagulation profile. A thorough evaluation of the cardiovascular and respiratory systems is essential. Table 1-36 summarizes the physiologic consequences of hepatic failure.

Little can be done to improve the overall condition of the patient who has end-stage liver failure, but if surgery is required, the preoperative preparation should correct any fluid, electrolyte, and coagulation abnormalities. The presence of ascites usually is associated with hypoproteinemia and hypoxemia, both of which can be treated. Esophageal varices are cause for concern, even if they are not actively bleeding, especially if surgery is planned to reduce portal hypertension. Temporary occlusion of the portal vein or vena cava often results in resumption of active

Table 1-35	Conditions Associated with Morbid Obesity

Pulmonary
  Increased work of breathing
  Restrictive lung disease
  Hypoxemia
  Pulmonary hypertension
  Periodic alveolar hypoventilation (sleep apnea)
  Pickwickian syndrome

Cardiovascular
  Increased circulating blood volume
  Increased cardiac output
  Systemic hypertension
  Biventricular failure
  Ischemic heart disease

Other
  Diabetes mellitus
  Hyperlipidemia
  Polycythemia
  Liver failure
  Increased gastric volume and acidity
  Psychological problems
  Anatomy: difficult airway, intravenous access, blood pressure
    measurement, etc.

Table 1-36	Conditions Associated with Liver Disease

Hepatic dysfunction
  Hyperbilirubinemia
  Altered drug metabolism and excretion
  Coagulopathy
  Hypoglycemia
  Electrolyte abnormalities
  Portal hypertension
  Ascites
  Variceal bleeding

Cardiopulmonary
  Peripheral vasodilation
  Decreased sensitivity to catecholamines
  Increased circulating blood volume
  Intrapulmonary and extrapulmonary shunting
  Increased cardiac output
  Cardiomyopathy

Renal insufficiency

Hepatic encephalopathy

bleeding, and major blood transfusions are required. The coagulopathy of liver failure can be treated with fresh frozen plasma and platelet transfusions. Support of the cardiovascular system requires monitored blood volume resuscitation to maintain urine output and tissue oxygenation. Because hypoglycemia is an ongoing concern, even in the early stages of liver disease, blood glucose levels are checked often before and during surgery. Because hepatic encephalopathy is accompanied by increased ICP, appropriate precautions must be taken to avoid further increases in ICP.

The chronically alcoholic patient, whether or not in hepatic failure, requires special consideration. This patient may have severe multisystem disease that may include cardiomyopathy, nutritional deficiencies, peripheral and CNS abnormalities, and often pulmonary dysfunction. Alcoholic cardiomyopathy causes cardiomegaly and CHF. Often it is not amenable to treatment. The patient who has a failing heart, no matter what the cause, should be prepared and managed as discussed in the section on the cardiovascular system. Nutritional deficiency often causes megaloblastic anemia, and the red cell mass may be severely deficient. Many alcoholics are cigarette smokers and have chronic lung disease. In patients who are cirrhotic, intrapulmonary shunting with hypoxemia may occur. Finally, because acute alcohol withdrawal may occur during surgery, prophylactic treatment with benzodiazepines may be warranted when a history of recent intake or past delirium tremens indicates the possibility of withdrawal perioperatively.

Hematologic Disorders

Anemia and Polycythemia

Both anemia and polycythemia must be corrected preoperatively, but there is controversy about the optimal hemoglobin and hematocrit levels. Patients with chronic anemia because of hematologic disease or renal failure do well with a hemoglobin level of 6 to 8 g/dL. There is no evidence that transfusing them up to a more normal level improves their perioperative course. On the other hand, if the anemia is acute or if the patient cannot compensate with increased cardiac output, the reduction in oxygen-carrying capacity that results from hemoglobin of less than 8 g/dL can be detrimental. A preoperative hemoglobin level of at least 10 g/dL was historically suggested as a cutoff point for elective surgery. However, no conclusive data show that this practice results in better patient outcome, and many anesthesiologists now allow patients to come to surgery with a hematocrit of 20% if they are otherwise normal. Current practice is to individualize therapy after the cause of anemia is discovered and the level of compensation assessed. Polycythemia of any cause reduces blood flow to tissues and increases the risk of thromboembolism. It is easily managed preoperatively by phlebotomy. The blood is stored in case the patient requires transfusion later.

Sickle Cell Hemoglobinopathy

Hemoglobin S (Hb S) causes erythrocytes to distort and aggregate in an environment of decreased oxygen. Patients with sickle cell trait are probably not at increased risk during anesthesia and surgery because their cells do not sickle until the hemoglobin saturation falls below 20%. Patients with sickle cell disease and sickle cell–thalassemia disease are anemic because the bone marrow cannot keep up with erythrocyte destruction. These patients have hemolytic crises and organ infarctions because of circulatory obstruction. Sickling occurs with decreased arterial oxygen content, acidosis, hypothermia, and blood stasis. It occurs in proportion to the level of Hb S. Preoperative preparation of patients who have sickle cell disease or sickle cell–thalassemia requires hemoglobin electrophoresis to determine the level of Hb S. Exchange transfusions are usually carried out until the proportion of Hb S to normal red blood cells is less than 30%, but few data link this practice to a better outcome. Intraoperative management includes keeping the patient oxygenated, warm, and hydrated. Measures to avoid venous stasis include elevating the legs and using sequential compression boots. Postoperatively, patients with sickle cell hemoglobinopathy are given supplemental oxygen until they have prolonged normal oxygen saturation on room air.

Coagulopathy

Specific coagulopathies are corrected preoperatively with replacement of the deficient factors. Platelet dysfunction is associated with many chronic medical conditions as well as with aspirin and other anti-inflammatory agents. Only approximately 30,000 to 50,000 functioning platelets/mm^3 are necessary for normal coagulation, but a platelet count does not assess platelet function. If a platelet abnormality is suspected, bleeding time or specific tests for platelet function should be obtained, with platelet transfusions administered as necessary. Patients with chronic liver failure and uremia often lack many coagulation factors. These patients are best evaluated by obtaining prothrombin time, international normalized ratio (INR), and partial thromboplastin time. They are also likely to have dysfunctioning platelets, although their counts may be normal. Fresh frozen plasma and platelet transfusions usually restore coagulation function to a level that allows surgical hemostasis.

SUGGESTED READINGS

Ang-Lee M, Moss J, Yuan CS. Herbal medicines and perioperative care. *JAMA* 2000;286:208–216.

ASA Task Force on Blood Component Therapy. Practice guidelines for blood component therapy. *Anesthesiology* 1996;84:732–747.

Auerbach AD, Goldman L. Beta blockers and reduction of cardiac events in noncardiac surgery: scientific review. *JAMA.* 2002;287:1435–1444.

Dolin SJ, Cashman JN, Bland JM. Effectiveness of postoperative pain management: I. Evidence from published data [Review]. *Br J Anaesth* 2002;89:409–423.

Eagle KA, Berger PB, Calkins H, et al. ACC/AHA guideline update for perioperative cardiovascular evaluation for noncardiac surgery update: a report of the American College of Cardiology/American Heart Association Task Force on Practice Guidelines. Committee to Update the 1996 Guidelines on Perioperative Cardiovascular Evaluation for Noncardiac Surgery, 2002. Available at: http://www.acc.org/clinical/guidelines/perio/update/periupdate_index.htm. Accessed March 23, 2006.

Hurford WE, Baillin MT, Davidson JK, et al. *Clinical Procedures of the Massachusetts General Hospital*. 6th ed. Boston: Little, Brown; 2002.

Mulroy MF. Regional *Anesthesia: An Illustrated Guide*. 3rd ed. Philadelphia: Lippincott Williams & Wilkins; 2002.

National Institutes of Health Consensus Conference: Perioperative red cell transfusion. *JAMA* 1988;260:2700–2703.

Roizen MF, Fleischer LA. *Essence of Anesthesia Practice*. 2nd ed. Philadelphia: WB Saunders; 2002.

PHILIP J. WOLFSON ■ DAN POENARU
BARBARA PETTITT ■ DAVID ROGERS

Pediatric Surgery: Surgical Diseases of Children

OBJECTIVES

Perioperative Management of the Pediatric Surgical Patient

1 Compare the intracellular and extracellular fluid compartments in children and adults. Calculate the daily fluid and electrolyte requirements for children based on maintenance requirements, preexisting deficits, and abnormal ongoing losses.

2 Compare the indications for enteral and parenteral nutrition in pediatric surgical patients, and explain how each type of nutritional support is provided.

3 Define respiratory failure, and describe how it is managed with supplemental oxygen, mechanical ventilators, and extracorporeal membrane oxygenation.

4 Outline the appropriate steps in the preoperative preparation of children, list the important components of their operating room environment, and discuss the important components of their postoperative care, including pain management.

5 Discuss the emotional needs of children undergoing operations. Describe various pain control measures that may be provided postoperatively.

Neonatal Surgical Conditions

1 Explain the pathophysiology, clinical presentation, and appropriate management of congenital diaphragmatic hernia and other neonatal thoracic mass lesions.

2 Describe the different anatomic configurations of esophageal atresia and tracheoesophageal fistula, and explain how they are diagnosed and treated.

3 List the clinical presentation of congenital intestinal obstruction, and describe the common causes of congenital obstruction at each level of the intestinal tract.

4 Describe the various types of anorectal malformations, and relate their anatomy to treatment and prognosis.

5 Discuss the pathophysiology, clinical presentation, and treatment of necrotizing enterocolitis.

6 Define short bowel syndrome and outline its pathophysiology and treatment.

7 Discuss the management of an infant with jaundice, particularly as it relates to biliary atresia.

8 Compare the embryology, clinical presentation, associated anomalies, and treatment of omphalocele and gastroschisis.

9 List the advantages, disadvantages, and contraindications to neonatal circumcision.

Surgical Conditions in the Older Child

1 Describe the anatomic differences between an inguinal hernia, a communicating hydrocele, and a noncommunicating hydrocele, and discuss the rationale for the treatment of each.

2 Discuss the proper timing for repair of umbilical hernias.

3 Discuss the treatment of a boy with an undescended testicle, including the optimal age and reasons for orchidopexy.

4 Describe the typical patient with pyloric stenosis, the optimal techniques of diagnosis, and the proper management of this condition.

5 Compare the presentation of acute inflammatory conditions of the abdomen in young children and in adults.

6 Describe the clinical presentation of a child with non-perforated appendicitis and with perforated appendicitis.

7 Describe the typical patient who has intussusception, the importance of early recognition, and the treatment.

8 Discuss the three common complications of a Meckel's diverticulum.

9 List the common causes and characteristics of gastrointestinal bleeding in children of different ages.

10 Describe the symptoms and potential complications of gastroesophageal reflux in infants and children, and outline the diagnostic workup and indications for surgery.

11 Describe the pathophysiology, clinical presentation, and treatment of children with pectus excavatum and carinatum.

12 List the characteristics of the common types of midline and lateral neck masses seen in children.

13 Contrast the appearance, natural history, and treatment of hemangiomas and vascular malformations.

Tumors

1 List the common malignancies of childhood and their relative incidence.

2 Describe the treatment options for chronic venous access in children.

3 Discuss the clinical presentation (including age of child), diagnostic workup, approach to treatment, and prognosis for each of the following pediatric tumors: neuroblastoma, Wilms' tumor, hepatic tumors, rhabdomyosarcoma, and sacrococcygeal teratoma.

Trauma

1 List the major differences between pediatric and adult trauma.

2 In order of priority, outline the principal steps in the resuscitation of the severely injured child.

3 Discuss the treatment of the pediatric accident victim who has injuries to the head, chest, abdomen, and urinary system.

4 Outline the characteristics of the pediatric trauma victim that raise the possibility of child abuse.

5 Describe the treatment of the pediatric burn patient, with emphasis on fluid resuscitation and care of the burn wound.

6 Outline the treatment plan for a child who may have aspirated or ingested a foreign object.

Although many of the principles involved in managing infants and children with surgical diseases are similar to those for adults, three important differences justify the special field of pediatric surgery:

1 Most of the congenital anomalies that require surgery in children have no counterpart in older individuals. In fact, many would be lethal if not corrected promptly in early childhood.

2 Physiologically, young children are not merely small adults! They have unique metabolic demands and often limited reserves that require special attention to maintain their physiologic parameters within the narrow range of normality. On the other hand, children have a tremendous capacity for repair and regeneration. They are usually not afflicted by many of the preexisting chronic illnesses that affect older people. If handled with great care and skill, these young patients have the resiliency to recover rapidly from even major surgical procedures and subsequently live long, productive lives.

3 Children with surgical illness, and often moreso their parents, have special emotional needs and require extra support during what is often a trying time for the entire family.

This chapter describes (a) the perioperative management of the pediatric patient, (b) surgical conditions common to neonates (apparent at birth or within the first 30 days), (c) surgical conditions common to older children, (d) malignancies found in children, and (e) principles of trauma care in children and how they differ from those in adults.

PERIOPERATIVE MANAGEMENT OF THE PEDIATRIC SURGICAL PATIENT

Fluids and Electrolytes

Fluid and electrolyte management in pediatric patients must be extremely precise because the margin between dehydration and fluid overload is narrow. Compared with adults, infants and children have greater metabolic demands, and because they turn over body water and electrolytes so rapidly, pediatric patients may undergo rapid, major shifts in body fluid compartments. The immature neonatal kidney has limited concentrating and diluting capacities and therefore cannot be entirely relied upon to compensate for a deficiency or overabundance of fluids and electrolytes. Although children's needs may be estimated according to standard formulas, there is no substitute for frequent adjustments based on careful monitoring of the patient's condition.

Neonates have a significantly greater proportion of total body water than do adults because newborn infants have a larger pool of extracellular fluid (ECF) (Fig. 2-1). This fluid compartment is increased further in extremely premature infants (<30 weeks' gestation). At birth the ECF is even more expanded, and as much as 10% of birth weight is lost during the first week as this surplus water is excreted.

In calculating fluid and electrolyte requirements for children who cannot receive enteral feeds, the following quantities must be considered:

1 Maintenance requirements
2 Replacement of preexisting deficits
3 Replacement of ongoing abnormal losses

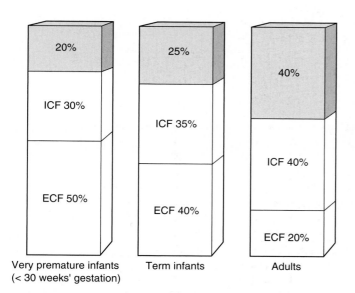

Figure 2-1 Body fluid compartments in very premature infants, term infants, and adults. Unshaded areas show the percentage of body weight as total body water. ECF, extracellular fluid; ICF, intracellular fluid.

Maintenance Requirements

Maintenance fluids and electrolytes are the quantities that must be provided to compensate for normal renal excretion and insensible losses through the skin and lungs. Table 2-1 provides guidelines for calculating the amounts of water and electrolytes required. In addition, a minimal quantity of glucose is included to provide for some protein sparing and to avoid hypoglycemia. These constituents can all be provided by D10% in 1/4 normal saline + 20 mEq/L KCl in infants and D5% in 1/2 normal saline + 20 mEq/L KCl in older children at the infusion rate calculated in Table 2-1. Calcium gluconate should be added for premature infants, who are calcium deficient.

Preexisting Deficits

Children with acute surgical illness may have significant fluid and electrolyte deficits from poor oral intake, vomiting, diarrhea, peritonitis, sepsis, burns, or hemorrhage. Intravascular volume must be rapidly restored to maintain adequate tissue perfusion for normal organ function, particularly if the child requires an urgent operation. Most surgical diseases cause isotonic dehydration. Instead of basing rehydration calculations on imprecise estimates of percentage of dehydration, fluid deficits are best corrected empirically in stages, as outlined in Table 2-2.

Children who are significantly anemic or actively bleeding may require blood transfusions. There is no arbitrary value of hemoglobin below which a transfusion is indicated, and each child must be individually assessed to optimize oxygen delivery. Volumes used for pediatric "units" are provided in Table 2-3.

Abnormal Ongoing Losses

Abnormal losses include measurable and immeasurable third-space fluid losses. Measurable losses refer to abnormal external drainage. In the surgical patient, these losses usually arise from the gastrointestinal tract or from various drainage tubes and are most accurately replaced on a vol-

Table 2-1	Fluids and Electrolytes: Maintenance Requirements	
	Weight (kg)	**mL/24 hr[a]**
Water	≤10	100 mL/kg
	11–20	1000 + 50 mL/kg for each kg >10
	>20	1500 + 20 mL/kg for each kg >20
Sodium	3 mEq/kg/day	
Potassium	2 mEq/kg/day	

[a]Exceptions: (1) Premature infants (<38 weeks' gestation) have increased evaporative losses because of their very thin skin and require up to twice the standard maintenance calculations; (2) during the first few days of life, the need to eliminate the surplus extracellular fluid lowers maintenance requirements to 65–100 mL/kg/day; (3) fever and various disease states (e.g., sepsis) elevate metabolic rate and increase fluid needs.

Table 2-2	**Fluids and Electrolytes: Replacement of Deficits**

Fluid deficit
Resuscitation stage (for initial rapid correction of isotonic, hypotonic, and hypertonic dehydration): lactated Ringer's solution[a] at 20 mL/kg every 10–20 minutes, with close monitoring, until clinical improvement occurs. Then:
Rapid infusion stage (for isotonic or mild hypotonic dehydration): D5% 1/2 normal saline at 2× the maintenance dose until the patient is clinically normovolemic.
Sodium deficit
If significant (Na <120), correct as: mEq Na required = (130 − serum Na) × 0.6 × weight (kg).
Potassium deficit
May add up to 40 mEq of KCl to each liter of intravenous fluid.

[a]Normal saline may be used instead of lactated Ringer's solution.

ume-for-volume basis. Gastric drainage is approximated as D5% in 1/2 normal saline + 10 mEq/L KCl. Alimentary tract losses distal to the pylorus are replaced as lactated Ringer's solution.

Immeasurable third-space losses are fluids and electrolytes that are pathologically sequestered within the body and are neither in equilibrium nor available to the intravascular space. In children with surgical diseases, such fluid can accumulate in the gastrointestinal tract from obstruction and inflammation, in body cavities as ascites and pleural effusions, and diffusely as edema from the leaky capillary syndrome that accompanies shock. Operative manipulation can cause edema in tissues as a result of direct trauma. Because third-space losses cannot be measured directly, their intravenous replacement is approximated. Sequestered fluid is almost always isotonic and is replaced as balanced salt solution. Although one common approach is to provide for the expected regional fluid loss from operative trauma by running intravenous fluids at 1.5 to 2 times the maintenance rate for the first 24 hours postoperatively, this method may give patients too much free water. It is preferable to administer boluses of isotonic normal saline or lactated Ringer's solution in 10 to 20 mL/kg aliquots as directed by the patient's clinical condition.

The adequacy of intravenous fluid therapy can be determined only by monitoring the patient's response. Useful parameters are level of activity, color, skin turgor and temperature, heart rate, and blood pressure. Most helpful is the urine output, which should exceed 1 to 2 mL/kg/hr in infants and 0.5 mL/kg/hr in adolescents. Children who

Table 2-3	**Blood Products: Equivalent "Units" for Pediatric Patients**

Packed red blood cells	10–20 mL/kg
Fresh frozen plasma	20 mL/kg (for coagulopathy and with massive transfusions)
Platelets	10 mL/kg

receive fluids solely as intravenous infusions should have serum electrolytes measured at least every other day.

Nutrition

The well-nourished child who will be eating within 3 to 4 days does not need nutritional support other than the basic fluids and electrolytes as outlined above. On the other hand, if feedings must be withheld longer, if the child is under significant stress, or if the child is premature, enteral or total parenteral nutrition (TPN) may be critical for survival. Compared with adults, growing children have increased nutritional demands, but often limited nutritional reserves. When compounded by the increased metabolic requirements imposed by surgical illness, the risks for malnutrition are considerable. Significant consequences of malnutrition include lack of growth, impaired organ function, immunologic incompetence, and the inability to heal wounds.

Enteral Nutrition

The provision of nutrients through the intestinal tract is ideal. Compared with TPN, enteral feeding is more physiologic, less prone to complications, and far less costly. A lack of enteral feeds leads to atrophy of the intestinal microvilli and to stagnation of the enterohepatic circulation. In critically ill patients it can also lead to translocation of bacteria across the intestinal mucosa, resulting in sepsis. Even if full enteral feeds cannot be tolerated, the provision of small, "trophic" amounts of enteral nutrition may counterbalance some of these problems. The common enteral feeds used for infants are summarized in Table 2-4.

If a baby cannot suck but has an otherwise functional intestinal tract, a small nasogastric or orogastric tube may be inserted for gavage feedings. Nasojejunal tubes may be used for individuals at high risk for aspiration (e.g., those with delayed gastric emptying or gastroesophageal reflux). A child who requires prolonged tube feedings (e.g. one who cannot swallow because of neurologic disease) is best served by a gastrostomy tube because nasogastric tubes are

Table 2-4	**Enteral Feeding in Infants[a]**
Breast milk	The "gold standard"; may be collected and stored for later use in surgical patients
Enfamil, Similac	Commercially available cow's milk formulas; contain constituents similar to those of breast milk
Isomil	Soy-based formula for infants with milk protein allergy or lactose intolerance
Pregestemil, Neocate	Elemental formulas with nutrients in their simplest form; indicated when normal absorption is impaired (e.g., short-bowel syndrome)

[a]Infants should receive at least 150 mL/kg/day of these formulas to obtain 100–110 cal/kg/day.

irritating, are easily displaced, and can promote aspiration. A number of Silastic low-profile tubes and buttons are available.

Parenteral Nutrition

Many children with major surgical disorders require TPN while the gastrointestinal tract is temporarily nonfunctional. All nutrient requirements are supplied intravenously by the administration of carbohydrates, proteins, fats, electrolytes, trace elements, and vitamins. Intravenous nutrition may be infused through either a peripheral or a central vein. Advantages of peripheral venous nutrition are ease of catheter placement and fewer catheter complications. Glucose can be administered up to a concentration of 12.5%. The rest of the required calories are supplied as emulsified fat. More hypertonic solutions (up to 25% glucose) may be delivered centrally through the superior or inferior vena cava. The umbilical vein can often be utilized for the first 1 to 2 weeks following birth. Thin, Silastic percutaneously inserted central catheters (PICCs) are inserted centrally through a percutaneously accessed extremity vein. When peripheral veins are scarce, central access is achieved percutaneously through the subclavian vein or by a cut-down procedure in the neck or groin. A silicone catheter with a tunneled Dacron cuff (of the Hickman or Broviac type) is preferred because it is minimally thrombogenic and tends to resist infection.

The nutritional needs of each child who is receiving TPN are calculated daily and the appropriate solution is prepared. TPN is infused at maintenance fluid rates by an infusion pump. Concentrations are gradually increased over several days until daily requirements are achieved. All children who receive TPN are monitored closely. Weight is recorded daily, urine is monitored for glucose, and blood is analyzed periodically for glucose, electrolytes, lipids, bilirubin, and liver enzymes.

Table 2-5 summarizes the complications of TPN. Mechanical complications are most common with centrally placed catheters. Catheter sepsis is also a major hazard with central catheters, and can be minimized by scrupulous surgical and nursing techniques. Bacterial contamination is often treated successfully with antibiotics administered through the catheter, whereas life-threatening infections or fungal sepsis usually necessitate catheter re-

moval. Liver damage may occur in any patient who is receiving TPN, but preterm infants are most susceptible. The precise etiology is unknown, but the cause is probably multifactorial and may include absence of enteral feeding, injurious components in the TPN, or essential components missing from TPN. Cholestasis is initially identified by rising serum bilirubin and alkaline phosphatase levels. It usually reverses when TPN is discontinued, but may progress to cirrhosis and hepatic failure.

Respiratory Management

Respiratory failure, or the inability to maintain adequate gas exchange through the lungs, is common in surgically ill children. Infants have high oxygen requirements, are obligate nasal breathers, and depend almost exclusively on their diaphragms rather than on chest wall muscles for air movement. As a result, they have a limited safety margin before respiratory insufficiency develops. Even moderate increases in intra-abdominal pressure can cause respiratory distress. Table 2-6 lists the common causes of respiratory

Table 2-5	Complications of Total Parenteral Nutrition

Mechanical	Metabolic
Catheter malposition	Hyperglycemia
Venous thrombosis	Hypoglycemia
Pneumothorax	Hyperlipidemia
Hemothorax	Electrolyte imbalances
Septic	Hepatic damage
Bacterial	
Fungal	

Table 2-6	Respiratory Failure in Children

Causes
  Hyaline membrane disease
  Meconium aspiration
  Congenital diaphragmatic hernia or pulmonary mass lesions
  Sepsis
  Pneumonia
  Pneumothorax
  Increased intra-abdominal pressure
  Hypoventilation due to anesthesia, narcotics, sedatives
Signs
  Apnea
  Agitation
  Nasal flaring
  Tachypnea
  Tachycardia
  Chest wall retraction
  Grunting
  Cyanosis
Evaluation
  Physical examination
  Chest x-ray
  Pulse oximetry
  Arterial blood gases
  Computed tomography scan (occasionally)
Management
  Airway maintenance, suctioning, chest physiotherapy
  Supplemental O_2 (nasal prongs, face mask, or hood)
  Endotracheal intubation and mechanical ventilation (indicated when Po_2 <60 or Pco_2 >60)
Mechanical ventilators: initial settings

Rate	25–40 breaths/min for infants
	15–20 breaths/min for children
Positive end-expiratory pressure	3–5 cm H_2O
Tidal volume	7–10 mL/kg (for volume ventilators)
Inspiratory pressure	18–25 cm H_2O (for pressure ventilators)

failure in children, the clinical signs, and the steps in management.

Endotracheal intubation provides the most secure airway. It is always necessary for prolonged mechanical ventilation, and it may facilitate pulmonary suctioning and physical therapy. The size of the tube to be inserted may be estimated from the diameter of the child's external nares or little finger, or for children over 2 years of age using the formulas Age (years)/4 + 4 for uncuffed tubes or Age (years)/4 + 3 for cuffed tubes. The pediatric airway is short; to avoid inserting the tube into a bronchus, bilateral equality of the breath sounds must be verified.

The two types of mechanical ventilators available are the volume- and pressure-modulated varieties. Volume ventilators deliver a preset tidal volume, regardless of pulmonary compliance, and are used in most patients beyond the newborn period. Pressure ventilators deliver breaths up to a preset pressure and are preferred for infants, in whom the very low lung volumes involved compared with the dead space would prevent accurate delivery of a preset volume to the lungs. The ventilator should be adjusted to its lowest possible settings consistent with adequate gas exchange. Oxygen levels must not be excessive, particularly in preterm neonates, who are at high risk for retinal damage and pulmonary toxicity that can lead to chronic fibrosis (bronchopulmonary dysplasia).

Pneumothorax is common in children who receive positive pressure ventilation and should be suspected whenever there is sudden deterioration in the respiratory status. The diagnosis is confirmed by chest x-ray or transillumination (a point source of light applied to the chest wall and lights up that entire side of the chest). Definitive treatment is the placement of an intercostal chest tube, but expeditious needle aspiration can provide immediate relief.

High-frequency ventilation is an innovation in which very low tidal − volumes are directed down the trachea at extremely rapid rates (150–2,500 breaths/min). When very high ventilatory settings are needed, this technique may allow adequate gas exchange to occur at lower airway pressures than with conventional rates, producing less trauma to the lungs.

Extracorporeal membrane oxygenation (ECMO) is a form of prolonged cardiopulmonary bypass in which gas exchange occurs in an external circuit that contains the patient's flowing blood and is utilized only when all forms of positive pressure ventilation are inadequate. ECMO can provide complete respiratory support, independent of the lungs, and thereby allows the lungs to rest and recover while organ function is well maintained. ECMO is reserved for the most desperately ill infants because it requires cannulation of major vessels and systemic anticoagulation. Overall survival in newborn infants treated with ECMO is approximately 80%, depending on the cause of respiratory failure. The survival rate for older children and adults is approximately 50%.

Preoperative Evaluation and Preparation

All children who undergo surgery require a careful history and a thorough physical examination, but laboratory studies are not routinely necessary in healthy children. When indicated, complete blood count (CBC), urinalysis, coagulation parameters, blood typing and crossmatching, serum electrolyte and arterial blood gas determinations, electrocardiogram, and x-rays films are obtained.

Children must be in the best possible condition at the time of operation. A child with an upper respiratory infection should have elective surgery postponed until the infection is resolved. A patient who is in shock should be resuscitated as completely as possible before even an urgent operation.

Many operations on infants can be performed on an outpatient basis, starting at 3 months of age for term babies and at approximately 52 weeks after conception for premature infants. Because the respiratory center is immature before that time and there is a risk of apnea after general anesthesia, elective operations should be delayed. After emergency procedures, close postoperative monitoring in the hospital for 24 hours or longer is mandatory.

Preoperative NPO guidelines differ from those of adults, and are outlined in Table 2-7.

Operative Care and Monitoring

The ability to perform major surgery successfully on preterm infants is a recent development and is largely the result of increased understanding of neonatal physiology and advances in technology. Even extremely premature neonates can be safely brought through surgery, provided that the anesthesiologist is knowledgeable and attentive to their special needs and the surgeon handles the fragile tissues with the utmost gentleness and skill.

Although general anesthesia is used for almost all children who undergo operations, supplementation with regional or local blocks (such as epidural, ilioinguinal/iliohypogastric, penile, and intercostal infusions) can lower intraoperative requirements of potent general agents and diminish postoperative pain and discomfort. Epidural catheters can be left in place for several days.

During the course of an operation, the clinical condition of a small child who is almost completely covered with drapes can change rapidly. The endotracheal tube can become blocked, slip out of the trachea, or migrate down a mainstem bronchus. Close monitoring is essential

Table 2-7	Preoperative NPO Guidelines for Children[a]	
	Type of Feeding	**Hours NPO**
<1 Year of Age	Clear liquids	2
	Breast milk	4
	Formula	6
	Solids, all else	8
>1 Year of Age	Clear liquids	2
	Milk, solids, all else	8

[a]Guidelines will vary by institution.

and should always include an electroencepahlogram (ECG), precordial or esophageal stethoscope, blood pressure cuff, temperature probe, pulse oximeter, and end-tidal CO_2 monitor for measurement of the adequacy of ventilation. Additional options can include a urinary catheter and arterial access (usually with an umbilical artery catheter in neonates) for frequent blood sampling and arterial pressure measurement. Central venous catheters (which may be inserted through the umbilical vein in neonates) can be used to estimate left ventricular filling pressures and help guide intravenous fluid requirements. Swan-Ganz catheters, which are more accurate in the presence of cardiopulmonary disease, are used much less often in children than in adults. They are cumbersome to insert and have relatively high complication rates in small patients.

Infants can rapidly become hypothermic in the operating room, leading to greatly increased metabolic demands, peripheral vasoconstriction, acidosis, and even death. Premature infants have a surface area that is up to 10 times that of adults per unit weight. In addition, they have little subcutaneous tissue for insulation and rely on the metabolism of brown fat for heat generation, which may be rendered inactive by anesthetic agents or depleted by poor nutrition. In the operating room, heat loss is exacerbated as body cavities are exposed and anesthesia abolishes muscular activity and causes vasodilatation. Children are kept warm by adequately heating the operating room; using radiant heaters, warming mattresses, and circulating warm air; covering the extremities and head; and warming all solutions and intravenous fluids used to prepare them for surgery.

Allowable blood loss is generally 15% to 20% of estimated blood volume, depending on patient stability. Greater losses generally require transfusions with packed red blood cells.

Postoperative Care and Pain Management

Close monitoring is most essential during the immediate postanesthesia recovery period, because children are especially prone to respiratory and cardiovascular complications at this time. Although most children can be extubated at the conclusion of the operative procedure, those who are critically ill or prone to apnea should remain ventilated until stabilized. Following extubation, supplemental oxygen should be given and pulse oximetry monitored to prevent hypoxia, which may temporarily occur postoperatively even after relatively minor operative procedures.

The most common cause of hypotension or oliguria in the postoperative period is hypovolemia secondary to inadequate resuscitation or third-space losses. A fluid challenge of 10 to 20 mL/kg of isotonic fluid should be given and the clinical response monitored.

Nutrition must be started postoperatively as soon as possible. In many situations, a regular diet may be offered as soon as the child is awake. Following gastrointestinal surgery or if the child is critically ill, parenteral nutrition may

be necessary until the gastrointestinal tract has recovered. Nasogastric tube decompression may avoid gastric distention, which can compromise respiration and lead to aspiration.

Postoperative pain is often inadequately managed because children may be unable to clearly express their complaints and because of exaggerated concerns by health care workers about narcotic addiction and respiratory depression. As mentioned, long-acting local nerve blocks can be given during general anesthesia to limit postoperative pain for hours, and epidural catheters may be left in place for several days. Narcotics should be administered intravenously rather than intramuscularly because of the pain and unpredictable pharmacokinetics of intramuscular injection. Because apnea is a concern in children younger than 6 months of age, narcotics should be given only in a carefully monitored setting. For children older than 5 years, patient-controlled analgesia, in which the patient triggers the infusion of intravenous medication within preset limits, provides superior pain relief with less total narcotic than with traditional pain control methods. Nonsteroidal anti-inflammatory drugs can be used to reduce narcotic dosages and side effects postoperatively. Table 2-8 provides dosages for commonly used analgesics.

Emotional Support

Even the most routine operation is often a major traumatic event for patients and their families. Children between the ages of 1 and 4 years are aware enough to be afraid, although they cannot understand the bewildering events going on around them. Older children and adolescents are particularly fearful of physical injury and mutilation. Parents are often devastated at the prospect of their child having to undergo an operation, with the dread of general anesthesia often superseding that of the operative procedure itself.

Much can be done to alleviate the anxiety of both children and parents. The approach must be individualized, depending on the age of the child and the temperament of the patient and family. Honest and open explanations

Table 2-8	Dosages of Local Anesthetics and Analgesics in Children
Bupivacaine (0.5% or 0.25%) with or without 1% epinephrine	Maximum of 3 mg/kg injected intraoperatively (or 0.5 mL/kg of the 0.5% solution)
Lidocaine	Maximum of 5 mg/kg without epinephrine (or 1 mL/kg of the 0.5% solution)
	Maximum of 10 mg/kg with epinephrine (or 2 mL/kg of the 0.5% solution)
Morphine	0.1 mg/kg intravenously every 1–2 hr
Fentanyl	1–2 μg/kg intravenously every 1–2 hr
Codeine (may be given with acetaminophen)	1 mg/kg orally or rectally every 4 hr
Acetaminophen	10–15 mg/kg orally or rectally every 4 hr

are best. The child should be included in the discussions and provided with ample opportunity for questions. Videos, booklets, and a tour of the clinical facility can transform an alien, hostile setting into a familiar, friendly one. Even when procedures are unpleasant or painful, children fare better when they know what to expect. For the parent, an excellent relationship with the surgeon and a clear understanding of the events is important because parents often transmit their own feelings to their children. Informed parents can do much to prepare children at home.

Separation from parents should be minimized. Preoperative workups are usually done before hospital admission, and children should be discharged postoperatively as soon as medically indicated. Parents can remain with their child until the last moment before the child enters the operating room and may be present in the postanesthesia care unit (PACU) when their child awakens.

Premedications are often given to allay anxiety and should be administered orally because an injection would defeat this purpose. In the operating room, anesthesia induction in younger patients is performed with a face mask, which can be flavored. Older children can choose between mask and intravenous induction.

NEONATAL SURGICAL CONDITIONS

Birth defects are the most common cause of perinatal mortality and a major source of morbidity in the United States. In most instances, the etiology of these malformations is unknown and likely results from a combination of genetic and environmental factors. Many of these defects require surgical intervention for either cure or palliation. With the increasing use of antenatal screening modalities, particularly ultrasonography, more anomalies are being discovered in utero. For a limited number of conditions (e.g., hydronephrosis, hydrocephalus, space-occupying lesions of the chest), intrauterine operations may be beneficial, but these are still experimental procedures and are performed in only a few specialized centers. Nevertheless, prenatal diagnosis allows for family counseling regarding management of the pregnancy and planning of the timing, mode, and location of delivery. Most important, personal relationships can be established between the parents and the health care team at an early stage.

Congenital Diaphragmatic Hernia

A **congenital diaphragmatic hernia** (CDH) is a condition in which the absence of a portion of the diaphragm can lead to life-threatening respiratory compromise. It occurs in 1:4,000 live births and serves as a prototype for surgical causes of neonatal respiratory distress. As a result of recent advances in management, the survival rate has steadily improved. The opening in the diaphragm can vary in location and size (Fig. 2-2). By far the most common type is the Bochdalek hernia, which is a defect of the posterolateral diaphragm, usually on the left. Morgagni hernias, which

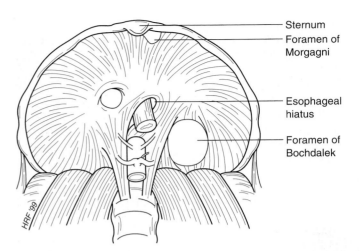

Figure 2-2 Locations of congenital herniations in the diaphragm.

are retrosternal defects, do not often present as emergencies in the newborn period.

Embryology

The etiology of CDH is unknown. Embryologically, the extruded midgut normally returns to the abdominal cavity between the 9th and 10th weeks of gestation. If the pleuroperitoneal canal through the posterolateral portion of the diaphragm remains open, the viscera will pass into the chest and compress the developing lungs. The resulting pulmonary hypoplasia and abnormalities of the pulmonary vasculature affect both lungs, but are more severe ipsilaterally. The timing and severity of the pulmonary compression determine the physiologic consequences.

Pathophysiology

A CDH causes respiratory distress by a combination of physical compression of the lungs by the herniated viscera, pulmonary hypoplasia, and pulmonary hypertension. Although the mechanical lung compression is relieved by surgery, the pulmonary hypoplasia can be fatal if severe. Pulmonary hypertension results from the abnormally high pulmonary vascular resistance caused by the paucity of pulmonary arterioles and the abnormal vascular reactivity of the vessels that are present. This increased pulmonary vascular resistance causes right-to-left shunting of desaturated blood across the foramen ovale and ductus arteriosus, exacerbating the hypoxemia.

Clinical Presentation and Evaluation

A newborn with a CDH has a variable degree of dyspnea and cyanosis. There are diminished breath sounds on the side of the hernia and a shift of the heart to the opposite side. The abdomen is characteristically scaphoid. The diagnosis is confirmed by a chest x-ray that shows air-filled loops of bowel in the chest (or opacity in the right chest if the liver is involved), loss of the diaphragmatic contour, and mediastinal deviation (Fig. 2-3).

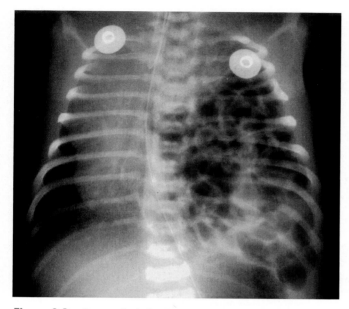

Figure 2-3 Congenital diaphragmatic hernia in a neonate. Intestinal loops are seen in the left side of the chest, with mediastinal displacement to the right.

Treatment

Initial resuscitation of a newborn with a CDH includes supplemental oxygen and usually endotracheal intubation with mechanical ventilation. Positive pressure ventilation through a face mask is contraindicated because gas will enter the gastrointestinal tract and further compress the lungs. A nasogastric tube is placed to minimize gastric distension.

The ventilatory management of CDH babies both preoperatively and postoperatively is most critical, as too-high ventilator settings will irreversibly damage the hypoplastic lungs. A strategy of "permissive hypercapnia" consists of strictly limiting the ventilatory pressures and oxygen concentrations while counterintuitively accepting some degree of hypercarbia and hypoxemia and has significantly improved survival. Adjuncts may include the administration of exogenous surfactant and inhaled nitric oxide (a pulmonary vasodilator) and the use of high-frequency ventilation. Finally, if all else fails, ECMO can provide complete respiratory support, allowing time for the pulmonary hypertension to improve while avoiding further lung damage by high ventilator settings.

The timing of the surgical repair of the CDH itself is no longer considered emergent, and there may be value in a delay of several days to stabilize the baby and improve the elevated pulmonary artery pressures. The operative approach is usually through the abdomen, although it may also be through the chest cavity. The viscera are reduced and the diaphragmatic defect is closed primarily or, if it is large, with a prosthetic patch.

Increasingly, CDH is being diagnosed by antenatal ultrasound. Delivery is then planned to take place in a spe-cialized center. Although antenatal repair of the defect has not been successful technically, inducing lung growth by fetoscopic tracheal occlusion or the administration of pulmonary growth factors is being evaluated experimentally.

Prognosis

The survival of babies with CDH has improved from 50% to 80% with a combination of permissive hypercapnia, delayed surgery, and the judicious use of ECMO. Although most survivors have had little disability because the lungs continue to grow postnatally, as more severely affected CDH babies survive, more are showing evidence of long-term problems with pulmonary function, poor growth, and developmental delay.

Neonatal Thoracic Mass Lesions

Mass lesions in the chest cavity of newborns are infrequent but not rare and may be life threatening. These conditions include congenital lobar emphysema, cystic adenomatoid malformation, pulmonary sequestration, bronchogenic cysts, and foregut duplication cysts. The lesions may be asymptomatic or they may cause symptoms as a result of a primary compressive effect or secondary infection, including chest pain, wheezing, dyspnea, and fever. The malformation is usually visualized on a chest x-ray performed to evaluate these symptoms or is discovered coincidentally for another reason if the chest mass is not symptomatic. A computed tomography (CT) scan should be obtained if the findings on chest x-ray are not definitive.

Patients with congenital lobar emphysema (which represents hyperinflation of normal lung tissue) who are not significantly symptomatic may be observed. All other mass lesions of the thoracic cavity should be excised, although it is sometimes not possible to arrive at an exact diagnosis until the time of operation. When the lesion is within the lung, the involved lobe is usually resected.

Unborn infants with cystic adenomatoid malformation that causes hydrops have a very guarded prognosis because of the high rate of fetal demise, although recently antenatal resection or maternal treatment with steroids has shown some success in salvaging these individuals. Otherwise, infants and children tolerate thoracotomy and lobectomy extremely well, with little of the morbidity seen in adults. Even after pneumonectomy, the remaining lung usually grows and develops with few long-term respiratory problems.

Esophageal Atresia and Tracheoesophageal Fistula

Esophageal atresia (EA) is a congenital interruption in the continuity of the upper and lower portions of the esophagus (Fig. 2-4A). A tracheoesophageal fistula (TEF) is an abnormal communication between the trachea and esophagus (Fig. 2-4E). Either condition may occur alone, but they usually appear in some combination (Fig. 2-4B–D). The

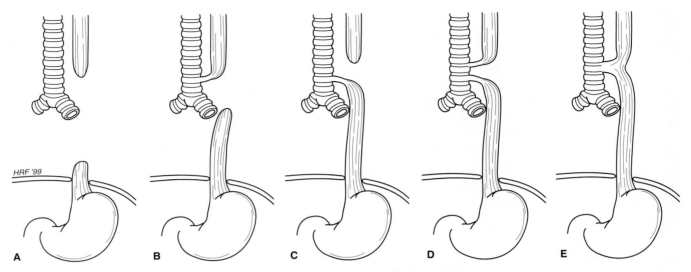

HRF '99

Figure 2-4 Anatomic patterns and approximate percentages of occurrence of esophageal atresia and tracheoesophageal fistula. **A,** Isolated esophageal atresia (8%). **B,** Proximal tracheoesophageal fistula (< 1%). **C,** Distal tracheoesophageal fistula (85%). **D,** Double fistula (< 1%). **E,** "H" type fistula (5%).

most common pattern is type C, in which the upper esophagus ends blindly and the lower portion communicates with the trachea. Overall, these anomalies are found in 1: 4,000 live births.

Pathophysiology

The etiology of EA and TEF is unknown, but it is believed that the septation process that normally divides the foregut into the trachea and esophagus by the seventh week of gestation is incomplete. In addition, the more rapidly growing trachea may partition the upper and lower esophagus into discontinuous segments. Neonates with EA and TEF often have certain other abnormalities, known as the **VACTER association** (vertebral, anal, cardiac, tracheal, esophageal, radial or renal). The presence of an anomaly of any of these structures should prompt a search for others.

Clinical Presentation and Evaluation

An infant with EA, with or without a TEF, immediately chokes and regurgitates with feeding, as the blind-ending upper esophageal pouch rapidly fills. An alert nurse usually notes excessive drooling even earlier because the infant cannot swallow saliva. An attempt should be made to pass a nasogastric tube. Resistance is encountered, and an x-ray confirms that the tip is in the upper mediastinum. Air visualized in the abdomen confirms the presence of a TEF, because an isolated EA is associated with no gas in the gastrointestinal tract because air cannot be swallowed. Although contrast material may be instilled carefully to outline the upper esophageal pouch, this study is not necessary.

An isolated TEF, the "H" type fistula (Fig. 2-4E), is more insidious because the esophagus is patent. These individuals have recurrent aspiration pneumonia, and the diagnosis is established by endoscopy or contrast swallow.

Treatment

Immediate measures are taken to prevent aspiration. The baby is kept with the head elevated to minimize reflux of gastric contents through the fistula into the trachea. To avoid the accumulation of oral secretions, a double-lumen tube is placed in the upper pouch for suctioning. Intravenous fluids and broad-spectrum antibiotics are administered.

Most neonates with EA and TEF undergo primary repair, with division of the fistula and anastomosis of the upper and lower esophageal segments through a right thoracotomy. If the infant is extremely premature or has other major illnesses and cannot tolerate a lengthy procedure, or if the gap between esophageal segments is long, a staged repair is preferable. In that case, a gastrostomy is performed initially to keep the stomach empty and prevent aspiration. It is subsequently used for feeding after the TEF is ligated. Upper and lower esophageal segments may require several months to grow close enough to permit approximation. Only in rare instances is a colon or gastric interposition necessary to bridge the gap.

Common Complications

Postoperative complications include anastomotic leak, stricture, recurrent TEF, gastroesophageal reflux, and tracheomalacia. Tracheomalacia is caused by underdevelopment of the cartilaginous tracheal rings and may be manifested by noisy respirations, a barking cough, and apneic spells. Reflux is especially common and may require subsequent fundoplication.

Prognosis

Most neonates with EA and TEF have excellent results. Mortality is usually limited to those who are extremely premature or have other major anomalies.

Congenital Gastrointestinal Obstruction

Congenital gastrointestinal obstruction refers to an obstruction that is present at birth. The site of the obstruction may be anywhere from stomach to anus, and it can result from a wide variety of causes. These disorders should be managed with some urgency because the obstructed neonate can rapidly develop fluid and electrolyte derangements, may aspirate vomitus, and can acquire sepsis from perforation of the distended bowel or necrosis from an underlying volvulus.

Clinical Presentation and Evaluation

The clinical manifestations of congenital intestinal obstruction will vary depending on the site of obstruction. The four key signs are listed below.

1 **Polyhydramnios.** The fetus swallows 50% of the amniotic fluid daily, which is largely absorbed in the upper intestinal tract. A high obstruction allows this fluid to back up and accumulate in excessive quantities.
2 **Bilious vomiting.** Nonbilious vomiting is common in infants; bilious vomiting is much more often pathologic.
3 **Abdominal distention.** Distention develops within 24 hours of birth in distal obstructions, as swallowed air accumulates above the blockage.
4 **Failure to pass meconium.** Within 24 hours of birth, 95% of term babies pass meconium. A delay may signify obstruction.

If obstruction is suspected following a careful history and physical examination, plain x-rays are performed because swallowed air is an excellent contrast material. If a few dilated loops of bowel with air-fluid levels and no distal air can be seen (Fig. 2-5A), complete, proximal obstruction is diagnosed and no further imaging studies are needed. If the obstruction appears to be partial or is questionable, with some distal air visualized, an upper gastrointestinal

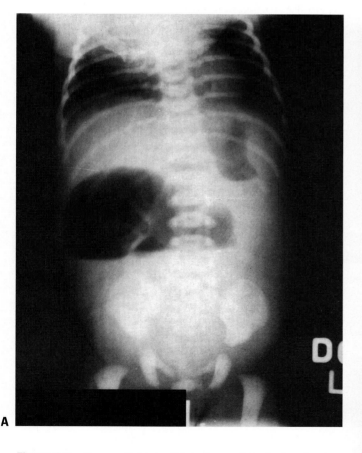

A

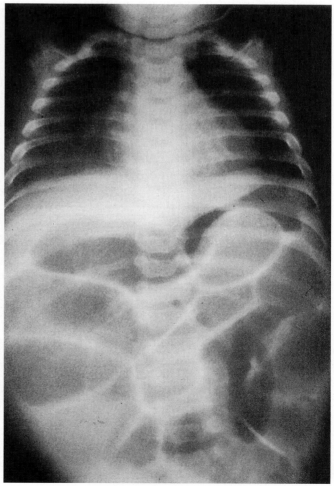

B

Figure 2-5   Congenital intestinal obstruction. **A,** Proximal obstruction from jejunal atresia. Air is visualized in the stomach and proximal jejunum only. **B,** Distal obstruction from ileal atresia. Multiple dilated bowel loops are seen.

Table 2-9	Neonatal Upper Intestinal Obstruction: Differential Diagnosis		
	Pyloric Stenosis	**Duodenal Atresia**	**Midgut Volvulus**
Onset of symptoms	1–6 wk	Birth	Any time (usually infancy)
Overall appearance	Hungry, dehydrated	Well	Well initially, then acutely ill; may be septic
Abdominal pain	None	None	+ + + (may be none early)
Vomiting	Nonbilious projectile	Bilious	Bilious
Abdominal distention	None	None	+ + + (may be none early)
Abdominal x-ray	Large gastric bubble	"Double-bubble" sign	Variable; may be normal early; may be gasless
Upper gastrointestinal study	Narrowed pyloric channel	Complete or partial duodenal obstruction	Distal duodenal obstruction; may have "corkscrew" appearance
Ultrasound	Enlarged pylorus	Dilated stomach	May show twisted superior mesenteric vessels ("whirlpool sign")
Treatment	Pyloromyotomy	Duodenoduodenostomy	Ladd's procedure with or without bowel resection
Urgency of surgery	Minimal	+	+ + +
Prognosis	Excellent	Good	May lead to short-bowel syndrome or death if treatment is delayed

contrast study is most useful. If many distended loops of bowel are seen, suggesting a distal obstruction (Fig. 2-5B), a contrast enema is indicated. Tables 2-9 and 2-10 compare features of the common causes of neonatal upper and lower gastrointestinal obstruction, respectively.

Treatment

Initial management should always include nasogastric tube decompression, intravenous hydration, and prophylactic antibiotics. The need for and timing of surgery then depends on the nature of the obstruction and the overall condition of the baby.

Duodenal Obstruction

Duodenal obstruction is commonly caused by (a) atresia and (b) **malrotation.** Most obstructions of this type are

distal to the ampulla of Vater, so the vomiting is bilious. Atresia may take several forms, including complete separation of the proximal and distal duodenal segments, stenosis, or a web across the lumen. During fetal development, the duodenal epithelium overgrows and transiently occludes the lumen. Failure of subsequent complete recanalization is believed to account for the various forms of atresia. There is a strong association of atresia with trisomy 21. An **annular pancreas** is frequently encountered, in which the ventral pancreatic bud fails to rotate around and become incorporated into the dorsal bud; the two instead fuse around the duodenum, creating a ring effect.

Rotation of the intestine normally occurs in the fetus after the midgut (i.e., the bowel from the duodenum to the transverse colon) has returned to the abdominal cavity from the yolk sac. The vertical midgut rotates 270 degrees

Table 2-10	Neonatal Lower Intestinal Obstruction: Differential Diagnosis			
	Intestinal Atresia	**Meconium Ileus**	**Meconium Plug**	**Hirschsprung's Disease**
Onset of symptoms	Birth	Birth	Birth	Any time (usually infancy)
Association	None	Cystic fibrosis	Prematurity	Trisomy 21
Abdomen	Distended if distal, soft	Distended, doughy feel, visible loops	Distended, soft	Distended, soft
Abdominal x-ray	Dilated bowel loops, air-fluid levels	Dilated bowel without air-fluid levels, "soap-bubble" appearance in right lower quadrant	Moderately dilated bowel loops, air-fluid levels	Dilated bowel loops, air-fluid levels
Contrast enema	Narrow colon, proximal obstruction and anastomosis	Narrow colon, meconium pellets in distal ileum	Normal colon with meconium plugs	Transition zone usually in rectosigmoid
Treatment	Bowel resection	Diatrizoate meglumine (Gastrografin) enema; laparotomy if unsuccessful	Contrast enema usually therapeutic	Pull-through procedure, often after an initial colostomy
Prognosis	Excellent	Poor (cystic fibrosis)	Excellent	Good

in a counterclockwise direction, placing the cecum in the right lower quadrant and the duodenojejunal junction in the left upper quadrant. Subsequently, the ascending and descending colon are fixed retroperitoneally by fibrous attachments that arise from the lateral abdominal wall. In malrotation, this process is incomplete. The cecum is located in the right upper quadrant or remains completely in the left abdomen, and the duodenojejunal junction is located to the right of the midline. This configuration allows the intestine, which is suspended between these closely fixed points, to twist as a midgut volvulus (Fig. 2-6A,B). Midgut volvulus may occur at any age in the presence of malrotation, but is most common in the first month of life. It is the most dangerous form of intestinal obstruction, potentially progressing to necrosis of the entire midgut if not urgently recognized and corrected.

In infants with malrotation, the peritoneal attachments to the lateral abdominal wall, which normally fix the cecum retroperitoneally, now cross over the duodenum to reach the high, malrotated cecum. These attachments are called **Ladd's bands** and may be another cause of partial or complete obstruction by compression of the duodenum. (Fig. 2-6C).

The diagnosis of complete duodenal obstruction at birth is established by visualizing a "double bubble" on x-ray, because air is present in the stomach and in the proximal, dilated duodenum, but none is seen distally (Fig. 2-7). If the obstruction is incomplete, some air will be noted below.

Duodenal obstruction demands expeditious surgery, unless midgut volvulus has been ruled out. For atresia with or without annular pancreas the obstruction is bypassed

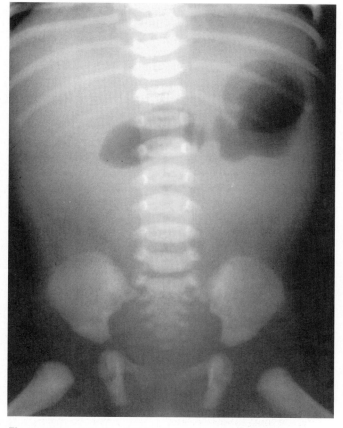

Figure 2-7 "Double bubble" sign in a neonate with duodenal atresia. Air is visualized in the stomach and proximal dilated duodenum only.

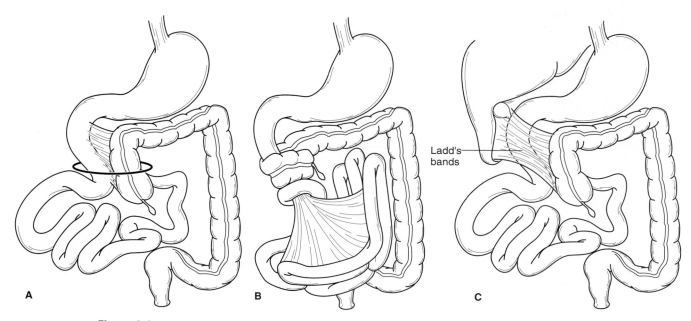

Ladd's bands

Figure 2-6 **A,** Congenital malrotation of the intestine with a high cecum and right-sided duodenojejunal junction forming a narrow pedicle. **B,** The midgut has twisted as a volvulus. **C,** Ladd's bands can also obstruct the duodenum in malrotation.

through an anastomosis between the proximal duodenal segment and the distal duodenum or a loop of jejunum (a gastrojejunostomy is poorly tolerated in infants). In malrotation, the volvulus (if present) is untwisted, Ladd's bands are divided, and the base of the small bowel mesentery is widened. Because the bowel must be returned to the abdomen in the malrotated position, an appendectomy is also performed to avoid misleading presentations of appendicitis. The entire operation (termed a Ladd's procedure) can now be performed laparoscopically.

Small Intestinal Obstruction

Congenital obstruction of the small intestine is usually caused by atresia, **meconium ileus,** and **intestinal duplication.** Like its duodenal counterpart, atresia of the small intestine may range from a web across the lumen (Fig. 2-8) to complete separation of the intestinal segments. The defects may be multiple. Unlike duodenal atresia, the proposed etiology is an in utero vascular accident, such as a localized twist or intussusception. Because there are no intraluminal bacteria antenatally, the resulting necrosis produces localized atrophy rather than bacterial peritonitis, occasionally leading to considerable loss of small bowel length.

Meconium ileus is caused by impaction of sticky, thick meconium in the distal ileum, the narrowest portion of the intestinal tract. It occurs in 15% of infants with cystic fibrosis, from the abnormally viscid enzymes secreted by the pancreatic and intestinal glands. A family history of cystic fibrosis, an autosomal recessive disorder, is suggestive, but is positive in only 25% of patients. X-rays often demonstrate a peculiar foamy appearance of the dilated meconium-filled bowel loops and a lack of air-fluid levels, as the thick meconium is mixed with air and fails to layer out. Calcification on abdominal x-ray indicates that an antenatal perforation has occurred.

Duplications are endothelial-lined cystic or tubular structures adjacent to any portion of the alimentary tract. They are found on the mesenteric side of the normal bowel, usually sharing a common wall with it, and may or may not communicate with the primary lumen. Mucous secretions or stool may accumulate in the duplication, causing it to distend. Obstructive symptoms from pressure on neighboring bowel or localized volvulus may appear during or after the neonatal period.

Atresias and duplications are managed surgically by resection and primary anastomosis. Meconium ileus can frequently be treated nonoperatively with diatrizoate (gastrografin) enemas. Gastrografin is a radiopaque fluid with a very high osmolarity that causes fluid to be drawn into the bowel lumen. The sticky meconium is hydrated and may be spontaneously evacuated. Intravenous fluids must be

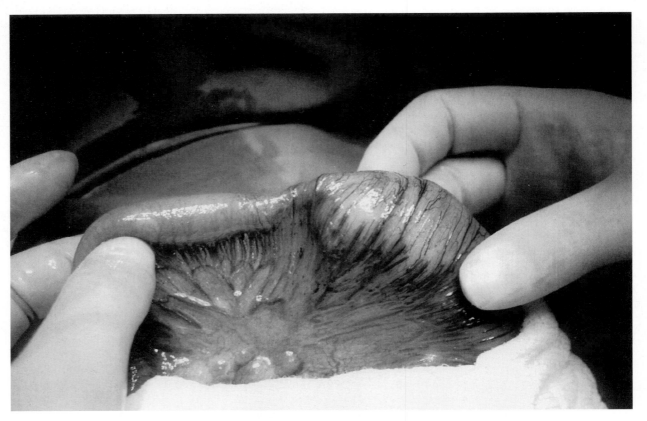

Figure 2-8 Atresia of the small intestine caused by an intraluminal web. A size discrepancy between the dilated proximal and contracted distal bowel is seen.

infused during the procedure, to avoid systemic hypovolemia. If the obstruction persists or if there is evidence of perforation, surgery is mandatory.

Colon Obstruction

Congenital colorectal obstruction may be due to: (a) **Hirschsprung's disease**, (b) **a meconium plug**, (c) neonatal **small left colon syndrome**, and, rarely, (d) atresia.

Hirschsprung's disease is a disorder in which ganglion cells of the parasympathetic nervous system are absent from the wall of the distal intestinal tract. Embryologically, these cells migrate from the esophagus to the anus; in Hirschsprung's disease they are arrested in their descent or development. The transition zone between the narrow aganglionic distal bowel and the dilated normal proximal bowel is usually in the rectosigmoid colon but can occur anywhere, with the entire colon or even the small intestine being aganglionic. The aganglionic bowel is not capable of normal peristalsis, producing a functional obstruction at the transition zone. The condition may first present in the newborn as a lower bowel obstruction or later in childhood as severe chronic constipation (Table 2-11). Boys are four times more frequently affected than are girls. A contrast enema usually demonstrates the transition zone (Fig. 2-9), and anorectal manometry will show absence of the internal sphincter relaxation reflex. A rectal biopsy will confirm the absence of ganglion cells.

The treatment for Hirschsprung's disease is classically staged with a temporary colostomy brought out proximal to the transition zone. This is followed several months later by a "pull-through" procedure, in which the ganglionic bowel is brought down and anastomosed to the anal canal. Increasingly, this traditional approach is being replaced by a transanal "incisionless" pull-through procedure during the first few days of life, with optional laparoscopic assistance.

Occasionally, patients with Hirschsprung's disease may develop a severe enterocolitis, with dehydration, peritonitis, and sepsis. This may be the first manifestation of the disease or may even occur after surgery. Treatment of

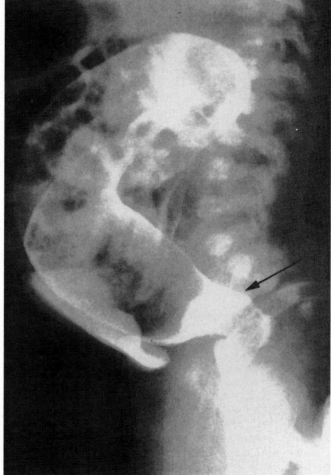

Figure 2-9   A 1-week-old boy with Hirschsprung's disease. Barium enema shows the transition zone (*arrow*) between the distal aganglionic rectum and the dilated proximal colon.

Table 2-11	Hirschsprung's Disease versus Functional Constipation	
	Hirschsprung's Disease	**Functional Constipation**
Age at presentation	Usually <2 yr	Usually >2 yr
Meconium passage	Delayed beyond 24 hr from birth	Within 24 hr of birth
Onset of symptoms	Birth	Usually after toilet training
Stools	Narrow caliber	Voluminous, "plug up toilet"
Weight loss	Present in late cases	None
Soiling	None	May be prominent
Rectal examination	Empty ampulla, with or witout explosive decompression	Full ampulla, may be impacted
Abdominal x-ray	Stool present in proximal colon	Stool present in rectosigmoid, fecaloma
Barium enema	Transition zone usually in rectosigmoid	Dilated rectosigmoid, no transition zone
Manometry	Absent internal sphincter relaxation reflex	Normal
Rectal biopsy	Absent gamglia, hypertrophied nerve fibers	Normal
Treatment	Colostomy; later pull-through procedure	Enemas, laxatives, diet, retraining

Hirschsprung's enterocolitis must be prompt with intravenous fluids, antibiotics, and colonic irrigations.

Meconium plug and small left colon syndrome are functional causes of large bowel obstruction, probably caused by transient motility disturbances of the immature colon. Meconium plugs frequently occur in premature babies, whereas small left colon syndrome is most common in infants of diabetic mothers. A contrast enema is generally both diagnostic and therapeutic. Babies are usually normal after treatment, but subsequent testing for Hirschsprung's disease or cystic fibrosis may be indicated.

Anorectal Malformations

Anorectal malformations (imperforate anus) represent a spectrum of disorders in which the rectum fails to reach its normal perineal termination. When the rectum ends above the levator muscles the malformations are classified as high, and when it passes through these muscles the malformations are low. High lesions are more frequent in males and low ones in females.

Pathophysiology

Although the rectum may end blindly in both types of defects, it usually terminates in an anterior fistulous tract. In high anomalies, the fistula communicates with the urethra or bladder in males (Fig. 2-10A) and with the vagina in females (Fig. 2-10B). In low malformations, the fistula drains externally in both genders, anterior to the normal anal site (Fig. 2-10C,D). Imperforate anus is part of the **VACTER association** (see earlier section on Esophageal Atresia and Tracheoesophageal Fistula) and associated abnormalities, particularly genitourinary, frequently occur.

Clinical Presentation and Evaluation

The diagnosis of an imperforate anus is usually obvious on inspection. Either no perineal opening exists (Fig. 2-11) or a fistula may be visible. In males, the external fistula is usually a small opening in the anterior perineum or as far forward as the scrotal raphe. Females may also have an external fistula draining into the anterior perineum, or else into the posterior vulva behind the hymen. A single perineal orifice in a female signifies a **cloaca,** where the

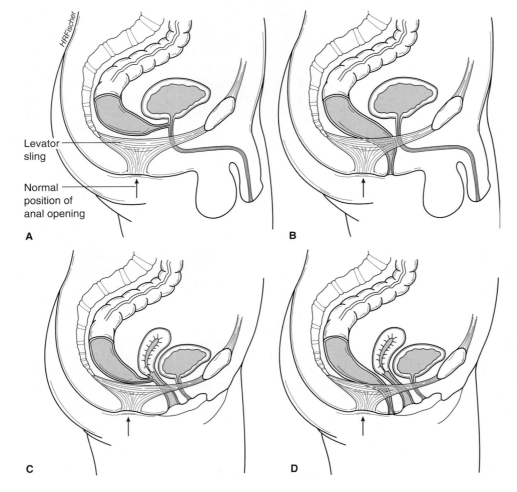

Levator sling

Normal position of anal opening

Figure 2-10 Congenital anorectal malformations. **A,** A boy with a high defect and a rectourethral fistula. **B,** A boy with a low defect and an anoperineal fistula. **C,** A girl with a high rectovaginal fistula. **D,** A girl with an anovulvar fistula. The normal location of the anal opening should be at the external sphincter (*arrows*).

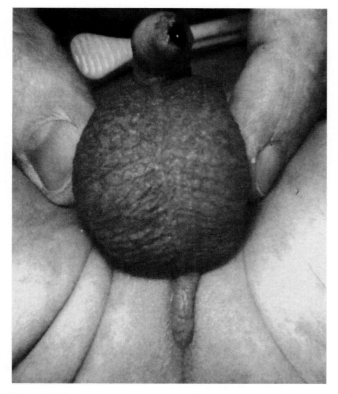

Figure 2-11 A newborn boy with a high anorectal malformation and a rectourethral fistula. The perineal opening is absent, and meconium is seen at the urethral meatus.

rectum, vagina, and urethra all open into one common chamber. This high anomaly is rare.

The management of babies with high and low anorectal malformations differs considerably, and it is therefore essential to distinguish between them. The presence of an external fistula *always* signifies a low lesion. In the absence of a visible fistula, most lesions are intermediate or high. If the level of the rectal termination is not clear, an "invertogram" is traditionally performed. The baby is held prone and head-down, and if on lateral x-ray air in the rectum rises to within 1 cm of the perineal skin, the lesion is low; if not, it is probably high. The invertogram is being replaced by ultrasound, computed tomography (CT), and magnetic resonance imaging (MRI) to identify the level of the rectum more precisely.

Treatment

Continence normally depends on the coordinated actions of the external sphincter, internal sphincter, and levator muscles. Because the levators are the most important, infants with low lesions in whom the bowel descends normally within the levator sling have an excellent functional outlook. A fistula only slightly anterior to the normal anal location (anterior anus) can often function normally and may therefore be left alone. Otherwise, a perineal an-

oplasty can be performed to establish an adequate communication between the rectum and the perineum, at the center of the external sphincter. This operation may be done in the newborn period or later, if the external fistula can be dilated sufficiently to permit the passage of stool.

Infants with intermediate and high malformations traditionally require an initial colostomy. Over the next several months a pull-through procedure is performed, in which the rectum is mobilized, brought through the center of the levator sling, and anastomosed to the perineum. Although various types of pull-throughs have been described, the Peña operation, in which all the muscles are divided posteriorly in the midline, has become the standard because of the excellent visualization that is obtained. More recently a laparoscopic approach has been advocated, with or without the utilization of a protective colostomy.

Prognosis

The functional prognosis for these children is mixed. Those with low lesions achieve excellent continence, although they often suffer from constipation and may require daily laxatives. Children with high anomalies often have difficulty toilet training, and the majority have at least occasional soiling. These patients often require a structured bowel management program, including daily enemas to achieve "functional continence."

Necrotizing Enterocolitis

Necrotizing enterocolitis (NEC) is an acquired ischemic necrosis of the intestine in neonates. It is primarily a disease of premature infants, but occasionally occurs in full-term babies. It is the most common indication for emergency surgery in neonates and is a major cause of death in premature infants who survive the first week of life.

Pathophysiology

NEC initially affects the mucosa but can extend to full-thickness injury and perforation. The precise pathogenesis of NEC is not clear but almost certainly involves an interaction between environmental stressors and unique responses of the gastrointestinal tract of premature infants. A number of conditions have been shown to increase the incidence of NEC, and all are related to a reduction in the perfusion of the gastrointestinal tract. Many types of bacteria are associated with NEC, including Gram-positive and Gram-negative aerobes and anaerobes. NEC is most common in babies who have already been fed, because feedings act as a substrate for bacterial proliferation in the intestinal tract. The ileocecal region is most often affected, but any portion of the gastrointestinal tract may be involved.

Clinical Presentation and Evaluation

Clinical signs of NEC are initially nonspecific and may consist of lethargy, feeding intolerance, temperature instability, and apnea. Gastrointestinal manifestations follow and include vomiting, bloody stools, and abdominal distention, and tenderness. Full-blown sepsis may supervene.

Abdominal x-rays may be nonspecific and show only dilated, air-filled loops of bowel. Pneumatosis intestinalis, the radiographic appearance of intramural gas produced by enteric organisms (Fig. 2-12), is pathognomonic for this disease. Portal venous air may be seen when the intraluminal gas enters the venous drainage system of the gastrointestinal tract. Laboratory findings are consistent with a systemic infection and include positive blood cultures, leukocytosis or leukopenia, thrombocytopenia, and acidosis.

Treatment

Most babies with NEC recover with medical management and do not need surgery. The goals of treatment are to maximize perfusion of the intestine and treat the infection. Fluid resuscitation is undertaken to restore intravascular volume, a nasogastric tube is inserted to decompress the intestinal tract, broad-spectrum antibiotics are adminis-

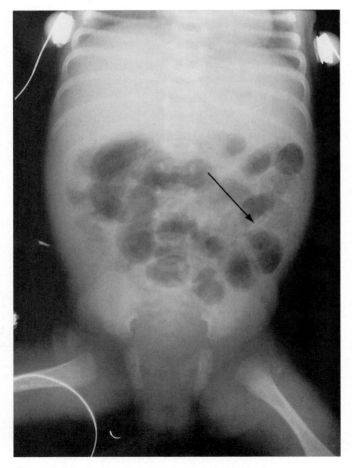

Figure 2-12 A premature infant with necrotizing enterocolitis and pneumatosis intestinalis. Intramural air (*arrow*) is seen.

tered, and the infant is observed closely. Indications for surgery are intestinal perforation and full-thickness necrosis. Perforation is usually identified by the presence of pneumoperitoneum (free air) on x-ray. Full-thickness necrosis without perforation and perforation without free air on x-ray are difficult to diagnose, but are suggested by systemic signs of progressive sepsis (e.g., worsening cardiorespiratory function, increased fluid needs, thrombocytopenia) or physical findings of peritonitis (tenderness, guarding, erythema or edema of the abdominal wall). In equivocal cases, paracentesis that yields peritoneal fluid containing intestinal contents or bacteria strongly suggests bowel necrosis. Surgical therapy usually consists of a laparotomy in which the entire intestine is inspected and all areas of necrosis are resected. The ends of the viable bowel are usually exteriorized as stomas, but a primary anastomosis may be performed if the disease is limited and the patient is otherwise stable. Alternatively, extremely small (<1,000 g), critically ill infants have been treated initially by the insertion of Penrose drains through a minilaparotomy, which can be performed at the patient's bedside. The patient is followed closely and laparotomy is undertaken if the clinical condition fails to improve.

Postoperatively, the same vigorous medical treatment is pursued as done preoperatively. The timing of stoma closure depends on the age, size, and stability of the child and the location of the stoma. A stoma in the proximal intestine is closed before the patient is discharged, but closure of a distal ileostomy or colostomy may be deferred for several months, allowing the baby to be discharged and grow.

Prognosis

The overall survival rate of babies with NEC is 80%. In those who require emergency surgery, the survival rate is 50% to 80%. Of those who are initially treated successfully nonoperatively, 10% later have a stricture and require an operation for intestinal obstruction.

Short Bowel Syndrome

Short bowel syndrome (SBS) occurs when there is insufficient small intestine to digest and absorb essential nutrients for growth and development. The incidence is increasing as more infants and children are surviving following the loss of massive lengths of small intestine from conditions such as necrotizing enterocolitis, midgut volvulus, and long-segment Hirschsprung's disease. The severity depends not only on the absolute length of the remaining small intestine but on the age of the child, the particular portion of small bowel remaining, the presence of an ileocecal valve and colon, and the degree of adaptation that has occurred. Although the term infant normally has 200 to 250 cm of small intestine, survival without intravenous nutrition has eventually been attained with as little as 15 to 20 cm with an ileocecal valve and 40 cm without one.

Malabsorption, along with the malnutrition and diarrhea that result, is primarily due to the loss of mucosal absorptive surface and a decrease in transit time through the foreshortened gastrointestinal tract. These problems may be compounded by an osmotic and secretory diarrhea that can be produced by insufficient absorption of digestive enzymes, fermentation of undigested sugars by colonic bacteria, the irritative effect of unabsorbed bile salts, and acid hypersecretion by the stomach due to elevated gastrin levels. Other major complications of SBS are sepsis from translocation of intestinal bacteria and liver failure. Fortunately, adaptation occurs over time as the intestine lengthens and dilates, villi hypertrophy, and transit time decreases. The ileum is more capable of undergoing adaptation than is the jejunum.

Treatment of SBS is primarily a delicate balancing act between intravenous and enteral feedings. Elemental formulas are employed initially and are often better absorbed when administered continuously than by bolus. These enteral feeds are gradually increased as adaptation occurs, and are slowly transitioned to more complex formulas. Medications may also be beneficial and can include drugs to decrease intestinal motility (e.g., loperamide, diphenoxylate); drugs to decrease gastric secretion (histamine-2 blocking agents such as ranitidine or proton pump inhibitors such as omeprazole); cholestyramine to bind bile salts; somatostatin to decrease biliary, pancreatic, and intestinal secretions; and antibiotics to inhibit bacterial overgrowth.

The goals of surgical therapy, employed when medical management and intestinal adaptation fail, are as follows:

1 **Reestablish intestinal continuity.** Close stomas when possible in order to maximize the absorptive surface and prolong transit time.
2 **Eliminate stasis.** Relieve any areas of intestinal obstruction; streamline dilated, stagnant segments of intestine by tapering or plication.
3 **Increase intestinal transit time.** Insert a nipple valve; interpose a reversed, antiperistaltic segment of small bowel or an isoperistaltic colon segment.
4 **Increase effective absorptive surface.** Double the length of dilated intestine by dividing it longitudinally between the leaves of the mesentery (the *Bianchi* procedure) or follow the ingrowth of an independent blood supply to the antimesenteric border by attaching it to the liver or rectus muscle.

Finally, if all other measures prove unsuccessful in managing SBS, particularly when accompanied by liver failure, intestinal transplantation should be considered.

Neonatal Jaundice: Biliary Atresia and Choledochal Cyst

Neonatal jaundice is usually caused by physiologic indirect hyperbilirubinemia and is self-limited. A direct bilirubinemia of more than 2 mg/dL that persists for more than 2 weeks warrants further investigation.

Pathophysiology

Biliary atresia is a progressive inflammatory obliteration of unknown etiology, which may affect part or all of the biliary ductular system. Infantile **choledochal cysts,** which usually consist of rounded, cystic dilatations of the common bile duct with distal narrowing, producing biliary obstruction, may be another manifestation of the same disease.

Clinical Presentation and Evaluation

An infant with biliary atresia has progressive jaundice during the first several weeks of life. The stools are pale, the liver is usually enlarged, and levels of serum conjugated bilirubin, alkaline phosphatase, and other liver enzymes are elevated. Choledochal cysts may present in a similar fashion. Other causes of neonatal jaundice include TORCH (toxoplasmosis, rubella, cytomegalovirus, herpes) infections, α_1-antitrypsin deficiency, galactosemia, and TPN or hypoxic injury to the liver. The usual evaluation includes ultrasound and hepatic scintiscan. Ultrasonography can identify a choledochal cyst, and the demonstration of bile flow into the duodenum on the scintican excludes the diagnosis of biliary atresia. A percutaneous liver biopsy may also be helpful.

Treatment

If biliary atresia is not excluded in the evaluation of persistant direct hyperbilirunemia, a laparotomy is performed, the hilum of the liver is inspected, and a cholangiogram is performed. The finding of a patent biliary system excludes the diagnosis of biliary atresia. If biliary atresia is confirmed, a Kasai portoenterostomy is performed. This procedure involves the excision of the atretic extrahepatic biliary system with creation of a jejunal conduit for bile drainage from the fibrous-appearing tissue in the hilum of the liver that contains microscopic biliary ductules. Success after this procedure is greatest if it is performed before the child is 8 weeks of age. In the usual case of choledochal cyst, the cyst is excised and the biliary system is reconstructed by anastomosing a defunctionalized bowel loop to the proximal hepatic ducts.

Prognosis

The success of the Kasai operation depends on the age of the patient, the diameter of the microscopic hepatic ductules, and the severity of hepatic fibrosis. Recurrent postoperative cholangitis is common and results in progressive deterioration of hepatic function. Portal hypertension with esophageal varices may develop even with restoration of bile flow.

Approximately 30% of infants ultimately do well after portoenterostomy and do not require additional surgery. Liver transplantation is the other available therapy and is generally reserved for patients with severe hepatic fibrosis at presentation or progressive liver disease. Infant livers are rarely available, so segments from adult donors are used.

In contrast to the prognosis for patients with biliary atresia, the prognosis for patients who undergo excision of choledochal cysts is excellent. Unresected choledochal cysts have significant potential for cholangiocarcinoma.

Abdominal Wall Defects: Omphalocele and Gastroschisis

Omphalocele and **gastroschisis** are congenital defects of the abdominal wall through which the abdominal contents variably protrude externally. The incidence of each is reported to be 1:5,000 births, although the number of babies with gastroschisis relative to those with omphalocele seems to be increasing. Although these conditions are in many ways similar, there are important differences.

Embryology

The abdominal wall is formed by four folds, the cephalic, the caudal, and two lateral folds that converge ventrally to form a large umbilical ring surrounding the umbilical cord vessels and yolk sac. During development, the ring contracts to close the abdominal wall. Between the 5th and 10th weeks of gestation, the rapidly growing intestine is extruded out of the umbilical ring and into the yolk sac.

It then returns to the abdominal cavity, where it undergoes rotation.

Pathophysiology

An omphalocele results when the lateral folds do not close and the extruded viscera remain in the yolk sac. Gastroschisis may be caused by an in utero perforation of the developing abdominal wall at the point where one of the paired umbilical veins undergoes atrophy, an area of relative weakness; alternatively, there is evidence that gastroschisis may be produced by the antenatal perforation of a small omphalocele sac.

Clinical Presentation

Babies with an omphalocele have an opening in the center of the abdominal wall and the protruding viscera are covered by a translucent membrane (Fig. 2-13). The umbilical cord inserts into the center of the omphalocele sac. In babies with gastroschisis, the opening is lateral to the umbilical cord, usually to the right (Fig. 2-14). The exteriorized viscera are not covered by a membrane and often become thickened and edematous. In both conditions, the size of the defect and the amount of protruding viscera are variable.

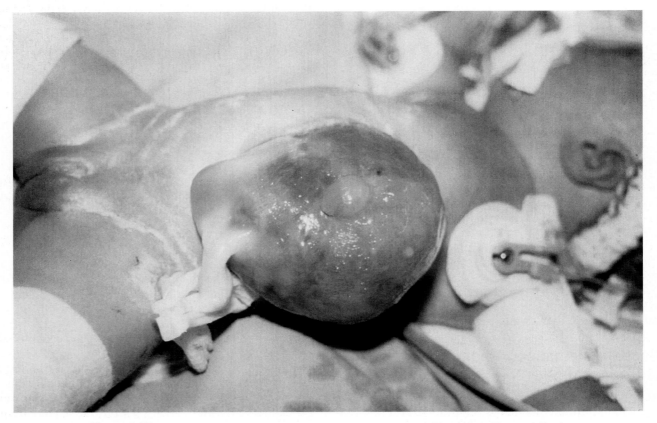

Figure 2-13 A large omphalocele that contains visible loops of intestine. The umbilical cord arises from the sac.

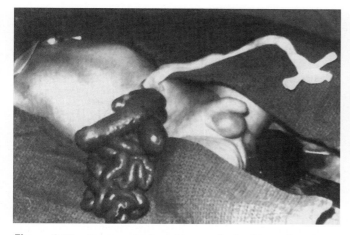

Figure 2-14   Gastroschisis, with exteriorized intestine that is not covered by a sac. The abdominal wall defect is on the right side of the umbilicus.

Babies with an omphalocele have a high incidence of associated congenital anomalies, including chromosomal defects. In contrast, the only associated disorder noted with increased frequency in babies with gastroschisis is intestinal atresia. These atresias are probably caused by in utero compression and vascular compromise of the bowel against the rim of the abdominal defect.

Treatment

Immediately after birth, infants with abdominal wall defects are at risk for fluid and heat loss from the exposed viscera; these should be kept moist with saline and the abdomen wrapped in plastic. Intravenous fluids and broad-spectrum antibiotics are given, and nasogastric decompression is instituted. In babies with gastroschisis, the viscera should remain on top of the baby or the baby turned on his or her side to avoid kinking the vascular supply of the protruding bowel. Cyanosis of the viscera mandates immediate enlargement of the defect at the bedside.

Babies with gastroschisis require emergency surgery to replace the viscera in the abdomen and close the defect. If the abdominal cavity is too small to allow primary closure without undue tension, a prosthetic covering is temporarily sutured to the edges of the defect (Fig. 2-15). A preformed spring-loaded silo is also available for this purpose. The silo is manually compressed daily to gradually reduce the viscera and expand the abdominal cavity. An omphalocele is treated in a similar fashion, except that surgery is not so emergent and time can be taken to evaluate associated anomalies. In cases of severe associated malformations or prohibitive operative risks, the omphalocele sac can be painted with an antiseptic (e.g., silver sulfadiazine [Silvadene] or povidone iodine). The sac eventually epithelializes and contracts, leaving a ventral hernia that can be repaired electively.

Atresias associated with gastroschisis are best repaired after the swelling and inflammation subside.

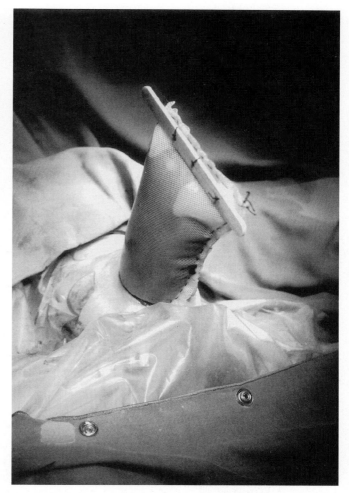

Figure 2-15   A giant omphalocele with a defect that is temporarily closed with a prosthetic silo of reinforced Silastic.

Prognosis

Infants with gastroschisis may have prolonged intestinal dysfunction after surgery as a result of chronic inflammation of the exposed bowel. However, the long-term outlook is generally good. The ultimate prognosis for babies with omphaloceles is usually related to any associated anomalies that may be present.

Circumcision

Circumcision, among the oldest surgical procedures known, is the most frequently performed operation on males in the United States. Although approximately 90% of boys in the United States undergo neonatal circumcision, routine circumcision is performed in only 40% of boys in Canada, 15% in Australia, and rarely in Europe. Circumcision remains a controversial topic, even within the medical profession. The American Academy of Pediatrics remains neutral on the subject, stating that the decision should be made by the parents, after the risks and

Table 2-12	Neonatal Circumcision: Advantages, Disadvantages, and Contraindications

Advantages
Prevents phimosis
Prevents paraphimosis (inability to pull the foreskin back over the glans after it is retracted)
Lowers the incidence of urinary tract infections in infancy
Prevents balanoposthitis (infection of the glans and foreskin from retained secretions)
Prevents cancer of the penis (uncommon; may also be prevented by proper hygiene)

Disadvantages
Medically unnecessary in most boys
Risk of painful complications (low, but may include bleeding, infection, meatal ulcers, postcircumcision phimosis, necrosis)

Contraindications
Anomalies of the external genitalia (e.g., hypospadias) because the foreskin may be needed for operative correction
Serious illness (including bleeding disorders)

benefits are explained. Effective analgesia, such as a penile nerve block, is strongly recommended for the procedure.

The prepuce, or foreskin, completely covers the glans, except for a small opening at the urethral meatus. The undersurface of the foreskin is fused with the glans at birth with congenital adhesions, and it is not until later in childhood that the foreskin is fully retractable. In uncircumcised boys, attempts at retraction should be avoided until 2 to 3 years of age. True phimosis is the inability to pull back the foreskin because of fibrotic narrowing at the preputial orifice, not these physiologic adhesions. Advantages, disadvantages, and contraindications to circumcision are listed in Table 2-12.

SURGICAL CONDITIONS IN THE OLDER CHILD

Inguinal Hernia and Hydrocele

Inguinal hernias and hydroceles are extremely common in children. Their repair is the most common operation performed by pediatric surgeons. Hernias occur in 3% of children overall. The incidence rises to 30% in very premature infants. Conditions that may increase intra-abdominal pressure or weaken connective tissues (e.g., ascites, connective tissue disorders) may also predispose to hernias. Boys are affected six times as often as girls. Inguinal hernias in children are virtually all indirect, with the hernia sac emerging through the internal inguinal ring. Direct and femoral hernias are rare.

Embryology

At 3 months' gestation, the processus vaginalis forms as an outpouching of the peritoneum and passes through the internal inguinal ring. This structure then migrates down the inguinal canal and into the scrotum, preceding the testicle, and comes to lie within the spermatic cord. The processus usually becomes obliterated around the time of birth, except for the most distal portion, which remains surrounding the testicle as the tunica vaginalis (Fig. 2-16A).

Pathophysiology

Continued patency of part or all of the processus vaginalis accounts for the development of hernias and hydroceles. If the processus remains widely open proximally, in continuity with the peritoneal cavity, the intra-abdominal contents may variably protrude into it, forming an inguinal hernia (Fig. 2-16B). If the processus remains open but is too narrow to admit any viscera, only peritoneal fluid may enter. Usually, this fluid surrounds the testicle within the widened tunica vaginalis, forming a communicating hydrocele (Fig. 2-16C). Less often, if the distal processus is obliterated, the fluid accumulates above the testicle as a hydrocele of the spermatic cord (Fig. 2-16D). Finally, with obliteration of the proximal processus, fluid may remain trapped distally in the tunica vaginalis, producing a noncommunicating hydrocele (Fig. 2-16E).

In girls, the round ligament is a vestigial structure analogous to the spermatic cord and has the same relation to the processus vaginalis. In addition to bowel, the ovary or Fallopian tube may enter a patent processus.

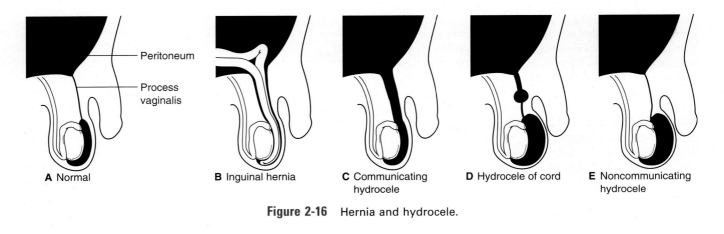

A Normal   B Inguinal hernia   C Communicating hydrocele   D Hydrocele of cord   E Noncommunicating hydrocele

Peritoneum
Process vaginalis

Figure 2-16 Hernia and hydrocele.

Clinical Presentation and Evaluation

Approximately half of all inguinal hernias appear during the first year of life. They occur twice as often on the right side as on the left because the right testicle descends later embryologically, and its processus is therefore less likely to have closed. Ten percent of inguinal hernias are bilateral. The hernia usually causes an intermittent bulge in the groin or scrotum, brought on by crying or straining. On examination, it is palpable as a firm mass that completely disappears with digital pressure (Fig. 2-17A). If not apparent, a hernia may be brought out by applying suprapubic

pressure in infants or by asking older children to jump or strain. Suggestive evidence of an inguinal hernia, if it still cannot be elicited, consists of a palpable thickening of the spermatic cord where it crosses the pubic tubercle (i.e., "silk glove" sign). A hydrocele usually causes diffuse swelling of the hemiscrotum (Fig. 2-17B). If it communicates with the peritoneal cavity, it fluctuates in size throughout the day as it fills and empties. Noncommunicating hydroceles remain fairly constant in size, but may gradually regress as fluid is absorbed.

Hernias can almost always be differentiated from hydroceles on physical examination. A hydrocele is more mobile, is not reducible, and does not extend upward into the internal ring. A hydrocele of the cord may be more difficult to distinguish from an incarcerated hernia because both are manifested as an irreducible mass above the testis. Hydroceles, however, produce no symptoms, whereas incarcerated hernias are quite painful and may produce intestinal obstruction. Transillumination is not particularly reliable, especially in infants in whom the thin bowel wall may transmit light readily. Table 2-13 summarizes the differences between hernias and hydroceles.

Treatment

Inguinal hernias in children never resolve and are at risk for incarceration and strangulation. The highest incidence of incarceration is in the first 6 months of life. Therefore, all inguinal hernias should be repaired by high ligation of the hernia sac at the internal ring. Repair of the floor of the inguinal canal, as is performed in adults, is unnecessary. The operation is usually carried out on an outpatient basis soon after diagnosis and can be performed via a small groin incision. Recently, some surgeons have adopted a laparoscopic approach. A dilemma is presented in the treatment of the very young and especially the premature infant because of the predisposition to postanesthesia apnea. If surgery is performed less than 52 weeks from conception, overnight monitoring in the hospital is necessary. Postoperative recovery is rapid in children, and complications (e.g., damage to the vas deferens) and recurrence are uncommon.

An incarcerated hernia is an emergency, not only because of the risk of strangulation of the hernial contents, but also because the testicle may become ischemic. An incarcerated hernia in a child can almost always be reduced. Slow, persistent pressure is applied bimanually on the mass. The child is often sedated with a narcotic (infants must be monitored for apnea). Following successful reduction, hernia repair is delayed for 24 to 48 hours until edema of the sac subsides. If reduction fails, surgery is performed without delay.

A child with one inguinal hernia has an increased risk of having another one on the contralateral side. Although opinions vary, many surgeons recommend exploration of the opposite side in children with a greater likelihood of bilaterality, such as in premature boys, as well as in young girls (in whom there is no danger of damaging the vas or

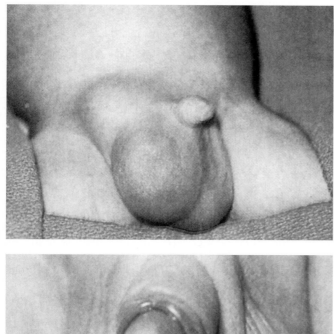

Figure 2-17   **A,** A right inguinal hernia in a 5-month-old boy. **B,** A right scrotal hydrocele in a 9-month-old boy.

Table 2-13	Differential Diagnosis of Groin Masses in Children		
	Hydrocele	**Reducible Inguinal Hernia**	**Incarcerated Inguinal Hernia**
Age	Most <1 yr	Any age	Any age
Overall state	Well	Well	Ill, anorexic, vomiting
Pain and tenderness	None	None	+ + +
Diurnal changes	None or fluctuates; usually increases in evening	Protrudes on straining	Always protruded
Site of swelling	Usually scrotum	Groin with or without scrotum	Usually groin and scrotum
Physical findings	Round, smooth, mobile	Firm elongated, disappears completely with pressure	Firm, fixed; cannot feel superior edge
Transillumination	+ +	None (except in infants)	±
Reducible	No	Yes	If possible, alleviates symptoms
Abdominal x-ray	Normal	With or without air in groin	All in groin; bowel obstruction
Treatment	Repair if persists >1–2 yr	Elective repair	Immediate reduction; urgent repair

spermatic vessels during surgery). Alternatively, if a unilateral hernia repair is performed via a groin incision, a small laparoscope can be inserted into the peritonial cavity through the hernia sac to visualize the opposite internal ring from above. Both internal rings are routinely examined in a primary laparoscopic approach.

Unlike hernias, most neonatal noncommunicating hydroceles resolve within the first year or two of life. Hydroceles that persist after that time or develop later are unlikely to resolve and should be electively repaired.

Umbilical Hernia

Pathophysiology

Umbilical hernias are caused by failure of the umbilical ring to contract completely. They are especially common in African American infants or children, in whom the incidence approaches 50%. Unlike inguinal hernias, most umbilical hernias resolve spontaneously during childhood. The risk of incarceration in infants is extremely low.

Clinical Presentation and Evaluation

The diagnosis is apparent by the presence of a bulge within the umbilicus. The fascial defect is readily palpable after the mass is reduced.

Treatment

Surgery is usually recommended when the hernia persists beyond 4 years of age. Parents are often anxious about these very visible protrusions. If the fascial defect remains larger than 1.5 cm by the time the child is 2 years old, spontaneous closure is unlikely and repair may be undertaken. Girls especially should have an umbilical hernia corrected before pregnancy, a time when increased intra-abdominal pressure could lead to complications. Skin excoriation over the hernia and pain from incarcerated fat are other rare indications for early operation.

Cryptorchidism

A cryptorchid testis is one that has not descended into the scrotum, an event that normally takes place between the seventh and ninth months of gestation. The incidence of **cryptorchidism** at the time of birth is 3% in term infants and up to 30% in preterm infants. Most testes that are cryptorchid at birth spontaneously descend within the first year.

Pathophysiology

Ultrastructural studies show that by the second year of a child's life, undescended testes already have histologic abnormalities. The fertility potential of an undescended testis is never 100%, but its repositioning in the cooler scrotal environment maximizes the potential for sperm production. Evidence even suggests that if a testis is left undescended, it may adversely affect spermatogenesis in the opposite, normally descended testicle.

The incidence of subsequent testicular malignancy in children with undescended testes is 10 to 40 times that of the general population. This risk begins to increase in young adulthood. Recent evidence, based on longitudinal studies of adults who had orchidopexy performed as young children, suggests that successful orchidopexy in young childhood reduces the risk of subsequent testicular cancer to that of normal controls. Orchidopexy performed in older children and adolescents does not decrease the risk of testicular malignancy, but it facilitates the early detection of testicular tumors on physical examination. Other problems encountered in boys with cryptorchidism include an increased risk of testicular torsion, more vulnerability to trauma, and psychological concerns.

Almost all undescended testes are associated with a patent processus vaginalis. This predisposition to the development of inguinal hernias is corrected at the time of orchidopexy.

Clinical Presentation and Evaluation

A cryptorchid testicle is absent from the scrotum and may be palpable in the groin. It must be differentiated from the much more common **retractile testis** that is pulled up transiently by an active cremasteric reflex. If the testicle can be manipulated into the scrotum without tension, even if it does not remain there, the parents can be assured that no abnormality is present and that observation alone is indicated. A cryptorchid testis may also be present ectopically. Therefore, examination should include careful palpation of the suprapubic, perineal, and upper inner thigh areas.

A testicle that is not palpable at all may be totally absent or may be located above the internal ring. Although ultrasound, CT, and MRI scanning have been advocated as imaging modalities, failure to visualize a testicle is not sufficient proof of its absence. Laparoscopy has become the procedure of choice because in many instances it allows both accurate diagnosis and treatment. In infants with bilateral nonpalpable testes, a human chorionic gonadotropin (hCG) stimulation test may be performed. If the serum testosterone level does not rise markedly in response to hCG administration, no testicular tissue exists.

Treatment

Hormonal treatment with hCG and, more recently, luteinizing hormone — releasing hormone has been advocated as initial treatment of cryptorchidism. However, the results are conflicting. Hormonal therapy may rationally be attempted in boys with bilateral cryptorchidism, in whom it is more plausible that an underlying hormonal deficiency is responsible for the undescended testes.

Orchidopexy is recommended for all boys whose testes remain undescended. It is usually performed during the second year of life. After appropriate dissection and closure of the patent processus vaginalis, the testicle is placed in a dartos muscle pouch (Fig. 2-18). Figure 2-19 shows an algorithm for the management of cryptorchidism. Orchiectomy, either laparoscopic or open, is indicated for atrophic testes and those first encountered in late puberty.

Prognosis

After early successful orchidopexy for unilateral cryptorchidism, 80% to 90% of boys are subsequently fertile. Only 50% of boys with bilateral cryptorchidism are fertile after bilateral orchidopexy. In contrast, testosterone production by the testes is unaffected by their location, and secondary sexual characteristics develop normally in all of these boys. Young men whose orchidopexy was performed in older childhood should be advised to do regular testicular self-examinations.

Pyloric Stenosis

Pyloric stenosis is a progressive hypertrophy of the musculature of the pylorus in infancy, leading to gastric outlet obstruction. It is a common disorder, occurring in 1:500 infants. It affects males four times as often as females, and it has a strong familial component.

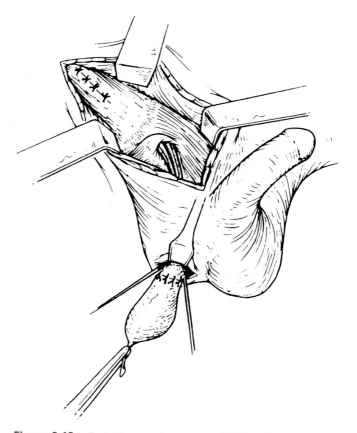

Figure 2-18   Orchidopexy for cryptorchidism. The undescended testicle is brought down and implanted into the scrotum between the dartos layer and the skin.

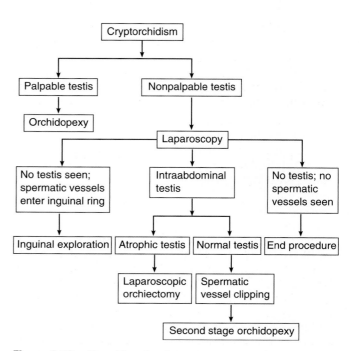

Figure 2-19   Algorithm for the management of a cryptorchid testis.

Pathophysiology

The etiology of pyloric stenosis is not known. One hypothesis suggests abnormal development of the ganglion cells in the wall of the pylorus. Another proposal is that milk curds propelled against the pylorus produce submucosal edema that initially blocks the gastric outlet, leading to subsequent work hypertrophy of the muscular pylorus.

Clinical Presentation and Evaluation

An infant with pyloric stenosis typically presents at 2 to 8 weeks of age with nonbilious vomiting after feeds. The vomiting, which may be projectile, becomes progressively worse until little is kept down. The infant remains hungry between vomiting episodes and sucks vigorously. Stool frequency and urinary output may diminish as less oral intake is retained.

On examination, the infant may appear irritable and dehydrated to a variable degree. Peristaltic waves are sometimes seen moving across the abdomen. The hallmark of pyloric stenosis is the palpable "olive," a hard, round, movable mass in the epigastrium. Success in palpating the pyloric mass depends on the examiner's experience and patience; an empty stomach and relaxed abdominal muscles are extremely helpful. The infant can be given an electrolyte and mineral supplement (Pedialyte) or a pacifier coated with sugar to promote relaxation. Then the stomach can be emptied with a nasogastric tube. When an olive is identified, no imaging studies are necessary.

If no palpable olive is found, ultrasonography is highly accurate in diagnosing pyloric stenosis because the length, diameter, and wall thickness of the pylorus are all increased (Fig. 2-20). If this study is equivocal, a barium swallow is obtained. It shows a narrowed, elongated pyloric channel.

Treatment

Appropriate preoperative rehydration is essential. These infants have been vomiting gastric contents and often have hypochloremic, hypokalemic, metabolic alkalosis. Depending on the extent of dehydration and alkalosis, D5% in $\frac{1}{2}$ normal saline or D5% in normal saline with 20 to 40 mEq/L KCl is administered at $1\frac{1}{2}$ to 2 times the maintenance rate. When urine output is 1 to 2 mL/kg/hr and serum electrolytes are normal, operative correction may proceed with a pyloromyotomy. This procedure involves a longitudinal split of the hypertrophic pyloric muscle that extends down to the mucosa, but does not enter it (Fig. 2-21A,B). Feeding is initiated 6 to 12 hours postoperatively and increased gradually until a regular schedule is tolerated.

Prognosis

Infants may have transient vomiting postoperatively, either as a result of a chronically overdistended stomach or from mucosal irritation. Significant complications are rare.

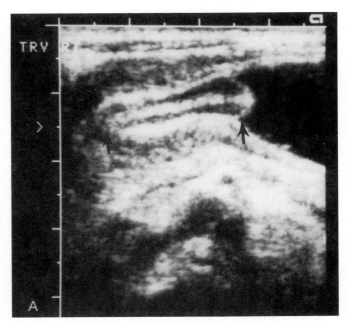

Figure 2-20 Ultrasound appearance of pyloric stenosis. The narrowed, elongated pyloric channel *(between arrows)* has thickened walls. (Reprinted with permission from Lesions of the stomach. In Ashcraft K, ed. *Pediatric Surgery.* Philadelphia: WB Saunders; 1994:292.)

Acute Abdomen

Children who have acute abdominal pain present a challenge for all physicians involved in their care. The diagnostic dilemma involves differentiating children who need immediate surgery from the many others who may be managed conservatively. Several factors contribute to the diagnostic challenge:

1. Young children tend to have a uniform response to infection. Whether they have streptococcal pharyngitis, pneumonia, viral gastroenteritis, or appendicitis, they often have fever, vomiting, and a stomach ache.
2. Most surgical diseases in children are age-dependent. The relative risks for various conditions vary significantly with age.
3. Children have a limited ability to express their symptoms. The younger they are, the less likely they are to have classic manifestations of various abdominal conditions.
4. A child who is in pain is not a cooperative patient, and even a simple abdominal examination can be a challenge. A child who is asleep or lying in his or her parent's arms should be first examined in that position. Waking the child or placing him or her in the supine position causes crying and voluntary guarding and significantly reduces the effectiveness of the examination. Building trust through patient interaction with the child and very gentle initial palpation is crucial.
5. Parental anxiety adds to the stress of the situation.

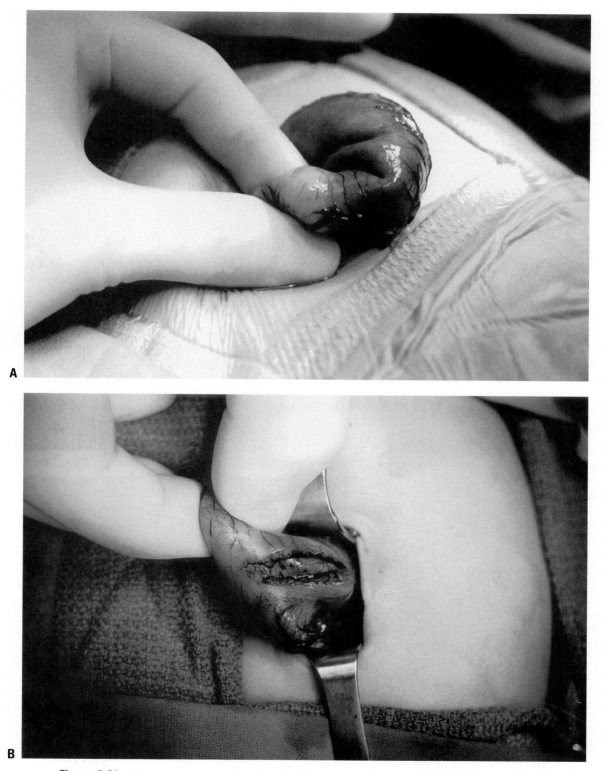

Figure 2-21   Pyloromyotomy. **A,** The hypertrophic pylorus is delivered. **B,** Longitudinal incision that extends down to, but not through, the mucosa.

Despite these factors, in most cases a diagnostic decision can be made, based chiefly on a thorough clinical assessment and a few simple added investigations. Although a pathologic diagnosis must be sought, the key decision in acute abdominal pain is whether the child warrants observation or requires immediate surgery. The index of suspicion must be high. In cases of uncertainty, overnight observation with serial examinations by the same observer is warranted.

Appendicitis

Acute appendicitis is the most common condition that requires emergency surgery in childhood. It is rare in infancy, but after that its incidence increases progressively, peaking in adolescents and young adults. Appendicitis is caused by obstruction at the base of the appendiceal lumen by a fecalith or lymphoid hyperplasia. Mucosal secretions distend the appendix and increase intraluminal pressure, leading to bacterial overgrowth and impairment of perfusion. Without prompt treatment, perforation occurs in 24 to 48 hours. Delayed recognition is much more likely in young children. In most cases of appendicitis in children younger than 5 years of age, perforation has already occurred on presentation.

Clinical Presentation and Evaluation

The initial symptom is almost always pain, although the classic progression from the periumbilical area to the right lower quadrant may not be elicited. Anorexia, nausea, and vomiting are common. The temperature is typically normal or mildly elevated. An early, high fever suggests another diagnosis. Later, it may signify a ruptured appendix. The cheeks are often flushed, and the child is unusually quiet, lying with the knees pulled up. Abdominal examination usually shows diminished bowel sounds and signs of localized peritonitis, with involuntary guarding, tenderness, and rebound in the right lower quadrant. Rectal examination may elicit tenderness on the right side if the appendix extends into the pelvis. Children with a ruptured appendix are often septic, have abdominal distention from an ileus, and have frank peritonitis. They also may have a right lower quadrant or rectal mass.

Laboratory studies should include a CBC and urinalysis. The white blood cell count is usually elevated or shifted to the left. The presence of many white cells in the urine suggests a urinary infection, although the finding of a few white or red cells is consistent with an inflamed appendix in contiguity with the urinary tract. β-hCG levels should always be obtained in adolescent girls to exclude ectopic pregnancy. Abdominal x-ray films are obtained only in patients in whom the diagnosis of appendicitis is questionable and in the very young, in whom the diagnosis is always difficult. The only pathognomic sign of appendicitis is a calcified fecalith that can be visualized in 5% to 15% of

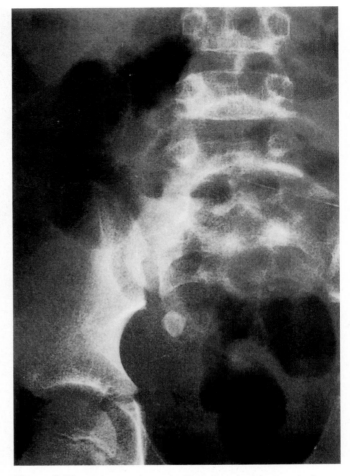

Figure 2-22   Calcified fecalith. (Reprinted with permission from Liebert PS, ed. *Color Atlas of Pediatric Surgery.* 2nd ed. Philadelphia: WB Saunders; 1996:188.)

cases (Fig. 2-22). Other radiographic findings are less specific. They include dextroscoliosis, obliteration of the right psoas shadow, and localized ileus. Ruptured appendicitis in children may lead to an incomplete small bowel obstruction; it is the most common cause of intestinal obstruction in school-aged children. CT scans are reported to be 95% accurate in identifying an acutely inflamed appendix but are associated with significant exposure to ionizing radiation (data suggest that 1 in 1,000 children who receive an abdominal CT scan will develop a life-threatening malignancy later in life as a result). In children in whom there is doubt about the diagnosis of appendicitis, ultrasonography is therefore preferred, and in expert hands it is more than 90% accurate. Ultrasound is particularly helpful in adolescent girls to rule out such entities as an ovarian cyst, adnexal torsion, and pelvic inflammatory disease. Laparoscopy is very accurate and again most useful in adolescent girls. It requires anesthesia and is both invasive and expensive.

The differential diagnosis of appendicitis in children is

Table 2-14	Differential Diagnosis of Acute Abdominal Pain in Children				
	Intussusception	**Appendicitis**	**Ruptured Ovarian cyst**	**Mesenteric Adenitis**	**Gastroenteritis**
Age	6 mo–3 yr	Any; usually older; rarely <4 yr	Postmenarchal	Any; usually 4–12 yr	Any age
Type of pain	Intermittent attacks	Gradual onset, increases	Sudden onset, constant	Fluctuating	Crampy
Stools	May have blood and mucus ("red currant jelly")	Normal or irritation diarrhea (frequent small amounts)	Normal	Normal	Often large-volume diarrhea
Overall appearance	Unhappy, lethargic between attacks	Ill, quiet, flushed cheeks	Unwell	Well	Well or sick
Fever	Variable	None or low-grade early; high later	Usually none	Often high	May be high
Abdominal findings	Tender; may be right upper quadrant mass	Localized right lower quadrant peritonitis (tenderness, guarding rebound)	Right lower quadrant and suprapubic tenderness, with or without guarding	Right lower quadrant or diffuse tenderness; soft	Diffuse tenderness, soft
White blood cell count	Usually normal	Mild increase; later significantly increased	Normal	Normal or decreased (viral leukopenia)	Normal, increased, or decreased
Abdominal x-ray	Right lower quadrant paucity of air; dilated bowel later	Fecalith, ileus, dextroscoliosis, loss of psoas shadow	Normal	Normal	Nonspecific small bowel air pattern; ileus
Ultrasound	"Donut," or "pseudokidney," sign	Noncompressible blind-ending tubular right lower quadrant structure, pericecal fluid or mass	Pelvic fluid; ovarian cysts	Enlarged mesenteric lymph nodes	Normal; some free fluid
Treatment	Contrast enema reduction; surgery if unsuccessful	Appendectomy	Analgesia	Reassurance	Hydration

extensive. Table 2-14 details the features of the key surgical and nonsurgical diagnoses.

Treatment

The standard treatment for acute appendicitis is urgent appendectomy performed after rapid intravenous hydration and the administration of broad-spectrum antibiotics. The procedure can be done laparoscopically, but the advantages in children are controversial. If the appendix is not ruptured, postoperative antibiotics are unnecessary. For perforated appendicitis, antibiotics are usually given for a minimum of 3 days postoperatively and discontinued when the patient has been afebrile for 48 hours and has a normal white blood cell count. Recovery from nonruptured appendicitis is rapid, and children are usually discharged within 24 to 48 hours.

Common Complications

Perforated appendicitis has a significant incidence of complications, particularly intra-abdominal abscesses and wound infections. Abscesses are often drained percutaneously or transrectally under ultrasound guidance. Wound infections are opened and drained. The high complication

rate has led to an alternative approach to the uncommon presentation of a nonseptic child with perforated appendicitis who has a localized mass without peritonitis. Intravenous antibiotics are given for several days, followed by oral antibiotics until symptoms completely resolve. There is evidence to suggest that this approach can even be used in selected cases of nonlocalized, perforated appendicitis, but this method of treatment is controversial and more study is needed. When the appendix has not been removed, an "interval" appendectomy is performed electively in 6 to 8 weeks, although recent evidence questions whether this operation is necessary.

Intussusception

Intussusception is a telescoping of one portion of the intestine into another. It is usually ileocolic, and the distal ileum invaginates and advances for a variable distance into the colon. Intussusception is an emergency condition, because the involved intestine can become strangulated.

Pathophysiology

Intussusception typically affects children between 6 and 18 months of age. Viral hypertrophy of Peyer's patches in the intestinal submucosa accounts for most cases. Less often, a pathologic lead point is found (e.g., **Meckel's diverticulum,** polyp, lymphoma, hematoma). These conditions are more prevalent in children who have intussusception at a later age.

Clinical Presentation and Evaluation

Intussusception often follows a viral illness and is seasonal. It is characterized by intermittent bouts of colicky abdominal pain during which the child cries and draws the knees to the chest. Between episodes the child is initially well, but becomes increasingly lethargic. Vomiting is common and eventually becomes bilious as intestinal obstruction develops. Blood and mucus may be passed rectally as "currant jelly" stools as a result of congestion and ischemia of the intestinal mucosa.

On examination, these children may be irritable or somnolent, as well as dehydrated. A tender, sausage-shaped mass can sometimes be palpated in the right upper abdomen. Digital rectal examination may yield blood and mucus. Abdominal x-rays may appear normal or show a paucity of air in the right lower quadrant. Eventually, dilated small intestinal loops consistent with obstruction develop.

Unfortunately, the diagnosis can be difficult because intermittent crying spells are very nonspecific in children and many more suggestive findings may be absent. If intussusception is suspected, the standard investigation is barium or air-contrast enema. Ileocolic intussusception appears as a filling defect in the colon, at which point the flow of contrast material stops (Fig. 2-23). Ultrasound can also be diagnostic by showing the intussuscepted mass in the right flank, with obstructed flow across the ileocecal valve. Ileoileal intussusception is rare and is associated with pathologic lead points or may occur after other abdominal operations. Nonoperative reduction is rarely successful in these cases, and surgery is necessary.

Treatment

The pressure of the barium or air during administration of the barium enema is used to reduce the intussusception and is successful in most cases. Some centers also use a saline enema under ultrasound guidance. After successful reduction, the child is admitted overnight for observation. Surgery must be performed promptly if nonoperative reduction fails. After expeditious hydration and antibiotics, the intussusception is manually reduced and the appendix is removed. If the intestine is necrotic or a pathologic lead point is identified, that segment of intestine is resected.

Prognosis

Recurrent intussusception occurs in 5% to 8% of children, regardless of the method of reduction.

Meckel's Diverticulum

A Meckel's diverticulum occurs in 2% of the population. It is located in the ileum, within 2 feet (100 cm) of the ileocecal valve.

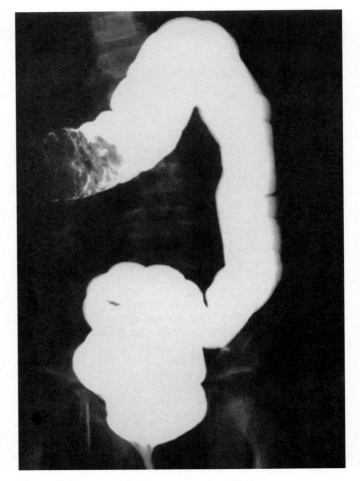

Figure 2-23 Ileocolic intussusception. Barium enema outlines a filling defect in the transverse colon.

Pathophysiology

A Meckel's diverticulum contains heterotopic tissue in 50% of symptomatic patients. It is most often lined with gastric mucosa. Embryologically, the yolk sac communicates with the intestine through the vitelline (omphalomesenteric) duct. If this structure does not involute and remains completely open, intestinal contents drain from the umbilicus after cord separation, and a vitelline fistula forms. Much more commonly, only the intestinal side of the vitelline duct remains patent and creates a Meckel's diverticulum. The distal end may lie freely or may be attached to the undersurface of the umbilicus by a fibrous band.

Clinical Presentation and Evaluation

Although most Meckel's diverticula remain asymptomatic, they may be complicated by bleeding, obstruction, and inflammation. Bleeding results from peptic ulceration adjacent to the ectopic gastric mucosa of the diverticulum. It usually occurs in children younger than 5 years of age. The bleeding is typically dark red and painless, and it may be massive. Contrast x-rays rarely visualize the diverticulum, but technetium pertechnetate scans, which show increased uptake in gastric tissue, are positive in 50% of cases.

A Meckel's diverticulum can cause intestinal obstruction by acting as the lead point of an intussusception or by allowing the intestine to twist around it as a volvulus when the diverticulum is fixed to the anterior abdominal wall.

Meckel's diverticulitis occurs in somewhat older children and is almost always misdiagnosed preoperatively because its manifestations are so similar to those of appendicitis. Whenever a normal appendix is found at laparotomy for presumptive appendicitis, the distal ileum must be inspected for the possibility of Meckel's diverticulitis.

Treatment

A symptomatic Meckel's diverticulum is resected by laparotomy or laparoscopic surgery. Asymptomatic diverticula found incidentally at surgery are usually resected if the child is young, if the diverticulum has a narrow neck, if it is attached to the abdominal wall, or if heterotopic tissue is palpable within its lumen.

Gastrointestinal Bleeding

Gastrointestinal bleeding may be frightening to parents, but is usually mild and readily managed. The most likely sources of bleeding in a child may be suspected by the patient's age, the level of bleeding (upper or lower), the color and amount of blood, and the associated findings. If the bleeding is massive and the child is hemodynamically unstable, rapid resuscitation is required, with insertion of large-bore intravenous catheters, fluid administration and blood transfusions, and prompt investigation of the cause. For smaller amounts of bleeding, which are much more common, outpatient evaluation is appropriate.

Table 2-15 lists the common causes of gastrointestinal bleeding according to age and the diagnostic modalities that are used in their evaluation.

Gastroesophageal Reflux

The reflux of stomach contents into the esophagus is known as gastroesophageal reflux (GER). GER is particularly common in infants and children who have neurologic impairments. Although most children with GER are managed successfully with medical measures alone, surgical procedures to combat reflux are now among the most common major operations performed in children.

Pathophysiology

GER is common in normal babies because the lower esophageal sphincter is relatively incompetent for the first few months of life. This type of GER is usually self-limited because its incidence and severity decrease with normal growth and development. Patients with neurologic disor-

Table 2-15	Causes of Gastrointestinal Bleeding by Age

Neonates (in a substantial number, the etiology is not found)
  Swallowed maternal blood (diagnosed by determining relative quantities of adult and fetal hemoglobin [Apt test])
  Anal fissure (can be visualized on inspection)
  Necrotizing enterocolitis
  Midgut volvulus
  Hemangiomas
  Clotting disorders
  Formula intolerance
Young children
  Intussusception
  Gastroenteritis
  Meckel's diverticulum
  Rectal prolapse (generally at the time of toilet raining; usually responds to conservative measures; evaluated for cystic fibrosis)
  Anal fissure (from hard stools; produces bright rd blood and pain; treat with stool softeners and local ointments; rarely needs surgery)
  Duplications
  Juvenile polyps (hamartomas, with no malignant potential, found most often in left colon; may be removed endoscopically or observed [often will autoamputate])
Older children
  Peptic ulcer
  Inflammatory bowel disease
  Peutz-Jeghers polyps (autosomal dominant, with melanin spots on lips and buccal mucosa and hamartomatous polyps in the small intestine; surgery reserved for persistent intussusceptions and major bleeding)
Evaluation
  Appropriate studies may include hemoglobin levels, coagulation tests, nasogastric aspiration for blood, upper and lower contrast studies, upper and lower endoscopy, Meckel's technetium scan, tagged red blood cell bleeding scan, and angiography

ders may have motor and reflex abnormalities of the entire foregut, including disordered swallowing, decreased esophageal clearance, an incompetent lower esophageal sphincter, and delayed gastric emptying. All of these predispose patients to GER and its complications at all ages.

Clinical Presentation and Evaluation

In most infants, GER is of minor consequence. It is responsible for the occasional regurgitations and "wet burps" seen. In some cases, vomiting is more severe and may even mimic pyloric stenosis. Clinically significant complications of GER include: (a) failure to thrive (inadequate growth and weight gain because of chronic regurgitation); (b) aspiration of gastric contents into the lungs, causing recurrent pneumonia or reactive airway disease; (c) apnea, probably because of reflux-induced laryngospasm or a vagal reflex (may be one cause of sudden infant death syndrome); and (d) peptic esophagitis, which can lead to gastrointestinal bleeding, stricture formation, and Barrett's esophagus (more common in older children). Patients who have certain underlying disorders, including chronic neurologic impairment, esophageal atresia, and diaphragmatic hernias, are more likely to have severe GER.

Evaluation of a child with significant GER is initiated with a barium swallow to rule out obstructive lesions and define the anatomy. If massive GER is observed, no further diagnostic studies may be necessary. If GER is suspected clinically but not documented radiographically, more sensitive tests (e.g., pH probe study, nuclear scintiscan of the esophagus) are indicated. Endoscopy is useful to demonstrate esophagitis and its complications, but it is used much less often in children than in adults. Manometry is rarely useful in children.

Treatment

GER is so common in babies that the diagnosis and initial treatment are often based on the clinical impression alone. Medical management, including upright positioning, thickening of feeds, and possibly agents to promote gastric emptying (e.g., metoclopramide), is usually effective for uncomplicated reflux. H_2 blockers or proton pump inhibitors are used to prevent or treat esophagitis.

Surgery is indicated if medical management does not control the complications of GER, or sooner for life-threatening complications (e.g., apnea). Surgery is more likely to be necessary if the child has an underlying condition that predisposes to GER. Many operative procedures have been devised, but the Nissen fundoplication, in which the gastric fundus is wrapped 360 degrees around the lower esophagus, is most commonly performed and may be done laparoscopically. If long-term access for enteral feeding is anticipated, a gastrostomy tube is placed at the time of the procedure.

Common Complications

Possible complications of antireflux procedures include inability to vomit and the gas-bloat syndrome, in which patients become distended after feeding because they cannot burp. Children usually outgrow these problems. Recurrence of GER after antireflux surgery is much more common in neurologically impaired children than in the general population.

Chest Wall Deformities

A variety of skeletal malformations of the chest wall may present at birth or in early childhood. The most common of these are pectus excavatum and pectus carinatum.

Pathophysiology

Pectus excavatum, or "funnel chest," is characterized by depression of the sternum and sharp angulation of the lower costal cartilages where they bow out over the upper abdomen (Fig. 2-24). It occurs in up to 1 in 400 births and has a strong familial component. Several theories exist to explain the pathogenesis of pectus excavatum, but none has been proven. The involved costal cartilages are abnormal, both on gross and microscopic inspection. **Pectus carinatum,** or "pigeon breast," is characterized by protru-

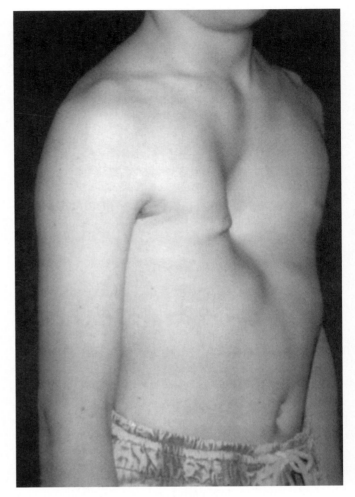

Figure 2-24 A 15-year-old boy with pectus excavatum. (Reprinted with permission O'Neill JA Jr, Rowe MI, Grosfelf JL, Fonkalsrud EW, Coran AG, eds. *Pediatric Surgery.* 5th ed. St. Louis: Mosby; 1998:788.)

sion of the anterior chest wall. It is believed to be due to overgrowth of the costal cartilages and is much less common than pectus excavatum.

Clinical Presentation and Evaluation

Young children with chest wall deformities are usually brought for evaluation by parents who are concerned about the obvious cosmetic problem. Boys may be unwilling to expose their chests while swimming or engaging in sports. Symptoms due to restrictive pulmonary changes are more common in older children and adolescents, and include easy fatigability, decreased stamina and endurance, and an increased incidence of respiratory illness. In severe forms of pectus excavatum, the heart is displaced into the left side of the chest, and inspiratory expansion of the lungs is inhibited. Thoracic CT scans provide information regarding displacement of the heart and assessment of lung volumes. Pulmonary function tests can be used to determine the physiologic abnormalities when symptoms are present. Most children with pectus carinatum do not have cardiopulmonary impairment, and consideration for operative correction is based on the severity of the deformity.

Treatment

The traditional operation for pectus excavatum involves resection of the involved costal cartilages for the entire length of the deformity and elevation of the sternum to a neutral position via a wedge osteotomy anteriorly. The sternum is then stabilized in this position using a stainless steel bar or wire, which is removed several months later when healing in the new position is complete. A similar procedure is performed for pectus carinatum. A newer procedure for pectus excavatum, the so-called "Nuss procedure," involves the insertion of a semicircular bar under the sternum and anterior ribs via small incisions on either side of the chest under thoracoscopic vision. The bar is left in place for 2 years, when permanent remolding of the sternum and costal cartilages has occurred.

Common Complications

Early postoperative complications of the traditional procedure for pectus excavatum and carinatum include pneumothorax; fluid accumulation in the pleural cavity, mediastinum, or subcutaneous space; and wound infection, dehiscence, and hematoma. Later complications include migration of the stabilizing bar and a 5% to 10% rate of recurrence after the bar is removed. Impaired chest wall growth has been noted in adolescents whose corrective surgery was done during young childhood. This has been attributed to intraoperative injury to the costochondral junctions, which are the longitudinal growth centers for the ribs. Identification of this late complication has prompted many surgeons who perform the traditional procedure for chest wall deformities to delay surgery until after the pubertal growth spurt or to perform the Nuss procedure. Complications of the Nuss procedure are similar to those of the traditional procedure and also include injury to thoracic organs during insertion of the bar.

Neck Masses

Neck masses are often found in children and seldom carry the same ominous import as they do in adults, although certain malignancies do occur. In most cases, neck masses are accurately diagnosed by history and physical examination alone. Surgical excision may be required for definitive treatment and occasionally for diagnosis. Neck masses are classified according to their location. Table 2-16 lists the most common types of neck masses in children.

Midline Neck Masses

Among the midline neck masses found in the older child are **thyroglossal duct cysts,** ectopic thyroid, dermoid or epidermoid cysts, enlarged lymph nodes, and thyroid

Table 2-16	Neck Masses in Children
Midline	Lateral
Thyroglossal duct cyst	Lymphadenopathy
Ectopic thyroid	Cystic hygroma
Thyroid masses	Branchial cleft cysts
Dermoid and epidermoid cysts	Torticollis
Lymphadenopathy	

masses. An ultrasound or thyroid scan should always precede surgical excision to ensure that there is a normally located thyroid gland.

Embryologically, the thyroid gland descends from the base of the tongue. If the thyroglossal duct, along the path of descent, does not obliterate, a thyroglossal duct cyst can result. This cyst usually appears between 2 and 10 years of age as a firm, round, midline neck mass (Fig. 2-25). It rises with swallowing and protrusion of the tongue. Infection often occurs. A thyroglossal duct cyst must be removed with its tract and the center of the hyoid bone, or most of these cysts will recur.

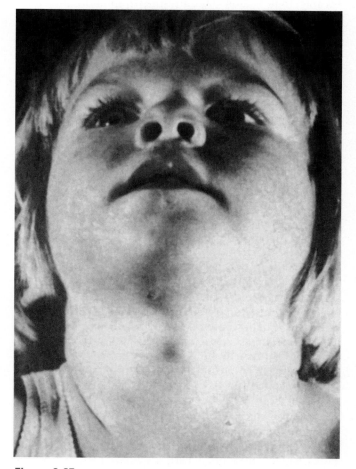

Figure 2-25   A thyroglossal duct cyst in a 5-year-old girl.

In an ectopic thyroid, the gland is arrested in its antenatal descent. It may present as a midline neck mass and is the patient's only thyroid tissue. An ectopic thyroid gland may be divided and moved bilaterally, or excised. The patient then receives thyroid replacement therapy.

A dermoid or epidermoid cyst arises from trapped epithelial elements and may present as a midline neck mass. It is usually more superficial than a thyroglossal duct cyst. Enlarged lymph nodes (lymphadenopathy) may also appear in the midline of the neck.

Thyroid masses are usually recognized by their location. Although uncommon in children, they may be caused by the same abnormalities as in adults. A thyroid nodule in a child is more likely to be malignant. Either lobectomy with biopsy or needle aspiration biopsy and an attempt at suppression with thyroid hormone (if the patient does not have hyperthyroidism) is recommended.

Lateral Neck Masses

Lateral neck masses in older children may involve the lymph glands, lymphatic vessels, branchial cleft cysts and sinuses, or the sternomastoid muscle.

Acute cervical lymphadenitis occurs predominantly in young children as a result of staphylococcal or streptococcal infection, usually after an upper respiratory infection. The child is febrile, and the swelling shows signs of inflammation, including erythema and tenderness. Antibiotics may be curative, but if the mass becomes fluctuant because of an abscess, incision and drainage are necessary.

Chronic lymphadenopathy is extremely common in the cervical region. It usually represents nonspecific benign hyperplasia. Other causes of chronically enlarged cervical lymph nodes are infections with mycobacteria (usually nontuberculous), cat scratch disease, and, rarely, lymphoma. Lymphoma is more likely if the nodes are hard or fixed, if the nodes continue to grow, and if the patient has systemic symptoms of fever, malaise, and weight loss. Open biopsy of enlarged cervical lymph nodes is indicated if they are larger than 2 cm and persist for 6 weeks, or sooner if malignancy is suspected based on physical findings.

Cystic hygromas, or lymphangiomas, are congenital malformations of the lymphatic vessels characterized by multiloculated cysts filled with lymph. They may occur anywhere, but are most common in the posterior triangle of the neck, followed by the axilla. They may be present at birth and almost always appear by 2 years of age. A cystic hygroma can usually be diagnosed by physical examination as a soft, compressible mass with ill-defined borders. It may become infected and rarely regresses. Resection is indicated, although there are recent reports of eradication of complex hygromas by the injection of sclerosing agents.

Branchial cleft cysts and sinuses arise when the various branchial clefts and arches do not completely resorb. Sinuses usually present in early childhood as small cutaneous openings that drain clear fluid. Cysts are noted as subcutaneous masses in older children, as fluid gradually accumulates within them. They are less complete abnormalities than sinuses, in that external closure has occurred. Skin tags and collections of cartilage may also occur. Remnants of the second branchial cleft are the most common and are located along the anterior border of the sternomastoid muscle. Remnants of the first cleft are found near the ear or the angle of the mandible. These cysts and sinuses may become infected, and resection is indicated as soon as infection is controlled.

Neonatal torticollis, or wry neck, is caused by fibrosis and shortening of the sternomastoid muscle. A traumatic cause is hypothesized, with hematoma formation and organization within the muscle. The infant has a firm neck mass. The face is rotated away from the affected side, and the head is tilted toward the ipsilateral shoulder. Ultrasound confirms that the mass is within the muscle. Passive rotational exercises by the parents are usually curative. Surgical division of the sternomastoid muscle is reserved for rare treatment failures. Untreated, torticollis may lead to permanent facial asymmetry.

Vascular Tumors

Vascular tumors are common in childhood and are found in 10% of children during the first year. The terminology used to describe them is variable and confusing. Biologic classification is the most useful. **Hemangiomas** are biologically active benign vascular tumors characterized initially by cellular proliferation and followed in most cases by involution. In contrast, vascular malformations are biologically inert errors of morphogenesis of vessels. They are not proliferative and only grow with the child.

Hemangiomas

Most hemangiomas appear within the first few weeks after birth as a small red spot that grows rapidly during the first year and then slowly regresses over the next several years. They are commonly located on the head and neck, but may be found anywhere. Hemangiomas may be superficial or deep and may involve the viscera. Superficial lesions, or capillary hemangiomas, are firm, bright red, and raised. They are the most likely to regress (Fig. 2-26A,B). Deep or cavernous lesions are softer and may have a blue discoloration. They may be less likely to resolve.

Most hemangiomas should be left alone because the overwhelming majority resolve spontaneously in early childhood. Indications for treatment include significant facial distortion, interference with function (e.g., as occurs with lesions of the eyelid or airway), thrombocytopenia from platelet trapping, and congestive heart failure. Management includes steroids (by intralesional injection or systemically), cyclophosphamide, α-interferon, emboliza-

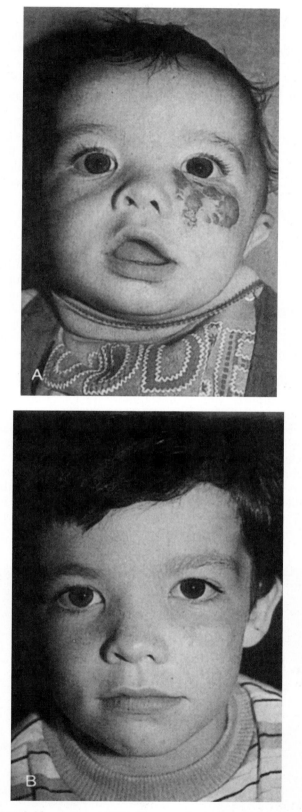

Figure 2-26   **A,** A superficial hemangioma in an infant boy.
B, Regression by 5 years of age.

tion, and surgical excision, depending on the location and characteristics of the hemangioma.

Vascular Malformations

Vascular malformations are much less common than hemangiomas and tend to remain stable over time. One such malformation, the port wine stain, is seen at birth as a red or purple nonraised lesion, usually on the face. Another vascular malformation is a congenital arteriovenous fistula. These anomalies are most common in the extremities and central nervous system (CNS). In the extremities, they are usually multiple and may cause heart failure and hypertrophy of the involved limb.

A port wine stain never regresses and is best treated with laser photocoagulation. Treatment of a congenital arteriovenous fistula, although not completely satisfactory, consists of elastic compression, ligation of the involved vessels, embolization, or surgical excision.

TUMORS

Few ordeals are more devastating for young people and their families than childhood cancer. Cancer accounts for 11% of all childhood deaths. The frequency distribution of malignant neoplasms in children differs markedly from that in adults. Leukemia (25%), CNS tumors (20%), and lymphoma (12%) predominate. Neuroblastoma and Wilms' tumors each account for 5% to 10% of pediatric cancers, followed by malignancies of the liver, bone, and other soft tissues.

Fortunately, the outlook for children with malignancies has improved markedly in the last two decades, largely as the result of multicenter clinical trials. The pediatric surgeon almost always treats children with solid malignancies as a part of a multidisciplinary team that combines the use of surgery, chemotherapy, radiation therapy, and sophisticated diagnostic imaging. Each of these modalities of therapy has side affects that affect surgical therapy. For example, chemotherapy may cause renal dysfunction that affects fluid and electrolyte therapy in the perioperative period. Radiation has an effect on wound healing that must be considered in surgical planning. Secondary malignancies can occur as a consequence of therapy, and pediatric surgeons are often involved in the management of these problems.

Vascular access devices offer a substantial advantage in children with many types of cancer. These catheters are used to administer chemotherapy and intravenous nutrition and blood products, as well as to sample blood. Some catheters (e.g., Hickman, Broviac) have a subcutaneous cuff and external tubing. Others (e.g., Port-A-Cath) are completely internalized and have implanted subcutaneous reservoirs that are easily accessed percutaneously with a special needle. These implanted devices are associated with a lower infection rate and are less limiting to patient activities when not in use.

Neuroblastoma

Neuroblastoma is the most common extracranial solid tumor of childhood. It has the unique ability to undergo maturation to a benign form, ganglioneuroma, or to spontaneously regress altogether.

Pathophysiology

The tumor is derived from embryonal neural crest tissue. It arises anywhere in the sympathetic nervous system. Three quarters of neuroblastomas are intra-abdominal. Of these, most arise from the adrenal medulla. Other sites include the posterior mediastinum, neck, and brain. Most children with neuroblastoma excrete catecholamines and their breakdown products in the urine.

Clinical Presentation and Evaluation

One half of neuroblastomas occur in the first 2 years of life, and 90% are found by the time a child is 8 years old. An abdominal mass is the presenting feature in most patients. Tumors of the mediastinum may produce respiratory distress, may cause Horner's syndrome because of involvement of the stellate ganglion, or may be noted incidentally on chest x-ray. Paraplegia can occur if there is extension through the intervertebral foramina with compression of the spinal cord. Systemic symptoms are common and include fever, weight loss, failure to thrive, anemia, and hypertension. Most children have metastases at diagnosis, with the most common sites of spread being bone, bone marrow, lymph nodes, liver, and subcutaneous tissue.

A child with a suspected neuroblastoma undergoes studies that include ultrasonography, CT or MRI scan, bone scan, bone marrow aspiration, and measurement of urinary catecholamines. An MRI is performed preoperatively if intraspinal extension is suspected. Several staging systems have been proposed to specify the extent of disease and the completeness of surgical resection. Tumor specimens are examined for histology, karyotype, and genetic analysis. Prognostically positive features include favorable nuclear and stromal histologic characteristics, DNA aneuploidy, and lack of amplification of the N-*myc* oncogene.

Treatment

Therapeutic protocols are based on the child's age, tumor location and characteristics, and extent of disease. Surgical resection remains the mainstay of treatment and is currently the only method of cure. In cases in which tumor recurrence is likely or there is residual cancer, postoperative radiation and multiple-agent chemotherapy are usually indicated. For advanced disease with an unresectable tumor, chemotherapy may be given initially to shrink the lesion and permit subsequent resection. Bone marrow transplantation rescue has been used after massive chemotherapy and total body irradiation, with prolonged relapse-free survival. Immunotherapy is being evaluated as well.

Prognosis

The overall survival rate is 40% to 50%, but it depends greatly on the age of the patient and the site and characteristics of the tumor. The survival rate for infants less than 1 year of age is 84%, but it is only 42% for children older than 1 year. Children with localized, completely resected disease have a 90% survival rate. However, for those with metastatic disease, the survival rate is less than 20%. An unusual form of this disease occurs in infants younger than 1 year of age who have metastases limited to the liver, bone marrow, and skin. The survival rate for these children is approximately 80%, even with little or no treatment.

Nephroblastoma (Wilms' Tumor)

Pathophysiology

Nephroblastoma, or Wilms' tumor, is an embryonal neoplasm of the kidney. It is often associated with other anomalies (e.g., hypospadias, hemihypertrophy, and aniridia [congenital absence of the iris]). The tumor occurs bilaterally in approximately 10% of patients, is often familial, and is associated with a deletion at the 11p13 and 11p15 chromosome site.

Clinical Presentation and Evaluation

Most children with Wilms' tumors are 1 to 5 years old. They usually have an asymptomatic abdominal mass. Occasionally, they have abdominal pain, hematuria, or hypertension, but systemic manifestations (e.g., fever, anorexia, weight loss) are much less frequent than in children with neuroblastoma. Metastases are also less common and tend to occur in regional lymph nodes and in the lungs. Wilms' tumors may also invade the renal vein and and extend into the inferior vena cava. Investigations include ultrasonography and CT scans of the abdomen and chest (Fig. 2-27).

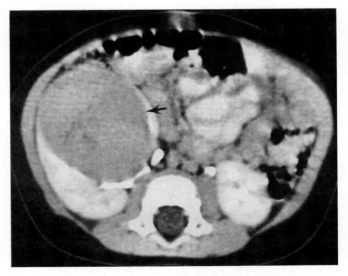

Figure 2-27 Large Wilms' tumor of the right kidney *(arrow)* seen on contrast-enhanced computed tomography scan.

Treatment

Resection of the tumor as a total or partial nephrectomy is the mainstay of treatment. Preoperative chemotherapy is given intially for unresectable tumors. All children receive chemotherapy postoperatively. Radiation therapy is added for those with unfavorable histology, residual tumor, or metastatic disease. Children with bilateral Wilms' tumors usually undergo partial nephrectomies and chemotherapy in an effort to preserve renal tissue.

Prognosis

Survival depends on the stage, size, and histologic type of the tumor, and on patient age. Younger children fare better, and the long-term survival rate for patients with localized tumors is more than 90%. Even for those with extensive disease and unfavorable histology, it is more than 50%.

Teratomas

Teratomas are neoplasms that originate early in embryonic cell division, yet can manifest at any age. It is unclear whether they arise from germ cells or from other totipotential embryonic cells. Teratomas often occur in the gonads or near the midline of the body, where undifferentiated cells might be found. They contain a wide spectrum of tissue types of varying degrees of differentiation, and they may be benign or malignant. Benign teratomas produce symptoms by compressing adjacent organs or by torsion. Malignant teratomas may invade and metastasize.

The most common locations for teratomas in children are the sacrococcygeal region and the ovary. Other sites are the neck, anterior mediastinum, retroperitoneum, testes, and CNS. Operative resection is curative for benign teratomas. Patients with malignant teratomas usually undergo resection followed by chemotherapy, but recurrences and metastases are common.

Sacrococcygeal teratoma is the most common tumor found in neonates. It occurs predominantly in girls and can be massive (Fig. 2-28A,B). It arises from the coccyx and usually has an external component that is covered with skin. It may also have a significant internal portion that extends in front of the sacrum and enters the pelvis. Rarely, the entire tumor is internal, with no visible abnormality. Initial treatment involves surgical resection, which is curative in benign sacrococcygeal teratomas. The outlook for cure and for normal function in these patients is excellent. However, survival after malignant transformation is unlikely. Sacrococcygeal teratomas are increasingly diagnosed in utero. Delivery by cesarean section is recommended for large tumors because rupture with exsanguination can occur during vaginal delivery.

Hepatic Tumors

Tumors of the liver are the third most common abdominal malignancy in childhood, after neuroblastomas and Wilms' tumors. Approximately three fourths of hepatic neoplasms in children are malignant.

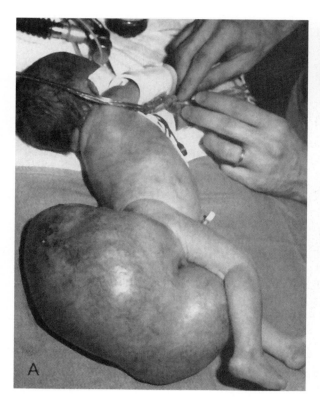

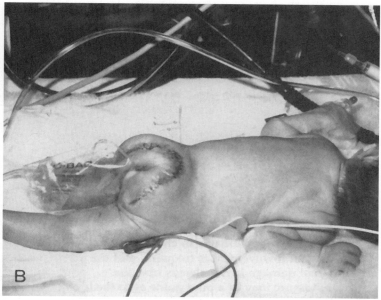

Figure 2-28 **A,** A sacrococcygeal teratoma in a newborn infant displacing the anus anteriorly. **B,** The same infant postoperatively.

Malignant Tumors

The most common malignant tumors are hepatoblastoma and hepatocellular carcinoma. Hepatoblastoma is more common and is found in children younger than 3 years of age.

Patients with liver tumors usually have an abdominal mass that is often associated with discomfort, anorexia, weight loss, and occasionally jaundice. Serum α-fetoprotein levels are usually elevated. Hepatocellular carcinoma usually occurs in older children, is more invasive, and is more often multicentric. Resection is the treatment of choice and may follow a course of chemotherapy if the tumor is initially unresectable. Liver transplantation should be considered for unresectable hepatoblastomas without metastases. The survival rate for patients with hepatoblastoma is more than 50%. It is substantially lower for those with hepatocellular carcinoma.

Benign Tumors

Hemangiomas are the most common benign tumors of the liver in children. Other benign liver lesions in children are adenomas and focal nodular hyperplasia. Hemangiomas appear as dilated vascular spaces and may be solitary or multiple. They are sometimes accompanied by cutaneous hemangiomas and may produce congestive heart failure and platelet trapping. Asymptomatic hepatic hemangiomas are best left alone; many spontaneously regress. Symptomatic lesions can be treated with steroids, embolization, ligation of the hepatic arteries, or surgical resection. Digitalis and diuretics may be beneficial for heart failure.

Rhabdomyosarcoma

Rhabdomyosarcoma is the most common soft tissue sarcoma in children, accounting for approximately 4% of pediatric malignancies. Rhabdomyosarcomas are a diverse group of tumors, derived from primitive mesenchymal cells that may occur anywhere in the body. The embryonal type, found mostly in infants and young children, tends to occur in the genitourinary tract, head and neck, and orbit. The alveolar type occurs in older children and usually involves the trunk and extremities. These tumors invade locally and metastasize by lymphatic and hematogenous spread. The clinical presentation depends on the site of disease, but often consists of an asymptomatic mass. Careful planning, including imaging studies, must be done before the biospy to allow for subsequent excision. Multimodal therapy now allows for much less radical therapy than was advocated in the past. Anatomic location, nodal status, and size are the important prognostic features of this tumor, with overall survival rates ranging from 90% for orbital lesions to 65% for extremity lesions.

TRAUMA

Trauma is by far the most common cause of death in children, accounting for more fatalities than all other causes combined. In addition to the over 10,000 children killed each year in the United States by injuries, over 50,000 are permanently disabled, and 10 million (representing 1 of every 6 children) are temporarily incapacitated and require emergency room evaluation. The cost of these injuries in 1999 was $347 billion, representing 3.8% of the gross domestic product! The automobile is responsible for 50% of accidental deaths in children. Child battering accounts for the majority of homicides in infants, whereas firearms are involved in most homicides in children and adolescents. Burns, firearms, drowning, poisoning, falls, sports injuries, and child abuse are also significant causes of childhood mortality and morbidity. The treatment that young trauma victims receive very often determines whether they survive and if they will have permanent disabilities. To ensure the best outcome, children with serious injuries should be transported to specialized trauma centers. The most effective means for reducing deaths and disability from childhood trauma is by prevention through education and legislation.

Differences in Trauma Care Between Adults and Children

Many of the basic principles of trauma care are the same in children and adults, but there are important differences, as follows:

1 Blunt trauma predominates in children, where there are often multiple injuries and the extent of internal damage is not always obvious on initial evaluation.
2 Hypoxia is the most common cause of cardiac arrest in the injured child; prompt management of the airway and breathing are of the highest priorities.
3 Hypotension is not a sensitive sign for shock. Children can compensate very effectively for hypovolemia by increasing their peripheral vascular resistance. Hypotension develops only after loss of 30% of the total blood volume.
4 Children are more vulnerable to head injury because the head is relatively large and poorly stabilized. The subarachnoid space is relatively smaller and less protective of the brain.
5 Children are at greater risk for hypothermia because of their proportionately larger body surface areas.
6 The young skeleton is quite flexible and more readily transmits applied forces. Children may therefore sustain major internal damage without overlying fractures.
7 Injury to the epiphyseal growth plate can result in growth inhibition and deformity.
8 Gastric distention is more common in children because they tend to swallow air. This may compro-

mise respiration, promote aspiration, or mimic significant intra-abdominal injuries.

9 Children are more likely to have long-lasting adverse psychological problems as a result of the pain, fear, and loss of function that accompany traumatic injury.

10 As a consequence of the difficulty in examining children, the high risk of multiple injuries with blunt trauma, and the success at managing many childhood injuries nonoperatively, imaging techniques have a particularly important role in the evaluation of injured children.

Evaluation of the Injured Child

The first priority of management involves the *primary survey* and ABCs of resuscitation, focusing on life-threatening conditions of the airway, breathing, and circulation. The *secondary survey*, which is a more complete evaluation, then follows.

Primary Survey

The initial ABCs include the following principles:

1 Airway evaluation and maintenance are the top priority. The airway is cleared of blood, vomitus, and debris and positioned so the tongue and soft tissues do not obstruct. A plastic airway or endotracheal tube may be required. Emergency nasotracheal intubation is contraindicated in children under 9 years of age because of possible penetration of the cranial vault; tracheostomy in the emergency setting also has a high incidence of complications. In the rare instance in which an airway is needed and orotracheal intubation is not possible, surgical cricothyroidotomy is recommended in children over 10 years of age and needle cricothyroidotomy in those under 10. (See also the Trauma chapter in *Essentials of General Surgery*, 4th ed, and Chapter 5 in the present volume.)

2 The neck must be immobilized until a cervical spine injury is ruled out.

3 Supplemental oxygen is provided, and breathing is supported by positive pressure ventilation if necessary. A tension pneumothorax should be decompressed immediately by needle aspiration, after which a chest tube is placed.

4 The circulation must be supported. External bleeding is controlled by direct pressure. Large-bore intravenous catheters are inserted percutaneously if possible or by cutdown if necessary. For children younger than 3 to 5 years of age in whom emergency intravenous access cannot be obtained, an intraosseous route below the tibial tuberosity or through the upper femur using a bone marrow or spinal needle is temporarily acceptable for fluid infusion. Blood samples are sent for type and cross-matching, a CBC, and an amylase level. Lactated Ringer's solution may be adminis-

tered rapidly in 20 mL/kg boluses. If the patient does not improve with three such infusions, blood transfusion is indicated and surgical intervention must be considered.

Further resuscitation at this time includes the placement of monitoring devices (ECG, pulse oximeter, temperature probe), a nasogastric tube to decompress the stomach (if there is a risk of cribriform plate injury, the tube may be placed through the mouth), and a Foley catheter to obtain urine for analysis and to monitor the output as a guide to further resuscitation. A contraindication to the insertion of a Foley is injury to the urethra, as evidenced by blood at the urethral meatus or a hematoma at the prostate on rectal examination. Unstable fractures are splinted and open wounds are covered.

Secondary Survey

Following the primary survey and general resuscitation, a more detailed, head-to-toe physical examination (the secondary survey) is completed. X-rays of the lateral cervical spine, chest, and pelvis are usually taken early in the resuscitation phase. Later, films may be obtained of the remainder of the spine, head, abdomen, and extremities, as indicated by the mechanism of injury and findings on physical examination. CT scans are obtained if needed (see later discussion). A decision must be made as to whether an urgent operation is needed or if the patient should be transported to a suitable facility for further support and monitoring.

Head Injuries

Head injury is the major cause of death of injured children. A CT scan provides excellent anatomic definition and should be obtained promptly for any suspected injury. Localized intracranial hematomas require immediate surgical drainage. More commonly, a cerebral contusion occurs that may result in diffuse edema that can raise intracranial pressure and impair brain perfusion. Oxygen delivery to the brain is optimized by maintaining good blood pressure and oxygen saturation and controlling the intracranial hypertension. Intracranial pressure is minimized by hyperventilation to produce hypocapnia (which limits cerebral vasodilation) and by fluid restriction and diuretics (to decrease brain swelling). Continuous intracranial pressure monitoring is helpful. Compared with adults, children have an enhanced ability to recover from severe head trauma (see Chapter 8, Neurosurgery).

Chest Injuries

Although thoracic trauma occasionally requires immediate, dramatic intervention, most injuries to the chest can be managed nonoperatively with chest tube drainage and supportive care. Indications for surgery are massive, continued blood loss or uncontrolled air leaks through chest tubes; pericardial tamponade; and suspected injury to the esophagus, diaphragm, and great vessels. Pericardiocentesis can be lifesaving for tamponade, but should always be followed by operative repair of the underlying cardiac injury. Pulmonary contusions are very common in children following blunt trauma and appear as focal or diffuse infiltrates on chest x-ray, often in the absence of rib fractures. Treatment consists of respiratory support as needed. (See Chapter 4, Cardiothoracic Surgery: Diseases of the Heart, Great Vessels, and Thoracic Cavity.)

Abdominal Injuries

Abdominal surgery following trauma is required for a child with a distended, tense abdomen or free intraperitoneal air on x-ray, because these findings indicate either massive intra-abdominal bleeding or a perforated viscus. In other injured patients, if abdominal injury is suspected, a CT scan is indicated (Fig. 2-29). CT scans can reliably identify intraperitoneal blood, intraperitoneal free air, and solid organ injuries that may be the source of bleeding. A laparotomy is not always necessary for intra-abdominal bleeding; if the child can be stabilized with intravenous fluids and transfusions, close observation with bed rest in a critical care unit is preferred. Diagnostic peritoneal lavage is used only if a CT scan is not available, because the presence of intraperitoneal blood does not mandate an operation. The utility of ultrasonography in children with abdominal trauma is undergoing investigation. Every effort should be made to salvage a ruptured spleen, whether surgery is required or not, because children are particularly susceptible to overwhelming postsplenectomy sepsis.

Urinary Tract Injuries

Trauma to the urinary tract usually produces hematuria, which is an indication to perform a CT scan. Most injuries

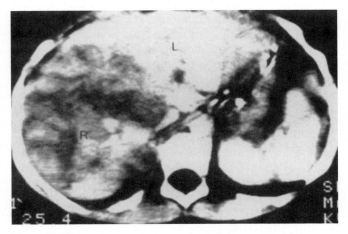

Figure 2-29 A 7-year-old girl with intrahepatic hemorrhage from an automobile accident. A contrast-enhanced computed tomography scan shows inhomogeneity, with irregular areas of low attenuation in the right lobe of the liver *(R)*. The left lobe *(L)* is normal.

are minor and resolve with observation. Surgical repair is necessary if there is any extravasation of urine from the kidneys or bladder and for injuries of the major renal vessels. The presence of gross blood at the urethral meatus requires the performance of a urethrogram to rule out a urethral injury before inserting a Foley catheter.

Burns

After the automobile, burns are the second common cause of accidental death in children. One third of burn injuries are due to child abuse. Major burns produce a profound physiologic insult to the child. The burned individual rapidly develops severe hypovolemia from evaporative loss through the damaged skin barrier and from the seepage of plasma into the tissues through leaky capillaries. There is a marked hypermetabolic state, and multiple organ failure frequently supervenes. Infection is a constant threat. Children with significant burns should be cared for in a specialized burn center. (See the Burns chapter in Lawrence et al., *Essentials of General Surgery*, 4th ed.)

Clinical Findings

Burns are classified according to their depth, as follows:

1 **First degree:** Involves epidermis only and produces erythema, as in sunburn.
2 **Second degree:** Involves partial thickness of dermis while sparing enough epidermal appendages to allow spontaneous healing; characterized by painful blistering.
3 **Third degree:** Necrosis of full-thickness dermis, including the epidermal appendages; skin is leathery with no sensation.

When calculating the percentage of body surface area burns in children, the "rule of nines" used for adults does not apply. The Lund and Browder chart (Fig. 2-30) may be used to estimate burn size according to the age of the child and should include all second- and third-degree burns. Hospital admission is advised if a second-degree burn involves more than 10% of body surface area or a third-degree burn covers more than 2%. Inpatient care is also recommended for significant burns of the hands, feet, face, or perineum and in children under 2 years of age.

Treatment

Minor burns are treated by debridement of devitalized tissue, antimicrobial cream, and occlusive dressings. Intact blisters are generally left alone. The wound should then be washed and dressed once or twice a day at home. Scrupulous care is necessary, because infection can convert a partial-thickness injury into full-thickness necrosis.

Major burns are treated with full-scale resuscitative efforts as for other pediatric trauma. In addition, the burns are cleansed and dressed. Bronchoscopy and pulmonary support may be needed for inhalational injuries. Analgesia

Estimation of Size of Burn by Percent

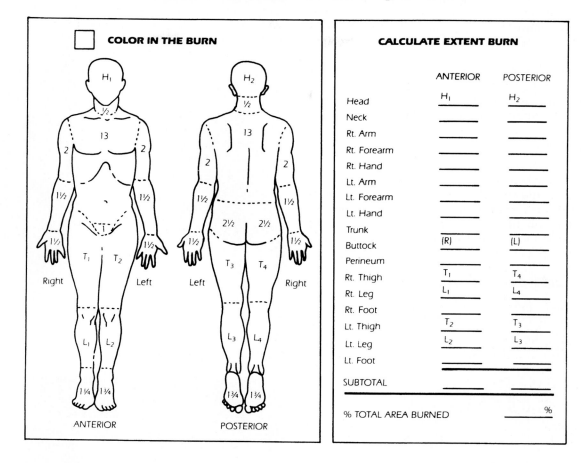

CIRCLE AGE FACTOR

	PERCENT OF AREAS AFFECTED BY GROWTH AGE					
	0-1	1-4	5-9	10-14	15	Adult
H (1 or 2) = ½ of the Head	9½	8½	6½	5½	4½	3½
T (1, 2, 3, or 4) = ½ of a Thigh	2¾	3¼	4	4¼	4½	4¾
L (1, 2, 3, or 4) = ½ of a Leg	2½	2½	2¾	3	3¼	3½

Figure 2-30   Modified Lund and Browder chart, which indicates the proportion of total body surface area of burn according to age and provides for an estimation of burn size; all second- and third-degree burns should be used in the calculation.

should be provided. If the burned, leathery skin constricts and impairs distal perfusion to an extremity or limits respiration, emergency escharotomy is necessary.

Fluid resuscitation should always be adjusted to the responses of the patient. However, several formulas provide initial guidelines. The Parkland formula is as follows:

- Lactated Ringer's solution is administered at 4 mL/kg/ % burn for 24 hours, with half being given in the first 8 hours.
- Colloid is usually started after 24 hours, when capillary integrity is improved.
- Enteral fluids and nutrition are administered as soon as the ileus resolves.

Full-thickness burns are often surgically excised and covered within several days of injury, to restore normal physiology and prevent infection. Coverage may be provided with partial-thickness autografts or temporarily with pigskin. For large burns, multiple staged excisions are necessary.

Rehabilitation may be prolonged and often includes a compressive, elastic garment that is worn for months in order to limit hypertrophy of the burn scar. Psychological problems are common and must be fully addressed.

Child Abuse

The incidence of child abuse is unknown but may be increasing. Certain elements of the history and clinical examination should raise the suspicion of intentional injury. These features are itemized in Table 2-17. The physician must not only treat the injuries medically but must admit the child to the hospital for protection and must contact the proper authorities.

Foreign Body Aspiration and Ingestion

Young children put all manner of objects into their mouths, some of which are aspirated or ingested. Among children under the age of 4 years, aspirated and ingested foreign bodies are among the top four causes of accidental death.

Aspiration

An aspirated object that completely obstructs the larynx will rapidly lead to suffocation unless it is coughed out or promptly removed. A smaller object that passes through the larynx usually lodges in a main bronchus. Complete obstruction will cause atelectasis as air is absorbed distally, and pneumonia often results. In contrast, partial obstruction of a bronchus produces hyperinflation distally through a ball valve effect, as the airway collapses around the object during expiration and excessive air is trapped.

Clinical Manifestations

Choking and coughing may or may not occur. Once these symptoms subside, the patient frequently evidences unilat-

Table 2-17	Child Abuse: Suspicious Clinical Features

History
  Discrepancy between history and physical findings
  Prolonged delay before seeking medical care
  Recurrent trauma
  Inappropriate response of parents to child or to medical advice

Examination
  Child is overly fearful or withdrawn
  Sharply demarcated burns in unusual areas
  Long bone fractures in children <3 yr
  Trauma in genital or perianal areas
  Multiple old scars or healed fractures
  Bizarre injuries (e.g., bites, cigarette burns, rope marks)

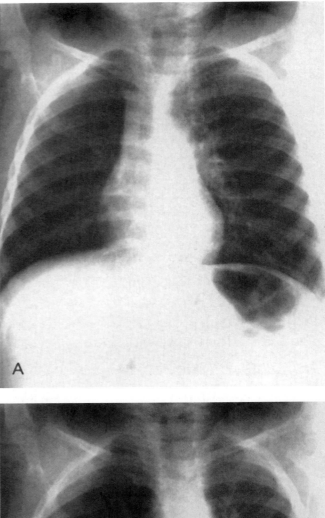

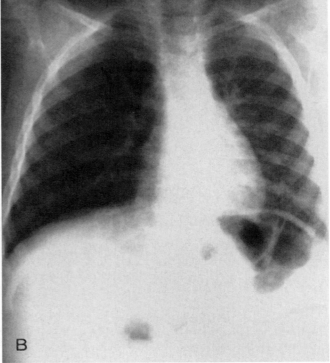

Figure 2-31 **A,** Normal inspiratory chest x-ray of a child with a radiolucent bronchial foreign body. **B,** Expiratory film of the same child, with increased lucency of the right lung and mediastinal shift to the left.

eral wheezing or decreased air entry on the affected side. A chest x-ray will rarely reveal a radiopaque foreign body but often demonstrates hyperaeration of the involved lung or lobe. Expiratory films and fluoroscopy are very helpful, because expiration exaggerates the hyperinflation and produces a mediastinal shift in the opposite direction (Fig. 2-31A,B). Other x-ray findings consistent with foreign body aspiration are persistent atalectasis and recurrent or nonresolving pneumonia.

Treatment

If there is any suspicion of foreign body aspiration, rigid bronchoscopy is performed under general anesthesia and any object identified is removed.

Ingestion

Most foreign objects that are swallowed and reach the stomach will pass unimpeded through the gastrointestinal tract (Fig. 2-32). Weekly x-rays are obtained; if a sharp object remains in the same position for a week, or a blunt object for a month, endoscopic or operative removal is considered. Symptoms of obstruction, perforation, or bleeding are indications for immediate intervention. If the swallowed object is seen lodged in the esophagus on x-ray, there is a significant risk of perforation and extraction, usually by rigid endoscopy, is necessary.

An exception to the above recommendations concerns swallowed alkaline disc batteries, which can leak and cause local necrosis. If they pass beyond the esophagus, expectant observation is still warranted, but if they fail to advance beyond the stomach for 24 hours, or the same area of intestine for a week in spite of purgatives and enemas, their removal is indicated.

Caustic substances may be ingested accidentally by young children or purposely by adolescents in a suicide attempt. Strong alkali (such as lye), which penetrates tissues deeply and produces liquefaction necrosis, predominantly injures the esophagus. Acid causes a surface coagulation necrosis that tends to limit deeper penetration of the esophagus and more frequently damages the stomach. All patients who have potentially ingested corrosive substances require prompt evaluation. For severe injuries, airway control and fluid resuscitation may be necessary. Rarely, emergency surgery is required for peritonitis or mediastinitis, which are indicative of full-thickness necrosis. Otherwise, endoscopy is indicated to assess the degree of injury. Although the approach is controversial, significant esophageal burns are usually treated with steroids and antibiotics. A feeding tube is passed for enteral nutrition and to maintain access through the length of the esophagus if subsequent stricture dilatation is necessary. The rare stricture that is resistant to dilatation is treated surgically by esophageal replacement with either a gastric or colon interposition. Patients who have sustained caustic strictures to the esophagus are at increased risk for later development of esophageal carcinoma.

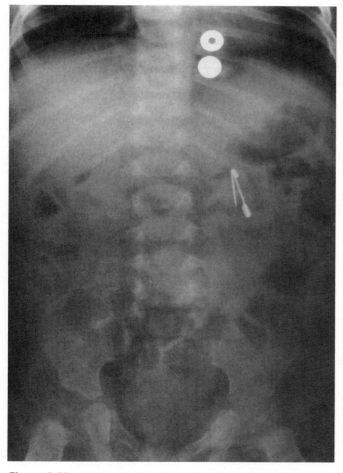

Figure 2-32 Abdominal radiograph of an infant with a swallowed sharp foreign object that passed uneventfully.

SUGGESTED READINGS

Colombani PM. What's new in pediatric surgery. *J Am Coll Surg* 2003; 197:278–284.

Dalla Vecchia LK, Grosfeld JL, West KW, et al. Intestinal atresia and stenosis: a 25-year experience with 277 cases. *Arch Surg* 1998;133: 490–496.

Herrinton LJ, Zhao W, Husson G. Management of cryptorchidism and risk of testicular cancer. *Am J Epidemiol* 2003;157:602–605.

Jain AM. Emergency department evaluation of child abuse. *Emerg Med Clin North Am* 1999;17:575–593.

Mattei P, ed. *Surgical Directives: Pediatric Surgery*. Philadelphia: Lippincott Williams & Wilkins; 2003.

O'Neill JA. Advances in the management of pediatric trauma. *Am J Surg* 2000;180:365–369.

Pena A, Hong A. Advances in the management of anorectal malformations. *Am J Surg* 2000;180:370–376.

Reilly JS, Cook SP, Stool D, Rider G. Prevention and management of aerodigestive foreign body injuries in childhood. *Pediatr Clin North Am* 1996;43:1403–1411.

Swenson O. Hirschsprung's disease: a review. *Pediatrics* 2002;109: 914–918.

Wolf SE, Debroy M, Herndon DN. The cornerstones and directions of pediatric burn care. *Pediatr Surg Int* 1997;12:312–320.

GARRETT A. WIRTH ■ **GREGORY R. D. EVANS**

Plastic Surgery: Diseases of the Skin and Soft Tissue, Face, and Hand

OBJECTIVES

1 Discuss the different types of wounds and their management.

2 Discuss the different types of skin grafts and flaps used in the reconstruction of soft tissue defects, and describe their appropriate applications.

3 Describe the clinical presentation and indications for treatment of benign skin lesions, including nevi, keratoses, hemangiomas, cysts, and lipomas.

4 Differentiate hypertrophic scar and keloid formation from normal wound healing.

5 Describe the initial assessment of a patient with facial trauma and the repair of soft tissue injuries.

6 Describe the evaluation, diagnosis, and treatment of facial fractures.

7 Discuss the examination of the hand and the diagnosis and initial treatment of acute hand injuries.

8 Describe the clinical features and indications for treatment of paronychia, felon, tenosynovitis, and human bites of the hand.

9 Discuss the evaluation and treatment of common tumors of the hand.

10 Describe the development of prepalatal and palatal structures and their relation to cleft lips and cleft palates.

11 Discuss the objectives and different types of post-mastectomy breast reconstruction.

12 Describe the different types of aesthetic operations and their appropriate uses.

The field of plastic and reconstructive surgery is concerned with the reconstruction or improvement of the form and function of many areas of the body. Rarely can either form or function be sacrificed for the other, but one is often of greater concern. This chapter concentrates on recon- structive surgery that is required because of abnormalities of the skin and soft tissues. These abnormalities may be caused by trauma, malignancies, congenital deformities, or other diseases.

Because plastic surgery almost always involves the skin, this chapter begins with a review of the structure of the skin, the process of wound healing, and the reconstruction of large defects. (For a more complete discussion of wound healing, see Chapter 8 in Lawrence et al., *Essentials of General Surgery*. 4th ed.) These discussions are followed by sections on benign skin lesions, facial trauma, hand surgery, congenital deformities, acquired deformities, and, finally, aesthetic surgery. This type of surgery differs from reconstructive surgery because it is directed at the cosmetic improvement of normal structures.

SKIN STRUCTURE

The skin, or integument, is the largest organ of the body and completely envelops its surface. The skin is both the primary defense against the environment and the principal means of communicating with it. The skin also serves important functions in terms of homeostasis and thermoregulation. The integument is an indispensable organ: total destruction of the skin is incompatible with life.

The skin is divided into two embryologically distinct layers: the epidermis and the underlying dermis (Fig. 3-1). The epidermis has five distinct strata, the cells of which all derive from the innermost of these strata, the stratum germinativum, or basal layer. Mitosis of this layer, with transformation of these cells as they migrate outward, forms the other strata of the epidermis. Located within the basal layer are the pigment-containing melanocytes. The epidermis is devoid of vasculature and receives its nourishment from the underlying dermis. Epidermal projections known as rete pegs extend down into the underlying dermis.

The dermis is 15 to 40 times thicker than the epidermis. It is divided into the thin papillary dermis, located beneath the epidermal rete pegs, and the thicker subjacent reticular dermis. The papillary dermis contains reticular and elastic fibers intermingled with a rich capillary network. The reticular dermis contains dense bundles of collagen parallel to the surface of the skin. This layer provides much of the tensile strength of the skin. Also contained within the dermis are pilosebaceous apparatus, eccrine and apocrine units, and important nerve end organs (e.g., pacinian and Meissner's corpuscles).

WOUND HEALING

Wound healing has three phases. The initial (inflammatory) phase is characterized by inflammation around the edges of the wound, a nonspecific reaction to any injury. Leukocytes remove debris and bacteria. Toward the end of this relatively brief phase, activated macrophages appear and direct the next phase. The inflammatory phase lasts approximately 4 days in wounds with little contamination, but may be significantly prolonged in contaminated wounds. The second (proliferative) phase is characterized by collagen production by fibroblasts. Tissue fibroblasts synthesize collagen at an increased rate for approximately 6 weeks in normal wound healing. This synthesis causes a rapid gain in wound tensile strength that peaks at the end of this phase (Fig. 3-2). The third (maturation) phase consists of the remodeling of collagen by the formation of intermolecular cross links. This phase, which lasts 6 to 18 months, leads to a flatter, paler scar, with little increase in tensile strength through a dynamic balance of collagenolysis and collagen synthesis.

Wound healing is classified as healing by primary, secondary, or tertiary (delayed primary) intention. Healing by primary intention involves recent, clean wounds that are managed by suture repair. These wounds are first gently irrigated and debrided to minimize the inflammatory process. Debridement consists of removing foreign material and devitalized tissue. After debridement, the tissue planes are approximated accurately to provide optimal healing. At the peak of collagen synthesis, the scar is mildly inflamed. It is raised, red, and often pruritic. Over time, the scar flattens, thins, and becomes much lighter. The process takes at least 9 to 12 months in an adult and somewhat longer in a child. The final appearance of a scar depends on the initial injury, the amount of contamination and ischemia, and the method and accuracy with which the wound was closed. Wound healing is delayed by multiple factors, including impaired circulation, immunosuppression, infection, or inadequate nutrition. Absorbable sutures are usually used below the skin surface. Nonabsorbable sutures are used for the outer closure because they are less reactive (Fig. 3-3).

Wounds that are left open to heal without surgical intervention heal by secondary intention. This secondary closure is characterized by a prolonged inflammatory phase that persists until the wound is covered with epithelium. Wounds treated in this manner eventually heal, unless factors such as infection and foreign bodies are present. Epithelialization from the wound margins proceeds at approximately 1 mm/day in a concentric pattern. Wound contraction greatly reduces the size of the wound, although it never approaches the final appearance of a primarily closed wound. Healing by secondary intention is indicated in infected or severely contaminated wounds because abscess or wound infection rarely develop in an open wound.

Delayed primary closure, or healing by tertiary intention, involves the subsequent repair of a wound that was initially left open or was not repaired. This method is indicated for wounds with a high ($>10^5$) bacterial content (e.g., human bite), a long time lapse since initial injury, or a severe crush component with significant tissue devitalization. Successful closure depends on the cleanliness of the wound, preparedness of the wound edges, and absence of significant bacterial colonization ($<10^5$ bacteria/g tissue).

Abnormal healing may take the form of **hypertrophic scars** or **keloids**. Hypertrophic scars are raised, widened, and red. They may be pruritic, with tissue remaining within the boundaries of the scar (Fig. 3-4A). Keloids have an abnormal growth of tissue that usually mushrooms over the edges of the wound and extends outside the boundaries of the scar (Fig. 3-4B). Keloids are more common in Afri-

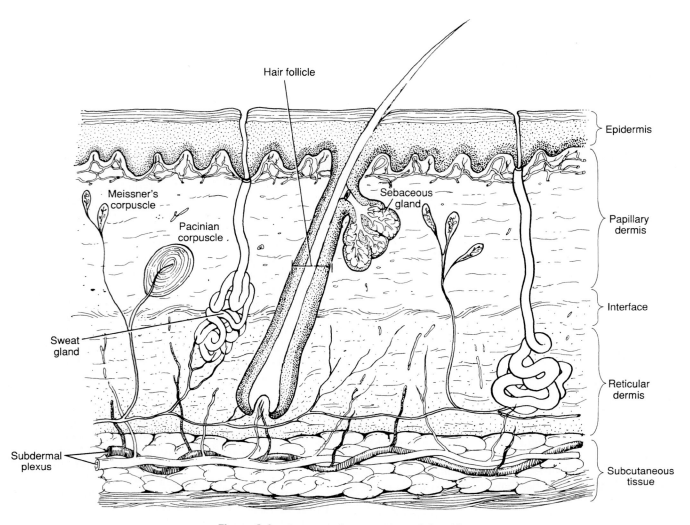

Figure 3-1 Cross-section anatomy of the skin.

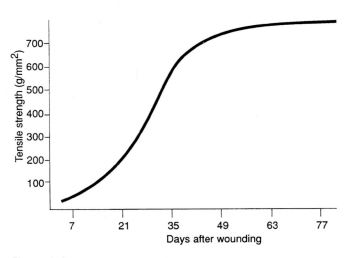

Figure 3-2 Wound tensile strength as a function of days.

can Americans and Asians. Differentiating between the two scars is important because their treatment differs. A hypertrophic scar often improves with time or may be improved by surgical revision. A keloid may be made worse by revision and is treated with intralesional steroids, external pressure, radiation, or a combination of modalities. (For further discussion of wound healing, see Lawrence et al, *Essentials of General Surgery.* 4th ed., Chapter 8, Wounds and Wound Healing.)

Suture Material

Suture material, suture placement, and knot-tying are fundamental elements to a successful surgical outcome. Understanding the properties of suture material and becoming proficient in knot-tying are critical skills for most physicians, not just surgeons. Properly tying sutures requires a great deal of practice. (A review of the various suture materials is provided in Chapter 8 in Lawrence's *Essentials of General Surgery,* 4th ed, Wounds and Wound Healing, Table 8-4, Suture Material.)

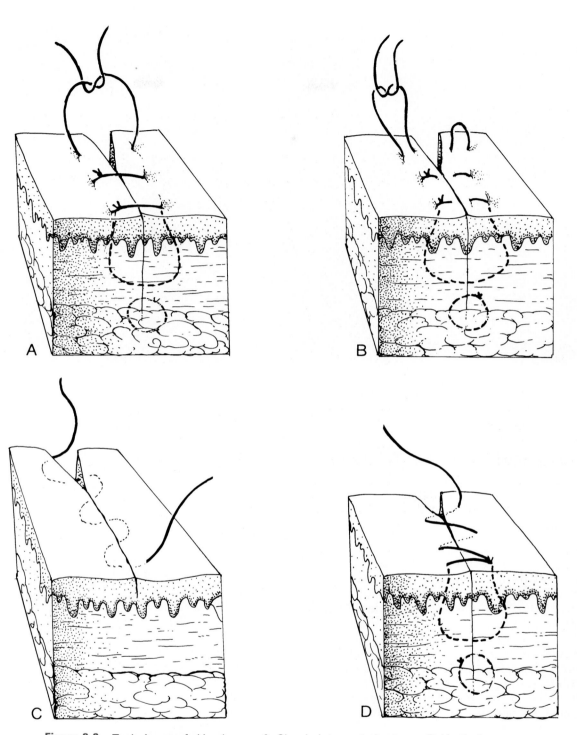

Figure 3-3   Techniques of skin closure. **A,** Simple interrupted sutures. **B,** Vertical mattress sutures. **C,** Running intracuticular (subcuticular) sutures. **D,** Continuous simple sutures.

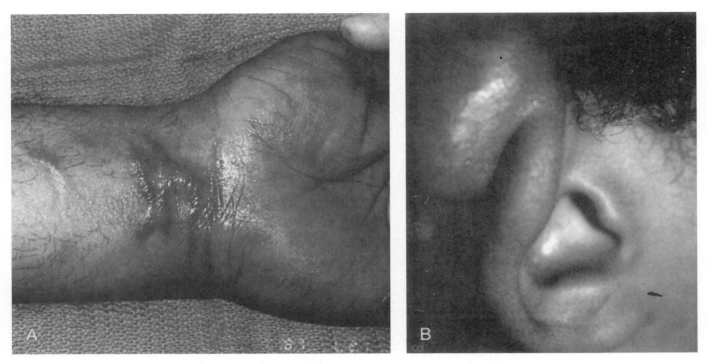

Figure 3-4   A, Hypertrophy of a scar on the volar wrist. The scar does not extend beyond the boundaries of the original scar. **B,** Keloid of a scar of the helical rim. The scar tissue mushrooms out beyond the boundaries of the original scar.

Types of Wounds and Their Treatment

Different wounds have specific causes and treatment guidelines.

Lacerations

Lacerations consist of cut or torn tissue. Care includes gentle handling of tissues. In addition, the wound should be cleansed of clots, foreign material, or necrotic tissue and irrigated with a physiologic solution (e.g., saline, lactated Ringer's solution). Administering a local anesthetic before the final cleansing is helpful. Once cleansed, lacerations are closed with an atraumatic technique, with care taken not to further crush or injure the tissues. Careful closure of wound margins gives the best chance for ideal healing with minimal scarring (Fig. 3-5). Dressings should consist of sterile material that will protect the wound and absorb some wound drainage. Immobilization is helpful in complex extremity wounds.

Abrasions

Abrasions are injuries in which the superficial skin layer is removed. They may be of variable depth. Abrasions should be gently cleansed of any foreign material. Occasionally, more vigorous rubbing with a scrub brush is appropriate. A local anesthetic can facilitate cleansing. Dirt and gravel are removed to prevent permanent discoloration (traumatic tattooing). The wound must be cleansed

within the first day after injury. After this cleansing, an abrasion can be cared for by any method that keeps it clean and moist. The use of topical antibiotic ointment or protective dressings is appropriate.

Contusions

A contusion is an injury that is caused by a forceful blow to the skin and soft tissues. The entire outer layer of skin is intact, although it is injured. Contusions require minimal early care. They should be evaluated early to diagnose a possible deep hematoma or tissue injury. Large or expanding hematomas may require evacuation, particularly if, through pressure, they threaten the viability of the overlying skin, cause vascular or neurologic compromise, or cause airway obstruction.

Avulsions

Avulsions are injuries in which tissue is torn off, either partially or totally. In partial avulsions, the tissue is elevated but still attached to the body. If this raised portion of tissue is adequately vascularized and appears viable, it is gently cleansed, irrigated, replaced into its anatomic location, and anchored with a few sutures. If the tissue is not viable but is still attached, the best approach is usually to excise the tissue and use an alternative method of closure (e.g., skin graft, local flap; discussed later). Completely avulsed tissue usually cannot be directly replaced as a graft because

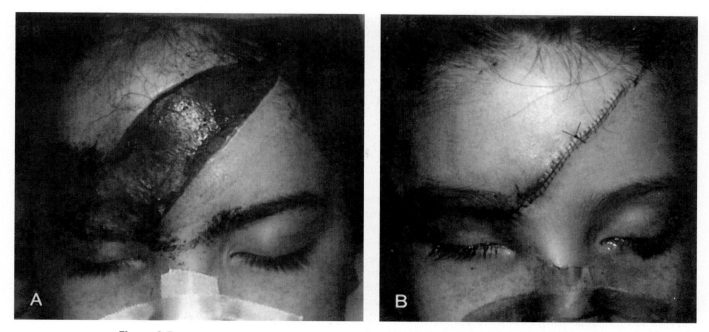

Figure 3-5 Complex laceration of the forehead and eyelid. **A,** Before debridement and closure. **B,** After debridement and closure.

it is too thick to permit reliable healing. In some cases, the skin is debulked, defatted, and used as a skin graft.

Major avulsions (e.g., amputation of extremities, fingers, ears, nose, scalp, eyelids) require specialty evaluation and care. Because replantation of some avulsed tissue is possible if it is handled appropriately, a replant team should be consulted promptly. For appropriate tissue preservation techniques, see the discussion of amputations.

Bites

Bites from animals and humans are a major problem because they are heavily contaminated by bacteria. Although dog bites may be appropriately left open for wound care, most, if handled appropriately, can be closed and heal without infection. Because of their much heavier bacterial contamination, however, human bites should be irrigated, debrided, and left open. In sensitive areas such as the face, thorough debridement and attempted closure may be appropriate. Broad-spectrum antibiotics should also be administered. Human bites to the hand are a special topic and are discussed later. Immobilization and elevation of extremity wounds aid in the healing of these heavily contaminated wounds.

Contaminated Wounds

A contaminated wound is one that has been exposed to bacteria from the body or local environment. The management of acute, significantly contaminated wounds consists of debridement, irrigation, and healing by secondary or tertiary intention. The use of antibiotics is reserved for severely contaminated wounds, wounds in immunocom-

promised patients, contaminated wounds that involve deeper structures (e.g., joints, fractures), and obvious infection. The choice of antibiotic depends on the most likely organisms given the cause of the injury. Broad-spectrum antibiotics with coverage of *Staphylococcus aureus* are usually recommended. Contaminated wounds are closed cautiously, depending on the degree of contamination and the location of the wound. Deep sutures should be kept to a minimum and should be monofilament. Patients with contaminated wounds are reevaluated within 24 to 48 hours. If any signs of deep infection are seen on reevaluation, at least a portion of the wound is opened by removing the sutures.

Contaminated Chronic Wounds

Lacerations and open injuries that are older than 24 hours require debridement and irrigation. With few exceptions, systemic antibiotics are not helpful in controlling bacterial colonization within a contaminated chronic wound. Antibiotic penetration into a chronic wound, with its granulating fibrous bed, is poor and unpredictable. Topical antibiotic cream (e.g., silver sulfadiazine [Silvadene], bacitracin, Neosporin) may be helpful in areas of partial-thickness skin loss. However, some of these topical agents inhibit epithelialization and the initial aspects of wound healing. Highly toxic solutions (e.g., alcohol, hydrogen peroxide) may adversely affect wound healing by destroying normal tissue. Contaminated wounds should be closed only after bacterial contamination is controlled. Chronic wounds that show no evidence of epithelialization or contraction or that are any color but the beefy red of a granulating bed usually have significant bacterial contamination and may be clinically infected. Although the type of organism is important, the principal determinant of wound sepsis seems to be the total bacterial load per gram of tissue ($>10^5$ bacteria/g tissue). Proteinaceous and necrotic debris may also be treated with enzymatic (e.g., collagenase, papain, and urea) as well as surgical debridement.

Wound Management

The initial care of the wound is a major determinant in healing. Methodical assessment of the injury, followed by meticulous closure, minimizes deformity and maximizes the functional result. Evaluation includes an assessment of tissue injury, amount of tissue lost, and degree of injury to deeper structures. Treatment of a wound begins after the patient is evaluated and stabilized. After careful debridement and hemostasis, the injury pattern and tissue deficit are defined before the appropriate reconstructive technique is selected. Bleeding within the wound is controlled by direct pressure. Random clamping of tissue with hemostats should be avoided because it can crush normal tissue or injure other structures (e.g., nerves). Because a tourniquet can increase venous bleeding or cause limb ischemia, it is used only to control life-threatening hemorrhage that cannot be controlled by other means. After bleeding is controlled, the wound is gently irrigated with a physiologic solution (e.g., normal saline).

After the wound is cleaned, the viability of the wound margins is assessed. Clean lacerations have minimal surrounding tissue injury. Contused, contaminated wounds have a crush component of surrounding ischemic tissue. In general, recent, clean wounds without tissue loss can be gently irrigated and closed. However, crushed, contaminated wounds have areas of tissue injury and devitalization that may require debridement and closure, delayed closure, or even the use of skin grafts or flaps to resurface injured areas that have inadequate overlying tissue. Specialized tissues (e.g., eyebrows, eyelids, ears, lips) and other tissues that are difficult to replace precisely should be debrided only by a physician experienced in complicated wound care. Some areas of the body (e.g., face) have a rich vascular supply and tend to heal well. However, the viability of portions of these wounds initially may be in

question. As a rule, any questionable tissue should be gently irrigated and reexamined 24 to 48 hours later. Although contused, crushed injuries predictably have a less favorable outcome, precise reconstruction can optimize the results.

A recent adjunct to wound management has been a vacuum-assisted closure device (V.A.C., Kinetic Concepts, Inc., San Antonio, TX). This device consists of a sponge that is placed in the wound bed, which is then sealed with a dressing and connected to suction. The ability to prescribe negative pressure wound therapy provides multiple benefits for wound management and closure. The V.A.C. system will assist in promotion of granulation tissue formation, aid in removal of interstitial fluid, and uniformly draw wound edges closer together through the use of the controlled, localized negative pressure.

For all penetrating injuries and many nonpenetrating injuries (e.g., abrasions, burns), the patient's tetanus immunization status must be determined. Guidelines for wounds that may be tetanus-prone should be followed (Table 3-1).

RECONSTRUCTION OF LARGE WOUNDS AND TISSUE DEFECTS

Wounds that cannot be repaired by simple approximation of the wound margins often require an alternative method of reconstruction (e.g., graft, flap). When choosing the appropriate method of reconstruction, the concept of a "reconstructive ladder" must be kept in mind (Fig. 3-6). This ladder is a classification of the methods of wound reconstruction in order of increasing complexity. Simpler methods are often best, but they do not always suffice. The different "rungs" of the ladder are discussed in this section (direct closure, where appropriate, was discussed previously under Types of Wounds and Their Management, Lacerations).

Skin Grafts

A skin graft is a portion of the skin (including the epidermis and a variable amount of dermis) that is completely removed from its original location (donor site) and trans-

Table 3-1	Immunization Recommendations				
	Tetanus Prone		**Nontetanus Prone**		
History of Immunization	Tetatnus Toxoid	Tetanus Immune Globulin	Tetanus Toxoid	Tetanus Immune Globulin	
Unknown or incomplete	0.5 mL[a]		0.5 mL[a]	No	
Complete, last booster >5 yr ago	0.5 mL	No	No[b]	No	
Complete, last booster <5 yr ago	No	No	No	No	

[a]In unimmunized children, DT (diphtheria, tetanus) or DPT (diphtheria, pertussis, tetanus) is used. Completion of immunizations is necessary.
[b]Yes, if booster >10 yr ago.

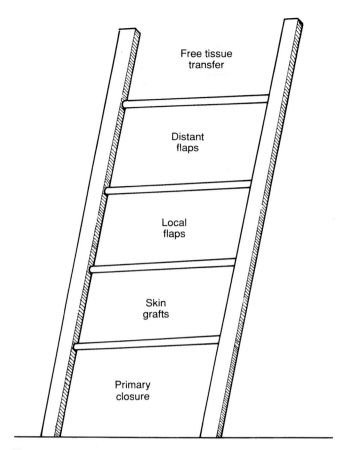

Figure 3-6 The reconstructive ladder.

ferred to another area of the body (recipient site). No underlying tissue is included. Because of its separation, a skin graft derives all of its nutritional supply from its recipient bed. It carries neither vasculature nor any lymphatic or nerve structures. Skin grafts are categorized according to species and thickness.

Species Classification

An autograft is a graft taken from one place on an individual and transplanted to another place on the same individual. Immunologic compatibility is ensured, and the graft is considered permanent. An **allograft** (homograft) is a graft taken from one individual (usually a cadaver) and transplanted to another individual of the same species. These grafts are useful for temporarily resurfacing defects. Rejection eventually occurs, except in cases of transplantation between identical twins or, potentially, in people who are permanently immunosuppressed. The third type of species graft, a xenograft (heterograft), is a graft from a donor of one species to a recipient of a different species. This type of graft, commonly used in clinical practice, entails the use of porcine skin to cover large skin and soft tissue defects on a temporary basis. A variety of new synthetic bilaminar products (e.g., Biobrane, Berthek Pharmaceuticals, Mor-

gantown, WV, or Transcyte, Smith and Nephew, La Jolla, CA) has been developed to assist in coverage of wounds. Although their long-term stability is less than that of autografts, they can serve a significant role for early wound coverage

Thickness Classification

A **split-thickness skin graft** includes the epidermis and a portion of the dermis (Fig. 3-7). The graft includes a variable number of dermal appendages, depending on the thickness of the dermis taken with the graft. The success of the skin graft increases with thinner grafts because less vascular ingrowth is required to maintain their viability. Thinner grafts can also be expanded to a greater degree than thicker grafts. They are used in areas of large skin loss (Fig. 3-8), over areas of granulating tissue, and in areas of marginal vascularity or potential contamination. These grafts are harvested with an air- or electric-powered dermatome or a specialized freehand knife. The donor site, which represents a partial-thickness loss, heals by reepithelialization from wound edges and from residual deeper skin dermal appendages scattered throughout the wound base. The donor site requires ongoing care to prevent secondary infection, which can create full-thickness loss. This care consists of keeping the wound moist while minimizing contamination, pressure, and desiccation. Split-thickness skin grafts are usually taken from the buttock or high thigh area because of the large amount of surface area available and the relatively inconspicuous location. Split-thickness skin grafts have an added benefit in that they can easily be "meshed" with an opertive device at various ratios (e.g., 2:1, 3:1, 4:1). This allows for gentle separtaion of the meshed tissue for greater surface area coverage.

A **full-thickness skin graft** consists of the epidermal layer and the entire thickness of the dermis (Fig. 3-7). In contrast to a split-thickness graft, it provides a more durable form of coverage, its appearance is more normal, and it carries an increased number of dermal appendages. However, because of its greater thickness and slower revascularization, it may be less likely to succeed than a split-thickness skin graft. The absolute thickness may vary according to the thickness of the dermis at the donor site. A thin full-thickness skin graft may be obtained from the eyelid or postauricular areas. Thicker full-thickness skin grafts can be obtained from the cervical and groin areas. Full-thickness grafts are usually used on the face because of their better color match, on the fingers to avoid joint contractures, and at any site where thicker skin or less secondary contraction is desired. Because the donor site is a full-thickness defect, it is managed by either primary closure or split-thickness skin grafting. This factor limits the size of full-thickness skin grafts. These grafts are usually taken from the groin, postauricular area, upper eyelid, supraclavicular area, or scalp. The last four locations are useful for reconstruction in the head and neck because of

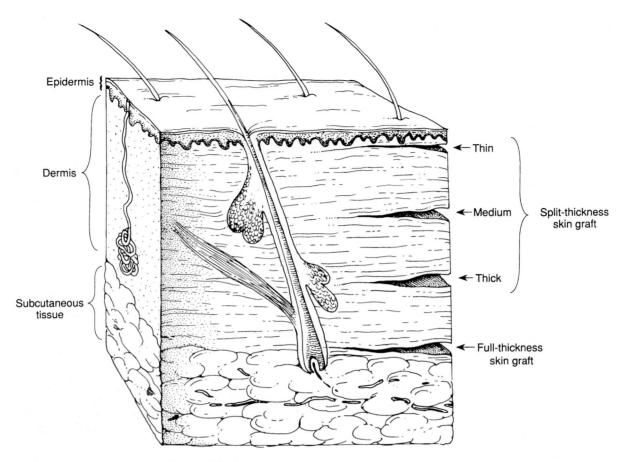

Figure 3-7   Different levels of thickness of skin grafts.

proper color match, but a limited amount of skin is available (Fig. 3-9).

When a graft is harvested, it contracts immediately after it is freed from the surrounding tissue. This primary skin graft contraction is related to the number of elastin fibers in the graft. Thus, the thicker the graft (because of the greater number of elastin fibers it contains), the greater the primary contraction.

Secondary contraction occurs during the healing phase (Fig. 3-9). As healing occurs, the graft contracts to leave a smaller surface area. The thicker the graft, the less secondary contraction occurs. This phenomenon is more closely related to the percentage of dermis in the graft than to the actual thickness. Consequently, a graft that includes 50% of the dermis would be predicted to contract less than a graft that contains 30%. Secondary contraction is mediated by myofibroblasts (specialized fibroblast-like cells that contain smooth muscle contractile elements) within the wound. The dermis suppresses the myofibroblast population. Greater suppression is seen with greater thickness of the dermis.

Contraction must be taken into account when planning reconstruction. Thus, reconstruction of defects or scar con-

tractures may need more graft placed than initially predicted. On the other hand, secondary graft contraction may be used to provide an advantage. A large defect can be surfaced with a thin split-thickness skin graft with the expectation that the total surface area will shrink with the skin graft contraction. A secondary procedure can be performed to excise a portion of the defect and leave a much smaller defect.

Skin Graft Healing

Because the skin graft is completely isolated from its original nutrient source when it is harvested, it must survive initially by diffusion of oxygen and nutrients from the recipient bed. The diffusion of nutritional elements and fluid from the recipient site and the subsequent diffusion back to the host bed of metabolic waste products is called plasmatic imbibition. This process allows the skin graft to survive for the first 48 to 72 hours after placement. Vascular ingrowth begins shortly after the skin graft is placed on the host bed. However, adequate nutritional exchange to maintain tissue viability does not occur until 48 to 72 hours after graft placement. The new ingrowth of capillary tissue

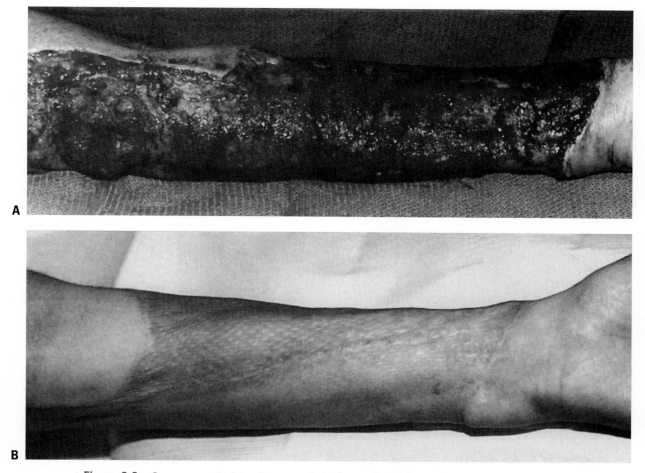

Figure 3-8   Open wound of the forearm. **A,** Before split-thickness skin grafting. **B,** After successful healing of a meshed graft.

Figure 3-9   Comparison of split-thickness and full-thickness skin grafts.

Split-thickness graft	Full-thickness graft
Success higher (more reliable)	Success lower
Less 1st degree contraction	Greater 1st degree contraction
Greater 2nd degree contraction	Less 2nd degree contraction
Donor site heals by reepithelialization	Donor site must be closed
May be used in most wounds	Used in specialized situations

into the graft (neovascularization) is known as inosculation. The recipient bed is prepared by minimizing the bacterial concentration and removing poorly vascularized tissue. Wounds may require debridement at grafting or even several days before grafting. An adequate vascular supply must be ensured, particularly in the compromised extremity. Physical examination is usually sufficient, but Doppler examination or arteriography may be necessary. If local blood flow is inadequate, vascular bypass or another procedure may be necessary. A well-vascularized recipient site, if kept clean, shows signs of local capillary proliferation. The mixture of capillary buds and connective tissue (granulation tissue) is usually beefy red and bleeds easily to touch. In most cases, it forms a good recipient bed for skin grafting, but because it is a chronic open wound, it also supports bacterial growth.

The graft should be immobilized on the recipient site to prevent shear forces from dislodging the tenuous ingrowth of new capillaries. Separation of the graft from its bed prevents both the diffusion of nutrients and the ingrowth of new vascular tissue, resulting in loss of the skin

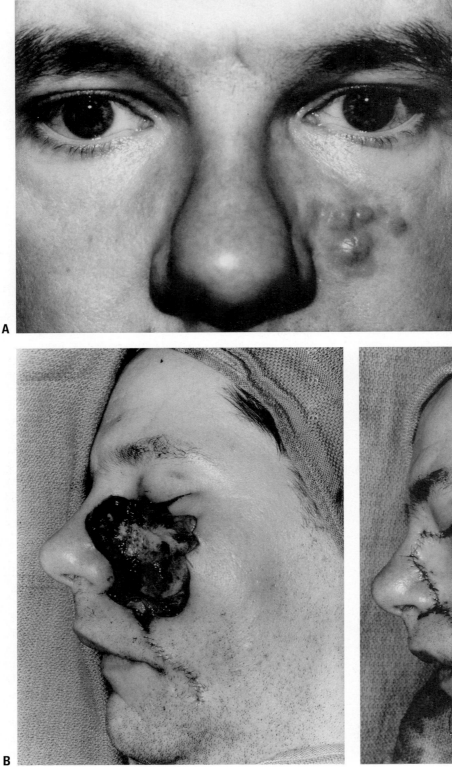

Figure 3-10   **A,** Patient with a dermatofibrosarcoma protuberans of the left lower eyelid and cheek. **B,** After radical resection. **C,** After coverage with a random-pattern skin flap of adjacent cheek and neck skin. The length-to-width ratio of the flap is approximately 1:1.

graft. Because skin grafts require a well-vascularized recipient bed, they do not take on relatively avascular structures (e.g., bone, tendon, heavily irradiated areas, infected wounds). However, skin grafts take well on periosteum, paratenon, and perichondrium.

Graft failure is usually caused by mechanical blockage of diffusion (e.g., hematoma or seroma under the graft), shearing forces that dislodge the graft from its recipient bed, or an inadequate recipient site (because of contamination or poor blood supply). Systemic factors (e.g., malnutrition, sepsis, medications) may also play a role in the success of the skin graft. Systemic steroids, antineoplastic agents, and vasoconstrictors (e.g., nicotine) may adversely affect skin graft survival and wound healing in general.

Flaps

Tissues that are transferred from one location to another and are supported by an intact blood supply are commonly known as flaps. They are typically used to replace tissue that is lost because of trauma or surgical excision. Flaps provide temporary or permanent skin coverage in critical areas that require good soft tissue bulk for underlying structures (e.g., tendons, joints). They also may provide increased padding over bony prominences (e.g., pressure sore reconstruction). They bring a better blood supply to relatively poorly vascularized areas and are occasionally used to improve sensation to an area by bringing in an accompanying nerve supply. In addition, they are used to carry specialized reconstructive tissue (e.g., bone, cartilage). Flaps may consist of skin, subcutaneous tissue, muscle, bone, cartilage, nerve, and such specialized tissues as jejunum, omentum, or fascia. Skin flaps are classified according to their vascular anatomy as random or axial and according to their anatomic location as local, regional, or distant.

A **random-pattern skin flap** is an area of skin and subcutaneous tissue that has no specifically defined vascular distribution (Fig. 3-10). For viability, the flap depends mostly on the random dermal and subdermal plexus of vascular structures. It has a limited length-to-width ratio to ensure that enough blood vessels are included to provide nutrition throughout its length. Random flaps may be raised in any location, assuming normal vascularity of the skin.

A **Z-plasty** is a specific use of random-pattern skin flaps. It involves raising two random flaps in a Z-shape. The flaps are interpolated and then interdigitated with one another (Fig. 3-11). In so doing, two things are accomplished. First, the scar is lengthened at the expense of width. Second, the direction of the scar is reoriented. Z-plasties are often used when scar contractures have developed. Varying the angle of the Z will vary the amount of lengthening of the skin. The normal angles are usually 60 and 120 degrees.

Axial-pattern, or arterialized, flaps differ from random-pattern flaps because they are based on a named blood supply (Fig. 3-12). The underlying vasculature must be well mapped, and the flap outline must be designed to maximize the vascular supply. The vascular supply must include a direct artery and accompanying veins. Specific axial-pattern skin flaps in different anatomic locations take advantage of known cutaneous arteries. Because of this known arterial supply, a greater length-to-width ratio (up to 5:1 or 6:1) is usually possible than with the random flap. Some axial flaps may be used as free flaps (see later discussion).

Tissue expansion is a comparatively new technique that uses the ability of skin to relax and expand as a result of tension applied to it. When local tissue directly adjacent to the wound is the best option for reconstruction (e.g., scalp defects), the two-stage process of tissue expansion is used. An inflatable prosthesis is placed beneath the skin or other tissue to be expanded. After initial healing occurs, the expander is serially inflated through a valve or injection port, usually weekly. When full expansion is achieved, the expander is removed at a second operation. The expanded tissue is used as a local flap to reconstruct the wound (Fig. 3-13).

Composite Flaps

Composite flaps offer another technique for reconstruction. In this technique, multiple tissue types such as skin, fascia, and bone are transferred to allow closure of critical defects with materials similar to those that were lost.

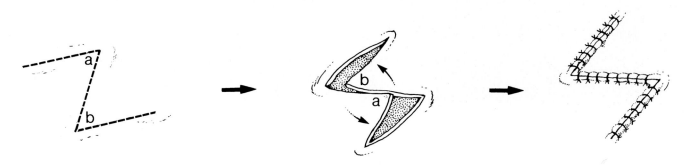

Figure 3-11   A Z-plasty is used to reorient and lengthen a scar (distance *a* to *b*) at the expense of width.

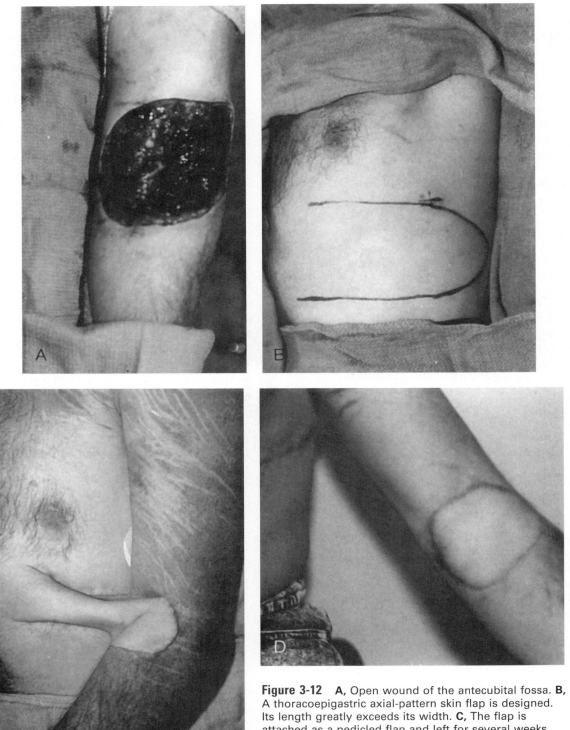

Figure 3-12   **A,** Open wound of the antecubital fossa. **B,** A thoracoepigastric axial-pattern skin flap is designed. Its length greatly exceeds its width. **C,** The flap is attached as a pedicled flap and left for several weeks before the pedicle is divided. **D,** After the pedicle is divided, is inset, and has healed.

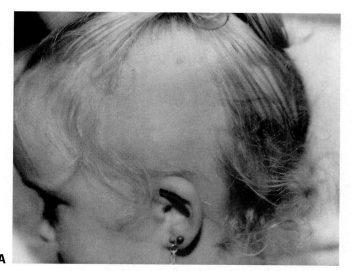

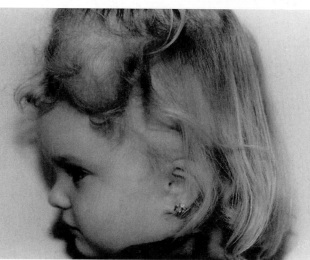

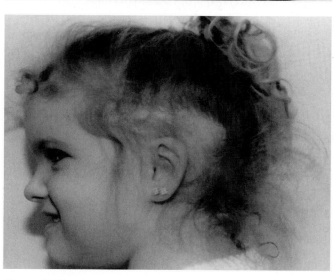

Figure 3-13   **A,** A young patient with a large sebaceous nevus of the scalp. **B,** A tissue expander is placed anteriorly and fully inflated. **C,** Result after resection of the lesion and coverage with the expanded scalp skin.

Myocutaneous flaps are the next most complex type of flaps used for reconstruction (Fig. 3-14). The skin overlying many muscles of the body is supported by vessels that course directly from the muscle to the skin (musculocutaneous perforators). Large amounts of skin left attached to the underlying muscle can be transferred from one location to another as long as the blood supply to the underlying muscle is preserved. Knowledge of the blood supply to these muscles allows rotation or transposition of the tissue from the donor site to the reconstructed wound. The location of the dominant vasculature is used as the pivot point for the arc of rotation. In some cases, a muscle alone is transferred and subsequent skin grafting is performed.

Fasciocutaneous flaps can also be used for coverage. These flaps are similar to myocutaneous flaps, except that the blood suppy to the skin does not course through muscle. Consequently, these flaps provide thin and well-vascularized coverage from a named artery to assist in covering defects.

Flaps Used in Microvascular Surgery

Free flaps raised from a distant site may be used if local skin flaps or regional myocutaneous flaps are not available for wound reconstruction. These flaps are transplanted from one site of the body to another by isolating the dominant artery and veins to a flap and performing a microscopic anastomosis between these and the vessels in or near the recipient wound. Muscle and skin are most commonly used, although bone, nerves, tendons, jejunum, and omentum may also be transferred. Although these flaps may be used in almost any reconstruction situation, they are predominantly used in lower extremity, breast, and head and neck reconstructions (Fig. 3-15).

MANAGEMENT OF BENIGN SKIN LESIONS

Types of Lesions

Skin lesions are either benign or malignant. Differentiation is important in providing appropriate care. Common benign lesions include the **nevus,** keratosis, verruca, fibroma, and **hemangioma.** Common malignant lesions include basal cell carcinoma, squamous cell carcinoma, and malignant melanoma. (Malignant lesions are discussed in Chapter 25 in Lawrence's *Essentials of General Surgery,* 4th ed.)

The nevus is the most common lesion in the adult. It is usually brown and slightly raised, and it may have hair (Fig. 3-16). Nevi are subclassified according to the appearance and depth of active proliferating cells. Dysplastic nevi have the potential for malignant transformation. They have irregular borders and varying shades of pigmentation. It is impractical to excise all nevi, but suspicious pigmented lesions that have had a recent change in size, ele-

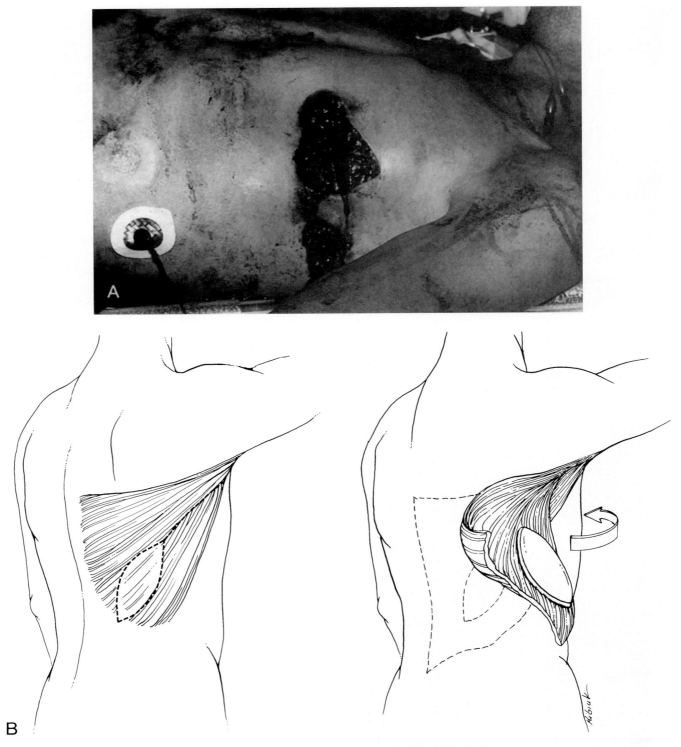

Figure 3-14   A, A patient who had a point-blank shotgun blast to the chest. **B,** The defect is closed with a latissimus dorsi myocutaneous flap. (*continues*)

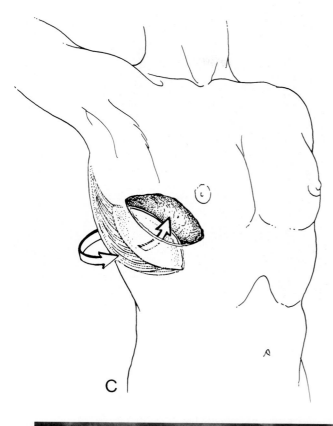

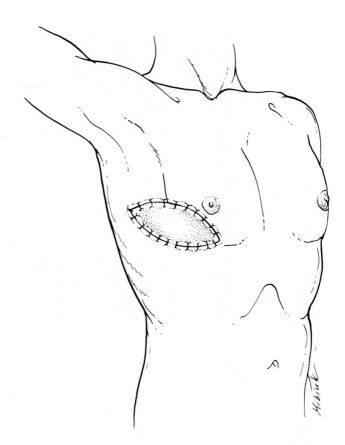

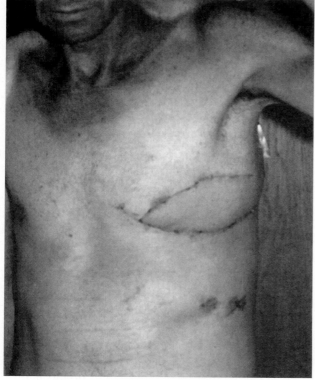

Figure 3-14 (*continued*) **C,** Once the flap is elevated, it is tunneled into the defect on the chest. **D,** The patient after successful reconstruction.

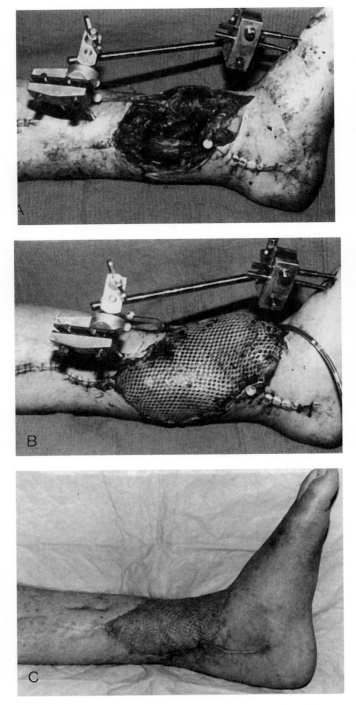

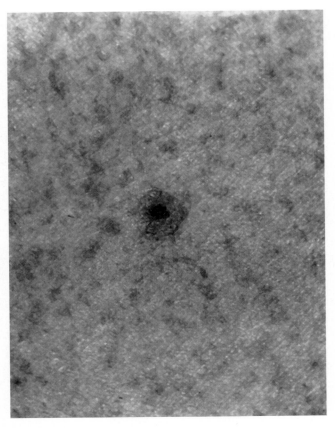

Figure 3-16   Benign nevus.

Figure 3-15   **A,** A close-range shotgun blast to the ankle required external fixation of the ankle and vascular reconstruction. **B,** The ankle immediately after reconstruction with a free muscle flap and a skin graft. **C,** Long-term result showing satisfactory reconstruction.

vation, color (brown to black or gray), or irregular borders (notching) should be excised. In addition, lesions that have a surface discharge, a tingling sensation, bleeding, or itching and those that are constantly irritated (e.g., those under a belt line or bra) should be excised. All significant nevi should be carefully observed.

The second most common type of benign lesion is keratosis. It is subclassified into seborrheic keratoses, actinic keratoses, and **keratoacanthomas.** A seborrheic keratosis is elevated, brown, and has a greasy feeling. It usually has a "stuck-on" appearance and can be treated by freezing, scraping, cauterizing, or excision. If the diagnosis is uncertain, it should be excised. An actinic keratosis is a rough, irregularly shaped, brownish patch, most commonly seen in the elderly. Because these keratoses may be premalignant, some may be removed at the discretion of the surgeon and patient. A keratoacanthoma is a rapidly growing, elevated lesion that may have a central crater or ulceration (Fig. 3-17). It usually resolves spontaneously in 4 to 6 months; however, concern over its growth and appearance often justifies excision for diagnosis.

A verruca (wart) usually has a viral etiology. It is characteristically self-limiting. Spontaneous disappearance after several years is the rule. Surgical excision is occasionally indicated, especially if the lesion occurs on pressure points and is symptomatic (e.g., soles of feet, palms of hands).

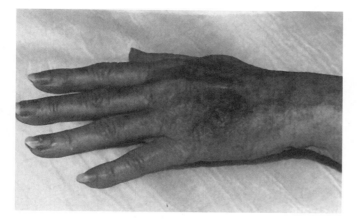

Figure 3-17 Keratoacanthoma of the hand, with a central crater or ulcer.

However, these lesions are usually removed with cryosurgery or laser vaporization. Persistently enlarging lesions may suggest verrucous carcinoma and require surgical excision.

Fibromas are solid lesions. They occur just below the skin surface and may involve skin structures. They are subclassified into fibromas, neurofibromas, and dermatofibromas. Large or symptomatic fibromas should be removed.

Hemangioma is the most common benign tumor of infancy. It consists of an abnormal collection of blood vessels. Several classifications exist based on the likelihood of proliferation or regression. Treatment consists of observation unless these tumors become physiologically or functionally important (e.g., causing visual or airway obstruction, bleeding, or ulceration).

Vascular malformations are the other classification of pigmented congenital lesions. They tend to grow with the child, with no regression being seen. A variety of options exists for these lesions, including laser therapy, embolization, and surgical excision.

Techniques for Excision

In excising small skin lesions or subcutaneous lesions, the goal is to completely remove the lesion while leaving as inconspicuous a scar as possible. Although the surgical technique significantly affects the final appearance of the scar, other factors (e.g., location, size, and orientation of the lesion; overall health; age) also influence the result. A spindle-shaped, or lenticular, incision is made. The total length of the spindle is approximately twice the diameter of the lesion. The long axis of the incision should parallel lines of relaxed skin tension. The incision is made distinctly into the subcutaneous tissue, but should not penetrate into the fascia or deeper structures. Gentle undermining can help decrease tension on the closure. Careful layered closure provides the best result. The specimen should always be sent to the pathologist, even when it appears to be benign.

FACIAL TRAUMA

The patient with facial injuries requires early wound care; accurate diagnosis by history, physical examination, and radiographic studies; and appropriate wound repair and fracture stabilization. Facial fractures should be reduced and stabilized within the first 5 to 7 days. If the patient's condition allows it and evaluation of the facial injuries is complete, early repair is preferable.

If the patient has other significant injuries (e.g., closed head, intrathoracic, cervical spine, or intra-abdominal injuries), medical attention to these injuries takes priority over repair of the facial fractures. However, fixation of facial fracture can be combined with neurosurgical, orthopedic, or other procedures without increased morbidity. This approach allows early or immediate repair of the facial injuries, diminishing the effects of soft tissue contraction, potential infection, and scarring. Secondary revision of facial injuries may be required, but should be delayed until scars mature and fractures heal (6–12 months). Occasionally, skin grafts and flaps are required for large soft tissue defects.

Emergency Care

The initial care of the patient with facial injuries focuses on managing the airway and controlling bleeding. Foreign material and blood are removed from the airway either by hand or by suction. Tracheostomy is seldom indicated when the injury involves only the facial soft tissues. However, for facial fractures, bleeding, and potential cervical spine injuries, cricothyroidotomy or early tracheostomy may be appropriate. After the airway is clear and adequate ventilation is established, bleeding should be controlled. Direct pressure is usually adequate. Dressings wrapped around the face rarely ensure prolonged control of bleeding. Vessels should not be clamped until the injury is adequately visualized because blind clamping can injure important structures (e.g., facial nerve).

After the extent of injury is assessed, the wound is carefully cleansed. All foreign material should be carefully removed. The wound is also palpated or gently explored to detect underlying injury to bony structures. Manual physical examination is the most sensitive means of detecting facial fractures. After initial wound care and hemostasis, the underlying structures can be repaired.

Soft Tissue Defects

As soon as the patient's general condition allows, soft tissue injuries are treated. Ideally, treatment occurs within the first several hours after injury. If the patient's general condition is not good, primary wound closure may be delayed. Because of the excellent vascular supply of the face, facial wounds can be closed up to 24 hours after injury if necessary.

Soft tissue repair of the face requires gentle cleansing,

minimal debridement, and restoration of all available parts. Most injuries cause little or no tissue loss once they are evaluated. The illusion of skin loss is the result of skin elasticity and retraction. Although nonviable tissue should be removed, questionable areas of skin should be replaced gently.

Early, skillful repair of soft tissue injuries provides the best result. Local anesthetics that contain epinephrine are used to allow adequate wound cleansing and hemostasis. After the wound is irrigated and debrided, it is carefully closed. The possibility of injury to deeper structures (e.g., facial nerve, lacrimal apparatus, parotid duct) is considered next (Fig. 3-18). Although rapid assessment of facial nerve function is possible in the awake, cooperative patient, it can be extremely difficult in the multiply injured or comatose patient. Ideally, facial nerve injuries should be identified on initial physical examination so that repair may be planned. Parotid duct injuries should be suspected when a cheek laceration crosses a line from the tragus of the ear to the base of the nose.

Injuries around the eyelids should be carefully evalu-

ated because of the precision of repair required and the possibility of injury to the lacrimal apparatus. Debridement must be conservative in areas as the eyebrows, eyelids, nose, ears, and lips. Because these areas are extremely difficult to reconstruct, it is better to repair questionably ischemic areas, even if a minor revision is required later, than to sacrifice large portions of usable tissue. However, obviously nonviable tissue must be debrided.

Treatment of specific injuries (e.g., abrasions, lacerations) is similar to that in other parts of the body. Lacerations around the lip and other such areas require independent reconstruction of the muscle layers. For most injuries, topical antibiotic ointments are adequate to keep the wound clean and moist. Their antimicrobial component has minimal effect. Systemic antibiotics are not routinely required in facial injuries unless there is massive gross contamination or open injury to deeper structures (e.g., cartilage, bone). Tetanus prophylaxis should always be considered. Sutures are left in place for 5 to 6 days. In significantly contused and crushed tissue, sutures may be left a few days longer. Although the initial injury and the

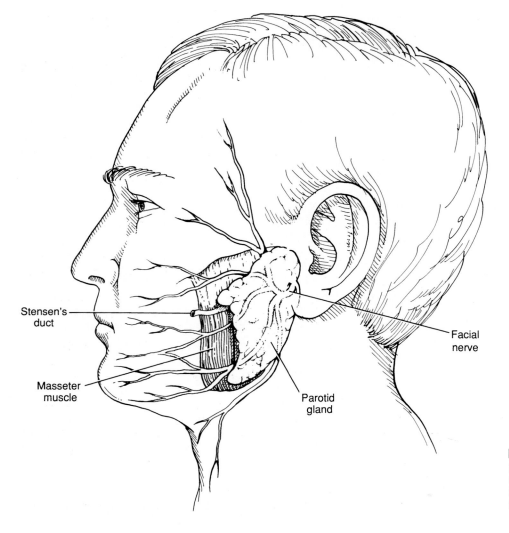

Stensen's duct

Masseter muscle

Parotid gland

Facial nerve

Figure 3-18 Anatomy of the parotid gland showing Stensen's duct and the relation of the facial nerve to the parotid gland and the face.

patient's genetic makeup are the main determinants in the outcome of healing, appropriate initial handling of the wound is also an important factor.

Simple lacerations are appropriately repaired by a generalist who uses careful technique. More complex injuries that involve stellate lacerations, crush injuries, or devitalized or avulsed tissue should be referred to a specialist. Likewise, significant injuries to the eyelids and injuries that involve deeper structures (e.g., nerve injury, parotid duct injury, fractures) require prompt referral.

Facial Fractures

General Principles

Facial fractures are common in patients who have traumatic injuries. Common causes include motor vehicle accidents, assaults, falls, and athletic injuries. These fractures may be open or closed. The overlying tissue may be significantly injured or contused in closed injuries. A history of the injury often indicates the facial area involved. The nasal bone and the zygomatic–malar area are the most commonly injured areas, followed by the mandible and the maxilla. Many patients have multiple facial fractures.

Most facial fractures can be diagnosed based on physical examination, which should include gentle examination and palpation of the facial bones. A fracture is suspected if there is any mobility of facial bones, asymmetry, palpable bony step-offs, extraocular muscle irregularities, sensory loss, localized pain or tenderness, or malocclusion of the teeth. This examination should be followed by radiographic evaluation after the cervical spine is cleared. Of patients with significant facial injuries, 15% to 25% have concomitant cervical spine injuries. The possibility of skull fracture and intracranial injury is also evaluated.

X-ray evaluation consists of a complete facial bone series, which includes the Water's, anterior–posterior, and lateral views. The Water's view, an oblique anterior–posterior projection, shows most clearly the entire facial complex and is most helpful. Currently, however, computed tomographic (CT) scans in both the axial and coronal planes are the most accurate method of visualizing complex fractures. Three-dimensional CT scans or reconstructions are available in many centers. However, they add little to the acute management of facial fractures over what can be learned from routine CT scans. Mandibular x-ray evaluation is best obtained with the Panorex (panoramic x-ray) view. This specialized x-ray is superior to plain films of the mandible. However, in most facilities, the patient must be upright, a difficult position for the patient with multiple injuries.

After facial fractures are identified, the urgency of their treatment is assessed. Urgency depends on the likelihood of continued bleeding, cerebrospinal fluid (CSF) leak, or loss of airway because of shifting oropharyngeal structures. Early consultation with all services that treat facial fractures should be made. If the patient is stable and treatment is not urgent, repair of the facial fractures may be appropri-ately delayed for up to 5 to 7 days without adverse effects. This interval allows adequate time for evaluation and treatment of other injuries and for reduction of facial edema. CT scan examination can also assess and evaluate mandibular injury.

The principal goal of facial fracture reconstruction is the restoration of normal (premorbid) function and appearance. This goal is achieved by precise, anatomic reconstruction of all fractured bone segments, usually by open reduction and internal fixation. Although closed reduction may be adequate for simple fractures, internal fixation with interosseous wires or with plates or screws is usually performed. The bony pieces should be replaced if possible into the defect. If these bony fragments are unusable, immediate bone grafts should be considered, providing there is adequate soft tissue surrounding the structures.

Mandibular Fractures

Mandibular fractures often occur in facial trauma. They are rarely isolated to one location. Because of the ring structure of the mandible, 94% of patients with mandibular fractures have associated fractures in a second area of the mandible. When sufficient force is applied at one point to produce a fracture, a second fracture site is likely because the force is transmitted to the entire ring. Some regions are more commonly associated with multiple fractures (Fig. 3-19). Fractures of the mandibular condyle are often associated with fractures of the symphysis and the corresponding condyle on the contralateral side. Mandibular body fractures are associated with fractures of the contralateral mandibular angle.

The classification of mandibular fractures is similar to that of long bone fractures. Closed fractures show no break in the overlying skin or mucosa. Open, fractures, extremely common in the mandible, involve an external or internal (intraoral) wound associated with the fracture site. Although the overlying skin may not be broken, fractures into the tooth-bearing area are essentially open and should be treated as such. Alveolar or dentoalveolar fractures involve the alveolar process, but no other portions of the main body of the bone. These fractures are more common in the maxillary than in the mandibular area. Multiple fractures are common. (Anatomically, most adult mandibular fractures occur in the condylar area. The mandibular body in the molar region is the next most common location, followed by the angle of the mandible.)

Dislocation of the mandibular condyle is occasionally seen and may be unilateral or bilateral. Signs are inability to close the jaw, malocclusion, and pain. The dislocation is reduced by pressing downward on the mandible and sliding it posteriorly into position. Because the muscles of mastication (primarily the masseter and temporalis) quickly go into spasm, reduction may require sedation and occasionally general anesthesia. Recurrence is common.

Evaluation

The first priority in evaluating the patient with a mandibular fracture is assessment of the airway. Manual displace-

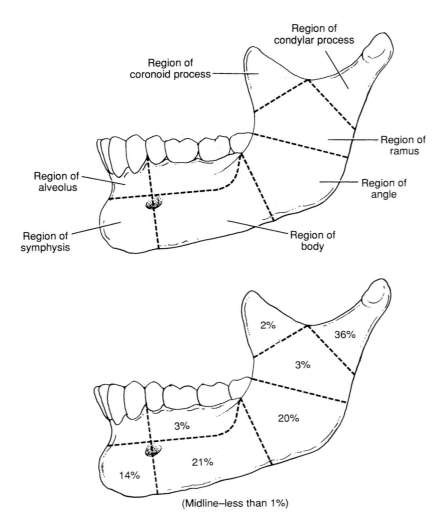

Figure 3-19   **A,** Anatomy of the mandibular regions. **B,** Frequency of fractures by mandibular region.

ment of the mandible forward usually relieves obstruction by the tongue. In some cases, emergent definitive airway management is needed. Routine complaints include alteration of normal **dental occlusion,** abnormal position of the teeth, and abnormal mobility of the mandible. Manual palpation shows disjointed movement of the mandible and some separation between mandibular fragments. Patients almost uniformly have pain. The presence of crepitus because of the fracture is unusual in mandibular fractures, but is virtually pathognomonic of a fracture. Patients may also have lacerated gingiva or mucosal ecchymosis. Occasionally, patients have anesthesia in the lower teeth secondary to injury or contusion of the inferior alveolar nerve.

Fractured mandibles are usually displaced. Appreciation of the normal pull of the muscle of mastication can be used to predict motion of the mandibular fragments. By evaluating the location of the mandible fracture and the angle of the fracture, and taking into account the location of muscle insertion and the vector of pull, it is possible to accurately predict the direction of displacement and estimate the ultimate stability of the fracture. If the normal muscle pull tends to reduce the mandibular fracture, the

fracture is favorable. If the normal muscle pull tends to distract the bony fragments, the fracture is unfavorable. This distinction can be helpful in determining whether a closed reduction is adequate or an open reduction is needed.

Treatment

Treatment methods include closed reduction (maxillo-mandibular fixation [MMF]), open reduction with internal fixation, and external fixation (primarily used for infected wounds or for significant loss of bony segments). A minimally displaced fracture can be treated by closed reduction (wiring the teeth together into normal occlusion). Good dentition, with reliable and stable occlusion, is necessary for this type of treatment. This method involves the placement of maxillary and mandibular arch bars that are wired or banded together in interdental fixation. In adults, 4 to 6 weeks of fixation is necessary; 2 to 4 weeks is necessary in children. Open reduction, with direct visualization of the fractures and wiring or plating in some configuration, is often necessary. This method provides better approximation of the fracture site. In addition, internal fixation prevents displacement and movement of the fracture, which provides more precise restoration of occlusion. Open reduction is accomplished either extraorally (through a neck incision) or intraorally. Interdental fixation is almost always used with internal fixation methods to help with fracture alignment. The concept is to align the fractured bone with stable, unfractured bone. This allows a stable platform to build on for fixation of the fractured segments. The open technique has a higher incidence of infection (4%–5%) than the closed technique. However, it allows earlier mandibular movement, with reduced morbidity from immobilization because of tightening of the muscles of mastication. External fixation with an external appliance may be used in complicated fractures, severely infected fractures, or fractures with significant bone loss.

During the period of interdental fixation, attention to oral hygiene is necessary. Although it is difficult to brush the teeth normally, frequent cleansing with a pulsatile water hygiene device and the use of mouthwash can be very helpful.

Complications

Mandibular fractures may have multiple complications. Delayed healing occurs in the presence of inadequate or loosened fixation, an infection, or a fault in the reduction and fixation technique. Loosened fixation is associated with initially poor technique, poor patient compliance, or secondary infection. Malunion is caused by lack of adequate treatment or lack of patient compliance with proper oral hygiene and wound care. Malunion essentially allows healing to take place in a nonanatomic position. It causes significant functional difficulty because of the resultant malocclusion. Malunion may require further surgery. Nonunion is caused by delayed healing, which often occurs secondary to inadequate fixation or infection. Nonunion may require secondary bone grafting, external fixation, or bone transport.

Special Cases

Mandibular condyle fractures deserve separate consideration. Patients routinely have tenderness and pain in the preauricular area. The mandible may deviate toward the fractured side on opening because of pterygoid muscle function. Mandibular movement is limited, and there may be malocclusion and preauricular swelling. On examination, there is pain on palpation of the anterior wall of the external auditory canal. Occasionally, hemotympanum or external auditory canal laceration is noted. (Radiographically, a Panorex view is the best diagnostic tool. CT scan is rarely helpful in evaluating a difficult mandibular fracture.)

Treatment of mandibular condyle fractures is usually by closed reduction, which is accomplished by interdental fixation with the patient in correct occlusion. When adequate occlusion cannot be obtained by closed reduction, open reduction of the condylar fracture is indicated. Complications of mandibular condyle fractures include ankylo-

sis, temporomandibular joint dysfunction, limited postoperative motion, malocclusion, occasional sequestration of a dislocated fragment, and chorda tympani nerve damage (especially with dislocation). In children, aseptic necrosis, with disruption of mandibular growth, may occur. Rarely, seventh nerve paralysis occurs in association with open reduction.

Edentulous patients with mandibular fractures present a therapeutic problem. Signs and symptoms are the same as for patients with dentition. However, bilateral body fractures are more common because of the atrophy of the mandibular segment in that area. Edentulous patients also have a much higher incidence of nonunion because of poor bone stock and decreased strength of the small atrophic mandible.

Zygomatic Maxillary Complex Fractures

The anatomy of the zygomatic and orbital regions has several important features. The orbit is composed of the maxilla, lacrimal, frontal, sphenoid, palatine, zygoma, and ethmoid bones. The orbital rims are composed of a confluence of bones that is relatively strong. By comparison, the floor and walls of the orbit are composed of bone that is thin and easily fractured. The eyelids are attached by ligaments at the medial and lateral canthi. The lateral canthal ligament is attached to the zygoma, and the medial canthal ligament is attached to the lacrimal bone. Each canthus may be displaced by certain fractures. The orbit also contains (and protects) many important structures. Cushioned within a layer of periorbital fat are the globe, optic nerve, ophthalmic artery, extraocular muscles, and their accompanying nerves. Injury to these structures in specific fractures is not uncommon.

Evaluation

Periorbital injuries and fractures are extremely common (Fig. 3-20). Patients routinely have chemosis (subconjunctival hematoma), which causes a ballooning effect of the conjunctiva and swelling over the cheek area. Palpation, however, shows flatness of the cheek bones (malar eminence) on that side. The injury may be missed if the examiner is unaware that overlying edema tends to mask this depression. Patients may have limited mandibular opening because the depressed zygomatic arch impinges on the temporalis muscle as it inserts on the choronoid process of the mandible. These patients may have anesthesia in the distribution of the infraorbital nerve, which traverses the floor of the orbit. Oblique canting of the eye may be caused by depression of the lateral palpebral fissure because of displacement of the lateral canthus (Fig. 3-21). Periorbital edema and ecchymosis are also present. Careful evaluation may show **enophthalmos**, diplopia (secondary to entrapment of periorbita), and step-offs at the inferior and lateral rims. The patient should be examined for intraoral buccal ecchymosis. Limitation of gaze in multiple planes is associated with corresponding entrapment of orbital contents. Loss of integrity of the orbital floor may

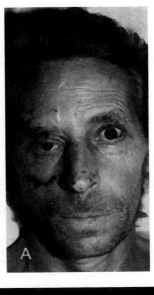

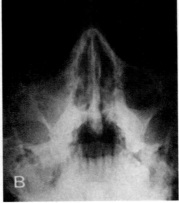

Figure 3-20   **A,** Grossly displaced right zygomatic maxillary complex fracture. **B,** X-ray showing the fracture lines and clouding of the right maxillary sinus.

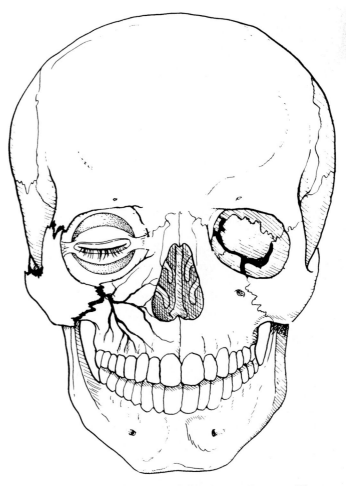

Figure 3-21   Zygomaticomaxillary complex fracture. The fracture through the infraorbital rim extends through the infraorbital foramen, where it can injure this sensory nerve.

allow herniation of orbital contents into the maxillary antrum, with downward displacement of the globe.

The patient should be evaluated with routine facial x-rays, which often show separation of the frontozygomatic suture, fractures or fragments of the lateral maxilla, orbital-rim discrepancies, and opacification of a maxillary sinus. Unilateral opacification of a maxillary sinus is considered a presumptive sign of a facial fracture until proven otherwise. A submental vertex view is important because it may show depression of the zygomatic arch. CT scans in the axial and coronal planes most clearly define the location of fractures.

Treatment

Treatment of zygomaticomaxillary complex fractures usually requires open reduction with internal fixation of the fracture segments at several locations. Orbital floor exploration may be necessary to rule out floor fracture. The infraorbital nerve is commonly contused. Consequently,

there is some anesthesia to the area of its distribution. Return of sensation may take several weeks or months, although in some cases, anesthesia of varying degrees may persist. However, this nerve is rarely lacerated.

Complications

Because of the possibility of ocular injury in any significant facial injury, ophthalmologic evaluation and consultation should be sought if an injury is suspected. Blood observed in the anterior chamber or retrobulbar hematoma, usually diagnosed by proptosis of the globe, occasionally occurs and should be treated immediately. In addition, the optic nerve may be involved, and loss of vision may occur. The presence of any of these symptoms requires immediate ophthalmologic consultation. Residual entrapment of orbital contents may occur after treatment. If residual entrapment occurs, reexploration is required. Late **enophthalmos** can occur and may be secondary to atrophy of periorbital fat with retrusion of the intraorbital structures. Surgical correction depends on the symptoms. It is crtical to assess vision before any type of reduction. Visual changes following surgery can occur because of bone fixation. Immediate evaluation is critical in order to prevent permanent injury.

Orbital Blow-Out Fractures

A **blow-out fracture** of the orbit is a relatively common fracture complex. It is an isolated fracture of the orbital floor. A segment of the orbital floor and a portion of the periorbital contents are displaced downward into the maxillary sinus, with or without extraocular muscle entrapment. In a pure blow-out fracture, there is no infraorbital rim fracture. However, a blow to the globe may transmit force to the orbital floor, causing the thin bone to break. Alternatively, a blow to the orbital rim may momentarily deform the rim, causing the floor to buckle and break without fracturing the rim. Either mechanism causes the floor to fracture into the maxillary antrum, creating a blow-out of the orbital region.

Evaluation

The patient may present with decreased extraocular muscle function and some diplopia. Evaluation may be difficult because of surrounding swelling, edema, and ecchymosis. There may be some evidence of enophthalmos, and anesthesia of the infraorbital nerve and some inequality in pupil height may be noted. Because these findings are relatively mild in most cases, radiographic confirmation is usually indicated. Plain radiographs rarely show any findings other than clouding of the maxillary sinus. CT scans more accurately show fractures (Fig. 3-22).

Treatment

Operative treatment of orbital floor fractures depends on the associated symptoms. Patients with minimal orbital floor fractures and who are asymptomatic or who report transient diplopia require no treatment. However, persistent diplopia, enophthalmos, displacement of the globe into the maxillary sinus, and a large fracture seen on CT scan are indications for operative repair. This repair involves exploration of the orbital floor, reduction of periorbital contents back into the orbit, and reconstruction of the orbital floor with bone grafts (usually autogenous cranial bone, rib, or allogeneic rib) or prosthetic materials (e.g., vitallium, titanium mesh, or resorbable plates). Long-term complications are usually posttraumatic enophthalmos or diplopia, especially if the fracture was inadequately treated.

Nasal and Nasoethmoidal Fractures

The nasal bone is the most commonly fractured bone of the face because of its relative weakness and prominent position. The thin nasal bones fuse laterally with the frontal process of the maxilla and superiorly with the frontal bone. Internally, the perpendicular plate of the ethmoid articulates posteriorly with the sphenoid and the vomer.

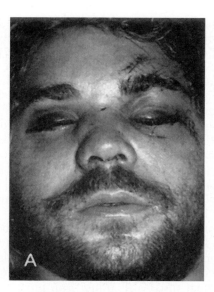

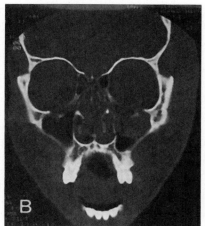

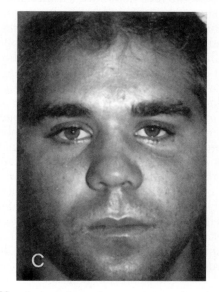

Figure 3-22   A, A patient who was beaten in an assault. **B,** Coronal computed tomography scans show bilateral orbital floor (blow-out) fractures. **C,** Only the left orbital floor fracture was symptomatic and required reconstruction.

In addition, the cartilaginous skeletal anatomy consists of upper lateral, lower lateral, septal, and accessory cartilages.

Evaluation

The mechanism of injury affects the nature of the fracture. Anterior blows usually produce a comminuted fracture, with flattening of the bridge or telescoping (shortening) of the nose. Lateral blows depress the affected side and cause a convex deformity on the other side. Patients always have significant swelling, which may make precise examination of nasal deformities difficult. **Epistaxis,** facial asymmetry, nasal airway obstruction, and periorbital ecchymosis are usually signs. However, crepitus over the nasal bones and septal hematomas are not uncommon.

Nasoethmoidal fractures cause all of the above symptoms as well as telecanthus (increase in the inner canthal distance) and severe depression of the nasal bridge, usually with telescoping of the nasal bones and fractures of the inferior orbital rims. CSF rhinorrhea, pneumocephalus, or anosmia may also be present. Simple nasal fractures are best evaluated by physical examination alone. Nasoethmoidal fractures require visualization by CT scans. Comparison of the patient's appearance with previous photographs is helpful in determining the extent of deformity.

Treatment

Treatment of nasal fractures can rarely be achieved early because of the amount of edema that rapidly develops. After the edema resolves (usually 3–4 days), operative repositioning of the nasal bones, or closed reduction, may be achieved. Delays of longer than 10 days make closed reduction difficult. Septal hematomas should be drained immediately, because undrained hematomas may produce pressure necrosis of the septum or such secondary problems as saddle nose deformity. Further description of septal hematoma can be found in the chapter on otolaryngology in this book. Repositioning of the nasal septum may be required. The nasal bones are usually stabilized with external splints and internal packs. Patients who have obvious nasal deformities and minimal or no acute swelling may have old nasal fractures that cannot be treated with closed reduction.

Nasoethmoidal fractures usually require open reduction and internal fixation. Although a number of approaches are used, the best is through a bicoronal incision that allows exposure of the glabellar, medial canthal, and superior orbital regions. Significant lacerations also may be used as an approach to the fractures. The goal of fixation is to reestablish or repair the nasal pyramid, medial canthal region, medial orbits, and normal restoration of the intercanthal distance. Interosseous wiring, plate-and-screw fixation, transnasal wiring of the medial canthal ligaments, and immediate bone grafting may be used.

Complications

Postoperatively, nasal and nasoethmoidal fractures may be complicated by residual nasal and septal deformities, with resultant nasal airway obstruction. Deformities of the medial canthi are common. They are usually caused by inadequate treatment and produce telecanthus, which requires secondary correction. CSF rhinorrhea may complicate more significant fractures. This rhinorrhea usually ceases after adequate fracture fixation, but complex neurosurgical procedures are occasionally needed. Damage to the lacrimal apparatus is common and is repaired secondarily.

Maxillary Fractures

Maxillary fractures may be subdivided according to the **LeFort classification.** Although not all fractures fit this classification, it remains useful.

LeFort I Fractures

A LeFort I fracture is a transverse fracture that extends through the maxilla and pterygoid plates above the floor of the maxillary sinus (Fig. 3-23A). The etiology is usually traumatic and most commonly involves a central midline blow. The patient has consistent findings of malocclusion and mobility of the maxilla. On examination, patients have ecchymosis in the buccal vestibule, some crepitus in the maxillary area, and false motion of the lower maxilla, with stability of the upper nose and orbits. Patients occasionally have airway obstruction, noticeable lengthening of the face, nasal septal deformities, and paresthesia in the distribution of the infraorbital nerve. The patient should be evaluated by routine facial x-rays and CT scans if appropriate.

Treatment of LeFort I facial fractures involves establishing the mandible as a foundation on which to base other repairs. Therefore, mandibular injuries are usually repaired before maxillary injuries. In most cases, intermaxillary fixation, with or without internal plate fixation, provides sufficient reduction and stabilization. Bone grafts may also be needed if severe comminution is present. Complications of LeFort I facial fractures often include malocclusion, paresthesia, nasal septal deformities, and facial asymmetry.

LeFort II Fractures

A LeFort II fracture is a zygomatic midfacial fracture with a floating, pyramid-shaped fragment (Fig. 3-23B), from which the term "pyramidal fracture" is derived. The central portion of the face is free-floating, but the lateral orbits and cranium are stable. The patient has flattening of the naso-orbital region and mobility across the nasal bridge. **Epistaxis** is common. The maxilla is mobile and moves with the nasal bridge and the medial component of the inferior rim. The lateral orbital rim and forehead remain stable. Open-bite deformities and malocclusion are also common. Palpation along the orbital rims and nasofrontal areas usually shows step deformities. CSF leaks are relatively common. The patient may also have some lengthening of the midface and paresthesia of the infraorbital nerve. Diplopia and decreased intraocular muscle function may occur when there is significant disruption of the orbital floor. Although most fractures are diagnosed on physical examination, a CT scan is usually indicated.

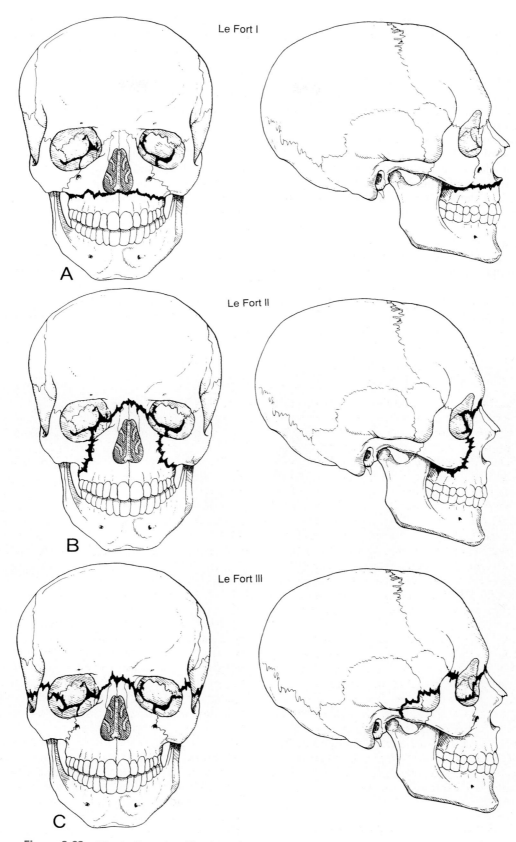

Le Fort I

Le Fort II

Le Fort III

Figure 3-23   The LeFort classification of maxillary fractures. **A,** LeFort I fracture. **B,** LeFort II fracture. **C,** LeFort III fracture.

Treatment involves restoration of the anatomic configuration and structure. Intermaxillary fixation is performed after stabilization of mandibular fractures. Direct fixation in the areas of the lateral maxilla, infraorbital rim, and nasofrontal angle is achieved with plate-and-screw fixation, which allows early motion and release of intermaxillary fixation. Bone grafts are used, if necessary, in cases of severe comminution or bone loss.

Basic complications of the LeFort II facial fracture are the same as those of the LeFort I fracture. If the fracture is incorrectly or inadequately corrected, the midface might be lengthened. There is a higher incidence of orbital injuries, CSF leaks, nasal deformities, and midface abnormalities involving the lacrimal system.

LeFort III Fractures

A LeFort III fracture is a severe fracture that completely separates the midface from the upper face (craniofacial disjunction) (Fig. 3-23C). Signs and symptoms of LeFort III fractures are similar to those of LeFort II fractures, with additional signs associated with basilar skull fractures. De-

pressed zygomatic arches are often found, with the inferior orbital rims intact. Relatively common findings are **Battle's sign** (ecchymosis in the mastoid region), bilateral orbital ecchymosis (raccoon eyes) (Fig. 3-24), CSF otorrhea, and hemotympanum.

Diagnosis depends on the facial examination. On manipulation of the maxilla, movement is felt at the frontonasal angle and frontozygomatic sutures. However, the entire midface remains intact. Zygomatic arch fractures are also palpated. Radiographic diagnosis is usually made by CT scans, which also evaluate cranial vault fractures and intracranial injuries.

As in other facial fractures, the goal is anatomic restoration of the fracture complex. The general treatment protocol is the same as that for LeFort II fractures, except that the inferior orbital rims are no longer available for superior stabilization. Thus, stabilization must be achieved at the frontozygomatic sutures and zygomatic arches. Complications of LeFort III facial fractures are the same as those of LeFort II facial fractures, with the possible addition of injuries to the cranial base, with neurologic damage.

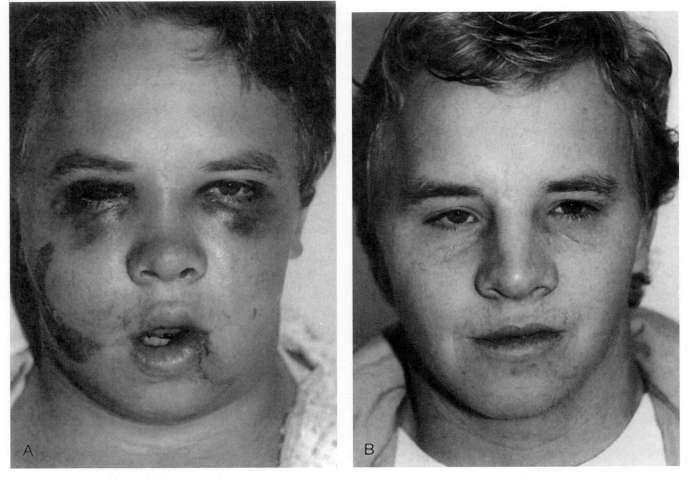

Figure 3-24 **A,** A patient with multiple facial fractures, including a LeFort III fracture. Note the raccoon eyes. **B,** After fracture fixation and facial reconstruction.

Pan-Facial Fractures

Patients who have facial trauma because of high levels of kinetic energy (e.g., high-speed motor vehicle crashes) often have multiple fracture complexes (Fig. 3-25). When they involve all areas of the face, they are known as pan-facial fractures. The same principles of diagnosis and treatment that are used in isolated fracture complexes are applied to these complex injuries. To avoid serious soft tissue contraction of the overlying facial skin, early fixation is usually indicated. Sequencing of fracture repair varies from physician to physician, but the concept of stable fixation to those structures that are not fractured is critical.

Cerebrospinal Fluid Rhinorrhea

CSF rhinorrhea occurs in as many as 25% of high-level midface injuries that involve the paranasal sinuses. Most of these cause leakage within the first 48 hours after injury. Less commonly, rhinorrhea occurs 5 to 7 days later. Clinically, CSF rhinorrhea is associated with a fracture of the cribriform plate and a dural tear in association with mid-face fractures. After this injury, the clear, watery CSF begins to leak out slowly. If the patient remains supine, fluid drains down the posterior pharynx and the patient may not be aware of any leakage. Nasal packing should be avoided, and any attempt at passing a nasogastric or nasotracheal tube is contraindicated.

Early reduction of facial fractures usually stops CSF leakage within a few days. Prophylactic antibiotics are used *only* perioperatively. If CSF rhinorrhea persists after fracture fixation, intracranial repair of the dural tear may be required. Accordingly, neurosurgical consultation is needed.

HAND SURGERY

The hand and upper extremity form a unique functional organ system that allows complex interaction between an individual and the environment. The hand both manipulates the external environment and receives sensations from it.

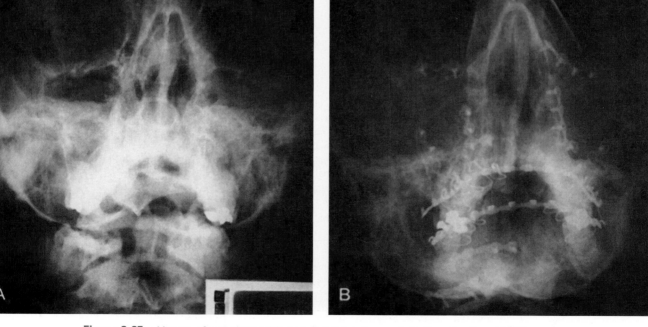

Figure 3-25   X-rays of a patient with pan-facial fractures. **A,** Before fixation. **B,** After fixation with both intermaxillary fixation and rigid internal fixation.

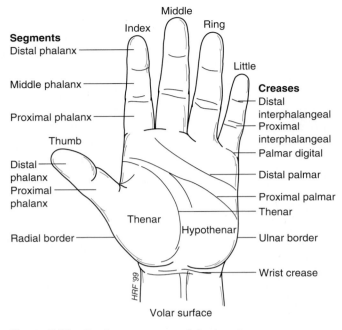

Segments

Distal phalanx

Middle phalanx

Proximal phalanx

Thumb

Distal phalanx

Proximal phalanx

Radial border

Index   Middle   Ring

Little

Creases
- Distal interphalangeal
- Proximal interphalangeal
- Palmar digital
- Distal palmar
- Proximal palmar
- Thenar
- Ulnar border
- Wrist crease

Thenar   Hypothenar

HRF '99

Volar surface

Figure 3-26   Surface anatomy of the hand.

Because hand injuries are often seen in clinical practice, all physicians should have a basic knowledge of hand anatomy and injuries to assess the need for primary treatment or referral. Because definitive treatment of the hand is usually performed by a specialist, emphasis is given to diagnosis and early treatment of the injured or diseased hand. Second only to back injuries, injuries to the hand and upper extremity are the most common reason for loss of workdays in the United States.

Functional Anatomy and Examination

The hand is composed of multiple finely balanced units. Its intricate anatomy allows specialized and refined func-

tions. Disturbance of these units, their interaction, or their innervation causes dysfunction and ultimate disability. To properly treat diseases and injuries of the hand, an understanding of its anatomy is essential. Hand anatomy is quite complex, but can be greatly simplified when broken down into its components. Therefore, hand anatomy is discussed in terms of its subsystems: nerves, muscles, tendons, bones, and blood vessels.

Terminology

In discussing hand anatomy, standard terminology should be used to avoid confusion. In addition, when describing hand injuries to a specialist, it is important to use a consistent, precise, and uniformly accepted vocabulary. In this way, injuries can be clearly delineated and safe treatment plans implemented.

The fingers should be named rather than numbered (i.e., thumb; index, long or middle, ring, and small fingers). The hand and digits have a dorsal and a volar, or palmar, surface. Each has a radial and an ulnar border (Fig. 3-26). The volar surface of the hand has a thenar and a hypothenar eminence and a midpalmar area between the two. The thenar eminence is the muscle mass overlying the thumb metacarpal. The hypothenar eminence is the muscle mass overlying the small finger metacarpal. Each finger has a proximal, middle, and distal phalanx. Each finger has a metacarpophalangeal (MCP) joint, proximal interphalangeal (PIP) joint, and distal interphalangeal (DIP) joint. The thumb has only a proximal and distal phalanx, an MCP joint, and a single interphalangeal (IP) joint (Fig. 3-27).

Nerve Anatomy and Evaluation

The hand is innervated by the median, ulnar, and radial nerves. The median nerve enters the hand at the wrist through the carpal tunnel accompanied by the nine extrinsic flexor tendons of the digits (Fig. 3-28). The median nerve motor branch to the thenar musculature arises

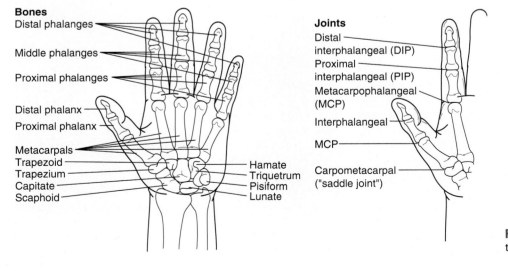

Bones

Distal phalanges

Middle phalanges

Proximal phalanges

Distal phalanx

Proximal phalanx

Metacarpals
Trapezoid
Trapezium
Capitate
Scaphoid

Hamate
Triquetrum
Pisiform
Lunate

Joints

Distal interphalangeal (DIP)

Proximal interphalangeal (PIP)

Metacarpophalangeal (MCP)

Interphalangeal

MCP

Carpometacarpal ("saddle joint")

Figure 3-27   Skeletal structure of the hand and wrist.

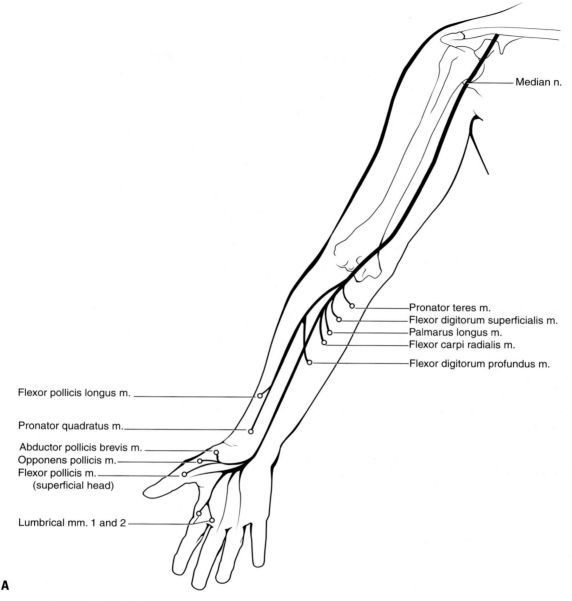

Median n.

Pronator teres m.
Flexor digitorum superficialis m.
Palmarus longus m.
Flexor carpi radialis m.
Flexor digitorum profundus m.

Flexor pollicis longus m.

Pronator quadratus m.

Abductor pollicis brevis m.
Opponens pollicis m.
Flexor pollicis m.
   (superficial head)

Lumbrical mm. 1 and 2

A

Figure 3-28   **A,** Muscles innervated by the median nerve in the forearm and hand. (*continues*)

within the carpal tunnel or just distal to it. The common digital branches innervate the lumbrical muscles to the index and long fingers. The median nerve divides into sensory branches that serve the volar aspect of the thumb, the index and long fingers, and the radial half of the ring finger (Fig. 3-29A). The ulnar nerve enters the hand at the wrist accompanied by the ulnar artery through Guyon's canal. Within the hand, motor branches to the intrinsic muscles arise from the ulnar nerve. Digital branches provide sensation to the volar and dorsal aspects of the ulnar half of the ring finger and to the entire small finger (Fig. 3-29B). The radial nerve (Fig. 3-29C) lies dorsally. It pro-

vides sensation to the dorsal aspects of the thumb, the index and long fingers, and half of the ring finger. The motor component of the radial nerve innervates the muscles that extend the wrist and MCP joints and abduct and extend the thumb. Significant anatomic variation may occur in these innervation patterns.

When examining the hand, tests of motor and sensory function of the nerves can be performed. Sensory function is usually tested by light touch from a wisp of cotton or fine filament, as well as by two-point discrimination. The patient is asked to look away from the hand during the examination. If it is not clear whether there is sensory loss,

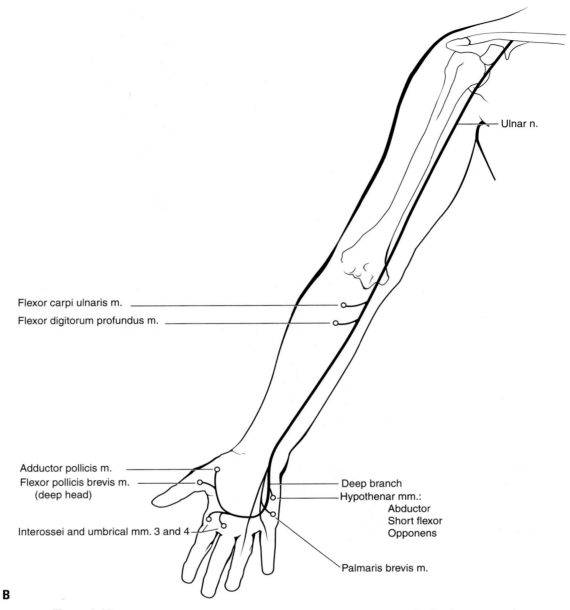

Flexor carpi ulnaris m.

Flexor digitorum profundus m.

Ulnar n.

Adductor pollicis m.

Flexor pollicis brevis m.
(deep head)

Interossei and umbrical mm. 3 and 4

Deep branch

Hypothenar mm.:
Abductor
Short flexor
Opponens

Palmaris brevis m.

B

Figure 3-28 (*continued*) **B**, Muscles innervated by the ulnar nerve in the forearm and hand. (*continues*)

the examination is repeated later. Median nerve motor function is tested by assessing the ability to flex the fingers and to oppose the thumb and small finger. Because the thenar muscles are innervated by the median nerve, asking the patient to touch the thumb to the small finger tests distal median motor function. The interosseous muscles, which abduct and adduct the fingers, are innervated by the ulnar nerve. The motor function of the ulnar nerve is tested by asking the patient to spread the fingers against resistance or to hold a piece of paper between opposing surfaces of adjacent fingers while the examiner attempts to withdraw it. The motor function of the radial nerve

is tested by asking the patient to extend the wrist against resistance.

Motor Unit Anatomy

The muscles of the hand can be divided into extrinsic and intrinsic muscle groups. Extrinsic muscles, both flexors and extensors, have their origins in the forearm and their tendon insertions in the hand. Extrinsic flexors are located on the volar aspect of the forearm and are responsible for flexion of the digits and the wrist. Extrinsic extensors are located on the dorsal aspect of the forearm and produce

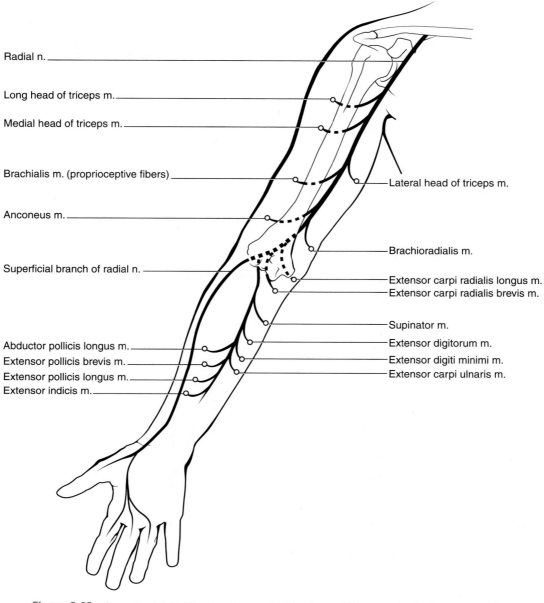

Radial n.

Long head of triceps m.

Medial head of triceps m.

Brachialis m. (proprioceptive fibers)

Anconeus m.

Superficial branch of radial n.

Abductor pollicis longus m.
Extensor pollicis brevis m.
Extensor pollicis longus m.
Extensor indicis m.

Lateral head of triceps m.

Brachioradialis m.

Extensor carpi radialis longus m.
Extensor carpi radialis brevis m.

Supinator m.
Extensor digitorum m.
Extensor digiti minimi m.
Extensor carpi ulnaris m.

C

Figure 3-28   (*continued*) **C,** Muscles innervated by the radial nerve in the forearm and hand.

extension of the wrist and digits. The intrinsic muscles have their origins and insertions completely within the hand.

Flexor Anatomy and Examination
Flexion of the MCP, PIP, and DIP joints are served by separate musculotendinous units. The lumbricals, which are intrinsic muscles, arise within the hand and insert into the proximal phalanges, crossing the MCP joint (Fig. 3-30). These, along with the interossei, are responsible for MCP joint flexion and for DIP and PIP joint extension. The extrinsic flexors, the flexor digitorum superficialis and the flexor digitorum profundus, are responsible for flexion at the PIP and DIP joints, respectively.

The flexor digitorum profundus muscle originates in the forearm and gives rise to four tendons that run through the wrist within the carpal tunnel to insert at the base of the distal phalanges of the fingers. Its function is tested by blocking flexion at the PIP joint of the involved finger and observing flexion at the DIP joint (Fig. 3-31). Because a single muscle gives rise to all four deep flexor tendons, the flexor digitorum profundus acts as a unit, and independent DIP flexion is not observed. PIP flexion is achieved through the action of the flexor digitorum superficialis.

Sensory Distribution of Median Nerve

Sensory Distribution of Ulnar Nerve

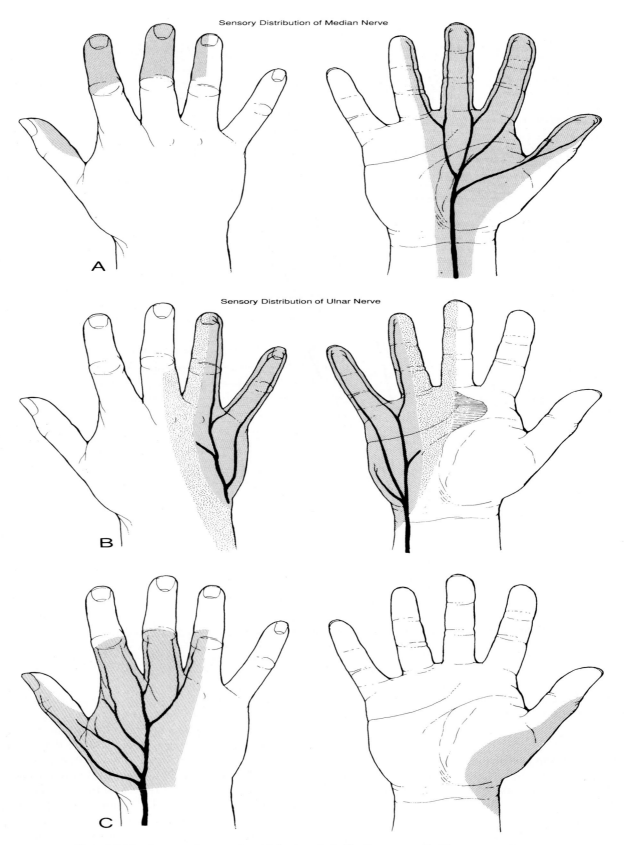

Figure 3-29   Sensory innervation of the hand. **A,** Median nerve. **B,** Ulnar nerve. **C,** Radial nerve.

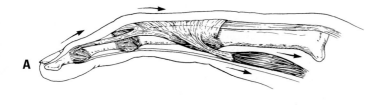

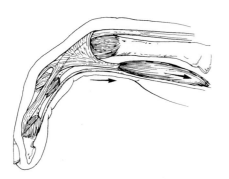

Figure 3-30   Anatomy and function of the lumbrical muscle. **A,** The insertion of the lumbrical muscle onto the extensor apparatus allows extension of the distal interphalangeal and proximal interphalangeal joints on contraction of the lumbrical muscle. **B,** Because the lumbrical tendon passes on the volar surface of the metacarpophalangeal joint, flexion of the metacarpophalangeal joint is achieved by contraction of the lumbrical muscle.

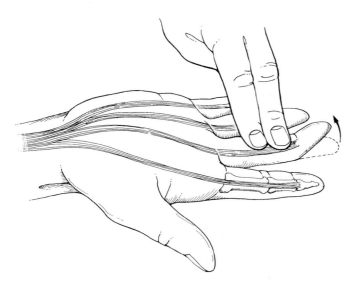

Figure 3-31   Examination of the flexor digitorum profundus. The integrity of the flexor digitorum profundus musculotendinous unit is examined by blocking flexion at the proximal interphalangeal joint and observing flexion at the distal interphalangeal joint of the finger.

This muscle is also located in the forearm and sends four flexor tendons through the carpal tunnel to ultimately insert on the base of the middle phalanges of the fingers. Separate muscle fibers give rise to each of the tendons, allowing independent flexion. To test the function of the flexor digitorum superficialis, passive extension of adjacent fingers is maintained (to block the deep flexor unit). Flexion of the PIP joint of the affected finger is observed (Fig. 3-32). The flexor pollicis longus muscle has its origin in the forearm, and it inserts on the volar base of the distal phalanx of the thumb. Flexor pollicis longus function is tested by asking the patient to flex the IP joint of the thumb against resistance.

Extensor Anatomy and Examination

Finger extension is achieved through the action of both intrinsic and extrinsic muscles that insert into a complex tendinous system on the dorsum of the fingers (extensor apparatus) (Fig. 3-33). The extensor digitorum communis is a common extrinsic extensor muscle that inserts onto the extensor apparatus and provides MCP extension, as a unit, of the index, long, ring, and small fingers. Independent extension of the index and small fingers is provided by two independent extensors (extensor indicis proprius and extensor digiti quinti minimi, respectively). PIP and DIP joint extension is achieved through an interplay of the common extensors and the intrinsic muscles of the hand (lumbricals and interossei). The intrinsic muscles travel volar to the axis of rotation of the MCP joint to insert into the lateral bands of the extensor apparatus (Fig. 3-30). This unique position allows the intrinsic muscles to act as flexors at the MCP joint and as extensors at the PIP and DIP joints.

Examination of the extensor function of the hand involves observation of extension, with or without resistance, of each of these elements. Because independent extension of the index and small fingers is provided, these digits must be evaluated both separately and as a unit with the long and ring fingers.

Thumb extension is also provided by extrinsic and intrinsic muscles. The extensor pollicis brevis and extensor pollicis longus are extrinsic muscles located within the forearm. They give rise to tendons that insert on the bases of the proximal and distal phalanges, respectively. These muscles provide extension at the MCP and IP joints of the thumb. The abductor pollicis, an intrinsic muscle of the hand, is innervated by the ulnar nerve and has tendinous insertions onto the extensor apparatus of the thumb. In this way, thumb IP extension is assisted by the intrinsic muscles. Thumb extension is also assisted by abduction of the thumb by the abductor pollicis longus, which crosses the wrist to insert on the thumb metacarpal. The area between the tendons of the extensor pollicis longus and the abductor pollicis longus on the radial aspect of the wrist is known as the anatomic snuff box.

The extensor tendons of the wrist and fingers are arranged in specific anatomic compartments on the dorsal surface of the wrist (Fig. 3-33B). Each compartment is a

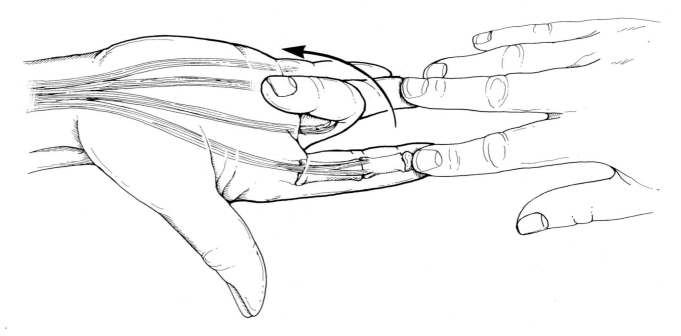

Figure 3-32 Examination of the flexor digitorum superficialis. Because the tendons of the flexor digitorum profundus have a common muscular origin, the action of this musculotendinous unit is blocked by maintaining adjacent fingers in extension. Flexion of the finger is then a function of only the flexor digitorum superficialis.

separate tunnel enclosed in a tough fibrous capsule through which the extensor tendons travel.

Thumb Opposition

Opposition of the thumb is the movement that allows the thumb to be approximated successively to the tip of each of the fingers. Specifically, the movement is described by radial extension, palmar abduction, and IP joint flexion. Thumb opposition, a unique ability of the hands, is provided by the muscles of the thenar eminence (opponens pollicis, flexor pollicis brevis, and abductor pollicis brevis). Opposition is assisted by flexion of the thumb IP joint, which is provided by the flexor pollicis longus, an extrinsic flexor whose tendon travels through the carpal tunnel and inserts on the base of the distal phalanx.

Bony Anatomy

The skeleton of the hand consists of 27 bones. It can be divided into three segments: phalanges, metacarpals, and carpal bones (Fig. 3-34). The fingers each have three phalanges; the thumb has two. The five proximal phalanges all articulate with their respective metacarpals. The metacarpals articulate with the carpal bones, which as a unit form the wrist joint. This joint articulates with the radial head. The carpal bones are arranged in two rows. The proximal row includes the scaphoid, lunate, triquetrum, and pisiform. The distal row includes the trapezium, trapezoid, capitate, and hamate. The wrist bones are interconnected through a complex of ligaments that also reinforce the articulations with the radius and ulna.

Vascular Anatomy

Both the radial and the ulnar arteries contribute to the blood supply of the hand (Fig. 3-35A). Usually, the ulnar artery is dominant. Together, these arteries form two arches, or arcades, within the hand. The common digital arteries arise from these arcades. Each common digital artery gives off "proper" digital arteries. The proper digital vessels travel along the radial and ulnar sides of the digits, and their respective digital nerves form neurovascular bundles. The integrity of the digital vessels may be checked by observing capillary refill in the fingers. The radial and ulnar arteries and their vascular arcades are examined with **Allen's test** (Fig. 3-35B). In this test, the radial and ulnar arteries are compressed at the wrist. The patient is asked to open and close the fist several times, thus exsanguinating the hand and leaving the skin blanched. The fingers are held extended while the radial artery is released from compression. If the radial artery is patent, with good collateral flow to the ulnar artery, the palm and all five digits turn pink. Arterial compression and exsanguination are repeated, but this time, the ulnar artery is released. If the ulnar artery is patent, with good collateral flow into the radial artery, the hand and all five digits turn pink. If vascular integrity is still uncertain, Doppler examination may be helpful.

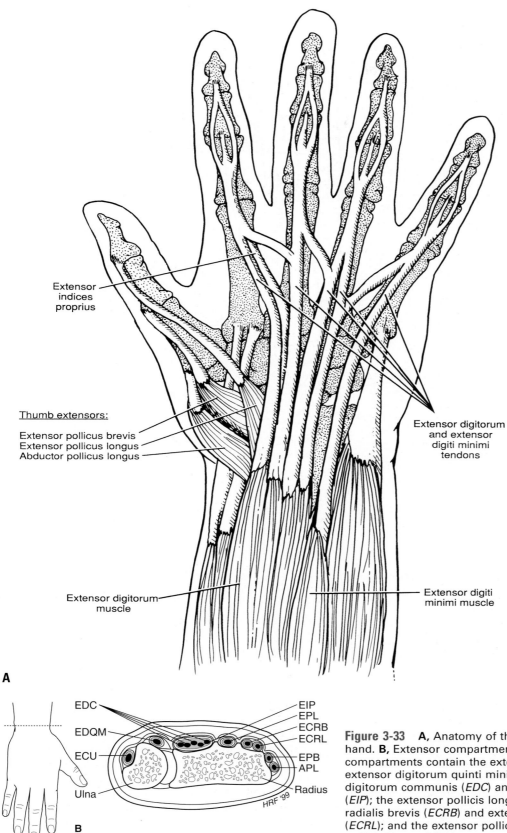

Extensor indices proprius

Thumb extensors:

Extensor pollicus brevis
Extensor pollicus longus
Abductor pollicus longus

Extensor digitorum
and extensor
digiti minimi
tendons

Extensor digitorum
muscle

Extensor digiti
minimi muscle

A

EDC
EDQM
ECU
Ulna

EIP
EPL
ECRB
ECRL
EPB
APL
Radius

HRF '99

B

Figure 3-33 **A,** Anatomy of the extensor tendons to the hand. **B,** Extensor compartments at the wrist. The six compartments contain the extensor carpi radialis (*ECU*); the extensor digitorum quinti minimi (*EDQM*); the extensor digitorum communis (*EDC*) and extensor indicis proprius (*EIP*); the extensor pollicis longus (*EPL*); the extensor carpi radialis brevis (*ECRB*) and extensor carpi radialis longus (*ECRL*); and the extensor pollicis brevis (*EPB*) and abductor pollicis longus (*APL*).

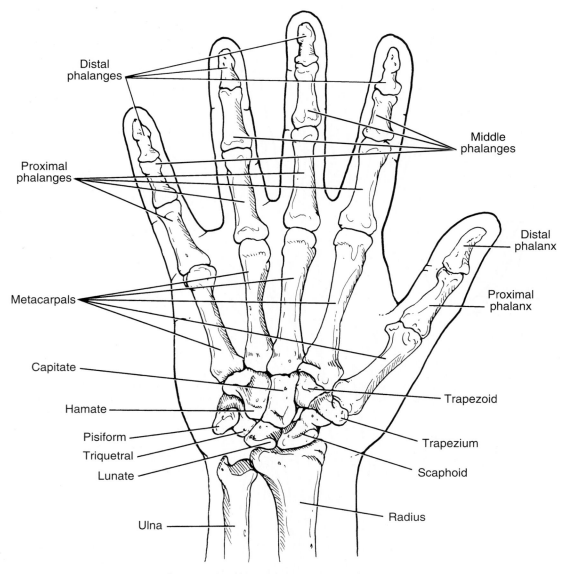

Figure 3-34 Skeletal anatomy of the hand.

Diagnosis of Hand Injuries

Because of the complex anatomy and function of the hand and the potentially severe consequences of hand injuries, most significant injuries should be treated by a hand specialist. However, the nonspecialist may be the first person to encounter these injuries and thus must be able to evaluate, initially treat, and, if appropriate, refer these patients for specialty consultation.

Evaluation of the hand begins with a proper history. The time and mechanism of injury and the environment in which the injury occurred are of paramount importance, particularly with open wounds. The patient's overall medical condition, allergies, medications, tetanus immunization status, and previous injuries are also documented. The patient's hand dominance, occupation, and avocations play an important role in therapeutic decision mak-

ing. They should be noted and communicated to the hand specialist.

Before the hand is examined in detail, its vascular integrity is evaluated so that if revascularization is needed, the patient can be referred immediately. Bleeding is controlled with direct pressure alone. Bleeding vessels are not clamped because of the risk of damaging accompanying nerves or further damaging reparable vessels. A pneumatic tourniquet is used only in extreme cases. The nail bed of each digit is examined for capillary refill, and the wrist and forearm are checked for pulse. Doppler examination can be used to confirm the patency of the ulnar and radial arteries, palmar arch, and digital arteries. If major portions of the hand appear ischemic, plans are made to transfer the patient to a replantation center with microvascular capabilities or to the operating room.

A careful examination of all motor and sensory units is

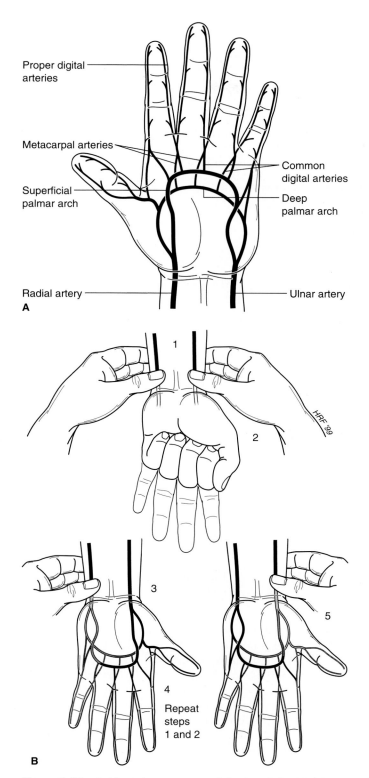

Figure 3-35　**A,** Vascular anatomy of the hand. **B,** Allen's test for vascular patency.

performed. The distribution of each major sensory nerve should be tested and recorded. Each flexor and extensor tendon should be individually examined, as previously outlined. When fractures are suspected, appropriate radiographs are obtained. Complex injuries that involve multiple tendons and nerves can be simply and well delineated with a thorough examination. Careful documentation of these injuries is required.

During the initial evaluation of the hand, fractures should be suspected and diagnosed. Inspection of the hand is often diagnostic when localized swelling, angulation, or rotational deformity is seen. Tenderness to palpation over the fracture site is the rule. In addition, there may be limitation of motion of the involved finger. A survey x-ray of the entire hand should be obtained, followed by anterior–posterior and lateral x-rays of the affected part. If suspected fractures are not well visualized, oblique views may be obtained.

Treatment of Hand Injuries

Soft Tissue Injuries

Open wounds of the hand should be copiously irrigated with a physiologic solution. For highly contaminated wounds, multiple liters of saline irrigation may be required. If no sensory or motor injuries are present, these wounds are simply closed in a sterile manner. Antibiotics are recommended for contaminated wounds or for open wounds with underlying bone, joint, or tendon injuries. Tetanus immunization status must be ascertained.

A lacerated nerve requires microscopic repair in the operating room. This type of injury does not require immediate repair if it is not convenient; it can be delayed for several days.

Flexor tendon injuries must also be repaired in the operating room. These injuries can be classified according to zone (Fig. 3-36). Injuries within Zone II (no man's land) can be the most difficult to manage. The deep and superficial flexor tendons run within the flexor sheath in this location. Once they are repaired, adhesions may form and restrict normal motion. A flexor tendon laceration can be repaired immediately or within several days. Simple skin closure and referral for repair within a few days is acceptable management of these injuries.

Many extensor tendon injuries can be repaired in the emergency room at the discretion of the hand surgeon. Injuries to the extensor tendon overlying the DIP joint cause **mallet finger** (Fig. 3-37A). Injuries to the central portion of the extensor mechanism at the PIP joint produce a boutonnière deformity (Fig. 3-37B). Laceration of the extensor tendon in the hand prevents extension of the finger (Fig. 3-37C).

Fractures of the Hand

Fractures of the hand are a common component of injury. The goal of treatment is proper reduction of the fracture

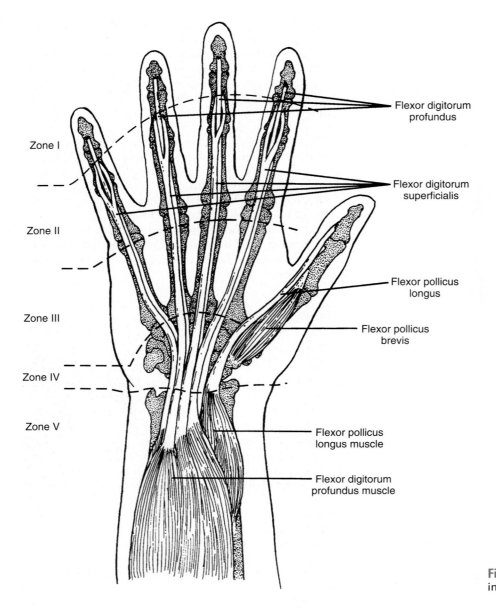

Zone I

Zone II

Zone III

Zone IV

Zone V

Flexor digitorum
profundus

Flexor digitorum
superficialis

Flexor pollicus
longus

Flexor pollicus
brevis

Flexor pollicus
longus muscle

Flexor digitorum
profundus muscle

Figure 3-36   Zones of flexor tendon
injuries.

and maintenance of the reduction with splinting, casting, or fixation (either internal or external). To achieve as near-normal function as possible, anatomic reduction of all fractures is ideal. In some fractures, minor discrepancy in final bone alignment can be tolerated. Because of the complexity of the hand and its fractures, nearly all fractures require the consultation of a hand surgeon.

Closed fractures are usually treated electively as the localized swelling allows. Proper splinting until fixation decreases patient discomfort and reduces swelling. All open fractures should be treated acutely as the patient's overall condition allows. With the exception of very minor fractures and those treated with casting alone, all definitive reduction and fixation should be done in the operating room. Although in-depth discussion of specific hand fractures is beyond the scope of this chapter, a few types are discussed here.

Probably the most common fracture is that of the end of the distal phalanx, or distal tuft. Because the fracture occurs distal to the insertion of the extensor and flexor tendons, precise anatomic reduction is not required. These fractures can be easily treated with splints for 2 to 3 weeks, usually without complications. Seriously crushed tips may require some molding during splinting to achieve the best result, and associated nail bed injuries require careful repair under loupe magnification. If the fracture involves the DIP joint space or any tendinous insertion, referral should be sought.

Fractures of the middle and proximal phalanges are also common. Stable fractures can be treated with splints or "buddy taping," whereby the injured finger is taped to an adjacent finger that functions as a splint. Unstable, comminuted, or spiral fractures and those that involve the joint space may require more complex fixation.

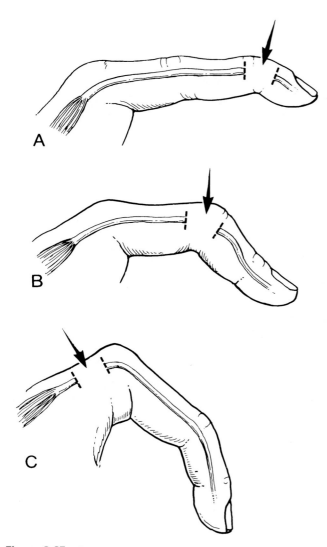

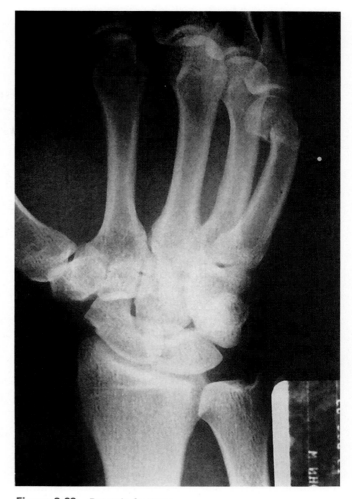

Figure 3-38   Boxer's fracture.

Figure 3-37   Extensor tendon injuries. **A,** Mallet finger deformity caused by a laceration of the extensor tendon at or just proximal to the distal interphalangeal joint. **B,** Boutonnière deformity caused by a laceration of the central slip of the extensor apparatus at or just proximal to the proximal interphalangeal joint. **C,** Extensor tendon laceration proximal to the metacarpophalangeal joint.

Fractures through the head or neck of the metacarpals often result from altercations. A **boxer's fracture** is a fracture through the fourth or fifth metacarpal neck, usually as a result of a blow to another object (e.g., an opponent's chin) (Fig. 3-38). Angulation or rotational deformity is often seen. Whereas 20 to 30 degrees of volar angulation of the fourth and fifth metacarpals may be acceptable, little or no angulation of the other metacarpals is acceptable. Likewise, rotational deformity is unacceptable because it interferes with normal motion. Boxer's fractures and other stable, nondisplaced metacarpal fractures may be treated with casting alone, but most others require additional methods of fixation.

Fractures of the scaphoid usually occur after a fall on the outstretched hand. This history and tenderness over the anatomic snuff box are key to making the diagnosis. Although initial radiographs may not show a fracture, repeat films in 1 to 3 weeks may. Because of the problems with nonunion in improperly treated scaphoid fractures, patients who are suspected of having such injuries, but whose initial x-rays are negative, should be casted and treated as though they have this fracture. Repeat x-rays are obtained 2 weeks later. Avascular necrosis is a common complication of the fractured scaphoid. This issue is further addressed in Chapter 6.

Splinting of the injured hand is important and deserves special note. Prolonged splinting in an inappropriate position may cause joint stiffness, shortening of musculotendinous and ligamentous units, and ultimate loss of some function. Although certain fractures or tendon injuries may require splinting in different positions, most injured hands should be splinted in the "safe" position to preserve function (Fig. 3-39). In this position, the wrist is in 20 to

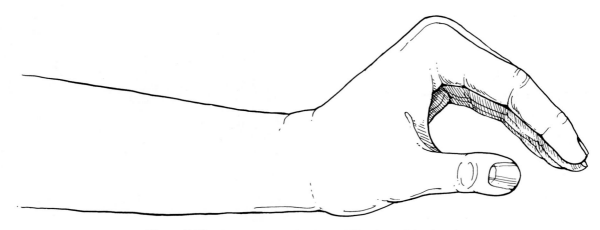

Figure 3-39 Safe position for immobilization of the hand.

30 degrees of extension, the MCP joints are flexed at 80 to 90 degrees, and the IP joints are straight or nearly so. The thumb is held in palmar abduction. Splints to maintain this position are usually placed on the volar surface of the hand, wrist, and forearm.

Special Injuries

Fingertip Injuries

Although fingertip injuries are common, their care can be very complex because of the structure and function of the fingertip. The goals of treatment are to maintain adequate length and normal sensibility. Simple distal skin losses can be treated with dressings alone and allowed to heal by contraction. However, injuries that involve the distal phalanx or nail bed require complex repairs. If the distal amputated part is available, it should be handled gently and cared for properly (see Amputations).

Amputations

Particular care is given to amputated parts. Digits or significant portions of digits are often amputated in industrial accidents that occur in unsanitary settings. The amputated part should be rinsed with saline to remove debris and gross contamination. The amputated part is then wrapped in moist gauze and placed in a watertight plastic bag. The bag is sealed and placed in a container filled with iced saline. The amputated part should not be allowed to become waterlogged by being placed directly in saline or frozen by being placed directly on ice. X-ray films of the amputated part should be obtained before it is transferred.

Although not all amputated parts can or should be replanted, the ultimate decision regarding replantation should be made by the replant surgeon. Replantation is always considered in thumb amputations, amputations distal to the PIP joint, multiple-digit amputations, bilateral amputations, hand or hemihand amputation, and in children. Replantation of severely crushed or avulsed parts usually is not indicated, nor is replantation of parts that have undergone warm ischemia for more than 6 to 12 hours.

Thermal Injuries

The thermally injured hand offers a challenge to the initial treating physician. Correct early treatment significantly improves outcome. The burned hand should be cleansed gently with physiologic solution and, if necessary, with mild soap. All foreign material (e.g., burned clothing) should be removed. Blisters should be left intact because they signify a second-degree burn and they protect the underlying tissue. When these blisters eventually break on their own, they should be gently debrided. Capillary refill of all burned digits should be checked because circumferential burns can interfere with distal circulation. This interference may take several hours to develop; if it does, escharotomy may be required.

After the hand is cleaned, an antibiotic ointment (e.g., Silvadene) is applied. The hand is placed in a bulky dressing and splinted in the safe position. Therapy consists of daily whirlpool baths, dressing changes, and aggressive range-of-motion exercises to prevent joint contracture. Patients who have significant partial-thickness burns or full-thickness burns that require skin grafting should be referred.

Burns represent a unique form of trauma. The role of the surgeon may involve patient care only for burn reconstruction or from the initial trauma all the way through reconstruction. The burned patient should be approached in the same logical and orderly manner as any other trauma patient at the onset, but a quality understanding of the unique characteristics of burn patients and burn care is critical to the near- and long-term successful treatment of that patient. An excellent review of trauma and burns can be found in Chapters 10 and 11 in Lawrence et al, *Essentials of General Surgery*, 4th ed.

Frostbite is a unique form of thermal injury classified as a local injury, and therefore separated from systemic hypothermia. The overall pathophysiology consists of the formation of ice crystals in the tissue fluid, leading to cellular injury. This injury must be recognized early and treated agressively. Successful treatment is based on rapid tissue rewarming in a 40°F waterbath. After this, the normal components of monitoring a burn patient (e.g., ABCs, urine output, monitoring for infection), wound management, and evaluation of tetanus status can be applied. Depending on the location of the injury and total areas involved, therapy for range-of-motion and strength exercises might be necessary.

Hand Infections

The complex structure of the hand offers multiple sites for infection. Although superficial cellulitis and subcutaneous abscesses can occur in the hand as in other locations, some infections are peculiar to the hand. Such infections can occur within the lateral nail bed (**paronychia**), at the finger pulp (**felon**), in the tendon sheaths (**tenosynovitis**), and in the deeper structures of the hand (deep-space infections). Human bites to the hand are a common infectious problem. Successful management of hand infections depends on a knowledge of both hand anatomy and the specific treatment of each infection

In the hand, infection usually progresses rapidly. Without prompt diagnosis and treatment, the infection can spread quickly along fascial planes, causing damage to adjacent structures. In addition, this rapid spread can lead to massive tissue necrosis, which may require amputation of the extremity. At a minimum, it can result in a stiff, nonfunctional extremity. Treatment of suppurative infections of the hand is based on adequate surgical drainage. Although systemic symptoms may be present, signs and symptoms are usually localized to the hand. Serious infections of the hand are usually treated in the operating room under regional or general anesthesia, with tourniquet control. Appropriate aerobic and anaerobic cultures are taken. After adequate surgical drainage, the hand is immobilized in the protective splinted position and elevated. Antibiotics are routinely administered (usually a first-generation cephalosporin or a penicillinase-resistant antibiotic). After surgical drainage, the hand is reevaluated frequently, and antibiotics are adjusted according to intraoperative culture results. Further extension of the infection is possible, and adequate drainage should be verified by progressive resolution of pain and swelling.

Paronychia

Paronychia, an infection of the lateral nail fold, usually presents as a small collection of purulent material at the side of the nail. If seen early, it is properly treated by elevating the skin over the nail or excising a small lateral, longitudinal portion of the nail to drain the purulent material (Fig. 3-40). More advanced infection may require incision within the nail fold for drainage. This procedure is followed by soaking the finger in warm water several times a day. Chronic paronychia suggests secondary colonization with more complex organisms. Antibiotic treatment for chronic paronychia should await results of cultures. Fungal nail infections or herpetic infection (herpetic whitlow) may be confused with chronic paronychia. Proper diagno-

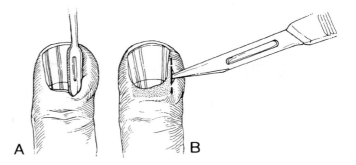

Figure 3-40   Treatment of paronychia. **A,** Elevation of the nail fold. **B,** Placement of an incision.

sis is vital because operating on a fungal or herpetic infection may worsen the condition by allowing secondary bacterial infection and delayed wound healing.

Felon

A felon, a purulent infection of the pad of the finger, is usually extremely painful. Fibrous septa within the tip of the finger allow a significant amount of pressure when only a minimal amount of purulent material is present. This condition also increases local tissue pressure to the point of interrupting capillary flow, which can produce ischemia and necrosis. The felon can be drained by various methods (Fig. 3-41). If skin necrosis is present, the incision can be made over it, or the incision can be made at a point of maximum tenderness. Alternatively, it is drained through a small stab incision laterally on the digit pad. In draining a felon, it is important to adequately disrupt the fibrous septa to provide enough drainage.

Tenosynovitis

Tenosynovitis is a painful inflammation of the tendon sheath. Suppurative tenosynovitis is usually caused by a puncture wound over the volar aspect of the hand. It can also develop from extension of a felon (Fig. 3-42). Diagnosis is usually made by observing four signs (**Kanavel's signs**): (a) finger held in slight flexion, (b) fusiform swelling of the finger, (c) tenderness over the tendon sheath, and (d) pain on passive extension. The fourth sign is usually the key to diagnosis.

Prompt and appropriate treatment is required to prevent complications. Some very early infections can be treated with intravenous antibiotics, elevation, and immobilization. However, for more advanced infections, surgical drainage of the tendon sheath is carried out in the operating room by a hand surgeon.

Deep-Space Infections

Infection of the deep spaces of the hand or thenar eminence can also occur. Patients usually have pain and swelling. Although the primary problem may be in a volar location, more dorsal swelling is almost always present.

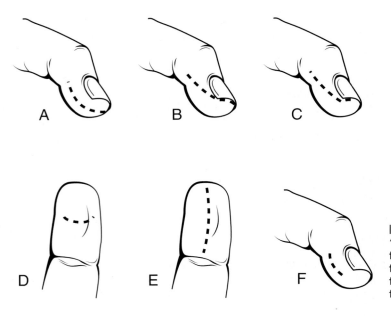

Figure 3-41   Drainage approaches for a felon. **A–C,** "Hockey stick" or "J" incision around the tip of the finger. **D,** Transverse incision across the pulp of the finger. **E,** Longitudinal incision down the center of the finger pad. **F,** Incision on the lateral aspect of the finger.

Treatment is surgical drainage of the affected spaces. The complexity of the anatomy of the deep spaces of the hand complicates their drainage. Referral to a hand surgeon is usually necessary. Deep-space infections of the hand initially involve specific sites (e.g., thenar, hypothenar, mid-palmar, parona's space). Infections are typically due to a penetrating injury, but the actual presence of a foreign body on radiographs is rare. Clinical examination is considered the hallmark of diagnosis. The space involved will generally show signs such as loss of palmar concavity (mid-palmar space), or wide abduction of the thumb and difficulty with opposition (thenar space). Urgent surgical intervention is required to provide adequate treatment of the infection, and frequently postoperative therapy is necessary to maintain range of motion and strength.

Human Bites

Human bites to the hand can produce devastating complications because of the degree of wound contamination from human saliva. The diagnosis is often complicated by an inaccurate or misleading history given by the patient. Lacerations overlying the dorsal MCP joint (knuckle) should always be suspected of being a "fight bite" (Fig. 3-43). Lacerations from human bites should never be closed, but must be left open to drain. Patients are admitted for 24 to 48 hours of intravenous antibiotics, with the hand elevated and immobilized. Bites that are not treated within 24 hours require longer hospitalization and more complex treatment. Those that are properly treated within 24 hours virtually always have a favorable outcome.

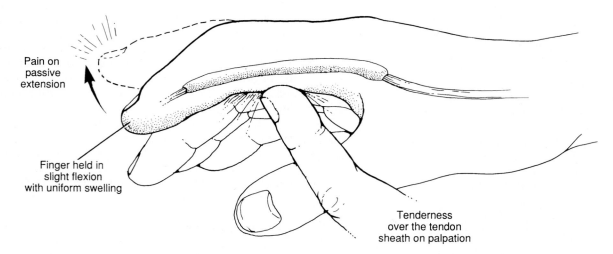

Pain on passive extension

Finger held in slight flexion with uniform swelling

Tenderness over the tendon sheath on palpation

Figure 3-42   Flexor tenosynovitis. The diagnosis is made by Kanavel's four signs: the finger held in slight flexion, fusiform swelling of the finger, tenderness over the tendon sheath, and pain on passive extension.

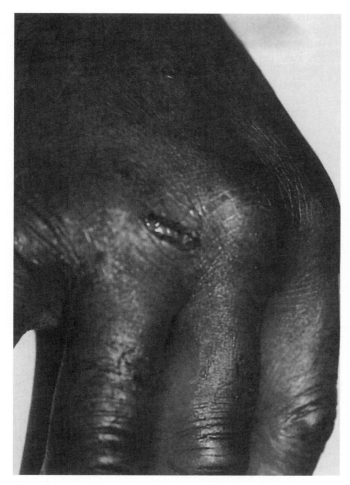

Figure 3-43   Human bite to the metacarpophalangeal joint. This is the typical appearance of a "fight bite."

Tumors of the Hand

Benign Tumors

Ganglion Cyst

The most common soft tissue mass of the hand is a **ganglion cyst.** These cysts occur in several anatomic locations. The ganglion is an outpouching of the synovium, usually of a joint or tendinous structure. The most common location is on the dorsal radial aspect of the wrist, where the cyst originates from the ligament joining the scaphoid and lunate bones. These cysts may also occur on the volar radial area of the wrist or along the palmar surface of the hand or finger overlying the flexor tendon sheath. Symptomatic ganglion cysts are surgically removed. Untreated, they tend to increase in size slowly but progressively. Other methods of treatment (e.g., digital rupture, aspiration, injection with steroids or sclerosing materials) are usually ineffective.

Mucous Cyst

A mucous cyst is not a true cyst, but a ganglion arising from the dorsum of the finger overlying the DIP joint.

Surgical resection is complicated by the need to excise the cyst, usually with some overlying skin and underlying periosteum. Small skin grafts or skin flaps may be required for closure.

Giant Cell Tumor

Another soft tissue tumor that occurs in the wrist or finger is the giant cell tumor (xanthoma). This slowly growing, yellow-brown tumor invades surrounding structures. It has a high recurrence rate after resection. Surgical excision is carefully performed under low-power magnification.

Malignant Tumors

Squamous and basal cell carcinomas of the skin are relatively common in the hands. They are usually caused by aging and sun exposure. As in other parts of the body, treatment is with wide local excision followed by soft tissue reconstruction. Malignant melanoma may be present under the nail bed, and the nails should be carefully examined.

Other Conditions That Require Surgery

Arthritis

Some common problems with the hands involve either degenerative or rheumatoid arthritis. These conditions are extremely debilitating and may cause permanent disability. The primary treatment of both diseases is medical. Surgical treatment is reserved for maintaining or restoring functional ability. In many patients, improvement is provided by early surgical intervention for joint reconstruction, muscle and tendon rebalancing, and synovectomy.

Dupuytren's Disease

Dupuytren's disease is progressive fibrosis of the palmar fascia of the hand. The etiology of the disease is unclear, but it has a definite hereditary pattern. It usually occurs after 40 years of age, is more common in men (7:1 ratio), and occurs bilaterally in more than 50% of cases. It causes increasing contraction of the fibrous palmar fascia that presents as nodules and bands in the hand. The natural course is progressive contracture of the hand and inability to fully extend the digits. There is no known medical treatment. Indications for surgery include limited finger extension, rapid progression of the disease, and painful nodules. The best surgical results occur when the patient is evaluated early and when surgical resection is performed before the formation of joint abnormalities or fixed joints. At surgery, the involved palmar fascia is removed, and the skin is repaired to alleviate scar contractures. Care must be taken because the neurovascular bundles may be encased in the diseased tissue.

Compression Neuropathy

Although compression neuropathy occurs in many locations of the upper extremity, the most common location is the carpal tunnel. The median nerve is compressed as it passes through the wrist within the carpal tunnel, which is bounded dorsally by the carpal bones and volarly by a tough ligament, the volar carpal ligament. Nine flexor tendons accompany the median nerve through the carpal tunnel (the four tendons of the flexor digitorum superficialis, the four of the flexor digitorum profundus, and the tendon of the flexor pollicis longus). Patients usually have numbness and tingling, particularly at night, within the median nerve sensory distribution of the hand. They may also have difficulty grasping objects. These patients often have occupations that require a large amount of repetitive manual work. Usually, pain and tingling can be reproduced by percussing the median nerve within the carpal tunnel (**Tinel's sign**). In advanced cases, atrophy of the thenar musculature can occur. Nerve conduction studies usually show delays.

Treatment is directed at relieving the compression and resultant inflammation of the median nerve. In early cases, splinting or alteration of work habits may be helpful. However, these measures usually provide only transient help. Definitive operative treatment involves division of the volar carpal ligament, and occasionally, internal neurolysis of the median nerve. Surgery should not be delayed until thenar atrophy develops because this condition can be permanent.

CONGENITAL DEFECTS

Congenital Defects of the Hand

Congenital defects of the hand can occur alone or in association with multiple other medical syndromes. Early diagnosis allows planned treatment. Common defects include webbed fingers (**syndactyly**) (Fig. 3-44) and extra digits (polydactyly). Syndactyly is routinely repaired before the infant is 6 to 12 months of age. Repair should not be delayed past 12 months of age unless other associated medical problems are present. If the two digits fused together are of unequal length (e.g., ring and small finger, thumb and index finger), progressive contracture and bony angulation will occur as the child grows. Another reason to proceed early with separation is the presence of complex syndactyly in which fusion of adjacent phalanges occurs. This fusion causes significant growth abnormalities if the phalanges are not divided early.

Surgical care of polydactyly usually involves amputation of the extra digits. Amputation should be done only after complete evaluation is made of the functional status and potential of all of the digits. Such an evaluation may require waiting for several months, or even more than a year, until it is evident which digit will be the most functional. Occasionally, combining some elements of one digit with those of the other is indicated.

Two congenital hand problems require early treatment. One is a constriction ring deformity, in which a band of amniotic tissue forms a tourniquet around a finger or another part of the body (e.g., wrist, leg, toe). The constriction must be at least partially relieved early because it tends

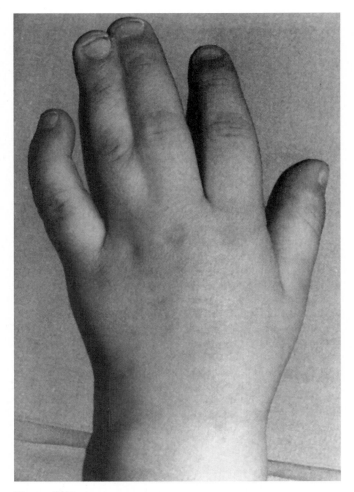

Figure 3-44 Simple syndactyly.

to limit circulation. A second defect that benefits from early treatment is the significantly deviated hand (e.g., radial clubhand). Very early splinting prevents increasing angulation and deformity.

Cleft Lip and Palate

The most common developmental anomalies of the face are cleft lip and cleft palate. The incidence of clefts is between 1:600 and 1:1000 live births. A cleft of the left lip and palate is more common in boys and has a hereditary component. A cleft palate alone is seen more often in girls and does not have a hereditary component. The etiology of clefts is not completely understood, but because heredity plays a significant role, many patients are concerned about the risk of clefts in their offspring. If one parent has had a cleft, a child has a 7% chance of having a cleft. This figure increases to 14% if there is already a sibling with a cleft. When two normal parents already have a child with a cleft, a second boy has a 4.5% chance of being born with a cleft.

The lip and palate structures are divided anatomically

into prepalatal (primary palate) and palatal (secondary palate) structures. The incisive foramen, located in the midline on the hard palate, just behind the alveolus, divides prepalatal and palatal clefts. The embryology of these clefts is different.

The prepalatal structures form between the fourth and seventh weeks of fetal life and arise from three mesenchymal islands (one central and two lateral). Incomplete migration of these elements can lead to clefts. Prepalatal clefts involve the lip, alveolus, nose, and nasal cartilage. Cleft lips may be unilateral or bilateral, and complete or incomplete. At 7 weeks, the palatal structures are composed of two palatal shelves that are vertically oriented along the sides of the tongue. As the neck of the fetus straightens, the tongue drops and the palatal shelves rotate upward to become horizontal by the 12th week. Palatal clefts are caused by incomplete fusion of the palatal shelves. They involve the hard palate, soft palate, and uvula. Various combinations of clefts of the prepalatal and palatal structures are seen.

Treatment of cleft lip is directed at returning the different lip elements to their normal position to improve appearance and correct such minor functional problems as lisping (Fig. 3-45). The timing of cleft lip repair is controversial. Repair is usually begun when the infant is 6 to 12 weeks of age and completed by 6 to 9 months of age. The ideal lip repair will establish symmetrical nostrils, alar bases, natural philtral columns and central dimple, as well as the Cupid's bow and vermilion tubercle. Functionally, the muscular repair will provide normal activity and lip competence. Although mutiple cleft lip repairs have been described in the past (e.g., Le Mesurier, Randall-Tennison) the most common unilateral cleft lip reconstruction is the Millard rotation-advancement. This repair advances a mucocutaneous flap from the lateral lip element into the cleft gap to approximate the rotated (inferiorly and into the cleft gap) medial segment.

Treatment of the nasal deformity is much more difficult because of the underdevelopment and malposition of the nasal cartilage. The cleft lip nasal deformity may require several revisions that extend into the teenage years. However, primary treatment of the nose at the time of lip repair is now commonly performed and provides either complete correction or significant improvement.

Whereas cleft lip is repaired primarily for the sake of appearance, cleft palate is repaired to ensure function, specifically, speech. The competent palate (or velum) elevates and meets the posterior pharyngeal wall (creating velopharyngeal closure) during speech and swallowing. The inability to elevate the palate produces abnormal speech, which can range from hypernasal to nearly unintelligible. The various cleft palate repairs are designed to reorient the musculature of the palate, close the cleft, and lengthen the palate. As with the lip, the timing of cleft palate repair varies. Many surgeons now prefer earlier closure (by 6–12 months of age) to allow for more normal speech development.

The cleft palate repair options are based primarily on

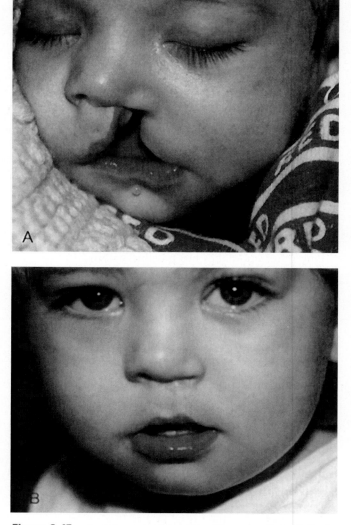

Figure 3-45 **A,** A 4-week-old child with a complete cleft of the left lip. **B,** The same child at 2 years of age, after lip repair with a rotation advancement method.

the anatomic defect to be corrected. Because no two cleft palates are exactly alike, the goal of the cleft palate repair must be correction of a functional defect. These repairs generally are accepted to include palatal closure alone, palatal closure in concert with palatal lengthening, or either of these with direct palatal muscle reapproximation. The techniques include a V–Y pushback, the von Langenbeck procedure, intravelar veloplasty, or even the double opposing Z-plasty technique. Future procedures may be indicated to correct speech abnormalities such as a pharygoplasty or pharyngeal flap.

Because of the abnormal orientation of the palatal musculature around the pharyngeal opening of the eustachian tube, middle ear infections are very common in these patients. Almost all of these children require myringotomy tubes to avoid long-term hearing problems. Another relatively uncommon cleft disorder is Pierre-Robin sequence, in which the palatal cleft is associated with a small or retropositioned mandible and a posteriorly displaced tongue. Emergency treatment may be required to maintain the airway.

A child with a cleft palate may have numerous developmental problems. Therefore, treatment should be conducted by a team of specialists under the direction of the plastic surgeon. The treating specialists should work efficiently to coordinate the integrated protocol of the Parameters of Care Guidelines, as established by the American Cleft Palate Craniofacial Association.

Other Congenital Head and Neck Anomalies

Branchial Cleft Cysts

Many other anomalies are possible within the head and neck area. The most common are variations of the **branchial cleft cyst** or sinus. This anomaly involves an epithelial tract along the *lateral* neck, which is seen along the anterior border of the sternocleidomastoid muscle. The cyst or sinus tract can range from a small blind pouch to a tract that extends completely into the oral cavity. Treatment consists of surgical resection. The timing may vary according to the symptoms.

Thyroglossal Duct Cyst

A **thyroglossal duct cyst** or sinus is an opening or defect in the absolute *midline* of the neck around the hyoid bone. The defect may be either a small blind pouch or a sinus tract that extends into the base of the tongue at the foramen cecum and is noted to move with protrusion of the tongue or deglutition. Occasionally, as in the branchial cleft cyst, infection occurs, and a brief course of antibiotics may be required. However, the definitive treatment is surgical excision. Because a thyroglossal duct cyst routinely goes through the middle of the hyoid bone, adequate resection requires removal of the central portion of the hyoid bone as well as the complete sinus, usually all the way to the base of the tongue.

Congenital Ear Deformities

Another type of congenital deformity is an ear deformity. Although complete absence of the ear (**anotia**) is rare, abnormally forming cartilage (e.g., protruding ears) and deficient cartilage (**microtia**) are relatively common. Anotia or microtia requires reconstruction of the cartilaginous framework of the ear. A large piece of cartilage is harvested, usually from the patient's rib, and carved to resemble the scaffolding of the ear. The cartilage is implanted and covered with adequate skin. Although the technique is difficult and demanding, in expert hands, it can produce excellent results. The amount of reconstruction depends on the severity of the defect. Routinely, three to four surgical procedures are required. Microtia repairs can be per-

formed after a child is 6 years old because the ear is almost adult size and adequate rib cartilage is available.

Congenital protruding ears are repaired by removing some of the conchal cartilage and plicating the remaining cartilage to the mastoid fascia. Acquired ear deformities, as in partial amputation, can be repaired with techniques similar to those used to reconstruct congenital defects.

ACQUIRED DEFORMITIES

Treatment of acquired soft tissue deformities often requires reconstructive surgery. Several factors are important to a successful reconstruction, beginning with careful consideration of the etiology of the deformity and the natural history of the disease that produces it. Next, the deformity itself is considered. The amount and type of missing tissue and the function of the tissue are important. Through this evaluation, the patient's reconstructive needs can be understood. Finally, the reconstructive surgeon must choose the most appropriate method of reconstruction, keeping in mind the reconstructive ladder.

In many cases, several reconstructive options are appropriate, or at least possible. A careful, comprehensive discussion of these options with the patient is important because the patient is an important part of the decision-making process. Further, because each patient has different needs, desires, and expectations, it is difficult to follow a "cookbook" approach that always treats certain wounds with specific operations. Each patient must be considered individually to appreciate his or her unique differences and needs.

Postmastectomy Breast Reconstruction

During the last 35 years, major advances have occurred in postmastectomy breast reconstruction. Technical advances include the development of tissue expanders, improvement in breast prostheses, and new methods of flap reconstruction. Psychological considerations have also come to be appreciated. The patient's psychological well-being and recovery may be significantly affected by proper breast reconstruction. As general surgeons have come to understand the methods of breast reconstruction, better collaboration with the reconstructive surgeon has resulted. Surgeons now understand that breast reconstruction can often be begun or completed at the time of mastectomy and that the method chosen must take into account the patient's body habitus, lifestyle, healing capabilities, adjuvant therapy (chemotherapy and radiation) and desires. The skin-sparing mastectomy, which preserves all or most of the breast skin (except the nipple–areola complex and the biopsy site), provides dramatic reconstructive results without compromising cancer cure.

Psychological Considerations

Because many options for breast reconstruction are available, adequate time must be spent with the patient to determine how to best suit her needs. All options must be discussed with the patient and the patient's preference elicited. When two options are equally appropriate or nearly so, the patient may choose the operation she prefers. The patient should also be counseled about what to expect regarding the operation, recovery, and ultimate aesthetic results. The reconstructed breast often looks as good as or better than the contralateral breast. In other cases, the reconstruction may appear only adequate (especially when the patient is fully clothed), but is superior to an external prosthesis.

Before undertaking breast reconstruction, the surgeon must determine whether the procedure should be performed, what the timing should be, and what method should be used. Although some form of reconstruction is possible for most patients, other patients, because of advanced disease, associated illness, or unrealistic expectations, should be counseled instead about external prostheses. Reconstruction can be immediate, starting with the mastectomy, or delayed, beginning after the mastectomy wound heals. Although a number of factors must be considered, the patient's desires are often the most important.

Reconstruction

Reconstruction of the breast can be divided into reconstruction of the breast mound and reconstruction of the nipple–areola complex. For the breast mound, local tissue with an implant or distant tissue, with or without an implant, may be used. A small or medium implant placed beneath the chest wall skin and the muscles of the chest wall (pectoralis major and serratus anterior) often gives an acceptable breast mound. If enough local tissue is not available to cover the implant chosen, a tissue expander may first be placed. The tissue expander is serially inflated during office visits to create enough soft tissue coverage to accommodate the appropriate permanent implant, which is placed at a second operation.

When local tissue is not available or not preferred, distant tissue can be used. The most common source is the soft tissue of the lower abdominal wall, or transverse rectus abdominis myocutaneous (**TRAM**) **flap** (Fig. 3-46). A transverse paddle of skin and fat from just above the umbilicus down to the pubic hairline can be elevated and supported by the deep superior epigastric vessels that lie within the rectus abdominis muscle. By maintaining the attachment to one or both rectus abdominis muscles, the tissue can be transferred to the chest to create a breast mound. This procedure not only provides the best breast reconstruction aesthetically but also improves the donor site by providing an abdominal lipectomy. Back skin and fat transferred with the underlying latissimus dorsi, supported by the thoracodorsal vessels, may also be used. This flap is exceedingly reliable and can be used when other options are unavailable. It is also used to salvage reconstructions by other methods when difficulties occur. A small breast implant can be placed beneath these flaps to provide the necessary breast mound projection. Free flaps are also used. A TRAM flap can be based on the deep or superficial

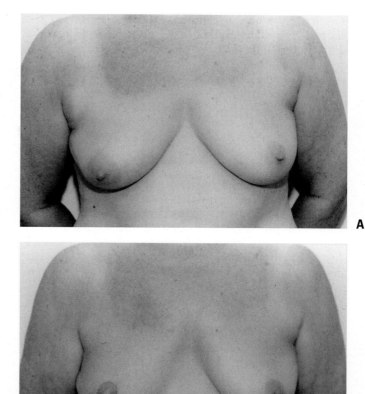

Figure 3-46   **A,** A woman with biopsy-proven carcinoma of the right breast before mastectomy. **B,** The result after skin-sparing mastectomy and immediate breast reconstruction with a transverse rectus abdominis myocutaneous flap, followed by nipple and areolar reconstruction.

inferior epigastric vessels and transferred as a free flap with only a small amount of underlying muscle. Newer techniques allow transfer of this abdominal skin with no sacrifice of muscle. Other potential donor sites are the buttock and lateral thigh.

Reconstruction of the nipple and areola, which completes breast reconstruction, is chosen by many patients. The nipple is created by a flap of local tissue folded on itself to give adequate projection or by a free graft from the contralateral nipple, if it is quite large. The areola can then be mimicked by intradermal tattooing to match the color of the normal areola or by a full-thickness graft of the contralateral areola if a breast lift (**mastopexy**) is being performed. The risk of transfering potential cancer cell should be considered with this technique, however. Full-thickness skin grafts from the groin or upper inner thigh can also be used for areolar reconstruction.

Lower Extremity Reconstruction

The soft tissues of the leg often require reconstruction of defects caused by trauma, vascular disease, or diabetes.

Trauma is the most common cause for reconstruction. High-energy blunt trauma (e.g., motor vehicle accident, crush injury, fall) is the most complex to repair. Wounds can involve the skin, bone, and vasculature of the leg. Loss of soft tissue causes exposure of fracture sites, orthopedic hardware, or vascular reconstruction, allowing infection. The infection can cause loss of fixation, disruption of vascular anastomoses, or osteomyelitis. Any of these complications may cause loss of the extremity.

Trauma

Because of the complex nature of traumatic wounds, a team approach that involves trauma, vascular, orthopedic, and plastic surgeons is used. The first priority is survival of the patient. Next, the viability of the leg must be ensured, with vascular reconstruction undertaken as necessary. Bony fixation or stabilization is achieved to ensure adequate limb length, proper orientation, and a stable skeletal platform for soft tissue reconstruction. Afterward, all efforts are directed at achieving adequate soft tissue coverage of open wounds and exposed fracture sites. Open fractures of the leg present the most challenging reconstruction problems. Some wounds can be managed with skin grafts, skin flaps, or fasciocutaneous flaps, but muscle flaps are usually required. These flaps can cover large areas of exposed bone, obliterate dead space, and provide a rich vascular coverage of exposed fracture sites to aid in bone healing.

In terms of available muscle coverage, the leg is divided into proximal, middle, and distal thirds. Wounds of the proximal third are usually reconstructed with the medial or lateral gastrocnemius muscles, usually covered by a skin graft. Likewise, the middle third of the leg is the domain of the soleus muscle flap. Because of the lack of local muscle flaps in the distal third of the leg, free muscle transfers are usually required (Fig. 3-15). Free flaps may also be required for more proximal reconstruction when local muscles are unusable because of trauma.

Systemic Disease

When systemic disease causes defects (usually ulcers) in the soft tissues of the leg, the underlying disease must first be treated. Ischemic limbs should be revascularized. When venous or lymphatic insufficiency is the underlying cause, patients should be put to bed with their extremities elevated. In addition to treatment of the underlying disease, infection should be treated and appropriate wound care administered. Wounds that result from these diseases usually can be reconstructed with skin grafts. Prolonged bed rest, elevation, and occasionally adjuncts (e.g., hyperbaric oxygen, pharmacologic agents, growth factors) are necessary. In other cases, more complex reconstructive methods are needed.

Pressure Sore Reconstruction

Pressure sores are caused by irreversible tissue damage that occurs if a patient—because of paralysis and insensitivity,

debilitation or disease—lies in a given position for more than 2 hours. Traditionally, the pressure required to induce these changes over this time frame is 30 mm Hg. Patients with spinal cord injuries are the most susceptible because of their insensibility in areas of pressure. These patients cannot feel pain caused by the evolving pressure-related wound or injury. Pressure sores can develop in any location, but they usually develop over a bony prominence. They are most commonly located in the regions of the ischial tuberosities, sacrum, and trochanter. Less commonly, they are found at the elbows, heels, and occiput. The muscle and subcutaneous tissues are most susceptible to pressure damage and are closest to the bony prominences. Most sores are larger at their base than at their visible surface, assuming the shape of an inverted cone.

Pressure sores add significant cost and complexity to patient care. Obviously, prevention is the best treatment. Patients who cannot turn themselves require frequent repositioning. Alternatively, patients at risk can be placed on a fluidized air bed, which distributes pressure evenly throughout the body.

Once a pressure sore forms, treatment is directed at caring for the wound and placing the patient on a fluidized air bed to prevent further pressure-related damage. After the wound is debrided and is sufficiently clean, reconstruction is considered. The best candidates for reconstruction are those who are alert and cooperative enough to prevent the recurrence of pressure sores. Patients who are likely to have pressure sores immediately after treatment should be managed with wound care alone. Likewise, patients who have malnutrition or other major systemic illnesses should have these problems addressed before they are considered for reconstruction.

Operative treatment is directed at total excision of the ulcer, removal of the underlying bony prominence, and coverage with healthy tissue. Although many sores can be covered with local skin flaps, muscle flaps are of great benefit and are most often used (Fig. 3-47).

In patients with spinal cord injuries, virtually any muscle or myocutaneous flap may be used for soft tissue coverage. Commonly used muscles include the gluteus maximus, gracilis, tensor fasciae latae, and hamstrings. However, in ambulatory patients, many of these muscles are needed for ambulation and their function cannot be sacrificed. In addition, because pressure sores may be a chronic problem, when possible, flaps should be designed to allow their reuse if another pressure sore develops.

Head and Neck Reconstruction

Malignancy involving the head and neck, often intraoral squamous cell carcinoma, is by far the most common disease for which tissue reconstruction in that area may be needed. Trauma and other diseases also produce defects that require reconstruction of the skin of the head and neck, of the intraoral mucosal lining, or of the bone (usually the mandible). In cancer resection, reconstruction is usually performed at the time of tumor ablation. A number

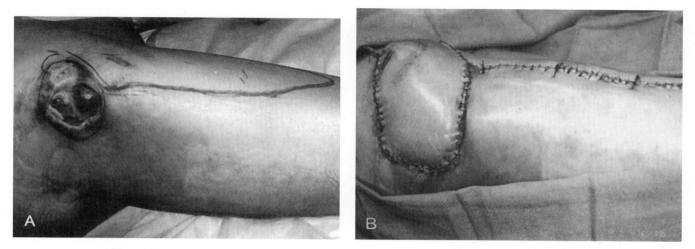

Figure 3-47   **A,** A paraplegic patient with a trochanteric pressure sore. **B,** The sore is closed with a tensor fasciae latae myocutaneous flap.

of axial-pattern skin flaps and myocutaneous flaps are useful in reconstructing some defects. The most common is the pectoralis major myocutaneous flap (Fig. 3-48). Because it is based on the thoracoacromial vessels, the flap can be elevated and tunneled through the neck for use in many areas of the head. Other myocutaneous flaps are also used (e.g., latissimus dorsi, trapezius). Free flaps can also provide excellent reconstruction. Osteocutaneous free flaps, or free flaps that include bone (e.g., radial forearm flap with a portion of the underlying radius, iliac flap with

a portion of the underlying iliac crest), may be used when mandibular reconstruction is desired.

AESTHETIC SURGERY

Aesthetic surgery involves improving the form of a normal structure. All aesthetic surgery is considered elective and should be undertaken only under optimal conditions and with the patient's clear understanding of all aspects of the

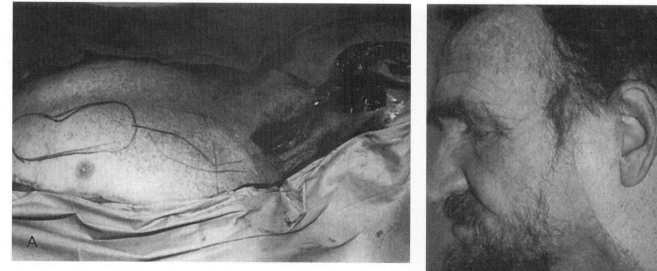
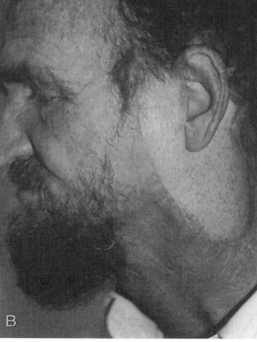

Figure 3-48   **A,** Radical resection for recurrent squamous cell carcinoma of the cheek and underlying parotid gland. **B,** After reconstruction with a pectoralis major myocutaneous flap.

surgery and recovery. Because these operations are directed at correcting perceived abnormalities, extensive preoperative consultation is required to understand such perceptions and how surgery will affect them. Aesthetic surgery is broadly divided into body-contouring surgery and surgery of the aging face. Some operations are performed for either aesthetic or reconstructive purposes (e.g., **rhinoplasty** can be performed to improve the nasal profile or to correct a nasal deformity caused by trauma).

Body-Contouring Surgery

Surgery of the Breast

Surgery of the breast involves changing both the shape and the size of the breast. It includes **reduction mammaplasty, augmentation mammaplasty,** and **mastopexy.**

Operations aimed primarily at decreasing the size of the breast (reduction mammoplasty) are reconstructive. Excessively large breasts create both physical and psychological problems. Physical problems include neck and back pain, posture-related problems, grooves in the shoulders created by bra straps, numbness of the arms, and skin problems within the inframammary fold. Psychological problems occur in adolescents who are teased by their peers for having ample breasts at a young age. The goal of reduction mammoplasty is to decrease the size of the breast, elevate the nipple position, and preserve the blood supply to the nipple–areola complex (Fig. 3-49). Most of these operations leave the nipple–areola complex attached to a pedicle of underlying breast tissue from which it receives its blood supply. These procedures are described by the orientation of the pedicle (e.g., inferior pedicle, superior pedicle, central pedicle). The correct nipple location must be chosen immediately preoperatively with the patient upright. At this time, all skin markings for the reduction are made.

Breasts that are considered too small can be enlarged through breast augmentation (augmentation mamma-

plasty). Breast implants are placed either directly beneath the breast tissue (subglandular) or beneath the pectoralis major (subpectoral or submuscular) by various approaches in skin incisions. Implants that are currently in use are constructed of an outer silicone shell filled with saline. The most common problem with implants is breast firmness, which can result from excessive scar tissue or from a capsule that normally forms around all implants. Capsular contractures cause symptoms in 15% to 20% of patients, and a few may require reoperation.

When breast size is adequate but shape is inadequate because of ptosis or sagging caused by pregnancy, aging, or weight loss, then a mastopexy, or breast lift, may be done. The nipple position is elevated by an appropriate skin excision. In some patients, breast augmentation is combined with mastopexy.

Abdominoplasty

Reshaping the abdominal wall usually involves the excision of abdominal skin and fat (abdominoplasty) and the repair or tightening of the rectus abdominis muscle (repair of rectus diastasis). The latter is considered reconstructive in women because it addresses abnormalities of the abdominal wall that result from pregnancy and childbearing and the resultant symptoms of back pain and inadequate abdominal support. Although a low abdominal incision is most commonly used, a vertical orientation or another orientation may be required if previous surgical scars are present. In general, the goal of skin excision is to remove the skin between the umbilicus and the pubic hair region. The abdominal skin and fat are elevated from the underlying musculature (from the pubic region up to the costal margin), the abdominal wall muscles are invaginated, the laxity is removed by sutures, and the excess skin is removed. The umbilicus is left attached to the underlying abdominal wall and is repositioned after skin excision (Fig. 3-50).

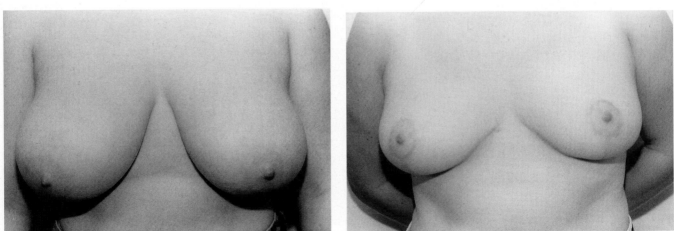

A   **B**

Figure 3-49 **A,** Mammary hyperplasia. **B,** After bilateral reduction mammaplasty.

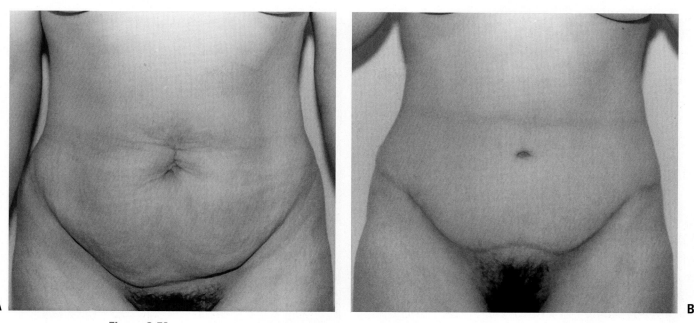

Figure 3-50 **A,** After her childbearing years, this patient underwent abdominoplasty. **B,** Six months after surgery.

Suction-Assisted Lipectomy

Suction-assisted lipectomy is directed at the removal of fat collections that are out of proportion to the patient's normal subcutaneous fat distribution. These procedures are not for obese patients, nor are they designed for weight reduction. Rather, they are performed on patients who are close to their ideal weight. In women, the lateral hips, thighs (saddlebags), legs, and abdomen are most commonly treated. In men, the hip rolls (love handles) and abdomen are often suctioned.

Through small incisions, suction cannulae are introduced. When connected to 2 atmospheres of suction, the normally solid fat can be aspirated as a semisolid material. Ultrasound assistance can be utilized for cavitation of the adipose tissue to aid in suction lipectomy. Important technical considerations include appropriate fat removal, preservation of a normal subcutaneous fat layer, and prolonged postoperative compression (6–8 weeks).

Surgery of the Aging Face

The effects of aging are often seen in the skin and underlying tissue of the face, including the eyelids, forehead, and neck. These changes are produced by a combination of factors, including gravity, atrophy or thinning of the skin, and sun damage. Although these processes are most evident in the skin, the underlying fat and musculature of the skin and neck are also affected. The signs of aging are predominantly sagging (ptotic) skin, wrinkles, and herniation of the underlying fat. The age at which these changes appear is variable. Some individuals in their 30s benefit from surgical correction of the aging process, particularly if they have a hereditary predisposition to early signs of aging or if they have had excessive sun damage. Most patients seek such surgery in the fifth, sixth, or seventh decade of life.

Facelift

A facelift, or **cervicofacial rhytidectomy,** is directed at correcting the effects of aging, generally below the level of the eyes and including the neck. Areas that are most affected include the nasolabial folds, jaw line (jowls), and neck. In this procedure, the skin of the face and neck is lifted from the underlying skin and facial musculature to a variable degree through an incision placed in front of, beneath, and behind the ear, and within the hairline. A small submental incision is also used. Usually, a deeper layer of facial muscle and platysma is also dissected. During the operation, this deeper layer (the superficial musculoaponeurotic system) is tightened, excess fat from the neck is removed, and the excessive skin is resected (Fig. 3-51). The most feared complication is injury to branches of the facial nerve that run beneath the superficial musculoaponeurotic system. Other complications include bleeding and skin slough, seen mostly in cigarette smokers.

Blepharoplasty

Recontouring of the eyelids is achieved with **blepharoplasty** because these structures are changed very little by a facelift (Fig. 3-51). This procedure removes excess skin from both the upper and lower eyelids. Fat pockets within the eyelids tend to become much more pronounced with age. Fat pockets in the lower eyelids give the impression of "bags" beneath the eyes. Some patients have a strong

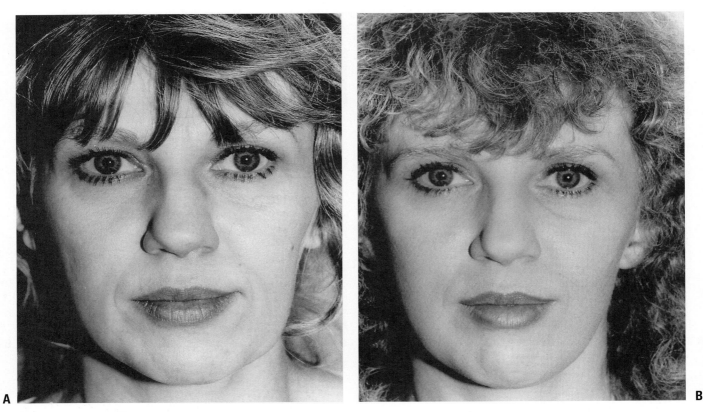

Figure 3-51 **A,** Before upper- and lower-lid blepharoplasty. **B,** After surgery

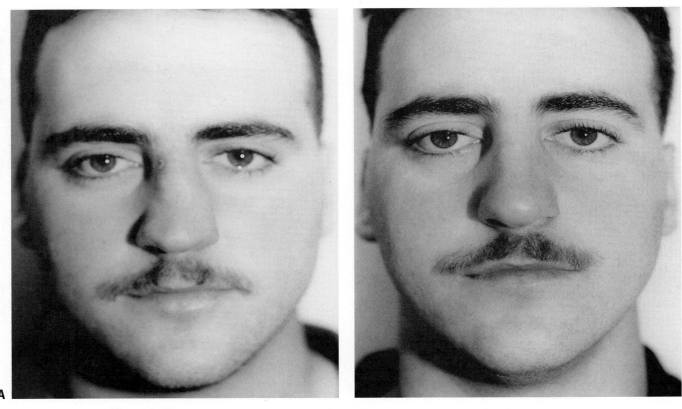

Figure 3-52 **A,** A young man with a posttraumatic nasal deformity. **B,** After reconstructive rhinoplasty.

family predisposition to lower-lid fat pockets and benefit from a lower-lid blepharoplasty at a young age.

For an upper-lid blepharoplasty, the incision is placed within the normal eyelid crease above the eye. In the lower eyelids, the incision is placed just beneath the eyelashes. Through these incisions, fat from the pockets is appropriately resected, and excess skin and muscle (orbicularis oculi) are removed. Newer concepts allow fat repositioning to obtain a more youthful appearance. Major complications result from bleeding or excess skin removal.

Laser-Assisted Skin Resurfacing

The carbon dioxide laser has been an important tool for the removal of fine lines and wrinkles from the face, with or without incisions to remove excess skin. The target of this laser is water within the skin. As the laser is applied to an area of skin, the superficial layers are vaporized as the water molecules absorb the energy from the laser beam. As these areas heal, the skin appears more taut and has fewer wrinkles. The development of a computerized pattern generator slaved to a CO_2 laser that allows a grid of laser points to be set down in a single burst allows the use of this technology for resurfacing of the entire face, segmental resurfacing of specific areas of the face, and blepharoplasty. Other ablative (surface-removing) and nonablative (surface-retaining) techniques can be used to tighten skin and treat other skin lesions. Lasers are also used for tattoo and vascular lesion removal.

Rhinoplasty

Patients seek changes in the shape of the nose because of trauma or a desire to improve the normal nasal profile. In cases of trauma, the operation is considered reconstructive (Fig. 3-52). In other cases the correction is considered aesthetic. In both cases, the rhinoplasty is performed in much the same way. While this complex operation is being performed, attention must be given to the nasal airway. When this airway is obstructed, surgery on the nasal septum, nasal value, or turbinates may be needed.

Through incisions that are usually placed within the nose, the nasal cartilage and bones are exposed. They are reshaped to give a better profile. Common areas of patient concern are a broad nasal bridge, a dorsal hump, or a bulbous nasal tip. Because the nasal bones are usually cut, postoperative support is required with a splint and nasal packs.

SUGGESTED READINGS

Achauer BM, Eriksson E, Guyuron B, et al, eds. *Plastic Surgery: Indications, Operations, Outcomes.* St. Louis: Mosby; 2000.

Ashton SJ, Beesly RW, Thorne CHM, eds. *Grabb and Smith's Plastic Surgery.* Philadelphia: Lippincott Williams & Wilkins; 1997.

Evans GRD. *Operative Plastic Surgery.* New York: McGraw Hill; 2000.

Green D. *Operative Hand Surgery.* New York: Churchill Livingstone; 1988.

Habal MB, Ariyan S. *Facial Fractures.* Philadelphia: BC Decker; 1989.

Lawrence PF, Bell RM, Dayton ME, eds. *Essentials of General Surgery.* 4th ed. Philadelphia: Lippincott Williams & Wilkins; 2006.

Mathes SJ, Nahai F. *Reconstructive Surgery: Principles, Anatomy, and Technique.* New York: Churchill Livingstone; 1997.

McCarthy J. *Plastic Surgery.* Philadelphia: WB Saunders; 1990.

Noone RB. *Plastic and Reconstructive Surgery of the Breast.* Philadelphia: BC Decker; 1991.

Plastic and Reconstructive Surgery: Essentials for Students. Chicago: Plastic Surgery Educational Foundation, American Society of Plastic and Reconstructive Surgery; 1979.

Smith JW, Aston SJ. *Plastic Surgery.* Boston: Little, Brown; 1991.

Yaremchuk MJ, Burgess AR, Brumback RJ. *Lower Extremity Salvage and Reconstruction.* New York: Elsevier; 1989.

ALAN SPOTNITZ ■ **MARSHAL L. JACOBS**
MANISHA R. SHENDE

Cardiothoracic Surgery: Diseases of the Heart, Great Vessels, and Thoracic Cavity

14 Describe the evaluation and treatment of traumatic rupture of the aorta, and discuss the complications of treatment.

15 Describe the evaluation and treatment of aortic dissection.

16 Describe the clinical manifestation, anatomy, and treatment of thoracic aortic aneurysms.

17 Discuss the diagnostic modalities available to investigate chest lesions (e.g., pulmonary mass, chest wall tumor, pleural disease).

18 Discuss the evaluation and differential diagnosis of hemoptysis.

19 Create an algorithm to evaluate a solitary lung nodule.

20 Describe the common causes of pleural effusion, and discuss the distinctions between exudate and transudate.

21 Discuss the etiology and management of lung abscess and empyema.

22 Define and discuss the management of various types of chest trauma, including open pneumothorax, tension pneumothorax, hemothorax, and flail chest.

23 Discuss the workup and management of patients with chest wall and mediastinal pathology.

24 Discuss the preoperative evaluation of patients for thoracic surgery.

25 Describe the common pathologic lesions of the anterior, posterior, and superior portions of the mediastinum.

26 Discuss the risk factors and symptoms of lung cancer.

27 Discuss the management of primary lung neoplasms.

28 Describe the preoperative preparation and assessment of patients who undergo pulmonary resection.

29 List the most common sources of metastatic lesions in the lung, and discuss the management of metastatic disease in the chest.

This chapter is divided into sections on the heart, the thoracic aorta and great vessels, and the thoracic cavity, which includes the chest wall, mediastinum, and lungs. Diseases of the esophagus that are treated by thoracic and general surgeons are covered in Chapter 13 of Lawrence et al, *Essentials of General Surgery*, 4th ed.

DISEASES OF THE HEART

This section discusses cardiac structure and function and demonstrates the surgeon's approach to ischemic heart disease, valvular heart disease, congenital heart disease, and disorders of the pericardium. Cardiovascular diseases are the most common causes of significant morbidity and mortality in all sectors of the population. Enormous resources are consumed in treating these diseases. Heart disease is of major concern to patients, physicians, and policy makers alike. According to the American Heart Association, in 2002 coronary artery disease, myocardial infarction, angina, and congestive heart failure affected 13,000,000, 7,100,000, 6,400,000, and 4,900,000 people, respectively, in the United States alone. Approximately 927,000 deaths occurred related to cardiovascular diseases. Congenital heart disease ranks as the second leading cause of death (following accidents) in children 15 years of age or less. Almost 210,000 cardiovascular procedures were performed on this younger age group. More than $383 billion were spent on treatment and prevention of cardiovascular diseases affecting all segments of the population.

Anatomy

The heart is a hollow, muscular organ that provides the physical force necessary to deliver oxygen-rich blood to the body and to return oxygen-poor blood to the lungs. The anatomy of the normal heart is well suited for this task, because blood destined for the lungs is kept separate from blood destined for the periphery. The atria receive blood from the peripheral or central circulation. They allow this blood to pass through one-way atrioventricular valves (tricuspid on the right; mitral on the left) into the primary pumping chambers, or ventricles. The left ventricle, which delivers blood against systemic vascular resistance, is more muscular than the right ventricle, which delivers blood to the lower resistance pulmonary circuit. The heart is an end-organ that receives its circulation from the epicardial coronary arteries that arise from the left and right sinuses of Valsalva, distal to the aortic valve (Fig. 4-1). The left main coronary artery branches into the left anterior descending coronary artery and the circumflex coronary artery. Each of these in turn may give off additional branches. The right coronary artery usually supplies the posterior descending coronary artery distally and a posterolateral branch. The blood supply to the sinus and atrioventricular nodes usually arises from the right coronary artery and often explains the occurrence of heart block in the presence of a right coronary occlusion or infarct.

As an end organ, the heart is affected by the same physiologic disturbances that affect peripheral organs. The ability of the heart to provide blood to the periphery may be

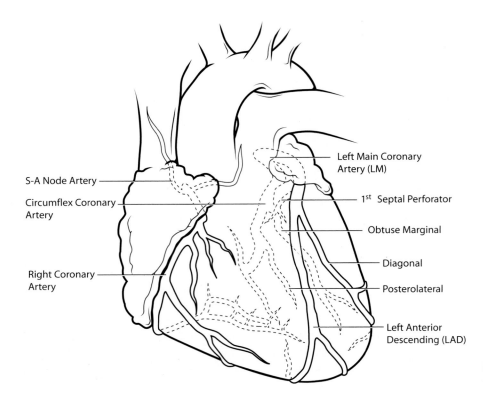

Figure 4-1 Diagram of heart and coronary arteries.

adversely affected by any alteration in the normal anatomy of the heart (e.g., defects of the atrial or ventricular septum, valvular incompetence or stenosis, coronary artery obstruction).

Physiology: Cardiac Function and Its Assessment

Physiologic manipulation of the circulation is essential for treating patients with cardiovascular disease (and therefore is covered here as well in the Critical Care chapter in Lawrence et al, *Essential of General Surgery*, 4th ed). It should always be recognized that cardiac function can be clinically assessed with simple parameters (blood pressure, urine output, skin color and texture, mental status, and heart rate). Unfortunately, these measurements do not always reflect changes in cardiac function until deterioration has occurred, sometimes irreversibly. Earlier detection of myocardial dysfunction is possible with both noninvasive and invasive techniques that permit pharmacologic and mechanical intervention to halt deterioration.

A catheter can be placed via a central vein so that its tip lies within the thoracic cavity to monitor **central venous pressure** (CVP). The limitation of the CVP is that it does not directly measure the function of the left side of the heart. It measures the ability of the right side of the heart to deal with the volume load delivered by systemic veins and can be useful in detecting compromised left ventricular function (in patients who do not otherwise have heart disease). When there is intrinsic cardiac disease, the re-

sponse of the left side of the heart will likely differ from that of the right side. Further, any clinical derangement that affects both the systemic volume and, indirectly, pulmonary vascular resistance may alter CVP without actually altering cardiac function. A single CVP measurement will probably overassess or underassess the dysfunction. A record of changes in CVP over time is more useful than an isolated measurement.

A flow-directed **pulmonary artery catheter** may be inserted into a large central vein and "floated" through the right heart and out into the pulmonary artery (Figs. 4-2 and 4-3). This is usually done with a Swan-Ganz catheter, which can be used to measure CVP, pulmonary artery pressure, **pulmonary capillary wedge pressure,** and cardiac output. When the balloon on the end of the catheter is inflated, the catheter can be wedged into a small pulmonary artery. The pressure measured in this position is called the pulmonary capillary wedge pressure (PCWP). By the laws of hydraulics, this will reflect left atrial pressure, which, in the absence of mitral valve disease, reflects pressure in the left ventricle at the end of diastole when the mitral valve is open (left ventricular end-diastolic pressure [LVEDP]). In turn, this pressure reflects the left ventricular end-diastolic volume component of cardiac output. According to Starling's law, left ventricular muscle contractile force is proportional to myocardial fiber stretch: the greater the volume of blood within the ventricle at the end of diastole, the greater is the force of contraction and therefore of cardiac output. Because rapid and accurate bedside methods to measure end-diastolic volume are not

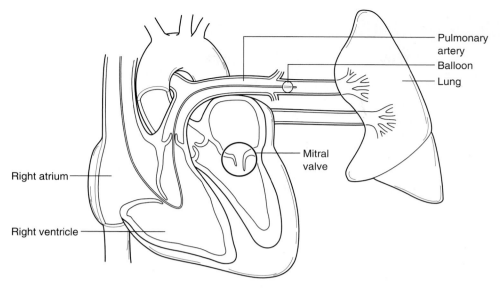

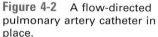

Figure 4-2 A flow-directed pulmonary artery catheter in place.

readily available, measurements of LVEDP are used instead. LVEDP is used as a guide to the volume status, or filling pressure, of the heart. The translation of left ventricular end-diastolic volume into a clinically useful pressure measurement (LVEDP) assumes that compliance of the ventricle remains constant. However, that is not always the case. Certain clinical conditions (e.g., left ventricular hypertrophy, acute myocardial infarction) that acutely alter left ventricular compliance can change the relation between left ventricular end-diastolic volume and pressure.

Cardiac output can be measured using the Swan-Ganz catheter by means of thermodilution techniques that use a thermistor at the tip of the catheter. This calculation is combined with blood pressure, CVP, and PCWP to calculate resistance and assess cardiac function. Adding a fiberoptic system that can provide real-time, on-line mea-

surement of oxygen saturation in the pulmonary artery allows further discrimination in such assessment. The mixed venous oxygen saturation (Svo_2) reflects cardiac index and systemic oxygen delivery as long as hemoglobin levels and oxygen extraction (metabolic activity and work) are accounted for. A decrease in Svo_2 can be caused by a decrease in cardiac output, a decrease in hemoglobin levels, or an increase in the amount of oxygen extracted at the cellular level. Careful assessment is necessary to decide which variable is operational in any given patient. The mixed venous oxygen saturation, although affected by hemoglobin concentration, is a clinically useful tool for moment-to-moment assessment of cardiac function. Table 4-1 shows the basic formulas used to assess myocardial function based on measurements available in an intensive care unit.

When these types of invasive monitoring are available,

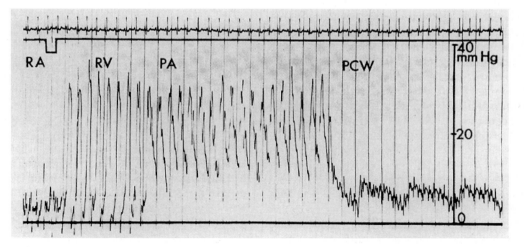

Figure 4-3 Tracings from a flow-directed pulmonary artery catheter. *RA,* right atrium; *RV,* right ventricle; *PA,* pulmonary artery; *PCW,* pulmonary capillary wedge.

Table 4-1	Assessment of Myocardial Function

Function	Normal Values
Arterial blood pressure	120/80 mm Hg
Mean arterial pressure (MAP)	
$\quad$ Pulse pressure + Diastolic blood pressure	70–90 mm Hg
$\quad\qquad\qquad 3$	
Heart rate	60–100 beats/min
Central venous pressure (CVP)	2–8 mm Hg
Pulmonary artery pressure (PAP)	25/10 mm Hg
Pulmonary wedge pressure (PWP)	6–12 mm Hg
Cardiac index (CI)	2.5–3.0 L/min/m^2
Systemic vascular resistance (SVR)	
$\quad$ MAP − CVP × 80	900–1,200 dyn/sec/cm^{-5}
$\qquad$ CO	
Peripheral vascular resistance (PVR)	
$\quad$ PAP (mean) − PWP × 80	150–250 dyn/sec/cm^{-5}
$\qquad$ CO	
Stroke volume (SV)	
$\qquad$ CO	60–70 mL/beat
$\quad$ Heart rate	
Stroke index (SI)	
$\qquad$ SV	35–45 mL/beat/m^2
$\quad$ BSA (body surface area)	
Left ventricular stroke work index (LVSWI)	
$\quad$ SI × MAP × 0.014	51–61 g/min/m^2
Arterial O$_2$ content (Cao$_2$) = % saturation	
$\quad$ (hemoglobin) × 1.39) + 0.003 (Pao$_2$)	18–20 mol/dL
Arterial O$_2$ delivery (Do$_2$) = CI × Cao$_2$	550–600 mol/min/m^2
Mixed venous O$_2$ saturation (Svo$_2$)	55%–70%

it is easy to distinguish the etiology of hypotension and shock. A patient who is in hypovolemic shock may be diagnosed by clinical signs (trauma, hemorrhage, vomiting, diarrhea, dehydration) and simple bedside measurements (assessment of mucous membranes, skin turgor, urine output, blood pressure, pulse rate). However, when clinical indicators are equivocal, invasive measurements that show low pulmonary artery wedge pressure (PAWP), CVP, and cardiac index usually confirm a low circulating volume. Appropriate therapy is transfusion with blood products or balanced electrolyte solutions. Both clinical and invasive measurements are used to gauge patient response.

Usually, patients who have heart failure because of chronic conditions (e.g., valvular heart disease) or acute problems (e.g., acute myocardial infarction) have elevated PAWP because of inadequate myocardial pump function and diminished cardiac index. However, the caution about the integration of myocardial compliance, wedge pressure, and cardiac index is often forgotten in the setting of acute cardiac dysfunction. For example, a patient who has an acute myocardial infarction, a cardiac index of 1.8 L/min/m^2, and a wedge pressure of 6 mm Hg is hypovolemic. The patient's edematous infarcted myocardium may require filling pressures greater than the "normal" wedge pressure of 12 to 15 mm Hg to stretch the myocardium sufficiently

to generate adequate cardiac output. Conversely, another patient who has an acute myocardial infarction may have a cardiac index of 1.8 L/min/m^2, but a wedge pressure of 25 mm Hg. This patient is clearly in pulmonary edema and will benefit from a reduction in the filling pressures of the left ventricle to allow improved coronary perfusion of the critical areas of subendocardial myocardial muscle mass. According to Laplace's law, wall tension is directly proportional to the radius of the heart chamber and the pressure within it. Therefore, a dilated left ventricle will have subendocardial perfusion deficits based on transmyocardial pressure gradients within the coronary circulation (especially during diastole, when most coronary perfusion occurs). Reducing the radius of the left ventricle with pulmonary vasodilators (e.g., morphine, nitroglycerin), diuretics (e.g., furosemide), or phlebotomy (actual or rotating tourniquets) will decrease wall tension and increase subendocardial perfusion and therefore improve overall cardiac function. In the presence of hypertension, afterload reduction is likewise helpful. Continued low cardiac output may require the use of inotropes, intra-aortic balloon, or emergency invasive intervention.

Vasodilatory shock can be associated with early sepsis or other causes leading to lowering of systemic resistance. In this situation, hypotension may in fact be associated with a high cardiac output and normal or elevated filling pressures. Vasoconstrictive agents are indicated in this situation to maintain adequate pressure to perfuse the end organs.

The shock associated with cardiac tamponade can be very difficult to assess and can lead to a delay in treatment that may be fatal. In this situation, low blood pressure is associated with a low cardiac output, elevated filling pressure and, usually, elevated systemic resistance. One of the hallmarks of tamponade is "equalization of pressures," that is, filling pressures on both sides of the heart tend to equalize, systemic pressure drops, pulmonary pressure rises, and pulse pressure may narrow. Treatment requires immediate relief of the tamponade by mechanical interventions such as pericardiocentesis or surgical drainage of the pericardium.

Although invasive monitoring devices provide valuable information, they can cause complications. Depending on the site of insertion, any central venous cannulation can cause hemorrhage and pneumothorax. In a critically ill patient whose condition is acutely deteriorating, proper insertion techniques must be used. The safest approach to introducing a pulmonary artery flotation catheter is a posterior-superior approach to the right internal jugular vein. In this approach, the introducer needle is never in contact with the lung. Lower jugular or subclavian approaches are more likely to cause pneumothorax. They are used especially cautiously in patients with blood dyscrasias and clotting abnormalities, because direct pressure cannot be applied to the subclavian vein or the internal jugular vein beneath the clavicle. In these patients, a high cervical approach to the central veins or the temporary use of the femoral vein is recommended. Perforation of

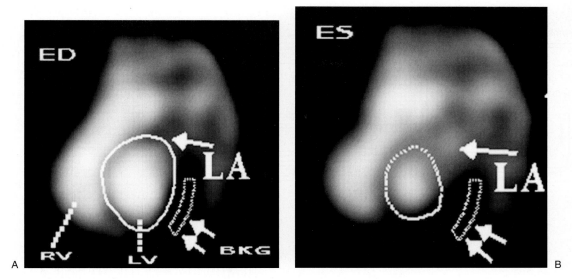

Figure 4-4   Radionuclide angiocardiography. Frames representing end-diastole (*ED*) and end-systole (*ES*). An automatic edge detection algorithm was applied for definition of the edges. Left atrium (*LA*) is correctly excluded from the left ventricular (*LV*) region of interest. Background region (*arrows*) is in standardized position and covers representative background area (*BKG*). Here the camera is positioned in left anterior oblique 45-degree position. *RV,* right ventricle. (Reprinted with permission from Images.MD, The Online Encyclopedia of Medical Images. Taken from Mannting F. *Atlas of Cardiac Imaging.* Edited by Richard Lee, Richard T. Lee, Eugene Braunwald. Current Medicine LLC: 1998.)

the pulmonary artery with massive **hemoptysis** may occur after insertion of a pulmonary artery catheter. In addition, cardiac arrhythmias can occur when the catheter is passed through the right ventricle. Infectious endocarditis is also a potential problem, especially when the catheter is in place for more than 3 days.

Additional noninvasive means of assessing cardiac function include radionuclide scanning, echocardiography, and cardiac magnetic resonance imaging (MRI). Multiple gated acquisition (MUGA) scans show ejection fractions quite accurately and therefore can categorize cardiac function (Fig. 4-4), but they are not easily performed at the bedside. Echocardiography and transesophageal echocardiography can be performed at the bedside, but must be interpreted by an experienced echocardiographer. Cardiac MRI is a newer method of cardiac evaluation and can be very accurate in the assessment of cardiac function, but again is not available at the bedside. During surgical procedures, a transesophageal echocardiogram (TEE) can be used to continuously monitor cardiac volume, function, and wall motion.

Cardiopulmonary Bypass and Myocardial Protection

Cardiopulmonary Bypass

The ability to perform surgery on the heart and great vessels awaited the development of a method to artificially

support the circulation and respiration while, at the same time, preventing significant damage to the heart. In the 1930s, Gibbon began work on a technique of circulatory support to allow pulmonary embolectomy; a procedure that he believed was inadequately dealt with by the closed techniques of Trendelenburg. It was not until the early 1950s that cooperation among Gibbon, the IBM Corporation, the University of Minnesota, and the Mayo Clinic produced the first clinically successful pump oxygenators. The heart–lung machine was used successfully for the first time in 1953 to repair a secundum atrial septal defect in a young girl. Numerous failures occurred before this case. The mortality rate for early open-heart surgery approached 40% to 50%. Over time, biomechanical improvements resulted in safer cardiopulmonary bypass.

There are multiple components to the heart-lung machine (Fig. 4-5). All of the "foreign" surfaces involved are thrombogenic and require the use of systemic heparinization in order to prevent thrombosis. Today, the roller pump and the vortex pump are the most commonly used devices to provide for the actual circulation of blood. Membrane oxygenators of various designs provide for gas exchange and take over the function of the lungs. Temperature regulation is maintained by a heater–cooler, and scavenging of blood from the operative field is done by suckers that return heparinized blood to the machine. Filtering devices are present, as are sensors and traps to prevent air embolization during the procedure. Blood is withdrawn from the venous circulation, either through a single

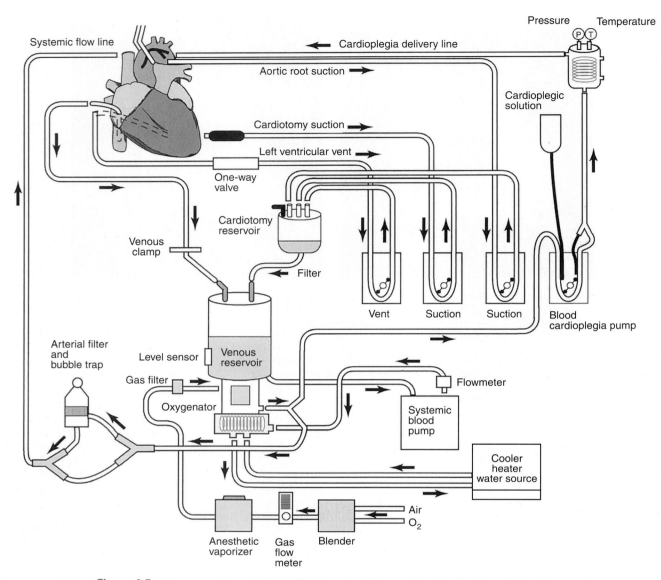

Figure 4-5 Diagram of a typical cardiopulmonary bypass circuit with vent, field suction, aortic root suction, and cardioplegic system. Blood is drained from a single "two-stage" catheter into the venous reservoir, which is part of the membrane oxygenator/heat exchanger unit. Venous blood exits the unit and is pumped through the heat exchanger and then the oxygenator. Arterialized blood exits the oxygenator and passes through a filter/bubble trap to the aortic cannula, which is usually placed in the ascending aorta. Blood aspirated from vents and suction systems enters a separate cardiotomy reservoir, which contains a microfilter, before entering the venous reservoir. The cardioplegic system is fed by a spur from the arterial line to which the cardioplegic solution is added and is pumped through a separate heat exchanger into the antegrade or retrograde catheters. Oxygenator gases and water for the heat exchanger are supplied by independent sources. (Reprinted with permission from Cohn LH, Edmunds LH Jr, eds. *Cardiac Surgery in the Adult.* New York: McGraw-Hill, 2003. Available at: http://cardiacsurgery.ctsnetbooks.org/cgi/content/full/2/2003/317#Pumps.)

cannula in the right atrium or through separate cannulae in the inferior and superior vena cavae. The blood passes through the oxygenator, where oxygen levels are replenished and carbon dioxide is removed. With the appropriate pump mechanism, blood is reintroduced into the circulation through either the ascending aorta or the femoral artery. Mild, moderate, or deep hypothermia is often employed because metabolic demands are diminished at lower temperatures. The responses of the body to this insult are manifest in many ways and are frequently characterized by a total body inflammatory response that can lead to or be associated with many of the complications of using the heart–lung machine, including organ failure and coagulopathy.

Myocardial Protection

The goal of myocardial protection is to provide a quiet, bloodless field, the optimal environment for working on or in the heart, without causing damage to the heart muscle. To achieve this, cardiac activity must be stopped, the coronary circulation occluded, and protection provided to the myocardial cells. The cells are protected by minimizing the metabolic demand of the heart while it is deprived of its normal circulation and oxygen supply. Recalling the determinants of oxygen demand (wall tension, heart rate, and contractility), this is achieved by emptying the heart, stopping the heart, and eliminating any work it must do (taking over its pumping function). A major improvement in the survival of patients undergoing cardiac surgery came with the introduction of potassium cardioplegia in the late 1970s. Since its inception, the principles of cardioplegic arrest have been adopted as the standard method of myocardial protection. The heart is stopped after initiating cardiopulmonary bypass by applying a cross-clamp to the aorta and delivering potassium cardioplegia into the aortic root and down the coronary arteries. The high potassium content (20–25 mEq/L) of the solution eliminates the concentration gradient of potassium across the myocardial cell membranes and induces electrochemical paralysis of myocardial cellular function. The composition of the cardioplegic solution varies among institutions, but it usually consists of a crystalloid or a blood carrier, a buffer to antagonize the ischemic acidosis, and a substance (e.g., mannitol) to render the solution hypertonic to the myocardial cell to minimize edema. Various modifications of this solution are used for cardioplegia induction and reperfusion. To overcome the heterogeneous distribution of antegrade cardioplegia because of coronary artery stenoses, some surgeons will instill cardioplegic solution in a retrograde fashion through the coronary sinus. The coronary venous system has no valves and is not subject to atherosclerotic obstruction, allowing homogeneous distribution of the cardioplegia. Periods of ischemic cardioplegic arrest lasting 1 to 3 hours are well tolerated. Cardiac activity resumes after normal perfusion is restored. Any damage that occurs during reperfusion after ischemic arrest can be aggravated by various electrochemical elements (e.g., oxygen free rad-

icals). Free-radical scavengers can improve cardiac performance after ischemic arrest.

Ischemic Heart Disease

Pathophysiology

The most commonly recognized cause of ischemic heart disease is the occlusion of large epicardial vessels in the heart by atherosclerotic cardiovascular disease. Other etiologies include valvular heart disease, vasculitis, congenital coronary anomalies, and dissection of the thoracic aorta if the ostia of the coronary arteries are involved. In all of these cases, the underlying pathogenesis is the mismatch of myocardial oxygen supply and demand. This mismatch is most commonly caused by the obstruction of flow through the coronary bed by a narrowing of more than 50% of the cross-sectional diameter of the vessel (Fig. 4-6). The usual manifestation of ischemia is **angina pectoris** characterized by substernal chest pain or pressure that may radiate down the arm. Other "anginal equivalents," however, may be present (e.g., jaw pain, throat pain, arm pain, dyspnea on exertion). Diabetics in particular are likely to manifest dyspnea on exertion as their anginal equivalent because of decreased neural sensitivity from the heart.

The physiology of oxygen supply to the heart is unique compared with that of other end organs. Although other organs are perfused mainly during systole, the heart receives most (approximately 80%) of its blood flow during diastole, when intracavitary pressure of the heart and the resulting transmural pressure gradient are low. The heart extracts 70% or more of the oxygen carried by capillary blood before the blood is returned to the venous system. Consequently, the heart cannot meet increased metabolic demands by increasing the extraction of oxygen from the blood, as most other organs do. Instead, it must rely on increased blood flow to the myocardium to meet these needs.

The supply of oxygen to the heart is determined by the duration of the diastolic interval (which decreases as heart rate increases or obstruction to left ventricular outflow occurs); the oxygen-carrying capacity of the blood (hemoglobin level and oxygen saturation); and the unimpeded flow of blood through the coronary arteries. Stenosis that narrows the cross-sectional area of a large epicardial coronary artery by more than 75% (50% cross-sectional diameter) impedes the required increase in blood flow to the bed supplied by that coronary artery when metabolic demand increases.

Demand of the heart for oxygen has three major determinants: (a) wall tension as measured by Laplace's law (tension = [pressure $\times$ radius]/2 $\times$ wall thickness); (b) heart rate; and (c) the level of contractility of the heart (Starling's law). Laplace's law summarizes the effects of preload (radius of the chamber and pressure in the chamber during diastole), afterload (pressure during systole), and wall thickness (compensatory changes to chronic increases in afterload).

Rest

Stress

Rest

Stress

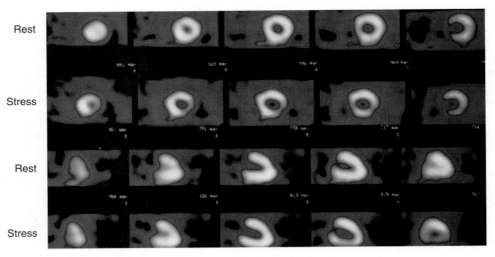

Figure 4-6   Myocardial perfusion imaging. Myocardial perfusion scan from a 61-year-old woman presenting with recurrent typical exertional chest pain (CP). Test stopped due to typical CD; electrocardiography shows 1-mm ST depression. Findings: No rest perfusion abnormalities. During stress, moderate severe ischemia in the lateral wall from apex to base (6 of 25 segments, typical left circumflex coronary artery [LCx] territory). Subsequent coronary angiogram: LAD 40% stenosis, LCx totally occluded distally, obtuse marginal branch 95% stenosis, right coronary artery small and totally occluded. Thus, LCx and RCA are both occluded. Both the lateral and the inferior still show normal perfusion at rest. This appearance can be explained by sufficient collateral flow at rest, but insufficiency of the collateral flow during stress first manifested in the lateral wall. (Reprinted with permission from Images.MD, The Online Encyclopedia of Medical Images. Taken from Mannting F. *Atlas of Cardiac Imaging.* Edited by Richard Lee, Richard T. Lee, Eugene Braunwald. Current Medicine LLC: 1998.)

The etiology of atherosclerotic cardiovascular disease is multifactorial. It is a progressive disease that can appear microscopically, even in infants. The lesions develop over time as a complex interaction of lipid deposition within the intima of the vessel wall, along with blood and blood products, fibrous tissue, and calcification. After significant stenoses occur, symptoms may ensue. In addition, dynamic plaques (intermittent closure), rupture of plaques with hemorrhage into the wall, or acute thrombosis superimposed on these plaques can contribute to episodes of ischemia or to the development of myocardial infarction, even if oxygen demand on the heart is not increased. More recently, factors associated with inflammation and the inflammatory response have been implicated in these changes.

Many factors are recognized as contributing to the development of atherosclerotic cardiovascular disease. These include genetic factors, hypertension, diabetes, obesity, hypercholesterolemia, stress, inactivity, and smoking. Many of these factors can be modified to alter the progressive course of the disease.

Clinical Presentation and Evaluation

The diagnosis of ischemic heart disease may be complex and depends on the presentation of the patient. Some patients come to the hospital with severe unstable angina or acute myocardial infarction that requires rapid diagnosis and treatment.

History

Patients may present emergently with acute onset of severe chest pressure or pain (often radiating down the arm), diaphoresis, nausea, and vomiting. Some patients have heart failure manifested by pulmonary edema or hypotension. Such patients are likely to be evolving an acute myocardial infarction or having severe unstable angina. These patients require hospitalization for further emergency diagnosis and treatment.

Other patients have more chronic forms of ischemic heart disease. They often have angina, especially associated with physical activity. A complete, careful history and physical examination often raise the suspicion of ischemic heart disease. The history should focus on defining the nature of the discomfort and identifying factors that bring on the symptoms (e.g., exercise, sexual intercourse, emotional stress) or other factors that significantly increase myocardial oxygen demand. Angina must be differentiated from other causes of chest pain, such as the epigastric discomfort of heartburn, the chest pain of pericarditis or pleuritis, or the discomfort of bursitis or inflammatory problems in the chest wall. Additional inquiries should be made regarding family history and personal history of myocardial infarction, heart murmur, hypertension, diabetes, or connective tissue disorders. Questions should be asked about smoking, exercise, dietary habits, and use of medication.

Physical Examination

The examiner should attempt to elicit signs of coronary artery disease or other diseases that may be associated with atherosclerotic disease of the heart. Peripheral signs of atherosclerosis include carotid bruits, abdominal aortic aneurysms, loss of peripheral pulses, and symptoms of leg ischemia and cerebral ischemia. Signs of heart failure include rales, peripheral edema, and hepatic enlargement. On cardiac examination, the patient may show signs of increased cardiac size and abnormal heart sounds that suggest heart failure. The presence of any cardiac murmurs should prompt a search for valvular lesions, usually by echocardiography.

Diagnostic Evaluation

In the emergency setting, acute changes are often noted on electrocardiogram (ECG), especially when there is ongoing pain. These changes may include Q waves that indicate myocardial cellular necrosis because of the inability of dead cells to become electrically excitable; ST segment elevations caused by the inability of the affected myocyte to repolarize normally; and T wave inversions and QT prolongations that reflect ongoing cardiac ischemia because of delayed repolarization. Creatine phosphokinase (CPK) isoenzymes and troponin levels are elevated when myocardial cellular damage has occurred.

In the more chronic situation, if the index of suspicion for ischemic heart disease is high, further diagnostic studies are often needed. The usual process is to proceed to stress testing. Stress is induced to increase coronary blood flow. This can be accomplished by physical exercise, increasing the heart rate by pacing, or coronary vasodilatation by dipyridamole or adenosine (strong coronary vasodilators.) The patient who is physically able exercises progressively to gradually increase heart rate and myocardial O_2 consumption, usually by walking and running on a treadmill at increasing rates and levels of inclination while blood pressure and ECG are monitored. The patient is questioned about any symptoms of angina. The onset of symptoms, especially when associated with significant ECG changes, is considered positive for ischemia. The development of hypotension associated with a stress test is an ominous sign that strongly suggests left main vessel or critical triple-vessel disease. The accuracy of a stress test alone is approximately 70%. The accuracy can be increased to approximately 90% with the addition of thallium or technetium. A stress thallium examination shows electrocardiographic changes of ischemia if they are present and graphically locates the ischemic myocardium by absence of tracer images in the ischemic area. In this test, the radioisotope is injected intravenously and the heart is scanned before and after stress is induced. Ischemic areas show diminished radiolabeled tracer activity (Fig. 4-7). Resting echocardiography easily shows regional wall motion abnormalities consistent with ischemia or infarction, and allows estimates of valvular dysfunction, pulmonary artery pressures, and chamber size. In patients with normal

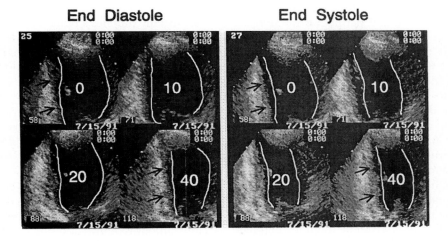

Figure 4-7   Dobutamine stress echocardiogram from a patient with prior inferior wall myocardial infarction. End-diastolic and end-systolic frames from the apical two-chamber left ventricular view are presented. End-diastolic and end-systolic screens are divided into four quadrants, with representative images at four dobutamine doses: 0, 10, 20, and 40 mcg/kg/min. Note decreasing chamber size with augmenting dobutamine stress. The inferior wall, indicated by *black arrows,* is akinetic at rest and remains akinetic at 40 mcg/kg/min dobutamine. At intermediate doses, there is no evidence for enhanced inferior wall systolic thickening, while the anterior wall, seen contralateral to the inferior wall, augments systolic motion with increasing dobutamine levels. Anatomically, the inferior wall should show extensive scar formation, with very little functioning or viable myocardium. Such a region would not respond favorably to revascularization.

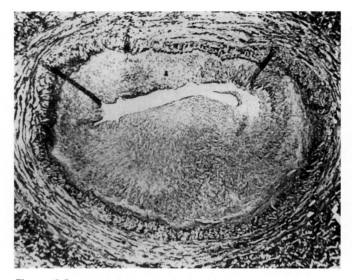

Figure 4-8 Atherosclerotic obstruction of a coronary artery that causes marked reduction of blood flow to the affected heart muscle.

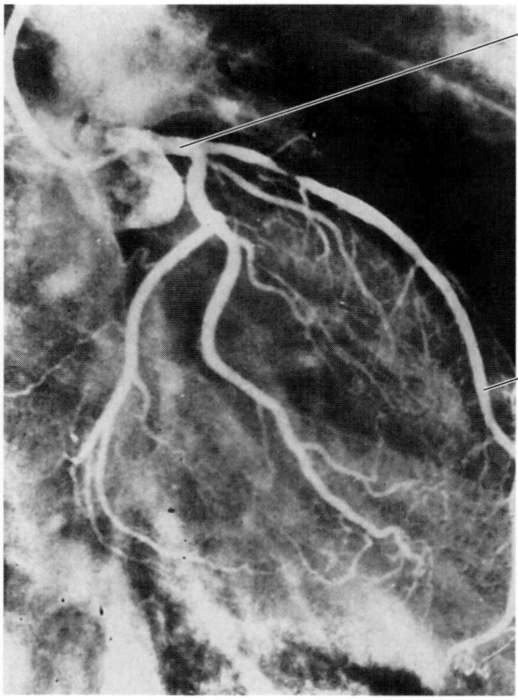

Figure 4-9 Coronary angiography showing an obstruction in the proximal left anterior descending artery.

resting values, an inotropic challenge with dobutamine may unmask an ischemic myocardium (Fig. 4-8).

The decision to proceed with more invasive testing depends on the index of clinical suspicion (even in the absence of a positive stress test), the severity of the disease, and the concern over impending cardiac events (e.g., myocardial infarction). Invasive testing is recommended for symptomatic patients with high-risk clinical indicators (e.g., ischemic abnormalities on ECG, ST depression during exercise testing, concomitant peripheral vascular disease, age, diabetes, smoking history, and family history of atherosclerotic heart disease). All patients in whom ischemic heart disease is suspected ultimately undergo cardiac catheterization to determine whether coronary artery or valvular heart disease is present. This test remains the gold standard in the diagnosis of ischemic heart disease, although MR angiography and CT angiography may replace diagnostic coronary angiograms in the near future. A catheter is placed through a large peripheral artery (usually femoral) and passed retrograde to the heart and coronary arteries (left heart catheterization), or through a large vein (again, usually femoral) into and through the right side of the heart and out the pulmonary artery (right heart catheterization). Left heart catheterization includes coronary angiography, in which dye is injected directly into the coronary arteries to define their anatomy (Fig. 4-9) and measurements of pressure in the aorta and left ventricle. Left ventriculography (in which dye is injected into the left ventricular cavity to evaluate left ventricular function) is usually performed and the results are reported as a global ejection fraction with additional description of regional wall motion abnormalities. If valvular lesions are suspected, more extensive pressure measurements may be required.

Coronary anatomy is commonly discussed in terms of the two major coronary arterial systems: the left main coronary artery and the right coronary artery. The left main divides into the left anterior descending (LAD) coronary artery and the circumflex coronary artery. The right coronary usually supplies a branch to the atrioventricular node and is the origin of the posterior descending coronary artery 80% to 85% of the time (right dominant system). Branches of the LAD are referred to as diagonal arteries and septal perforators. Obtuse marginal arteries are branches of the circumflex coronary artery. Obstruction of the left main coronary artery carries a significantly worse prognosis because both the circumflex and the anterior descending systems are included within its watershed. A 50% stenosis of a coronary artery visualized in two planes at angiography is a hemodynamically significant lesion. Studies of the natural history of coronary artery disease show that the prognosis worsens as the disease increases from one to three vessels, as would be expected when larger amounts of myocardium are placed in jeopardy. It is not enough, however, to denote single-, double-, or triple-vessel disease without allowing for variations in the amount of myocardium served by each vessel (i.e., myocardium at risk). For example, high-grade stenosis of a nondominant right coronary artery is not an indication for coronary revascularization, but high-grade stenosis of a large, dominant right coronary artery would be likely to require revascularization of some kind.

The presence of left ventricular dysfunction is significant in terms of prognosis, with and without further therapy, and may dictate treatment. When ventricular dysfunction is associated with large areas of scarred myocardium, revascularization may be of no value. However, "hibernating" myocardium that is nonfunctional because of chronic ischemia or "stunned" myocardium that is nonfunctional because of an acute ischemic episode from which it has not recovered may benefit from revascularization and may have improved long-term outcome. Current strategies allow safe coronary revascularization for patients with a very low (20%) ejection fraction when ischemic myocardium is present, but patients with ejection fractions of less than 20% often are not candidates for revascularization.

Treatment

Three types of therapy are available to patients with ischemic heart disease: medical, percutaneous interventions, and surgery. Treatment decisions must be individualized and are based on the symptoms, the anatomy, and the risks of the selected therapy. In all patients, however, risk factor modification of lifestyle and dietary habits may be of considerable benefit, especially when coordinated with smoking cessation, cholesterol-lowering strategies, and medical regimens selected on an individual basis.

Medical Management

When the risk of impending myocardial infarction is low, medical therapy to control symptoms may be appropriate. Medical therapy includes treatment with β-blockers to minimize increases in heart rate in response to physical and emotional demands, calcium channel blockers to decrease afterload and prevent coronary spasm, and nitrates to decrease preload and dilate the vessels that supply ischemic coronary beds. In theory, only after all three modes of medical therapy have been used simultaneously and at maximally tolerated doses is a patient considered to have "failed medical therapy" and to be a candidate for another more invasive mode of treatment.

Percutaneous Interventions

Percutaneous transluminal coronary angioplasty (PTCA) was first introduced in the United States by Gruntzig in the early 1980s and radically changed the approach to coronary artery disease. PTCA also led to the further development of many procedures performed in the cardiac catheterization laboratory to open partially occluded coronary vessels percutaneously. In addition to PTCA, these procedures include laser angioplasty, directed atherectomy, and the placement of intracoronary stents. With techniques similar to cardiac catheterization, a guidewire is directed across the coronary lesion under fluoroscopic control. A PTCA balloon is passed over the guidewire and across the lesion. After the balloon is inflated, it compresses the lesion against the walls of the vessel (Fig. 4-10). Intracoronary stents made of fine metal mesh have been developed, and results show an increased likelihood of longer patency after angioplasty, as well as decreased risk of emergency surgery at the time of the procedure.

Patients who undergo these procedures usually suffer

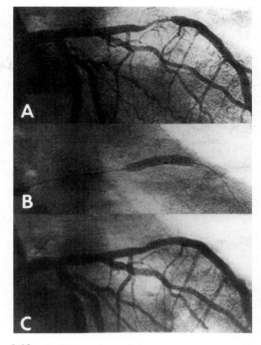

Figure 4-10   A, Narrowing of the coronary artery. **B,** Balloon inflated across the obstruction. **C,** The end result is near-normal diameter at the site of the previously obstructing lesion. (Reprinted with permission from Vogel JHK, King SB III. *Practice of Interventional Cardiology,* 2nd ed. St. Louis: Mosby-Year Book; 1993:84.)

little disability, and hospitalization is usually quite short. Return to normal activities within 1 to 2 weeks is not uncommon. There are some potential disadvantages, however. Recurrence rates of 25% to 30% are not uncommon within 6 months of the procedure, even when stents are used. In many cases, PTCA can be repeated. A new generation of "drug-eluting" stents to prevent local recurrence is being developed and may result in better long-term patencies. During 1% to 3% of all PTCA procedures or stent insertions, a patient may require emergency surgery because of a complication. In these cases, the surgical results are not as good as those for elective surgery. The rates of perioperative myocardial infarction and mortality are both higher.

Surgical Treatment

The decision to use **coronary artery bypass grafting** (CABG) to treat patients with ischemic heart disease is based on the anatomy, the symptoms, and the potential risks to the patient, as well as the long-term benefits of the operation. The American Heart Association and the American College of Cardiology have developed specific guidelines for the selection of patients being considered for CABG. Certain anatomic situations alone (e.g., left main artery disease, left main equivalent, proximal LAD, and circumflex occlusions) may warrant surgery, even in the absence of symptoms, because of the large amount of myocardium in jeopardy and the recognized high mortality rate without surgical treatment (especially sudden death). Patients with stable angina that is unresponsive to medical therapy, unstable angina (e.g., pain at rest, preinfarction angina, postinfarction angina), or double- or triple-vessel disease with diminished left ventricular function are likewise candidates for surgical intervention. In these patients, surgery usually relieves symptoms, prevents myocardial infarction, and prolongs life. In addition, concomitant CABG may be indicated for patients who undergo surgery for complications of myocardial infarction (e.g., acute mitral regurgitation, ventricular septal defect, free rupture of the heart) or those who undergo elective valve replacement procedures when critical vessel occlusions are present. Recent comparisons of PTCA alone and CABG, when both are feasible, have favored surgery for patients with long life expectancies.

CABG can be performed with or without the use of the heart–lung machine and its potential complications. Traditionally, cardiopulmonary bypass has been used to provide a stable, bloodless field in which to perform the precise distal anastomoses to the coronary arteries required for successful long-term results. Off-pump coronary artery bypass surgery (OPCAB) has been introduced as a method of performing CABG without the use of cardiopulmonary bypass in the hope of reducing some of the complications (especially neurologic) associated with its use. OPCAB is done through a standard median sternotomy or, in certain circumstances, via a limited thoracotomy. Once the technique has been mastered and the "learning curve" has been passed, many centers report excellent results, especially with the use of new stabilizing devices developed specifically for this procedure. Long-term results of OPCAB must be evaluated and compared with the standard techniques of coronary bypass surgery before they can be readily accepted.

For some patients, the risks of surgery far outweigh its benefits. For example, patients with limited life expectancy from other diseases, the very elderly, and the physically impaired might not be surgical candidates because of associated conditions. In these cases, further medical treatment or attempts at partial revascularization with PTCA may be more appropriate. Although the benefits of CABG to patients with decreased ventricular function and double- or triple-vessel disease are well recognized, poor ventricular function adds to the mortality of patients who undergo the operation. Other factors that increase the mortality and morbidity rates associated with CABG and other open-heart procedures include age greater than 70 years, morbid obesity, diabetes, chronic obstructive pulmonary disease, hypertension, history of myocardial infarction, reoperation, chronic renal insufficiency or failure, peripheral vascular disease, and, possibly, female sex.

On the day of surgery, the patient receives preoperative medications, including prophylactic antibiotics to minimize the risk of perioperative infection. In many cases, the morning dose of cardiac drugs is given, especially if the patient has been taking a β-blocker. Monitoring devices (Swan-Ganz catheter, CVP, arterial line) are inserted and the patient is anesthetized. Once the patient has been prepped and draped, the incision used to expose the heart (usually a median sternotomy) is performed. For almost all CABG procedures, one or both of the internal mammary arteries is harvested from beneath the chest wall. The other conduits to be used for bypasses (saphenous veins from the leg or radial artery from the forearm) are harvested simultaneously under direct vision or using endoscopic techniques to minimize the extent of the skin incisions. The patient is heparinized and cardiopulmonary bypass is initiated with the heart–lung machine. The aorta is cross-clamped and the heart is arrested with cardioplegia to provide a stable, bloodless field in which to perform the distal microsurgery and to protect the heart during these periods of global ischemia. Bypasses are then performed. While using surgical loops to magnify the operative field, the surgeon makes a small opening in the native coronary artery. The size of the opening is approximately twice the diameter of the artery. The conduit used to bypass the obstruction in the coronary artery is then sutured to it. The bypass is completed by suturing the proximal end of the conduit to the aorta with the cross-clamp still in place or with a side-biting clamp after the cross-clamp has been removed. The proximal end of the mammary artery, where it branches from the subclavian artery, is left intact. After the patient is weaned from the heart–lung machine, the heparin is reversed with protamine, hemostasis is obtained, and the incisions are closed. Temporary pacing wires are usually placed on the atrium and ventricle, should they be needed. Chest tubes are placed to drain blood from around the heart and from the pleural space.

Preoperative and Postoperative Care. After the decision is made to proceed with surgery, appropriate preparation is necessary. Most elective CABG and valve procedures are now performed with the patient admitted to the hospital on the morning of surgery. Anticipated discharge home for low-risk patients is on the fourth or fifth postoperative day. Consequently, almost all preparations are made on an outpatient basis. Other patients with acute symptoms or unstable coronary syndrome (as many as 50% in some institutions) will require surgery while in the hospital following catheterization. Regardless of their status, a complete history and physical examination is required. In addition, attention is directed to documenting the absence of associated carotid disease, which could increase the risk of stroke at the time of CABG. The finding of significant carotid stenosis may prompt pre-CABG carotid endarterectomy or a simultaneous approach to decrease the risk of perioperative stroke. The presence of suitable conduits for the procedure must be verified, especially in patients with varicose veins, a history of deep-vein thrombophlebitis, a previous operation, or severe peripheral vascular disease. The patient and the family are given extensive education about the short- and long-term risks and benefits of the procedure, about the hospitalization itself, and about the postoperative recuperation. Many centers promote autologous blood donation in elective cases to reduce the need for homologous blood transfusion.

Years of experience and attention to detail in the preoperative, intraoperative, and postoperative care of patients who undergo CABG has resulted in almost routine care of these patients postoperatively. Many patients are extubated shortly after they return to the recovery unit. They are often transferred from the intensive care unit in less than 24 hours. Early mobilization is emphasized, as are the prevention of pulmonary problems and the prophylactic treatment of atrial fibrillation (incidences of up to 40% are reported) with β-blockers or other drugs. Aspirin is prescribed to increase long-term bypass graft patency, unless contraindicated. Because of the fluid weight gained during the surgery, aggressive diuresis to return patients to their preoperative weight is emphasized. Discharge from the hospital on the fourth or fifth postoperative day is not uncommon, especially for patients younger than 65 years of age who do not have associated disease.

Patients who are discharged from the hospital usually return to a lifestyle similar to the one they had before the onset of the ischemic syndrome. At discharge, they are likely to feel somewhat weakened, as though they had a "bad case of the flu." These patients should be ambulatory, however, soon after they return home. Early complications of heart failure, leg wound infection, or sternal infection are not common, but must be recognized and treated appropriately. Recovery over 4 to 6 weeks is one of gradually increasing ambulation and activity. At some point, most patients undergo a repeat stress test. If the stress test documents the absence of ongoing ischemia, most patients are enrolled in an exercise rehabilitation program for rapid reconditioning. Most patients can return to work within 6 to 8 weeks of discharge from the hospital, especially if their work is primarily sedentary. Patients whose work requires heavy physical activity may need to wait 3 to 6 months after discharge to permit the sternum to heal completely.

Postoperative Complications. Some patients who undergo CABG, as well as other cardiac surgery procedures, have a course that is far from routine. The care of these patients can be a challenge to the surgical team. The survival of these patients is based on rapid recognition of problems as they develop and rapid and appropriate responses to them. Close monitoring with invasive devices (e.g., arterial line, Swan-Ganz catheter) and appropriate therapeutic interventions can prevent many complications. Monitoring of blood pressure, pulmonary capillary wedge pressure, CVP, and cardiac output has made it easier to differentiate among the many major early postoperative complications. Hypotension caused by volume loss, cardiac tamponade, low peripheral resistance, or cardiac failure can be diagnosed and treated. Hypovolemia requires rapid replacement of blood volume. Signs of tamponade necessitate early return to the operating room or emergency opening of the median sternotomy incision in the intensive care unit to relieve the tamponade and correct the source of bleeding. Low resistance may require α-adrenergic agents

to improve vascular tone. Myocardial failure requires treatment with inotropic agents. Agents that have direct β-adrenergic effects on the heart are most appropriate and include dopamine, dobutamine, and epinephrine. The newer phosphodiesterase inhibitors (e.g., milrinone) are also helpful agents to increase cardiac contractility.

If these interventions do not reverse a low-output state due to cardiac failure, the use of an **intra-aortic balloon pump** is indicated. This pump is normally inserted percutaneously through the femoral artery to lie in the descending thoracic aorta. A cylindrical balloon mounted on the end of the catheter is positioned just distal to the left subclavian artery. It inflates and deflates synchronously with the ECG. Inflation occurs during diastole and results in high augmented diastolic pressure that causes increased coronary blood flow. Deflation of the balloon is actuated by a vacuum. Deflation occurs just before systole, causing significant afterload reduction resulting in decreased myocardial oxygen requirements. These two factors (increased coronary perfusion and decreased afterload) combine to increase cardiac output. However, the intra-aortic balloon pump is not an innocuous intervention. The most frequent complication is compromised flow to the lower extremity. Simple removal of the balloon may restore adequate flow, but limb-salvaging procedures may be required. If these procedures are unsuccessful, amputation may be necessary. In addition, removal of the balloon may leave the patient in a hemodynamically compromised state. Infection is reported, as is rupture of the balloon.

When the heart fails completely, the intra-aortic balloon pump alone is not sufficient. Complete support of the failing myocardium is required with a ventricular assist device. These devices assume 100% of the pumping function of the left or right side of the heart. The heart may recover function over time when extensive myocardial stunning occurs and sufficient time for recovery is provided. Failure to recover function within 1 week usually requires implantation of a more permanent assist device as a "bridge" to heart transplantation, if the patient meets the criteria for transplantation.

There are many potential complications in the early postoperative period. Essentially, any organ system can be affected by complications of CABG and the physiologic disruptions associated with the use of the heart–lung machine. Heart failure is only one of these complications. As in all surgical patients, infection may occur, such as pneumonia, urinary sepsis, or superficial or deep infection in surgical wounds. The most catastrophic complication is mediastinitis with true infection of the mediastinum and associated osteomyelitis of the sternum. This complication requires major revision of the incision, with extensive debridement and either a repeat closure, or, more likely, closure with vascularized muscle flaps or omentum.

Although there is controversy about the significance of perioperative microembolization, clinically evident stroke occurs in 1% of all patients undergoing CABG. Stroke is usually related to unrecognized carotid stenosis, intravascular air, or particulate embolization from the aorta. In patients who are older than 70 years of age, the incidence is as high as 6% to 8%. Manipulation of the ascending aorta by a cross-clamp or side-biting clamp is increasingly recognized as the major source of gross neurologic damage at the time of any heart surgery. Respiratory failure may occur, especially in patients with underlying pulmonary disease, those who have received large amounts of blood products, and those who have undergone bypass for prolonged periods. Renal insufficiency or failure can occur, especially in patients with preexisting renal problems or diabetes. These patients may require temporary or permanent dialysis.

The desire to minimize the possibility of any of these complications was a major motivation to explore less invasive methods of coronary revascularization, such as OPCAB, by eliminating the use of cardiopulmonary bypass. The results have been mixed but seem to demonstrate a decreased incidence of stroke (but only when aortic clamps are avoided), decreased renal insufficiency, and a decreased use of blood and blood products.

Minimally invasive approaches have been applied to CABG and valve replacement surgery. These efforts have usually been confined to making smaller incisions and limiting the length of the sternotomy, while applying general standard techniques of bypass and cardioplegia. Robotic techniques and other specially developed instruments have seen limited use. The purported advantages of these techniques are decreased pain, less bleeding, shorter recovery time, and decreased incidence of wound infection.

Prognosis. Although CABG produces excellent results, many factors contribute to operative mortality and morbidity. At most major centers, the mortality rate for all patients who undergo CABG is 2% to 4%. Survival rates of 95%, 88%, 75%, and 60% at 1, 5, 10, and 15 years, respectively, are reported. Freedom from angina is reported as 95%, 83%, 63%, and 37% at 1, 5, 10, and 15 years, respectively. Freedom from myocardial infarction approaches 99%, 96%, 85%, and 64% at 1, 5, 10, and 15 years, respectively.

The importance of the conduit used for revascularization appears to be of crucial importance for the long-term benefits of surgery. The most common conduit used is the greater saphenous vein. The patency of this vein varies from 50% to 70% at 10 years (Fig. 4-11). The internal thoracic artery (internal mammary) has a much better patency (>90% at 10 years) and has resulted in improved survival. In addition, the reoperation rate is halved (from 10%–15% to 5%–10%) within the first 10 postoperative years when at least one mammary artery is used. Because of the apparent benefit of using an arterial conduit, many investigators have attempted to use other arteries, including both internal mammary arteries, the gastroepiploic artery, the radial artery, and the epigastric artery. Early results appear favorable, but no long-term studies have been completed to verify their benefit and long-term patency.

Complications of Myocardial Infarction

Patients who survive the initial phase of a myocardial infarction remain at risk for a subsequent catastrophe that can occur up to 2 weeks following the infarct, but usually occurs within the first few days following infarct. Acute ventricular septal defect and free-wall rupture are manifestations of a similar mechanism: transmural infarction and subsequent rupture of the myocardium. Papillary muscle rupture and associated acute mitral regurgitation, on the other hand, can be associated with a limited infarction, where complete necrosis is limited to the papillary muscle alone. Each of these catastrophes will occur with similar symptoms and must be recognized as a mechanical defect that can be corrected only by emergency surgery. The typical patient will have recurrent pain within days of the original infarction, which will be associated with severe congestive heart failure or cardiogenic shock. Free-wall rupture may present with a picture of acute cardiac tamponade. Emergency resuscitation is often required, and diagnosis is made by echocardiography or the insertion of a Swan-Ganz catheter. Echo Doppler imaging will show a left-to-right shunt, acute mitral regurgitation, tamponade or

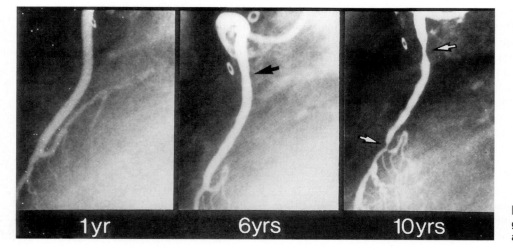

Figure 4-11   Saphenous vein graft: progression of graft atherosclerosis and obstruction.

pseudoaneurysm, or the actual defect. A Swan-Ganz catheter can show a step-up of oxygen saturation drawn from the CVP and pulmonary artery ports (a left-to-right shunt of the ventricular septal defect), pulmonary hypertension, acute V waves when the wedge pressure is obtained, or signs of tamponade with pressure equalization. Inotropic support, afterload reduction, and insertion of an intra-aortic balloon may help acutely, but surgery should be performed emergently and is associated with a high operative mortality but improved long-term survival.

Valvular Heart Disease

Surgical interventions to repair damaged or structurally deficient heart valves have been available since the early 1950s and 1960s, but these techniques did not become generally acceptable until the heart–lung machine was developed. Harken in Boston and Bailey in Philadelphia achieved modest success with valve repair of mitral stenosis in the late 1940s and early 1950s. This operation was referred to as a closed mitral commissurotomy and was performed through a thoracotomy. Starr in Oregon performed the first prosthetic replacement of a valve in 1961. Since that time, progress has been made in the surgical techniques used to treat these problems, but the ideal valvular prosthesis has yet to be developed. An ideal prosthesis should have lifelong durability, should not require the use of anticoagulants, should have excellent hemodynamics, should have a low risk of infection, and should be silent.

Because there is no ideal prosthesis, all decisions about surgical intervention in patients with valvular heart disease must be made carefully. The natural history of the disease, the risks associated with establishing a diagnosis, and the risks associated with the surgical procedure must all be carefully considered. In addition, the inherent advantages and disadvantages of each prosthetic device must play a role in this decision. The natural history of valvular heart disease has not changed, although rheumatic valvular disease is now far less prevalent in this country than in the past. Diagnostic methods have improved dramatically. Echocardiography and echo Doppler imaging permit noninvasive screening and diagnosis without the risks and expense associated with cardiac catheterization. Improvements in surgical techniques and myocardial protection have reduced the risks of the operation. Likewise, newer valves have decreased (but not eliminated) the risks and complications associated with valvular prostheses. In some cases, methods of valvular repair rather than replacement have excellent long-term results and permit earlier intervention.

Aortic Valve Disease

The etiology of aortic valvular disease is varied. Combined stenotic and regurgitant lesions are usually related to a history of rheumatic fever. Isolated aortic stenosis usually occurs because of progressive narrowing of a congenitally bicuspid valve or because of senile degeneration and calcification of an otherwise normal trileaflet valve. Aortic stenosis is progressive and is usually clinically silent until symptoms begin to develop as the degree of obstruction to left ventricular outflow increases. The left ventricle hypertrophies to overcome outflow obstruction. Eventually, however, the ventricle begins to dilate, and signs of congestive heart failure develop. The onset of the classic triad of symptoms (i.e., angina, heart failure, syncope) portends a poor prognosis without surgical intervention. The mortality rate approaches 100% within 5 years of the onset of symptoms. Congestive heart failure is the poorest prognostic sign, and the presence of all three symptoms should lead to prompt evaluation and surgery.

Aortic regurgitation can be an even more indolent disease, without the development of significant symptoms, even in the presence of massive cardiac enlargement. Volume overload of the ventricle associated with regurgitation causes dilation of the ventricle and significant cardiomegaly. Causes of aortic regurgitation include aortic annular dilation (usually attributed to Marfan's syndrome), scarring from the valvulitis of rheumatic heart disease, and valvular damage from bacterial endocarditis. Acute regurgitation related to aortic dissection or acute bacterial endocarditis is poorly tolerated and can lead to fulminant heart failure and death without early or even emergent treatment. All symptomatic patients with aortic regurgitation should be offered surgical treatment. Likewise, surgery should be performed on asymptomatic patients with cardiomegaly, especially when it develops under therapy. The mortality rate associated with aortic valve replacement is closely related to the degree of ventricular dysfunction present at the time of surgery. Echocardiogram is the ideal noninvasive measurement tool used to follow patients with aortic disease and to pinpoint timely surgical intervention.

Mitral Valve Disease

Mitral stenosis is caused by rheumatic valvulitis with scarring and fusion of the leaflets, scarring of the chordae tendineae, and shrinking of the subvalvular apparatus. Although the resulting obstruction to flow across the valve causes no recognized damage to the left ventricle, it causes distention of the left atrium, pulmonary hypertension, and signs of left and subsequently right heart failure (Fig. 4-12). The atrial dilatation often leads to atrial arrhythmias, especially atrial fibrillation. The resulting stasis in the atrium may lead to thrombosis and subsequent systemic embolization.

Chronic mitral regurgitation is caused by rheumatic valvular disease, myxomatous degeneration of the mitral leaflets, previous myocardial infarction, or endocarditis. Acute fulminant mitral regurgitation can be related to myocardial infarction, rupture of the papillary muscle, or acute bacterial endocarditis with valve disruption. These conditions may require lifesaving emergency valve surgery. Mitral regurgitation can lead to signs of pulmonary hypertension, atrial arrhythmia, and left and right heart failure. In mitral regurgitation, the left ventricle may be

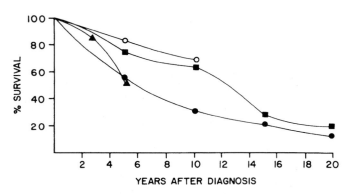

Figure 4-12 Natural history of mitral stenosis. *Black square,* data of Rowe JC et al.; *black circle,* data of Oleson KH; *black triangle,* data of Munoz S et al.; *open circle,* data of Rapaport E. (Reprinted with permission from Starek P. *Heart Valve Replacement and Reconstruction.* St. Louis: Mosby-Year Book; 1987:32.)

damaged because of the associated volume overload. This regurgitation into the low-resistance left atrium may lead to gross underestimation of the injury to the left ventricle. Patients who have major damage to the ventricle face a very high operative mortality rate and a poor prognosis, even when the operation is successful.

All patients with mitral valve disease (except perhaps those with end-stage mitral regurgitation) should be offered surgical intervention once symptoms of heart failure develop. When repair of the mitral valve (commissurotomy or valvuloplasty) is believed to be technically possible, earlier intervention may be indicated. Some patients with mitral stenosis, especially younger women, may be candidates for balloon valvuloplasty performed in the catheterization laboratory with techniques similar to PTCA, but with much larger catheters and balloons.

Tricuspid Valve Disease

Isolated disease of the tricuspid valve is not common. These patients usually have regurgitation secondary to pulmonary hypertension associated with mitral valve disease, which dilates the tricuspid annulus. Annuloplasty of the tricuspid valve, a procedure in which the dilated annulus is narrowed back to its normal size, is usually performed in conjunction with repair or replacement of the left-sided valves. Patients with tricuspid endocarditis (often drug addicts) may have recurring sepsis or septic pulmonary emboli. Excision of the valve without valve replacement, in the absence of pulmonary hypertension, is the usual treatment.

Treatment

The primary treatment for patients with valvular heart disease is surgery, once significant symptoms have developed or other signs for surgery exist. Aortic valve surgery almost always requires a valve replacement, although a few repairs of insufficient valves have been performed with varying success. Aortic stenosis in the adult is not amenable to valvuloplasty of any form and will recur within a year if this approach is taken. Mitral valve surgery, on the other hand, has been evolving into much more of a reparative field. Closed and open mitral commissurotomies can be performed for mitral stenosis. Percutaneous techniques can be applied as well. As many as 50% of patients with mitral regurgitation now undergo valve repair (valvuloplasty) with retention of the normal valve apparatus, eliminating the chronic risks of the prosthetic valve.

Since the first successful replacement of a mitral valve was performed by Starr in 1961 using a ball-and-cage Starr-Edwards valve, many designs for artificial heart valves have been attempted. Today, two types of artificial valves are most commonly used: mechanical prostheses and bioprostheses (Fig. 4-13).

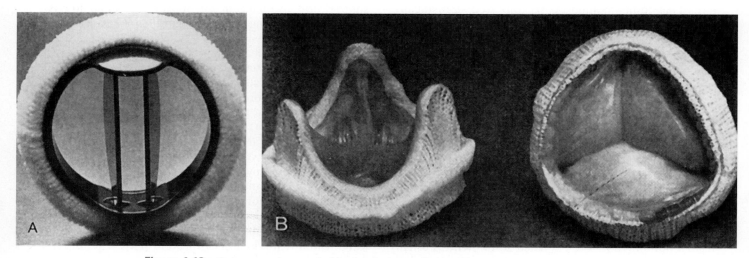

Figure 4-13 Valve prostheses. **A,** Mechanical prosthesis: bileaflet St. Jude. **B,** Bioprosthesis: porcine.

Mechanical prostheses are made of pyrolytic carbon, metal, and cloth. Examples include ball-and-cage valves, tilting disc valves, and bileaflet valves. Bileaflet valves dominate the market because of their low profile and relatively low thrombogenicity. The leaflets of these valves are made of pyrolytic carbon and the housings are made of titanium. They may not be visible on chest x-ray unless they are made lucent by metallic rings or other material added to the pyrolytic carbon.

Bioprostheses are either xenografts or homografts. Xenografts are made from the aortic valve of a pig. They are either mounted on a metal stent for suturing or inserted freehand into the aortic root. Xenografts are also made from the pericardium of a pig or cow and mounted on stents for insertion. All of these xenografts are treated with glutaraldehyde and sterilized before packaging. Consequently, they can be stored on the shelf at room temperature for many years. Homografts are harvested from cadavers within 24 hours of death. The ascending aorta and aortic valve are removed as a whole. They are then sterilized and frozen for storage (cryopreserved). They are thawed later for an isolated valve or root replacement of the aorta. More recently, autografting of the pulmonary valve into the aortic position (Ross procedure) with homograft replacement of the pulmonic valve has proved successful, especially in younger adults and children. Insertion of homografts and autografts is technically more challenging than that of mechanical valves or stent-mounted xenografts.

Each type of valve has advantages and disadvantages (Table 4-2). Mechanical prostheses are the most durable. They rarely require replacement for mechanical problems. However, they can be noisy and thus disturbing to the patient. They uniformly require anticoagulation, usually with warfarin (Coumadin). Lower levels of anticoagulation have been used in recent years without an increase in the risks of thromboembolism and with a decrease in the rate of anticoagulant-associated hemorrhage. Xenografts normally do not require anticoagulation in the aortic position, but their durability is lower, especially in younger patients. Autografts and homografts fall somewhere in between in durability. They also offer low thrombogenicity and have the lowest incidence of prosthetic endocarditis. The current advice given to most patients who are younger

than 70 years of age is to have a mechanical prosthesis implanted unless anticoagulants are contraindicated. Older patients, especially those with a life expectancy of 10 years or less, are offered a xenograft or homograft. Women of childbearing age who plan to have children should have a tissue valve implanted because of the potential teratogenic risk to the fetus while the mother is taking Coumadin, although they must anticipate a second operation in the future.

Valve replacement is not curative; it merely substitutes one disease (the problems associated with the prosthesis) for another (the diseased valve itself and the secondary physiologic derangement of the heart.). Common sequelae of valve replacement are thromboembolism (2%–6%), mechanical failure (including valve thrombosis if inadequately anticoagulated), prosthetic endocarditis (1%–2%), and bioprosthetic deterioration (30% at 10 years). The newest generation of bioprosthesis appears to have a greater duration without deterioration. In contrast to valve replacement, valve repair (when properly performed) is safe, effective, and durable, especially for mitral stenosis and regurgitation.

Antibiotic Prophylaxis for the Prevention of Bacterial Endocarditis

Antibiotic prophylaxis for patients with heart disease is problematic for many reasons. It is unclear whether it is completely effective in preventing endocarditis. It is also unclear how many patients are at risk for endocarditis with bacteremia and which regimens are most effective. Bacteremia can occur after tooth extraction, periodontal surgery, tooth brushing, urologic manipulation, endoscopic procedures on the bronchial and gastrointestinal systems, and normal obstetric delivery. Antibiotic prophylaxis is considered for patients who have prosthetic heart valves because foreign materials often serve as a nidus for bloodborne infections. This is also true for patients with deformed native heart valves with stenosis or regurgitation. Patients with mitral valve prolapse and regurgitation should also receive prophylaxis (Table 4-3). Prophylaxis is tailored to the individual risk factors. For example, patients who have artificial valves and undergo dental manipulations receive antibiotics (e.g., penicillin) that are active against oral anaerobes and microaerophilic organisms. Patients who undergo manipulation of the urinary tract receive antibiot-

Table 4-2	Comparison of Prosthetic Heart Valves	
	Mechanical Valves	**Bioprosthetic Valves**
Durability	+ +	±
Thromboembolism	−	+
Obstruction in small sizes	+	−
Calcification with age	+	−
Calcification with dialysis	+	−

+, valve compares favorably; −, valve compares unfavorably.

Table 4-3	Patients at Increased Risk for Developing Endocarditis

Prosthetic valve
History of endocarditis
Previously damaged heart valve (rheumatic or other scarring)
Congenital heart or heart valve defects
Hypertrophic cardiomyopathy

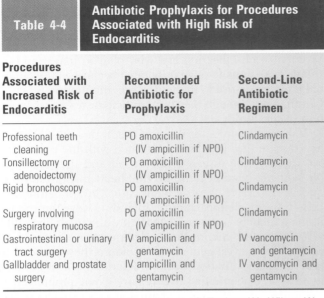

Table 4-4	Antibiotic Prophylaxis for Procedures Associated with High Risk of Endocarditis	
Procedures Associated with Increased Risk of Endocarditis	Recommended Antibiotic for Prophylaxis	Second-Line Antibiotic Regimen
Professional teeth cleaning	PO amoxicillin (IV ampicillin if NPO)	Clindamycin
Tonsillectomy or adenoidectomy	PO amoxicillin (IV ampicillin if NPO)	Clindamycin
Rigid bronchoscopy	PO amoxicillin (IV ampicillin if NPO)	Clindamycin
Surgery involving respiratory mucosa	PO amoxicillin (IV ampicillin if NPO)	Clindamycin
Gastrointestinal or urinary tract surgery	IV ampicillin and gentamycin	IV vancomycin and gentamycin
Gallbladder and prostate surgery	IV ampicillin and gentamycin	IV vancomycin and gentamycin

Adapted with permission from Dajani AS, Taubert KA, Wilson W, et al. Prevention of bacterial endocarditis: recommendations by the American Heart Association. *Circulation* 1997;96:358–366.

ics that are active against common urinary pathogens. Similar applications should be followed for surgery on the lungs, extremities, and gastrointestinal tract. Prophylaxis against rheumatic fever should continue as before because the purpose is to prevent reinfection with the ubiquitous streptococcal organisms.

Because of the potential complexity of this problem, the American Heart Association has published guidelines for the prevention of bacterial endocarditis (Table 4-4). (Endocarditis prophylaxis is also discussed in Lawrence et al, *Essentials of General Surgery*, 4th ed, Chapter 2 and Table 2-4.)

Pacemakers

Cardiac pacemakers use electrical power to substitute for an abnormal cardiac conduction system to preserve an adequate heart rate or atrioventricular synchrony. Pacemakers consist of the following components:

1 A power source (usually lithium-based and of varying size and composition)
2 Circuitry (sophisticated analytical electronic components to ensure variability in rate, power applied, sensing capabilities, telemetry, and all parameters within the system)
3 Housing (hermetic sealing of the electronic components to prevent body fluids from leaking into the battery and disabling the circuit)
4 Electrodes that provide the conducting mechanism from the power source and circuitry to and from the myocardium; may be unipolar or bipolar; the stimulating electrode is always negative (cathodal stimulation).

In general, candidates for pacemaker insertion include all patients with correctable symptomatic bradyarrhythmias and those with other conduction abnormalities that may intermittently lead to sudden death. Specifically, these include the following:

1 Complete heart block
2 Mobitz II second-degree heart block
3 Bradycardia associated with syncope, dizziness, seizures, confusion, or heart failure (correlation of symptom and bradycardia is needed)
4 Bradycardia caused by necessary drug therapy for which there is no alternative
5 Bradycardia associated with symptomatic supraventricular tachycardia or malignant ventricular arrhythmia
6 Bifascicular or trifascicular heart block with syncope
7 Complete heart block after myocardial infarction

To simulate normal cardiac electrophysiologic activity, the pacemaker must be able to sense intrinsic cardiac electrical activity, integrate that activity into a preprogrammed algorithm, and dispense appropriate electrical discharges to one or both cardiac chambers. Patients with complete heart block, for example, have atrial electrical discharges (P waves) at appropriate rates, but because they are not conducted to the ventricles and do not incite sequential ventricular contractions, atrioventricular synchrony is lost. The pacemaker must conduct the atrial activity (P wave) through its atrial electrode to the generator for analysis. At appropriate programmed intervals, it stimulates a ventricular contraction through the ventricular electrode. Therefore, it also senses the absence of ventricular activity after the P wave.

Some pacemakers are used in the atrium or ventricle alone. The majority are dual-chamber devices with sensing and pacing capabilities in both chambers. Pacemakers are classified according to a three-letter code (with some modifiers) as follows:

1 The first letter indicates the chamber that is paced: A = atrium, V = ventricle, D = both
2 The second letter indicates the chamber that is sensed: A = atrium, V = ventricle, D = both
3 The third letter indicates the function: I = inhibited, T = triggered, D = both, O = neither

Consequently, a simple ventricular demand pacemaker, which is inhibited when it senses an intrinsic beat, is classified as VVI. An atrial pacemaker with similar function is classified as AAI. A dual-chamber pacemaker that performs both sensing and pacing in both chambers, mimicking normal atrioventricular electrophysiology, is classified as DDD.

Advancing technology has permitted transvenous introduction of endocardial electrodes for automatic internal cardioverter defibrillators. Initially, these devices were affixed to the epicardium through surgical access (e.g., thoracotomy, sternotomy). Electrodes sense the electrical activity of the heart and its arrhythmias and deliver a shock of 20 to 35 J to the endocardium to terminate those arrhythmias. Studies show decreased cardiac death rates for patients who have a variety of electrophysiologic disturbances, including out-of-hospital arrests and inducible ventricular tachycardia or fibrillation.

Congenital Heart Disease

Congenital heart defects occur in 1 out of 125 live births. Although the spectrum of congenital heart defects includes an enormous number of individual anatomic diagnoses, congenital heart disease is generally classified in one of several ways. The simplest classification (Table 4-5) is based on the relative frequency with which various congenital heart lesions are detected in a given population. With respect to medical and surgical management of congenital heart defects, a system of classification based on pathophysiology is more useful (Table 4-6). Acyanotic heart defects are characterized by a normal level of oxyhemoglobin saturation in the systemic circulation. Cyanotic lesions are characterized by the presence of an abnormal amount of deoxyhemoglobin in the systemic circulation. This may be the consequence of right-to-left shunts, overall diminished pulmonary blood flow, or mixing lesions, where there is abnormal admixture of systemic venous blood together with pulmonary venous blood contributing to systemic perfusion. Obstructive lesions in the cardiovascular system generally result in increased pressure work for one or both ventricles. Left-to-right shunt lesions result

Table 4-6	Pathophysiologic Classification of Lesions in Congenital Heart Disease and Approximate Relative Incidence	
Classification		**Incidence (%)**
Acyanotic		
Left-to-right shunts		
Ventricular septal defect		20
Atrial septal defect		10
Patent ductus arteriosus		10
Atrioventricular septal defect		2–5
Aortopulmonary window		Rare
Left-sided obstructive lesions		
Aortic coarctation		10
Congenital aortic stenosis		10
Interrupted aortic arch		1
Mitral stenosis		Rare
Cyanotic		
Right-to-left shunts		
Tetralogy of Fallot		10
Pulmonary stenosis		10
Pulmonary atresia		5
With intact ventricular septum		
With ventricular septal defect		
Tricuspid atresia		3
Ebstein's anomaly		0.5
Complex mixing defects		
Transposition of the great arteries		5–8
Total anomalous pulmonary venous connection		2
Hypoplastic left heart syndrome		2

in increased ventricular volume work and may result in increased pressure work. The associated increase in pulmonary blood flow can affect the physiology and the development of the pulmonary vasculature. Cyanosis can result in decreased systemic oxygen delivery and eventually in the development of polycythemia. Surgery for congenital heart defects is generally indicated to normalize ventricular pressure and volume work in order to treat or prevent the development of congestive heart failure, and to achieve normal systemic oxygen delivery by optimizing cardiac output and by normalizing the oxygen content of systemic arterial blood.

Acyanotic Heart Disease

Ventricular Septal Defect

The most common congenital heart defect, ventricular septal defect (VSD), is an abnormal communication between the right and left ventricles. There are four fundamental types of ventricular septal defect, which are classified according to location (Fig. 4-14). The type I VSD, also referred to as conal, supracristal, infundibular, or subarterial, results from maldevelopment of the outlet septum. The adjacent leaflet of the aortic valve may prolapse into the defect. The type II VSD, also referred to as paramembranous, perimembranous, or conoventricular type defect, is the type most frequently encountered at surgery. These defects are generally adjacent to the aortic valve

Table 4-5	Common Lesions in Congenital Heart Disease and Approximate Relative Incidence	
Lesion		**Incidence (%)**
Ventricular septal defect		20
Atrial septal defect		10
Patent ductus arteriosus		10
Aortic coarctation		10
Congenital aortic stenosis		10
Tetralogy of Fallot		10
Pulmonary stenosis		10
Transposition of the great arteries		5–8
Pulmonary atresia		5
With intact ventricular septum		
With ventricular septal defect		
Atrioventricular septal defect		2–5
Tricuspid atresia		3
Truncus arteriosus		3
Total anomalous pulmonary venous connection		2
Hypoplastic left heart syndrome		2
Interrupted aortic arch		1
Ebstein's anomaly		0.5
Mitral stenosis		Rare
Aortopulmonary window		Rare

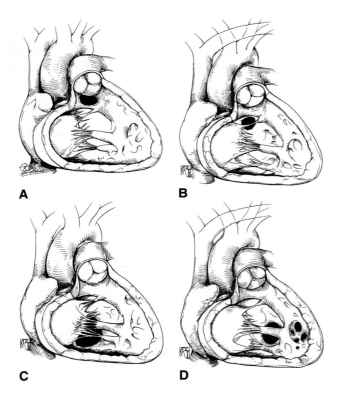

Figure 4-14   Classic anatomic types of VSD. **A,** Type I VSD (conal, supracristal, infundibular, subarterial). **B,** Type II or paramembranous VSD. **C,** Type III VSD (atrioventricular canal type of inlet septum type). **D,** Type IV VSD (single or multiple), also called muscular VSD. (Reprinted with permission from Mavroudis C. *Pediatric Cardiac Surgery*. St. Louis: Mosby-Year Book; 2003:299.)

just beneath the right and noncoronary cusps. The type III VSD is also known as atrioventricular canal type or inlet VSD. Type IV VSDs, also called muscular VSDs, are located in the trabecular portion of the ventricular septum, where they may be single or multiple. These may be difficult to visualize from the right side of the heart because of the coarse nature of right ventricular trabeculae.

The principal physiologic consequence of a ventricular septal defect is left-to-right shunting at the ventricular level during systole. The magnitude of the shunt depends on the size and location of the VSD, and on the pulmonary vascular resistance. Anatomically large defects (physiologically nonrestrictive) not only result in large shunts but also transmit systemic level pressure to the right ventricle and pulmonary circulation. Many small VSDs (particularly of the muscular type) close spontaneously within the first 2 years of life. Surgical intervention, however, is indicated in an infant with congestive heart failure that is poorly controlled on medication or with failure to thrive in the setting of a large VSD with significant pulmonary artery hypertension. Beyond infancy, closure is generally indicated in children with elevated pulmonary artery pressure, or with a ratio of pulmonary-to-systemic blood flow that

approaches 2:1. With the increasing safety of pediatric cardiac surgery, many centers are now more aggressive and require less stringent physiologic criteria for closure. Occasionally, an untreated nonrestrictive VSD may be associated with the development of irreversible pulmonary vascular obstructive disease as early as 2 years of age. In this situation, closure of the VSD might prove fatal to the child from right heart failure. Ultimately, pulmonary vascular disease can lead to a reversal of the shunt such that blood flows from the right to the left side of the heart (Eisenmenger's syndrome).

Historically, sick infants with VSD were often treated by banding of the main pulmonary artery to diminish pulmonary blood flow and delay the necessity of VSD closure. Such a palliative strategy is rarely used today because VSD closure with cardiopulmonary bypass in infants and young children is now accomplished at very low risk. With cardiopulmonary bypass support, most VSDs can be closed relatively easily. Only rarely is a right ventriculotomy incision required to close single or multiple muscular VSDs. Potential complications of VSD closure include low cardiac output, residual defect resulting in persistent shunt, and complete heart block resulting from suture trauma in the region of the penetrating conduction system.

Atrial Septal Defects

An atrial septal defect, the second most common congenital heart problem, is an acyanotic lesion associated with increased pulmonary blood flow. Because the compliance of the right ventricle is generally greater than that of the left ventricle, the direction of blood flow through an atrial septal defect is generally from left to right. Rarely in infancy is the shunt large enough to produce congestive heart failure or failure to thrive. Most children remain asymptomatic, but may develop fatigue, right-sided heart failure, recurrent pulmonary infections, arrhythmias, and, rarely, pulmonary vascular obstructive disease. The average life expectancy in the untreated patient is 45 years of age. Elective surgical repair is often undertaken as early as 1 to 2 years of age and most often before school age. Elimination of the atrial level shunt prevents further volume overload and enlargement of the right ventricle and prevents the risk of late ventricular failure or pulmonary artery hypertension. Repair is generally accomplished using cardiopulmonary bypass through a median sternotomy or a small right anterior thoracotomy. Incompetent foramen ovale and small ostium secundum types of atrial septal defects may often be closed by direct suturing. These can sometimes be closed in the catheter laboratory with catheter-delivered devices. Larger defects are generally closed with a patch of autologous pericardium or synthetic fabric (Fig. 4-15). Surgical mortality is less than 2%. Potential postoperative complications include atrial arrhythmias.

Patent Ductus Arteriosus

The third most common congenital heart defect, patent ductus arteriosus, is an acyanotic lesion generally associ-

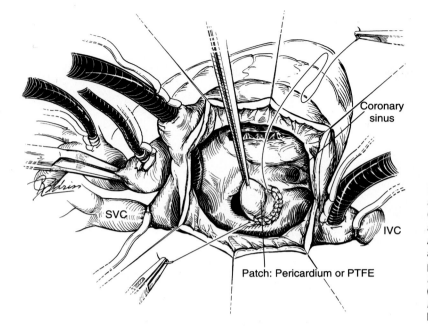

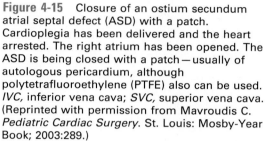

Figure 4-15 Closure of an ostium secundum atrial septal defect (ASD) with a patch. Cardioplegia has been delivered and the heart arrested. The right atrium has been opened. The ASD is being closed with a patch—usually of autologous pericardium, although polytetrafluoroethylene (PTFE) also can be used. *IVC,* inferior vena cava; *SVC,* superior vena cava. (Reprinted with permission from Mavroudis C. *Pediatric Cardiac Surgery.* St. Louis: Mosby-Year Book; 2003:289.)

ated with increased pulmonary blood flow. During fetal life, the ductus arteriosus conducts desaturated blood from the pulmonary artery to the descending thoracic aorta, bypassing the lungs. Normally, within hours to days following birth, the ductus closes spontaneously. If the ductus remains patent, the diminishing pulmonary vascular resistance allows reversal of blood flow, so that saturated blood from the aorta passes through the ductus into the pulmonary artery, thus increasing pulmonary blood flow. Especially in premature infants, this increased pulmonary blood flow may be associated with respiratory difficulties, early congestive heart failure, and suboptimal systemic perfusion. In older patients, a very large patent ductus arteriosus may be associated with congestive heart failure or pulmonary hypertension. Even a very restrictive patent ductus arteriosus is thought to be associated with an increased risk of infective endocarditis (endoarteritis). Aneurysm formation is a rare but important complication of untreated patent ductus arteriosus.

Although the patent ductus may close at any time, it is unlikely to do so after the first year of life. If used within the first several weeks of life, indomethacin, a drug that acts on smooth muscle fibers, will close the ductus in most cases. Surgical ligation is indicated when significant heart failure persists or the ductus remains patent beyond 3 to 6 months of age. Ligation is generally performed through a fourth interspace left posterolateral thoracotomy (Fig. 4-16). Ligation with multiple ties or metallic clips is routine, although division and oversewing the ends may be indicated for a wide, short ductus. Except in very low birth-weight premature infants, mortality rates are below 0.5%.

Coarctation of the Aorta

The fourth most common congenital heart defect, coarctation of the aorta, is an obstructive narrowing in the de-

scending thoracic aorta, usually just distal to the left subclavian artery. All patients with coarctation of the aorta are at risk for eventual development of left-sided heart failure as a consequence of the abnormally increased pressure work of the left ventricle. The defect may present early in life, especially when associated with such other defects as VSD or severe aortic stenosis. Late complications of coarctation of the aorta include hypertension, stroke, aneurysm formation, subacute bacterial endocarditis, and paralysis. The average life expectancy of a patient with untreated coarctation of the aorta is 35 years.

Coarctation repair is indicated in the newborn period or early in infancy whenever significant heart failure is present or if the systemic circulation is dependent on flow through the ductus. Otherwise, elective repair is generally undertaken at age 1 year or shortly thereafter. Although there is some evidence that early repair lessens the likelihood of persistent hypertension, it is nonetheless true that the risk of recurrent coarctation is greater for patients who require surgery during the newborn period. Primary repair of coarctation is generally accomplished by resection of the coarctation segment with end-to-end anastomosis (Fig. 4-17) or by subclavian flap arterioplasty. In selected instances, particularly in older patients, synthetic patch aortoplasty or even interposition grafting may be indicated. Surgery is generally performed through a left posterolateral thoracotomy in the fourth interspace. The most dire operative risk associated with coarctation repair is paraplegia from ischemic spinal cord injury. Fortunately, with current operative and anesthetic methods, this is an exceedingly rare complication. Mesenteric vasculitis, occasionally with gut ischemia and bowel perforation but more often manifested as simple ileus, is another increasingly rare postoperative complication. Paradoxical hypertension

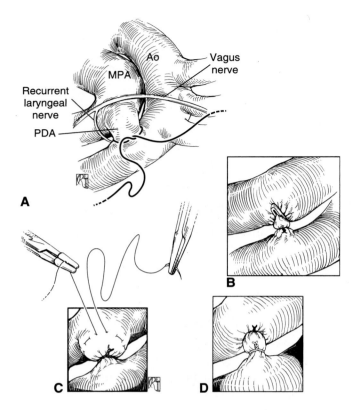

Figure 4-16   Techniques for ligation, multiple ligation, and ligation and hemoclip of patent ductus arteriosus (*PDA*). Exposure is via a left muscle-sparing thoracotomy. **A,** Ligation with a single 2-0 silk ligature. **B,** Ligation with a 2-0 silk ligature *and* placement of a hemoclip. **C** and **D,** Ligation with a 2-0 silk ligature *and* a 5-0 polypropylene adventitial purse-string suture. *Ao,* aorta; *MPA,* main pulmonary artery. (Reprinted with permission from Mavroudis C. *Pediatric Cardiac Surgery.* St. Louis: Mosby-Year Book; 2003:227.)

occurs commonly in the postoperative period and may require pharmacologic treatment. As noted, the likelihood of persistent late hypertension appears to be inversely related to the age at repair.

Cyanotic Heart Disease

Tetralogy of Fallot

The sixth most common congenital heart defect, tetralogy of Fallot, is generally classified as a cyanotic lesion with decreased pulmonary blood flow. Its four components are *ventricular septal defect, pulmonary stenosis (right ventricular outflow tract obstruction), right ventricular hypertrophy,* and *overriding of the aorta* (Fig. 4-18). The degree of cyanosis is related to the degree of right ventricular outflow tract obstruction and associated right-to-left shunting through the ventricular septal defect. Obstruction may be so mild that the patient remains acyanotic (pink tetralogy) or may be so complete as to cause pulmonary atresia. Cyanosis may also be episodic, occurring as "tetralogy spells." Still incompletely understood, these spells may be the consequence of increased dynamic obstruction of the right ventricular outflow tract, or of increased right-to-left shunting due to periods of decreased systemic vascular resistance. True tetralogy spells result in profound cyanosis and are associated with an altered level of consciousness. They may be associated with a mortality rate as high as 10%. In advanced cyanotic cases, patients with tetralogy are at risk for strokes, brain abscesses, and bacterial endocarditis.

Decades ago, it was quite usual for patients who developed symptoms or increasing cyanosis in the first year of life to undergo creation of a systemic-to-pulmonary artery shunt in order to augment pulmonary blood flow and prevent cyanotic spells. Definitive intracardiac repair would then generally be deferred until the child was several years of age. Contemporary management generally consists of definitive corrective open heart surgery for tetralogy of Fallot at the time that a child presents with symptoms of increasing cyanosis. If surgery must be delayed, the favored shunt procedure is the interposition of a small polytetrafluoroethylene (PTFE) graft between a subclavian artery and the ipsilateral branch pulmonary artery.

Corrective surgery for tetralogy of Fallot is accomplished through a median sternotomy incision using cardiopulmonary bypass support. The malalignment VSD is closed with a prosthetic patch, and the right ventricular outflow tract obstruction is relieved. In many instances, this can be accomplished by resection of muscle bundles and by a thorough valvotomy and valvuloplasty of the pulmonic valve. If either the pulmonary valve annulus is very small or the right ventricular infundibulum is very hypoplastic, complete relief of right ventricular outflow tract obstruction may be best accomplished by means of transannular patch augmentation of the right ventricular outflow tract. Effective elimination of the ventricular level shunt and relief of pulmonary outflow tract obstruction are imperative. Complications of surgery include bleeding, heart block, or low cardiac output syndrome. Mortality

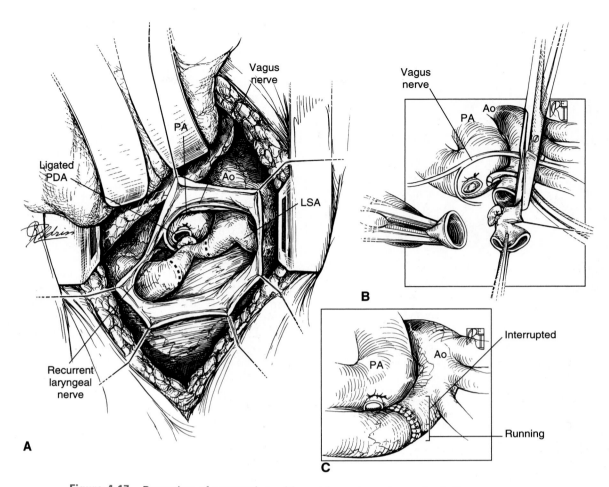

Figure 4-17 Resection of coarctation with end-to-end anastomosis. **A,** Exposure through a left thoracotomy. The patent ductus arteriosus (*PDA*) had been ligated and divided. *Dotted lines* show the area to be resected. **B,** Clamps have been applied and the coarctation segment is being resected. **C,** Anastomosis has been constructed with running suture for the back wall and interrupted suture anteriorly. *Ao,* aorta; *LSA,* left subclavian artery; *PA,* pulmonary artery. (Reprinted with permission from Mavroudis C. *Pediatric Cardiac Surgery.* St. Louis: Mosby-Year Book; 2003:257.)

is approximately 3% to 5%. Incomplete relief of right ventricular outflow tract obstruction, or failure to completely close the VSD, may necessitate reoperation.

Transposition of the Great Arteries

Transposition of the great arteries, the eighth most common congenital cardiac defect, consists of concordant atrioventricular connection and discordant ventriculoarterial connection. In the most common form, the aorta arises anteriorly from the right ventricle and the main pulmonary trunk arises posteriorly from the left ventricle. In the simplest form of transposition, the ventricular septum is intact. Many patients, however, have a VSD. Transposition of the great arteries is a cyanotic lesion with increased pulmonary blood flow. Because the defect consists of two circulations arranged in parallel fashion (as opposed to in series), survival is dependent on mixing at the intracardiac or great vessel level. Affected infants present with severe

cyanosis in the first days of life. Without treatment, 50% will be dead by 1 month and 80% by 1 year. Initial stabilization of the infant can be accomplished by improving mixing either at the arterial level by ensuring patency of the ductus arteriosus with an infusion of prostaglandin or at the atrial level by means of a palliative balloon atrial septotomy (Rashkind procedure). These procedures increase mixing and are associated with improved systemic arterial saturation and oxygen delivery.

Surgical therapy for transposition of the great arteries has changed significantly over the last several years. In the past, an intra-atrial baffle repair (either a Mustard or Senning procedure) was performed in the latter portion of the first year of life. Toward the early 1980s, these baffle procedures were more often performed in neonates. The atrial baffle procedures result in redirection of venous blood by a baffle of cloth, pericardium, or atrial tissue, allowing the blue systemic venous blood to flow from the

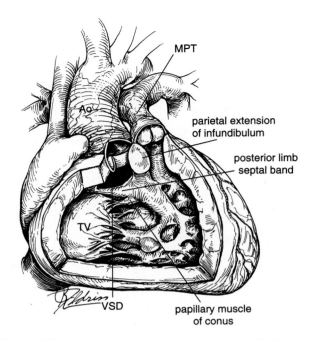

Figure 4-18 Pathologic anatomy of tetralogy of Fallot. A nonrestrictive malalignment ventricular septal defect (*VSD*) with aortic override is evident. The papillary muscle of the conus is shown along with the hypertrophied parietal and septal bands, which cause right ventricular outflow tract obstruction. An infundibular "chamber" and a stenotic, hypoplastic main pulmonary trunk (*MPT*) and valve are shown. *Ao,* aorta; *TV,* tricuspid valve. (Reprinted with permission from Mavroudis C. *Pediatric Cardiac Surgery.* St. Louis: Mosby-Year Book; 2003:384.)

inferior and superior vena cavae underneath the baffle to the mitral valve. The left ventricle would eject this desaturated blood to the pulmonary arteries, from whence it would return as oxygenated blood by way of the pulmonary veins. It would then be directed from the pulmonary veins through the tricuspid valve to the right ventricle and out the aorta to the body. Overall survival rate with this type of surgical procedure was excellent, with mortality less than 5%. However, late complications were common, including arrhythmias, systemic right ventricular failure, and baffle obstruction. In the last two decades, these atrial level repairs have largely given way to anatomic repair of transposition of the great arteries by means of the Jatene procedure, also known as the arterial switch operation. This technically demanding operation is generally undertaken within the first 2 weeks of life and includes switching of the pulmonary trunk and ascending aorta together with translocation of the origin of the coronary arteries to the neoaorta (Fig. 4-19). When performed by an experienced surgeon, this procedure carries a risk of less than 10%.

Tricuspid Atresia

Tricuspid atresia, although it accounts for only 3% of congenital cardiac defects, is representative of the important class of congenital cardiac anomalies characterized by univentricular-atrioventricular connection or functional single ventricle. Tricuspid atresia is absence of the right atrioventricular connection. There is no patent tricuspid valve. The only outlet from the right atrium is through the atrial septal defect. The left ventricle is generally well developed or large. The right ventricle is rudimentary, having no sinus or inlet portion. The small outlet portion of the right ventricle receives blood through a VSD of variable size. It is a cyanotic lesion usually associated with diminished pulmonary blood flow. Occasionally, however, it is associated with either a sufficiently large VSD or with transposition of the great arteries, in which cases pulmonary blood flow may be generous or excessive.

In the common form of tricuspid atresia with diminished pulmonary blood flow, palliation during infancy by means of construction of a systemic-to-pulmonary artery shunt is usually the initial form of therapy. In the cases with increased pulmonary blood flow, congestive heart failure may be present and the infant may require either banding of the main pulmonary artery trunk or creation of pulmonary atresia together with a systemic-to-pulmonary artery shunt. In any event, definitive repair generally consists of separation of the systemic and pulmonary circulations by means of a modified Fontan operation. This depends on unimpeded passive flow of systemic venous return through the lungs and to the systemic ventricle. The first stage, which is called the hemi-Fontan operation or bidirectional Glenn procedure, consists of a superior vena cava–to–pulmonary artery anastomosis. This diverts all systemic venous return from the upper body to the pulmonary circulation before it reaches the systemic ventricle. It results in normalization of the volume work of the systemic ventricle, but persistence of a degree of cyanosis (systemic arterial saturation around 80%–84%). Later in childhood, the completion Fontan procedure is undertaken. This second stage results in the diversion of inferior vena caval return as well to the pulmonary circulation. Thus, the completed Fontan procedure establishes pulmonary and systemic circulations in series. In the case of tricuspid atresia, the systemic ventricle is a morphologic left ventricle. In other univentricular anomalies, the same type of Fontan procedure can be accomplished utilizing a morphologic right ventricle as the systemic ventricle.

Although overall management of lesions characterized by a functional single ventricle has improved considerably in the past decade, mortality still remains a challenge. But for tricuspid atresia, the risk of the ultimate Fontan operation for appropriately palliated and prepared patients is now as low as approximately 5%.

DISEASES OF THE GREAT VESSELS

The thoracic aorta and the great vessels (i.e., innominate, intrathoracic carotid, and subclavian arteries) are subject to the same pathology as blood vessels elsewhere. Because of their size and propensity for exsanguinating hemorrhage and visceral ischemia, recognition of the disease processes of these vessels is extremely important.

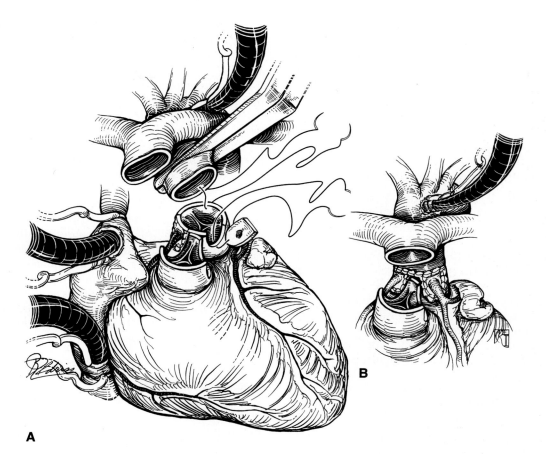

Figure 4-19 **A,** Arterial switch operation. After the coronary patches are mobilized, they are sutured to the facing sinuses of Valsalva of the old pulmonary artery (neoaorta). **B,** Neoaortic construction is completed with the end-to-end anastomosis between the proximal neoaorta and the ascending aorta. Coronary artery reperfusion is established after the cross-clamp is removed. (Reprinted with permission from Mavroudis C. *Pediatric Cardiac Surgery*. St. Louis: Mosby-Year Book; 2003:454.)

Anatomy

The aorta traverses the mediastinum from the aortic valve cephalad, arches posterolaterally, and finally descends through the thorax in a paravertebral location. It transverses the diaphragm into the abdomen. The brachiocephalic branches (i.e., innominate, left common carotid, left subclavian) arise from the transverse arch of the aorta. The innominate branch bifurcates into the right subclavian and right carotid arteries at the base of the neck, behind the sternocleidomastoid muscle.

Pathophysiology

The great vessels are subject to diseases similar to those of other organ systems, including trauma, congenital diseases, and degenerative (atherosclerotic) diseases. Laceration can cause exsanguination, luminal obstruction, or retrograde dissection with intrapericardial bleeding and tamponade.

Trauma

Traumatic rupture of the aorta (TRA) or great vessels is a potentially life-threatening injury. It is usually caused by rapid deceleration forces that occur on impact. Motor vehicle accidents and motorcycle trauma are the most common causes, and young people are most often affected. Because the surrounding pleura, adventitia, and mediastinal tissues can contain a free rupture, there may be no immediate physiologic consequences of great vessel transection. Many patients die at the scene because of rapid exsanguination. However, for those who survive initially, physiologic derangement may be absent or delayed in onset. Tears just above the aortic valve are almost uniformly fatal. Surviving patients nearly always have tears distal to the left subclavian artery. These traumatized tissues give way over time, and they cause exsanguinating hemorrhage and death in 95% of untreated patients.

Approximately 5% of patients develop chronic false aneurysms. These are noticed months to years later, as they expand. Because a false aneurysm has few immediate physiologic consequences, a heightened awareness of the possibility of aortic disruption is needed when treating patients with a history of traumatic injury. Knowledge of the mechanism of injury is important. History of a decelerating injury or a fall from a great height should prompt a search for the injury as soon as possible. (Traumatic aortic rupture is also covered in the Trauma chapter in Lawrence et al, *Essentials of General Surgery*, 4th ed.)

Clinical Presentation and Evaluation

Many patients with TRA have multiple system injuries. Because TRA may be physiologically silent (before rupture), attention may be easily diverted from this injury. Occasionally, the transection produces intimal or luminal obstruction that causes a blood pressure differential between the upper and lower extremities (e.g., pseudocoarctation). Because TRA is physiologically silent, a high index of suspicion is necessary to recognize it. Failure to recognize TRA subjects patients to the high mortality rates associated with nonoperative treatment.

Chest x-ray remains the most important initial screening tool (see also Lawrence et al, *Essentials of General Surgery*, 4th ed, Table 10-4). Radiologic findings on a supine anterior-posterior portable chest x-ray include widening of the mediastinum to more than 8 cm at the level of the aortic knob, an apical pleural cap (indicating the presence of an extrapleural mediastinal hematoma at the apex of the right hemithorax), loss of the contour of the aortic knob and aortopulmonary window, depression of the left mainstem bronchus, and rightward deviation of a nasogastric tube (indicating displacement of the esophagus).

All of these findings on chest x-ray indicate the presence of a mediastinal hematoma and are not specific for great vessel injury. The trauma surgeon must distinguish between great vessel injury, which requires immediate treatment, and mediastinal hematoma of another cause, which does not. Mediastinal hematoma is largely the result of injury to small arteries and veins in the mediastinum. An aortogram remains the best diagnostic study for delineating aortic trauma (Fig. 4-20). Plain computed tomography (CT) scans have a high false-negative rate that is unacceptable in this highly lethal injury. Additionally, an improper scan may delay aortogram, and a positive aortogram mandates immediate surgery. Recent advances in CT technology have led to the development of CT angiography (CTA), which has become useful as a screening tool when available because many patients with normal chest x-ray films, despite having a TRA, have an abnormal CTA film. Delineation of the false aneurysm is diagnostic and mandates surgical intervention.

Although chest radiography and knowledge of the mechanism of injury are quite sensitive (>90%) but not very specific (<10%) screening tools for TRA, approximately 90% of aortograms are negative. A useful screening tool that would allow patients to avoid the morbidity, expense, and time required by an aortogram would be ex-

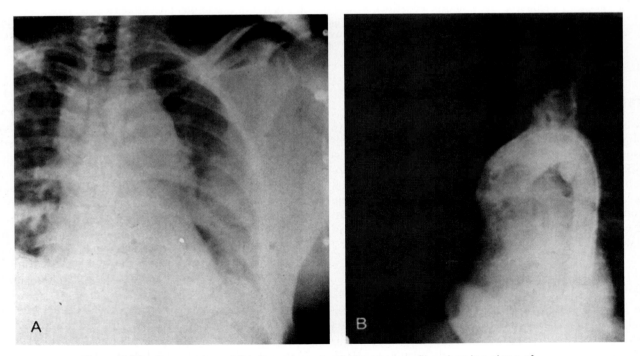

Figure 4-20   Transection of the thoracic aorta. **A,** Chest x-ray film showing signs of mediastinal hematoma. **B,** Aortogram showing a false aneurysm distal to the left subclavian artery.

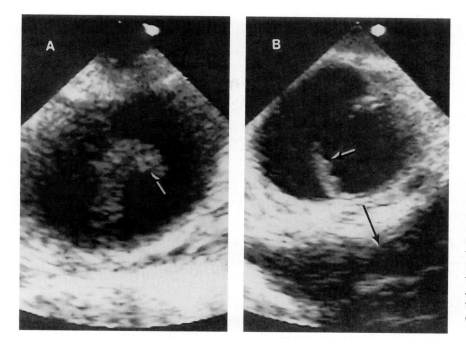

Figure 4-21   **A,** Characteristic ultrasonographic appearance of aortic disruption (*short arrow*). **B,** This patient also has the characteristic ultrasonographic appearance of aortic disruption. In addition, the *long arrow* shows a periaortic hematoma. (Reprinted with permission from Buckmaster MJ, Kearney PM, Johnson SB, et al. Further experience with transesophageal echocardiography in the evaluation of thoracic aortic injury. *J Trauma* 1994;37:990–992.)

tremely valuable. Transesophageal echocardiography is one such tool that can be used in the intensive care unit, operating room, or emergency department (Fig. 4-21). This technique provides an excellent image of the ascending and descending aorta, and it is quite specific for TRA when performed by experienced echocardiographers. Figure 4-22 shows an algorithm for the evaluation of TRA. Institutional capabilities often determine which test is definitive for confirming the diagnosis of TRA.

Treatment

Nonsurgical Treatment

The indications for nonsurgical treatment are few and specific because the mortality rate is high without surgical repair. Some patients with an associated severe pulmonary contusion may be unsuitable candidates for urgent repair because of the need for one-lung anesthesia. Similarly, a devastating head injury with a prohibitive surgical risk may justify a delay in aortic repair until they are corrected. Treatment with β-blockers and antihypertensives is appropriate in these situations

Surgical Treatment

Treatment of this injury depends on the extent of aortic injury. Partial disruptions can be repaired with simple suture techniques that avoid the use of prosthetic grafts; however, most patients incur total transection of the aorta, with retraction of the edges for a distance of 2 to 6 cm. Interposition of a prosthetic graft is usually necessary. Graft interposition requires cross-clamping of the thoracic aorta, usually between the left subclavian and left carotid arteries proximally, and just beyond the aortic tear distally. Problems caused by cross-clamping include proximal hypertension

and inadequate flow to the spinal cord and visceral arteries distal to the clamp. Surgical approaches include a clamp-and-sew technique, which may suffice if there has been no preoperative hypotension and if the cross-clamp time can be held to less than 30 minutes. Other techniques include left atrial–femoral bypass with a pump and an oxygenator to provide distal perfusion. Heparin-bonded, large (9 mm) plastic shunts can be placed proximal and distal to the area of clamping to provide flow to the lower body. Contraindications to heparinization (and therefore to bypass with an oxygenator) include severe head trauma and massive retroperitoneal injury. Newer cardiopulmonary bypass circuits coated with bonded heparin compounds may permit the use of the bypass technique with little or no systemic heparin. Because the incidence of spinal cord ischemia seems to be reduced by maintaining adequate distal perfusion pressures with shunts or bypass, this is useful in minimizing this devastating complication.

Complications associated with the treatment of thoracic aortic injuries are spinal cord ischemia and renal ischemia. Because it is difficult to determine which segment of the aorta gives rise to the anterior artery of Adamkiewicz, which supplies the anterior spinal artery, spinal cord ischemia occurs during aortic cross-clamping in 5% to 15% of cases. Perfusion of the lower body should be protective. Renal failure is unusual after these operations if the patient is adequately rehydrated and hypotension and acidosis are avoided after the aorta is unclamped. Because the recurrent laryngeal nerve courses through the exact location of aortic injury around the ligamentum arteriosum, care is taken to seek out the nerve and protect it. Loss of the recurrent laryngeal nerve may predispose the patient to airway compromise because of vocal cord paralysis. How-

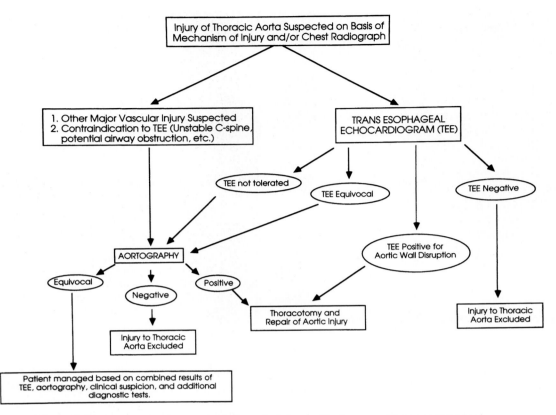

Figure 4-22 Algorithm for suspected aortic injury with the use of transesophageal echocardiography. (Reprinted with permission from Buckmaster MJ, Kearney PM, Johnson SB, et al. Further experience with transesophageal echocardiography in the evaluation of thoracic aortic injury. *J Trauma* 1994;37:990–992.)

ever, long-term sequelae are few if there are no early perioperative complications.

Great vessels other than the aorta may also be injured. Aortography should include the origins of the brachiocephalic trunks; overlooking injuries to these vessels may result in stroke and extremity ischemia. Intimal flaps may lead to thrombus formation or arterial occlusion. Repair techniques for these vessels are similar to those for the thoracic aorta, except for the incisions used. Injuries to the innominate artery are approached through a median sternotomy, with extension into the base of the right side of the neck. Similarly, injuries to the left common carotid artery or the subclavian artery may be approached through a sternotomy for proximal control, with extension into the left neck or left hemithorax for distal exposure. Bypass techniques are seldom necessary for brachiocephalic injuries and sequelae are few.

Degenerative Disease: Aortic Dissection

Pathophysiology

Dissection of the thoracic aorta originates from a tear in the intima of the aorta. It causes a dissecting hematoma between the intima and media of the vessel. This dissecting hematoma may occlude and compromise visceral circulation (e.g., coronary, carotid, and splanchnic vessels). It also may rupture into the pleura or peritoneum (causing exsanguinating hemorrhage) or into the pericardium (causing tamponade and death). The underlying pathogenesis is an abnormal aortic intima caused either by hemorrhage into atherosclerotic plaques or by cystic medial degeneration of the vessel caused by a connective tissue disorder (e.g., Marfan's syndrome).

Clinical Presentation and Evaluation

The patient describes an excruciating "tearing, ripping" pain, the worst pain imaginable, usually originating in the precordium and radiating to the back and flanks. This pain may be confused with the pain of coronary ischemia, but careful questioning can usually elicit the difference between the chest pressure of angina and the tearing pain of aortic dissection. Vascular occlusion caused by obstruction by the "false channel" may produce signs of end-organ ischemia (e.g., syncope, oliguria, stroke, coronary ischemia, abdominal pain, or leg numbness and pain). Chest or back pain in combination with these findings suggests aortic dissection until proven otherwise. New onset of aortic insufficiency associated with this pain is pathognomonic of the diagnosis. A decreasing blood pressure with rising central venous pressure and a small, silent heart on physical examination (Beck's triad) will suggest tamponade, as will a rise in jugular venous pressure on inspiration (Kussmaul's sign). Pulse differentials between the arms and/or the legs, bloody diarrhea, hemiparesis, and abdominal tenderness are diagnostic clues that are observable on physical examination.

A normal ECG and an abnormal chest x-ray film that shows a widened mediastinum may help in differentiating aortic dissection from angina or myocardial infarction. The diagnosis may be confirmed by echocardiogram, transesophageal echocardiogram, CTA (Fig. 4-23), or angiography.

When readily available, TEE has proved to be the most expeditious and useful modality in recent years because it can be performed in almost any location, with conscious sedation if necessary. It also obviates the need to send patients from the emergency department or intensive care unit for diagnostic studies (Fig. 4-24). If this modality is not available, thoracic CTA is most expeditious.

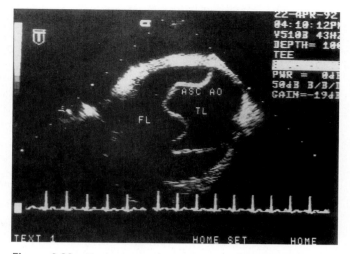

Figure 4-24   Transesophageal echo evidence of ascending aortic (*ASC AO*) dissection. *FL,* false lumen; *TL,* true lumen. (Reprinted with permission from Bave ER, Geha AS, Hammond GL, et al, eds. *Glenn's Thoracic and Cardiovascular Surgery.* Stamford, Conn: Appleton & Lange; 1995:2267.)

Treatment

The classification of aortic dissection depends on its anatomic location. According to a classification method from Stanford University, all dissections that involve the ascending aorta, regardless of origin, are considered type A. These dissections require immediate surgical intervention. Dissections that are confined to the descending thoracic aorta, distal to the left subclavian artery, are classified as type B. They should be treated nonoperatively if indications for surgery are not present. The rationale for this treatment algorithm stems from the fact that retrograde dissection into the ascending aorta may lead to rupture within the pericardial cavity, immediate tamponade, and death. The outcome is dismal for patients with nonoperatively treated type A dissections. Therefore, urgent surgery is mandatory. On the other hand, in the absence of indications for surgery (rupture into the pleural space—hemothorax), vital

organ ischemia, ongoing pain despite adequate blood pressure control, inability to control the blood pressure over time (24 hours), or evidence of ongoing bleeding into the mediastinum (widening mediastinal shadow on plain chest x-ray), patients with dissection of the descending thoracic aorta are best treated nonoperatively. In either case, once the diagnosis is made or is highly suspected, immediate early treatment may begin with drugs that decrease the force of left ventricular contraction and control blood pressure. The drugs that minimize the force that propels the dissecting hematoma (Dp/Dt) are primarily β-blockers. Unless significant contraindications exist, they are started intravenously to lower the pulse rate into the 60s. If hypertension persists, antihypertensive agents (e.g., intravenous sodium nitroprusside, nitroglycerine, or hydralazine) are used to further control the pressure. Additional antihypertensive agents may be added as necessary. Patients who are treated nonoperatively must be monitored closely in the intensive care unit. Arterial blood pressure, urine output, and central venous or pulmonary artery pressure must be measured frequently. Again, surgery is indicated if there is a change in clinical status that indicates visceral artery occlusion (e.g., splanchnic ischemia or renal failure), enlargement of the dissection based on CT or chest x-ray, unremitting and uncontrollable pain, or evidence of leakage of the dissection into the pleural space, with resultant hemothorax. If nonoperative treatment is continued, medications are switched to oral agents or antihypertensive cutaneous patches.

Operative techniques are similar to those used for other types of aortic surgery in terms of bypass, blood salvage, and perfusion of the lower body. Repair or replacement of an incompetent aortic valve may be necessary. Because the aorta is friable, methods to bolster suture techniques

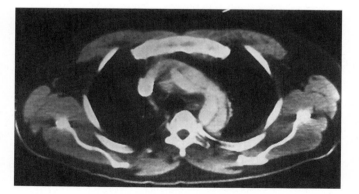

Figure 4-23   Computed tomography scan with contrast showing true and false lumens with an intervening intimal flap in the aortic arch.

and graft interposition must be used. Pledget material is used to distribute the force of the sutures and prevent them from tearing through the aortic wall. Newer "biologic" glues may be very helpful in controlling bleeding from suture lines. Closing or obliterating the site of the intimal tear, excising the dissected aorta, and obliterating the false lumen are the goals of surgery. The operative mortality rate is 5% to 20% and is highest when the tear originates in the aortic arch. Dissection at a site distal to the original tear is the most common cause of late death.

Atherosclerotic Disease: Aneurysm

Atherosclerotic, posttraumatic, chronic dissection with dilatation and infectious aneurysms may affect the thoracic aorta. Recognizable symptoms (e.g., chest and back pain caused by enlargement of the aneurysm against the vertebral column) and discovery on routine chest x-ray are common presentations. Indications for treatment include symptomatic aneurysms, enlarging aneurysms, aneurysms larger than 5 cm in diameter, and leaking aneurysms. Bypass and perfusion techniques are similar to those described previously and vary with the location of the aneurysm. Aneurysms in the ascending aorta and aortic arch are approached through a median sternotomy and usually necessitate femoral artery perfusion. The patient is often placed in hypothermic total circulatory arrest to protect the brain and viscera. Numerous grafting and repair techniques are used; most include resection and grafting of the aneurysmal tissue with Dacron grafts.

An alternative approach to resection and grafting is an endovascular technique that involves placement of an endovascular stent to exclude the aneurysmal segment of the diseased aorta. Early results have been successful in a selected group of patients when the aneurysm is confined to the descending thoracic (or abdominal) aorta. Larger, long-term reports to assess the safety and efficacy of this technique are needed (Fig. 4-25).

DISEASES OF THE THORACIC CAVITY: CHEST WALL, MEDIASTINUM, AND LUNGS

Thoracic surgeons treat a large number of patients with both benign and malignant disease processes (e.g., lung and esophageal cancer, pleuropulmonary infection, chest trauma). An understanding of the anatomic structures of the thoracic cavity and familiarity with respiratory physiology are crucial elements for a thorough understanding of this field.

Anatomy

The thorax is a flexible cage whose framework is made up of the ribs, sternum, vertebrae, scapula, and clavicles. Its main function is to facilitate the mechanics of ventilation.

These structures also protect the heart, lungs, and great vessels. The inside of the pleural cavities is lined by a layer of parietal pleura and the lungs are covered by the visceral pleura. These linings allow frictionless movement of the lungs with normal respiration.

The trachea bifurcates into the right and left mainstem bronchi; subsequent branching results in a total of 23 generations of airways. The right lung is made of three lobes: upper, middle, and lower; the left has two lobes, upper and lower. Each lobe is further subdivided into bronchopulmonary segments. These are the anatomic units of the lung with an individual blood supply and bronchus. There are generally 10 segments on the right and 8 on the left.

The last generation of the airway is the terminal bronchiole, which ends in alveolar ducts and sacs. This is where gas exchange occurs between the sacs and the capillaries, which are the terminal decisions of the pulmonary arterial system.

Physiology

Inspiration is an active process caused by coordinated muscular contraction (mainly the intercostal muscles and diaphragm, and to a lesser extent the sternocleidomastoid and serratus posterior). This process decreases the intrathoracic pressure and leads to inflow of air. At the end of inspiration, elastic recoil of the chest wall and of the lungs increases the intrathoracic pressure and forces air out. Thus, expiration is a passive process.

The alveoli are held open by a balance between the outward elastic recoil of the chest and the inward collapse of the lung. Pulmonary surfactant, which is secreted by type II pneumocytes, helps keep alveoli open by decreasing the surface tension within the alveoli.

Pathophysiology

Pathology of the thoracic cavity includes anything that disrupts the normal respiratory function and includes a variety of inflammatory, infectious, and neoplastic processes. Details are discussed under specific disease processes.

Clinical Presentation and Evaluation

Thoracic pathology presents in a number of ways, from an asymptomatic abnormality detected on chest x-ray to life-threatening hemoptysis. The workup is influenced by the presentation.

History

A thorough history is part of the workup of any thoracic problem. The history emphasizes the following elements:

1 Past illnesses (episodes of pneumonia, bronchitis, asthma, or other related illness)
2 Allergies that affect the respiratory system

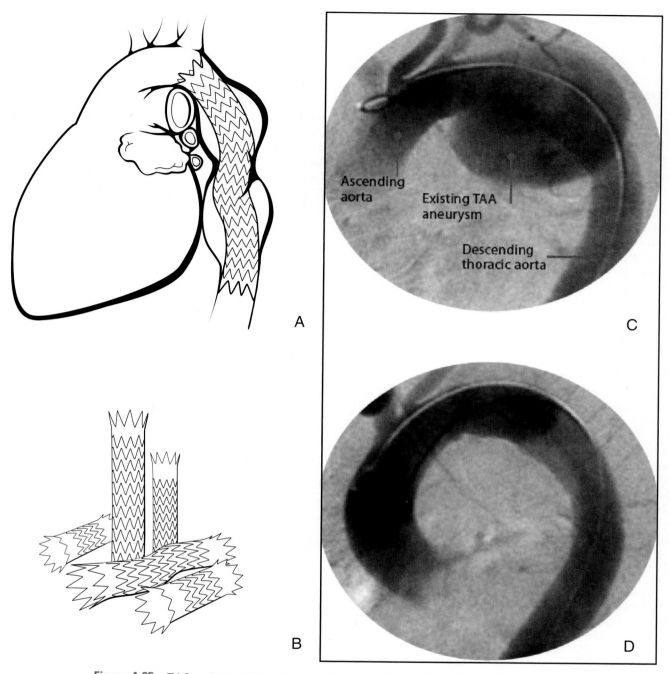

Figure 4-25   TAG endovascular graft. **A,** Artist's rendition of the delivery of a TAG thoracic endoprosthesis, allowing for endovascular repair of a thoracic aortic aneurysm (TAA). **B,** TAG thoracic endoprosthesis. **C,** Preoperative TAA. **D,** Postoperative TAA. No blood flow to the aneurysm. All blood follows through the TAG thoracic endoprosthesis. (Adapted with permission from W.L. Gore & Associates, Inc., Medical Products Division. *An Endovascular Treatment for Thoracic Aortic Aneurysm.* Flagstaff, Ariz; 2005.)

3 Exposure (occupational or other, including ionizing radiation, asbestosis, or other chemical exposure)
4 Habits (smoking or exposure to secondhand smoke)
5 Previous chest x-rays or their interpretation

Physical Examination

A thorough, complete physical examination is an essential part of the thoracic workup. The examination should focus on the integrity of the chest wall, auscultation and percussion of the lungs, and drainage of the lymph nodes in the axilla, neck, and scalene area.

Laboratory and Diagnostic Evaluation

Initial tests include posteroanterior and lateral chest x-rays and laboratory tests (e.g., complete blood count, blood chemistry). More specialized tests include sputum culture and sensitivity, cytology, arterial blood gases, and pulmonary function tests. Further radiologic evaluation is done most often by CT scans, positron emission tomography (PET) scans, MRI, and radionuclide studies. Direct evaluation of the airways is done with bronchoscopy.

Treatment

After a thorough workup that includes diagnostic tests, at least a tentative diagnosis can usually be made. Some pathology, especially infectious and inflammatory diseases, may be managed nonoperatively. The details of treatment of these medical diseases are beyond the scope of this chapter, but some of the basic principles are discussed later. Other types of pathology (e.g., neoplasm) are managed primarily with surgery. This treatment is more fully described.

Hemoptysis

The principal causes of hemoptysis have changed over the last two decades from tuberculosis and bronchiectasis to bronchitis and cancer. Bronchitis and other inflammatory and infectious processes now account for approximately 50% of cases of hemoptysis. Tumors account for almost 20%. Most hemoptysis is treated with bed rest, humidification, antitussives, antibiotics, and sedation.

Any patient who has persistent, recurrent, or massive hemoptysis should undergo a thorough workup. If the hemoptysis is not massive (<600 mL/24 hr), the workup can be done electively. If it is massive, the patient requires immediate diagnostic and therapeutic intervention. In approximately 90% of cases, posteroanterior and lateral chest x-rays followed by bronchoscopy show the cause of hemoptysis. Bronchoscopy is necessary to identify the site of bleeding. The patient is positioned with the side of the bleeding dependent, to minimize aspiration of blood into the other lung. Endobronchial occlusion of the appropriate bronchus is then performed. If bleeding is massive, an aortogram with bronchial arteriography facilitates management because bronchial artery embolization temporarily

controls hemoptysis in some patients. Determining the site of bleeding can be difficult because blood may collect throughout the endobronchial tree. Diligent bronchoscopy with occluding catheters and angiography may be necessary.

Surgical treatment is based on the etiology of the hemoptysis. In benign disease, as little lung as possible is resected. For any potentially curable malignancy, more extensive anatomic resection is necessary. The photocoagulating yttrium-argon-garnet (YAG) laser is used with some success to control hemoptysis from proximal endobronchial tumors.

Solitary Pulmonary Nodule

Some pulmonary masses are first noted as incidental findings on chest x-ray. If the radiograph shows a solitary pulmonary nodule or coin lesion, a workup is required to formulate a management plan (Fig. 4-26). The importance of previous chest x-rays cannot be overstated. Management decisions are greatly affected by knowledge of prior lesions and estimates of growth rates. Stable lesions are usually benign. New or enlarged masses must be presumed malignant until proved benign.

Pleural Effusion

For diagnostic and therapeutic reasons, pleural effusions (fluid in the pleural space) are divided into two types: transudates and exudates. Transudates originate from some external cause that upsets the normal balance of fluid secretion and absorption in the pleural space, allowing fluid to accumulate. Common causes include congestive heart failure, cirrhosis, and atelectasis. Exudates are caused by primary disease processes of the pleural cavity (e.g., malignancies that exude fluid or block lymphatic channels).

Symptoms of pleural effusions include shortness of breath, pleuritic pain, and a sense of fullness in the chest. Decreased breath sounds and dullness to percussion are noted on physical examination. Thoracentesis is the primary diagnostic procedure. The fluid is analyzed to determine whether it is a transudate or an exudate (Table 4-7). Gram stain and culture are also routinely performed. Usually, removal of as much fluid as possible allows subsequent chest x-rays to detect otherwise hidden lesions.

Treatment of a pleural effusion depends on its cause (Table 4-8). Transudates rarely require chest tube drainage. They are treated by addressing the underlying cause (e.g., congestive heart failure). Exudates usually require chest tube drainage. Malignant effusions often recur after thoracentesis alone. They require chest tube drainage. Drainage of the pleural space with a chest tube until the space is dry and instillation of a chemical sclerosing agent (e.g., tetracycline, bleomycin, talc) prevents reaccumulation in 60% to 80% of cases. For sclerosis to be effective, the underlying lung must reexpand and allow apposition of the visceral and parietal pleura. Occasionally, mechanical abrasion or excision of the pleura (pleurectomy) is indicated.

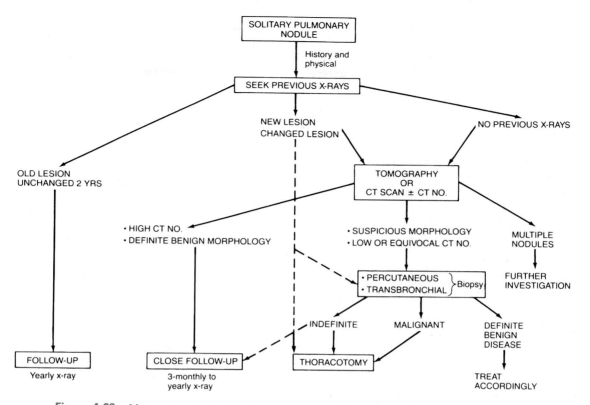

Figure 4-26   Management plan for the assessment of patients with an asymptomatic solitary pulmonary nodule. *CT,* computed tomography.

Lung Abscess

A lung abscess is suspected in any patient who has a fever and an air–fluid level seen within the lung parenchyma on chest x-ray. CT scan usually permits differentiation between a lung abscess (parenchymal process) and an empyema (extraparenchymal process). The most common cause of lung abscess is aspiration pneumonia. Persistent pneumonia can evolve into a lung abscess, as can pulmonary infarction. A bronchial neoplasm or an aspirated foreign body may also be the cause and can be excluded by bronchoscopy.

Treatment of a lung abscess consists of prolonged antibiotic therapy and vigorous respiratory physiotherapy.

Until the pathogen is identified, broad-spectrum antibiotics are indicated. An abscess caused by aspiration may include *Staphylococcus* species, fusiform bacilli, α-hemolytic streptococcus, and *Bacteroides fragilis*. Patients who are immunocompromised because of acquired immune deficiency syndrome, chemotherapy, or malignancy may harbor Gram-negative organisms, such as *Proteus, Pseudomonas, Escherichia coli*, and *Klebsiella*.

In most patients who have a lung abscess, bronchoscopy is indicated to obtain cultures, promote drainage, and rule out an endobronchial tumor or foreign body. Surgery is indicated only if the patient continues to be septic, has an enlarging cavity, or has a resectable endobronchial lesion. Resection and tube drainage of the abscess are the principal surgical treatment techniques.

Table 4-7	Tests to Differentiate Transudative from Exudative Pleural Fluid		
Test		**Exudate**	**Transudate**
Protein (g/dL)		>0.3	<03
Pleural fluid/serum protein (g/dL)		>0.5	<0.5
Lactate dehydrogenase (international units/L)		>200	<200
Pleural fluid/serum lactate dehydrogenase		>0.6	<0.5

Table 4-8	Common Causes of Pleural Effusion	
Transudates		**Exudates**
Congestive heart failure		Infection
Cirrhosis		Malignancy
Hypoalbuminemia		Chylothorax
Nephrotic syndrome		Tuberculosis

Pneumothorax

Pneumothorax is partial or total collapse of the lung due to air collecting in the pleural space. It eliminates the normal negative intrapleural pressure that counteracts the elastic recoil of the lung and prevents lung collapse. Spontaneous pneumothorax may be caused by rupture of subpleural blebs. Sometimes it occurs for no apparent reason (primary) or is caused by lung pathology (secondary). The diagnosis is made by history (chest pain or pressure) and physical examination (decreased breath sounds on auscultation and tympany on percussion). The diagnosis is confirmed by chest x-ray. Care is taken to differentiate a pneumothorax from an area with no lung markings (e.g., giant bulla), which would result in rupture of the bulla, pneumothorax, and potential bronchopleural fistula.

A significant or symptomatic pneumothorax usually requires a chest tube. The tube is placed in the fourth or fifth interspace in the midaxillary line, unless the pneumothorax is loculated. In this case, the tube may be more appropriately directed. The tube should reach the apex of the thoracic cavity, where most blebs are located. When anesthetizing the area for tube insertion, the needle is passed into the pleural space to ascertain that air can be freely aspirated. If air cannot be aspirated, either the diagnosis or the location of the pneumothorax should be reassessed. Once the diagnosis is confirmed by needle aspiration, blunt dissection with a hemostat through the muscles, over the top of the rib, and into the pleural cavity allows easy placement of the tube. For spontaneous pneumothorax, a 28-French tube is adequate. The tube is placed to −20 cm H_2O suction. A lung that reinflates too rapidly may cause significant transient pain that requires analgesia. The chest tube usually can be removed after the air leak stops. Occasionally, patients who have prolonged air leaks are discharged with chest tubes in place, connected to a one-way valve.

Surgical intervention should be considered for patients who have an air leak that persists for more than 7 to 10 days, recurrent pneumothorax, or bilateral simultaneous pneumothoraces. Surgery is considered for an initial pneumothorax in certain patients whose occupations put them at risk, such as deep-sea divers or airline pilots. Surgery consists of closure and exclusion of the ruptured bleb or any other large blebs with surgical staplers and mechanical pleurodesis. Pleurodesis, the creation of a fibrous adhesion between the visceral and parietal layers of the pleura, is accomplished by rubbing the parietal pleura with dry gauze to create an inflammatory reaction. This reaction, when coupled with complete lung expansion, ensures obliteration of the pleural space and prevents recurrence of pneumothorax. Mechanical pleurodesis is preferred over pleurectomy (removal of the pleura) because it has a much lower complication rate. A newer surgical approach is video-assisted thoracoscopic surgery (VATS). VATS allows resection of blebs, lysis of adhesions, and sclerosis through multiple small (about 1 cm) incisions on the chest. The thoracoscopic approach permits earlier mobilization, discharge, and return to normal activity.

Empyema

Empyema is an abscess of the pleural space; it usually occurs in conjunction with an underlying bronchopulmonary infection such as pneumonia. The fluid is initially thin and watery and over the course of a few days to 2 weeks changes to a thick fibrin purulent fluid. The fluid usually must be drained with a large chest tube. Indications for drainage include organisms seen on Gram stain, pH less than 7.1, glucose less than 40 mg/dL, and lactate dehydrogenase greater than 1,000 IU/L, all of which are indicative of a cellular exudate. The chest tube can be removed once the space is evacuated, the lung has reexpanded, and the fluid is no longer purulent. The tube may be left in place for several weeks and may be allowed to extrude over several more weeks. If treatment is delayed, tube drainage will not suffice because the thick fluid in later stages of empyema will not be completely evacuated with a chest tube alone. In these cases, more invasive methods may be needed. VATS can be used to drain loculi and remove the fibrinous exudates (called a *peel*). This process is called *decortication*. Complex empyemas may require further procedures (e.g., additional chest tubes, rib resection and drainage, decortication) (Fig. 4-27). Obliteration of the pleural space is the single most important principle that guides therapy for empyema. Once adherence between the parietal and visceral pleural surfaces occurs, resolution is all but ensured. If the lung cannot expand adequately to fill the space, the space must be obliterated by other means. One method includes transposing thoracic muscles into the pleural cavity (commonly used muscles are the serratus anterior or latissimus dorsi). Another method is to collapse the chest wall by excising ribs (called a *thoracoplasty*) This latter option is quite disfiguring and is rarely used.

Trauma

Although chest trauma accounts for 25% of all trauma deaths, fewer than 15% of patients who have chest trauma require thoracic surgery. It is important for all physicians to understand thoracic trauma. Chest trauma causes a wide variety of conditions. The most common are discussed here.

Open Pneumothorax

In open pneumothorax, the integrity of the chest wall is disrupted by an opening into the thorax. This opening interferes with respiration because it disrupts the negative pressure that is normally present for lung expansion. It is corrected with an occlusive dressing over the hole and a chest tube, or conversely, by endotracheal intubation with positive pressure breathing, which obviates the need for an intact chest wall. Definitive treatment requires operative debridement and wound closure, often with muscle flaps.

Tension Pneumothorax

A tension pneumothorax develops when a pneumothorax causes pressure to build within the thorax, as with a one-

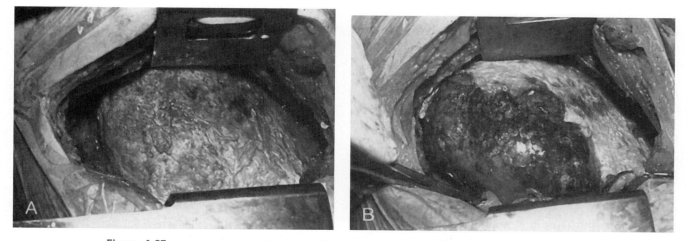

Figure 4-27 **A,** Lung trapped by exudative rind. Note the space between the lung and the chest wall. **B,** Partial decortication. The lung is released from entrapment and is beginning to expand.

way valve effect. A tension pneumothorax is often an emergency, with acute, severe shortness of breath. Decompression with a chest tube or a large-bore needle (inserted over the second or third rib in the midclavicular line) is followed by a confirmatory chest x-ray. The tension is the result of positive pressure in the chest, which causes the lung to deflate and mediastinal structures to shift. This shifting of structures can kink the superior and inferior vena cavae, leading to a relative obstruction of venous return to the heart. Symptoms include shortness of breath and light-headedness. Signs include absent breath sounds, hypotension, and often jugular venous distention. Cardiovascular collapse may occur. Placement of a chest tube rapidly alleviates this condition.

Massive Hemothorax

Significant bleeding into the thoracic cavity can interfere with respirations by limiting the volume available for lung expansion. Most cases are treated with chest tube drainage. Operation is indicated for a continued drainage rate of greater than 200 mL/hr for 4 hours or more, or its equivalent, rather than a predetermined amount of initial drainage.

Flail Chest

Fracture of a rib or ribs in more than one location may cause a portion of the chest wall to move paradoxically to the rest of the chest. On inspiration, as the rest of the chest expands, this segment is pulled in by the intrathoracic negative pressure. On expiration, as the normal chest wall collapses inward, this segment bulges outward because of the positive intrathoracic pressure. If physiologically severe compromise is demonstrated, the patient may require mechanical ventilation until the chest wall is stabilized by surgery or fracture healing. The most significant pathology is usually not the flail segment of chest wall, but damage to the underlying lung.

Neoplasms

Chest Wall Tumors

Half of all chest wall tumors are primary tumors. Of these, 60% are malignant. The other half are metastatic, arising mainly from lung, thyroid, gastrointestinal, or genitourinary tumors. Both types usually cause enlarging chest wall masses. Malignant lesions are more often painful, perhaps because of rapid expansion. The most common primary malignant tumor is chondrosarcoma. The most common benign tumor is fibrous dysplasia (Table 4-9).

All chest wall tumors should be considered malignant until they are proved benign. A careful history and physical examination may show a source of metastatic disease. Posteroanterior and lateral chest x-rays and CT scan of the chest are performed to further define the tumor. CT scan details whether the mass is solitary and provides an assessment of the underlying lung parenchyma and mediastinal structures. A bone scan helps to determine other sites of osseous involvement.

With the exception of plasmacytoma, which is treated as systemic myeloma, most solitary primary malignant tumors are removed with a wide excision that encompasses involved soft tissues, rib, sternum, and underlying lung or pericardium. Margins of 2 to 4 cm are recommended, and a variety of muscle pedicle flaps are used for reconstruc-

Table 4-9	Chest Wall Tumors	
Benign		**Malignant**
Fibrous dysplasia		Chondrosarcoma
Chondroma		Osteogenic sarcoma
Osteochondroma		Plasmacytoma
Eosinophilic granuloma		Ewing's sarcoma

tion. Patients who have Ewing's sarcoma, osteogenic sarcoma, or other soft-tissue sarcomas are candidates for postoperative adjuvant therapy with radiation therapy, chemotherapy, or both.

Mediastinal Tumors

A number of benign and malignant tumors, both primary and metastatic, occur in the mediastinum. Although most tumors are first found on standard posteroanterior or lateral chest x-rays, CT scanning is essential to localize the tumor accurately. MRI offers no significant advantages over CT scanning, except in posterior paraspinal tumors.

Mediastinal tumors are divided according to their location (Fig. 4-28). The anterior mediastinum is defined by an imaginary line that extends along the anterior wall of the trachea and down over the anterior pericardium. The posterior mediastinum is defined by an imaginary line that extends from the anterior border of the vertebral bodies to the costovertebral sulci. The middle mediastinum is the space in between. Tumors occur most often in the anterior mediastinum and least often in the middle mediastinum.

The most common tumors of the anterior mediastinum are thymoma, substernal thyroid tumor, teratoma (germ cell tumor), and lymphoma. Symptoms in patients with malignant lesions include chest pain, dyspnea, fever, chills, and cough. Patients who have benign lesions are usually asymptomatic and the lesions are found only on routine chest x-ray. A careful history and physical examination can give clues as to the type of tumor present.

Lymphoma can cause night sweats, weight loss, and peripheral adenopathy. Lymphomas are best treated with chemotherapy and radiation. A mediastinal germ cell metastasis can appear as a testicular mass. A thymoma can cause symptoms of myasthenia gravis. A substernal thyroid tumor often partially compresses the trachea, one of the few tumors to do so. Excision is the best treatment, except for lymphoma, which usually requires anterior mediastinotomy and biopsy to make the diagnosis if no extramediastinal adenopathy exists. Almost all substernal thyroids can be removed through a cervical incision. Resection of all other anterior mediastinal tumors is best approached with a median sternotomy.

The most common masses in the middle mediastinum are enterogenous cysts and metastatic lymph nodes from lung cancer. Asymptomatic mediastinal adenopathy can be a manifestation of sarcoidosis and can be diagnosed by mediastinoscopy. Middle mediastinal cysts (bronchogenic, esophageal, and pleuropericardial) are removed by lateral thoracotomy to rule out a malignancy that has similar radiographic findings.

The most common tumors of the paravertebral sulci are of neurogenic origin: neurilemoma, neurofibroma, ganglioneuroma, and neuroblastoma. Tumors in this location must be evaluated by MRI to determine whether there is extension into the spinal canal. If they extend into the canal, a combined neurosurgical–thoracosurgical approach is essential to ensure complete removal. Failure to remove the spinal canal component can cause paralysis years later, as the residual tumor slowly grows and presses against the spinal cord.

Lung Cancers

Lung cancer is the most common nondermatologic cancer in North America. It accounts for 14% of all new cancers and 30% of cancer deaths and is now the leading cause of cancer death in both men and women. More than 85% of patients with lung cancer have a significant smoking history. Other reported causative exposures are to radioactive materials, including asbestos dust and fluorspar, and secondary cigarette smoke.

The pathology of lung cancer may be either primary or secondary. Primary lung cancer progresses from dysplastic changes to in situ changes to frankly invasive carcinoma. It develops from two distinct cell lines, large cell lines (e.g., squamous cell, adenocarcinoma, mixed cell type) and small cell lines (e.g., oat cell, intermediate cell type, mixed cell type). Information about cell type is obtained from a variety of diagnostic procedures. These include cytologic evaluation of sputum and bronchial washings, and histologic and cytologic evaluation of tumor tissue obtained by direct or transpulmonary biopsy. The biopsy is performed through the bronchus or the chest wall by fine-needle aspiration. Identification of the originating cell line is important in determining treatment. Because tumors from the small cell line tend to metastasize earlier, they are often managed systemically with a combination of chemotherapy and radiation therapy rather than with a primary surgical approach. However, surgery may play a

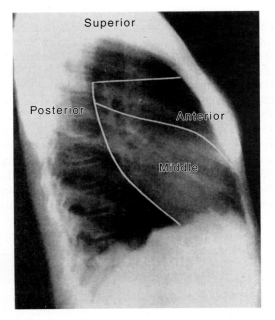

Figure 4-28 Lateral film of the chest showing the anatomic divisions into four subdivisions of the mediastinum. (Reprinted with permission from Sabiston DC, Spencer FC, eds. *Surgery of the Chest*. Philadelphia: WB Saunders; 1990: 872.)

role in selected early lesions that have no evidence of metastasis. Patients with neoplasms of large cell origin are always evaluated with resection in mind because surgical removal offers the best chance for cure.

Secondary lung cancers are caused by metastasis of lesions elsewhere in the body. These lesions usually originate in the breast, gastrointestinal system, genitourinary tract, or soft tissue. Surgery is an option when there is no evidence of other distant metastatic lesions. In some cases, surgical removal of solitary or well-localized metastatic lesions in the lung is justified by improvement in the survival rate. The development of metastatic lesions to the lung carries a generally poor prognosis. However, aggressive combination therapy can produce long, disease-free intervals and, in some cases, improve survival rate.

The clinical presentation of lung cancer is varied. Approximately 5% of patients are asymptomatic, and a lesion is discovered incidentally by chest x-rays performed for some other reason. Because the yield is low, especially in nonsmokers, routine screening chest x-rays usually are not recommended, although screening of selected populations may be revisited. If radiographs show a solitary pulmonary nodule (coin lesion), a workup is required to formulate a management plan (Fig. 4-26). Stable lesions are usually benign. New masses and those that show enlargement are presumed malignant until proven benign.

The other 95% of patients are symptomatic, with signs and symptoms that can be categorized as bronchopulmonary, extrapulmonary, metastatic, nonspecific, or nonmetastatic (Table 4-10). Extrapulmonary signs and symptoms suggest advanced disease. Paratracheal lymph node metastases may produce hoarseness because of involvement of the recurrent laryngeal nerve. Superior vena caval obstruction may occur with right-sided nodal enlargement or direct invasion. Pleural effusion may be caused by metastatic disease in the pleura, obstructive pneumonia, or lymphatic obstruction. Neurologic changes, abnormal liver function test results, and bone pain suggest metastases. A thorough search for metastases must be undertaken with CT scans of the brain and abdomen and bone scans. Nonmetastatic symptoms (paraneoplastic syndromes) occur in a small percentage of patients and may be very early signs of primary lung cancer. These include hypercalcemia and inappropriate secretion of antidiuretic hormone.

Once the possibility of bronchogenic cancer is raised, the physician must formulate a management plan. The plan depends on a precise diagnosis, the stage of the disease, and the ability of the patient to undergo operative treatment. The following three questions must be answered:

1 What is the diagnosis?
2 Can the patient undergo an operation?
3 Can the patient tolerate the maximally anticipated lung resection?

Table 4-10	Signs and Symptoms in Patients with Lung Cancer

Bronchopulmonary
  Cough (most common symptom)
  Chest pain (may indicate involvement of chest wall)
  Dyspnea (due to airway obstruction, or pleural effusion)
  Hemoptysis
Extrapulmonary
  Superior vena caval obstruction
  Hoarseness (recurrent laryngeal nerve invasion)
  Pleural effusion
Metastatic
  Neurologic (headache, change in mental status)
  Skeletal (bone pain)
  Visceral (liver or adrenal metastases are often asymptomatic)
Nonspecific (usually occur late in the course of the disease)
  Weight loss
  Anemia
  Fatigue
Nonmetastatic
  Dermatologic (hyperpigmentation, dermatomyositis)
Endocrine (some tumors secrete hormone-like substances causing hypercalcemia or SIADH)
  Vascular (lung cancer patients may become hypercoagulable)
  Neurogenic (Eaton-Lambert syndrome, autonomic neuropathy, etc.)
  Metabolic (hypercalcemia, Cushing's syndrome, carcinoid syndrome, etc.)
  Hematologic (anemia, thrombocytosis, etc.)
  Skeletal (pulmonary osteoarthropathy, clubbing)

Diagnosis. The diagnosis of bronchogenic carcinoma is confirmed by bronchoscopy or percutaneous needle biopsy. Flexible or rigid bronchoscopy is used to visualize proximal tumors. Direct biopsy (or the use of washings and brushings) provides a precise diagnosis in more than 90% of patients. Even patients with peripheral lesions that are not directly visible endoscopically can undergo biopsy with fluoroscopic guidance into the appropriate bronchopulmonary segment. Lesions that are not amenable to bronchoscopic biopsy are evaluated with percutaneous needle biopsy guided by either fluoroscopy or CT scan. Cytologic analysis is also performed, although some needles yield only a small histologic specimen. In most cases, clinical management is properly guided by the findings of needle biopsy.

The stage of the tumor determines the treatment. The size and spread of the tumor are important elements of staging. The most widely used classification is the TNM system of the American Joint Committee for Cancer Staging and End Results:

T = Size and location of the tumor
N = Presence and location of lymph node metastases
M = Presence of distant metastases

The TNM classification allows the surgeon to provide a stage grouping for the patient. Based on this stage, statistical prognostication can be made for most patients.

After the tumor is localized by bronchoscopy and radiologic evaluation, its resectability is determined. With rare exceptions, tumors at or near the carina are not considered resectable. The proximity of the tumor to vital structures can be determined with bronchoscopy and CT scanning with contrast.

In a patient who has lung cancer, the search for metastatic disease must be as complete as possible before pulmonary resection is performed. Pulmonary resection that leaves malignancy behind is both fruitless and dangerous. Suspected lymph node involvement should be confirmed by biopsy, not x-ray. Biopsy of the hilar and paratracheal lymph nodes is performed at mediastinoscopy. Specimens also undergo microscopic and histochemical evaluation. The presence of metastases in these nodes reduces the surgical cure rate to a level at which few centers attempt surgical resection. With rare exceptions, patients with a tumor limited to the ipsilateral hemithorax, with no evidence of mediastinal lymph node metastases and no involvement of other vital structures, are considered surgical candidates (Fig. 4-29).

Preoperative Evaluation. The decision to perform elective thoracotomy with resection is based on the patient's ability to tolerate a thoracic operation. This judgment is based on an assessment of comorbid conditions (e.g., age; cardiac, renal, hepatic, or neurologic conditions that may adversely affect operative risk). Cardiac reserve is evaluated by history, physical examination, ECG, and, occasionally, stress testing (Fig. 4-30). Pulmonary reserve is estimated by history, physical examination, and exercise testing. Evaluation is best done with pulmonary function tests, measurement of arterial blood gases, and sometimes selective ventilation–perfusion scanning. Spirometry evaluates a number of components of respiration. It is used to measure the volume of gas expired within

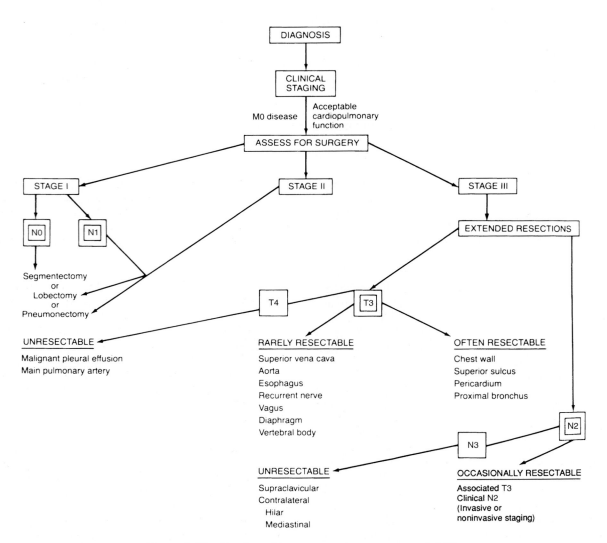

Figure 4-29   Staging of lung cancer to assess resectability.

PREOPERATIVE ASSESSMENT OF CARDIAC RISK

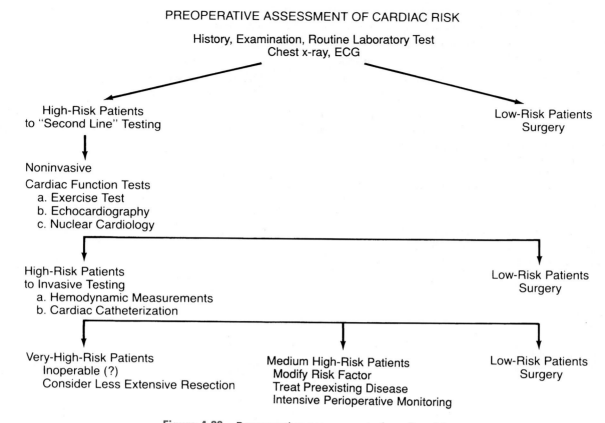

Figure 4-30 Preoperative assessment of cardiac risk.

a specific period (forced expiratory volume; FEV), the volume expired in the first second (FEV_1). The FEV_1 helps to identify patients who cannot tolerate pulmonary resection. An FEV_1 greater than 800 to 1,000 mL is needed to avoid chronic respiratory insufficiency after surgery. Maximal voluntary ventilation is another value that is used to assess a patient's ability to tolerate thoracic surgery. Diffusion of carbon monoxide helps to evaluate the alveolar–capillary membrane and its function. Preoperative assessment of respiratory risk is outlined in Figure 4-31. Measurement of arterial blood gases is also useful in predicting pulmonary reserve. The concentration of carbon dioxide in the blood (Pco_2) indicates the adequacy of alveolar ventilation. Carbon dioxide retention, particularly after exercise, may preclude pulmonary resection. Usually, a Pco_2 greater than 50 mm Hg contraindicates resection. Interpretation of the oxygen concentration in the blood (Po_2) is more difficult. Many believe that a Po_2 of less than 50 mm Hg, or less than 90% saturation, is usually associated with such severe dysfunction that pulmonary resection is not advisable.

Aggressive perioperative management of patients who undergo thoracotomy plays a crucial role in their recovery. In addition to careful patient selection as outlined earlier, this management involves pulmonary physiotherapy and pain control. Factors that seem to favorably influence peri-operative outcome are smoking cessation, bronchodilators, pulmonary physiotherapy, and short-term corticosteroids in patients with asthma or bronchitis. Epidural anesthesia seems to greatly facilitate pain management and postoperative respiratory function in thoracotomy patients. It is now used routinely.

Treatment. Surgical treatment is indicated after a patient is deemed operable and the tumor is deemed resectable. Usually, stage I and some stage II tumors can be resected completely. Extensive resection can be accomplished by ligating the pulmonary vessels within the pulmonary cavity to avoid hilar involvement with the tumor and by excising segments of the chest wall, provided complete tumor removal is anticipated. The goal of anatomic resection is to completely remove the tumor, yet leave enough lung tissue to permit satisfactory respiration. Lung resection may involve a segment (segmentectomy), a lobe (lobectomy), or the whole lung (pneumonectomy). A more proximal lesion requires lobectomy or pneumonectomy for complete removal. More complex operations became possible with the advent of bronchoplastic procedures and reconstruction of the tracheobronchial tree.

Resection is the best treatment for patients who have localized non–small cell primary lung cancer. The risk of death at resection is 2% to 5%, depending on the extent

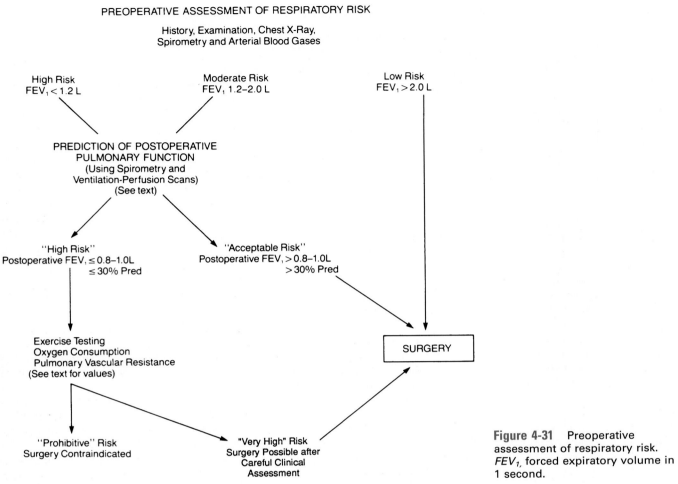

PREOPERATIVE ASSESSMENT OF RESPIRATORY RISK

History, Examination, Chest X-Ray,
Spirometry and Arterial Blood Gases

High Risk
$FEV_1 < 1.2$ L

Moderate Risk
FEV_1 1.2–2.0 L

Low Risk
$FEV_1 > 2.0$ L

PREDICTION OF POSTOPERATIVE
PULMONARY FUNCTION
(Using Spirometry and
Ventilation-Perfusion Scans)
(See text)

"High Risk"
Postoperative $FEV_1 \leq 0.8$–1.0L
$\leq 30\%$ Pred

"Acceptable Risk"
Postoperative $FEV_1 > 0.8$–1.0L
$> 30\%$ Pred

Exercise Testing
Oxygen Consumption
Pulmonary Vascular Resistance
(See text for values)

SURGERY

"Prohibitive" Risk
Surgery Contraindicated

"Very High" Risk
Surgery Possible after
Careful Clinical
Assessment

Figure 4-31 Preoperative assessment of respiratory risk. FEV_1, forced expiratory volume in 1 second.

of the resection and the age and underlying condition of the patient (Table 4-11). The long-term survival of patients who undergo pulmonary resection depends on the stage of the tumor and its cell type. In patients who have a well-differentiated squamous cell carcinoma that is completely resected, the 5-year survival rate is 60% to 70%. Patients who have more advanced or less well-differentiated tumors carry different prognoses (Table 4-12). A small number of patients have totally resectable small cell lung cancer. Accepted primary treatment for most patients with small cell carcinoma is a combination of chemotherapy and local radiation.

Table 4-11	Postoperative Mortality Rate after 2,220 Pulmonary Resections for Lung Cancer	
Type of Resection and Age of Patient	**Number of Resections**	**30-Day Mortality Rate**
All resections	2,220	3.7
Pneumonectomy	569	6.2
Lobectomy	1,508	2.9
Segmentectomy or wedge resection	143	1.4
60 yr	847	1.3
60–69 yr	920	4.1
70 yr	443	7.2

Table 4-12	Analysis of Survival According to Stage and Histology from the Lung Cancer Study Group[a]		
Stage	**Subset**	**Cell Type**	**4-Yr Survival Stage Subset (%)**
I	T_1N_0	Squamous cell	85
		Adenocarcinoma	72
	T_1N_1	Squamous cell	80
		Adenocarcinoma	63
	T_2N_0	Squamous cell	65
		Adenocarcinoma	60
II, III		Squamous cell	37
		Adenocarcinoma	25

[a] Postoperative mortality is excluded.

Common Complications After Pulmonary Resection

Postoperatively, early mobilization and full expansion of the lungs appear to favorably influence recovery. Patients require a variety of types of perioperative analgesia. Modalities that appear to help include local intercostal blocks, epidural analgesia, and systemic opioids, especially patient-controlled analgesia. Postoperative bleeding, pneumonia, wound infection, and cardiac events are rarely seen. The most common complication after lung surgery is atelectasis. Adequate analgesia and incentive spirometry can be helpful in its prevention. About 30% of patients may develop atrial fibrillation in the postoperative period.

Newer Surgical Procedures and Techniques

Lung Reduction Surgery

Lung reduction surgery is an innovative procedure that involves excision of a bullous portion of the lung in patients with severe emphysema. After this procedure, it is anticipated that the remaining, more normal lung will expand and that lung mechanics, including chest wall compliance, will improve, thereby palliating the severe symptoms of dyspnea. Some reported results are quite promising, but the exact indications and long-term results are still under investigation. For selected patients, lung reduction surgery is considered an alternative to lung transplantation.

Thoracoscopic Surgery

With the increasing use of minimally invasive surgery, there has been renewed interest in thoracoscopic surgery. This technique was first described in 1910. Endoscopic surgery is performed through transthoracic ports as a video-assisted procedure. There is markedly decreased postoperative pain and interference with respiratory mechanics. Often referred to as VATS, the basic technique consists of creating several small openings in the chest and using video imaging and specialized instruments similar to those used in laparoscopy to perform the necessary diagnostic or therapeutic maneuvers (Fig. 4-32).

This approach offers the advantage of minimal invasiveness. The small openings that are needed cause little disruption in the mechanics of respiration, and pain control is much easier than with other techniques. VATS also permits accurate diagnosis by directed biopsy. However, the size of the lesion and the presence of adhesions may limit the usefulness of this procedure. Patients who have VATS must undergo preparation for open thoracotomy, which is necessary if bleeding occurs or if the surgeon cannot accomplish the surgical objectives.

Thoracoscopy and diagnostic or therapeutic procedures are being performed in the following areas:

1 Pleural diseases: Video-assisted debridement and decortication, pleurodesis, and pleural biopsy.
2 Parenchymal diseases: Lung biopsy, management of spontaneous pneumothorax, and management of bullous disease.
3 Pulmonary nodules: Investigation of the indeterminate solitary pulmonary nodule (if it is accessible). Definitive treatment for lung cancer is also being done by VATS lobectomies.
4 Mediastinal procedures: Investigation of primary lesions of the mediastinum (thymectomy, biopsy of me-

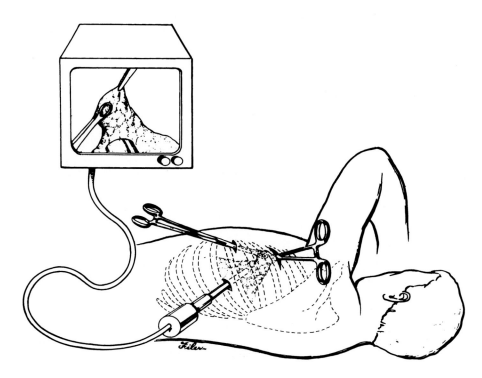

Figure 4-32 Video-assisted thoracic (thoracoscopic) biopsy of the lung with video assistance. (Reprinted with permission from Bave ER, Geha AS, Hammond GL, et al, eds. *Glenn's Thoracic and Cardiovascular Surgery,* 6th ed. Stamford, Conn: Appleton & Lange; 1996:192.)

diastinal masses, excision of bronchogenic or esophageal cysts).
5 Thoracic sympathectomy for hyperhidrosis.

SUGGESTED READINGS

American College of Cardiology, American Heart Association. 2004 guideline update for coronary artery bypass graft surgery: summary article. *Circulation* 2004;110:1168–1176.

American College of Cardiology, American Heart Association. Guidelines for the management of patients with valvular heart disease: executive summary. *Circulation* 1998;98:1949–1984.

American Heart Association. Diagnosis and management of infective endocarditis and its complications. *Circulation* 1998;98:2936–2948.

American College of Cardiology, American Heart Association, National Association for Sports and Physical Education. 2002 guideline update for implantation of cardiac pacemakers and antiarrhythmia devices: summary article. *Circulation* 2002;106:2145.

Eagle KA, Guyton RA, Davidoff R, et al. ACC/AHA 2004 guideline update for coronary artery bypass graft surgery: summary article — a report of the American College of Cardiology/American Heart Association Task Force on Practice Guidelines (Committee to Update the 1999 Guidelines on Coronary Artery Bypass Graft Surgery). *Circulation* 2004;110:1168–1176.

Feins RH, Watson TJ. What's new in general thoracic surgery. *J Am Coll Surg* 2004;199:265–272.

Gott VL, Alejo DE, Cameron DE. Mechanical heart valves: 50 years of evolution. *Ann Thorac Surg* 2003;76:S2230–S2239

Lawrence PF. *Essentials of General Surgery*, 4th ed. Philadelphia: Lippincott Williams & Wilkins; 2006.

Noonan JA. A history of pediatric specialties: the development of pediatric cardiology. *Pediatr Res* 2004;56:298–306.

Reitz BA. What's new in cardiac surgery. *J Am Coll Surg* 2004;198:784–797.

GERALD BERKE ■ ANDREW CELMER ■ JOSEPH VALENTINO
RICHARD C. HAYDON ■ TONI M. GANZEL

Otolaryngology: Diseases of the Head and Neck

Otolaryngology is the study of organ systems connected by the upper aerodigestive tract: the ear, vestibular system, cranial nerves, nose, paranasal sinuses, oral cavity, pharynx, larynx, esophagus, neck, and salivary and thyroid glands. These regions are critical for human interaction and communication, as well as functions rudimentary to sustain life (i.e., breathing and eating).

The disorders discussed in this chapter have a great impact on cost of health care and quality of life. More than 60% of all primary care visits for childhood illness and more than 50% of all adult primary care visits are for disorders of the ear, nose, and throat. Rhinosinusitis has the greatest financial impact to the economy of the United States through loss of job productivity and health care costs. The most common operation performed in the United States is placement of tympanic ventilation tubes.

THE EAR, THE VESTIBULAR SYSTEM, AND THE FACIAL NERVE

Anatomy

The ear is divided into the external, middle, and inner ear (Fig. 5-1). The external ear includes the auricle, which has a cartilaginous framework, and the external auditory canal, which is cartilaginous in one third of its lateral aspect and bony in two thirds of its medial aspect. The skin of the cartilaginous external canal contains hair follicles and the cerumen glands.

The middle ear is an air-containing space consisting of the eustachian tube, the tympanic membrane (ear drum), the middle ear cavity, the ossicular chain (malleus, incus, and stapes bones), the stapedius and tensor tympani muscles, and the mastoid sinuses (collections of air-containing sinusoids connecting to the middle ear cavity).

The inner ear consists of the cochlea, the semicircular canals, and the internal auditory canal. The inner ear is divided into the auditory and vestibular systems. These systems are composed of petrous bone, inside of which are tubular chambers that house delicate gelatinous and membranous structures submerged in fluid. Three types of sensory organ transducers are found in the inner ear: the organ of Corti (Fig. 5-2), located in the cochlea; the macula, located in the utricle and saccule; and the crista, located in the semicircular canals.

The internal auditory canal, located on the posteromedial aspect of the temporal bone, houses cranial nerves VII (innervates the muscles of facial expression) and VIII (innervates the vestibular and cochlear portions of the inner ear). It also houses the nervus intermedius, which carries taste fibers from the tongue and parasympathetic secretomotor fibers from the brain stem to the sublingual, submandibular, and mucosal glands of the nose and palate and to the lacrimal glands. The facial nerve, lying just superior to the auditory portion of the eighth nerve in the internal auditory canal, runs from the pons in the brain stem through the middle ear cavity and the mastoid, innervating the stapedius, postauricular, and digastric muscles. It emerges from the stylomastoid foramen and goes through the parotid gland to innervate the muscles of facial expression (Fig. 5-3).

Physiology

The adnexal and ceruminous structures of the outer portion of the external auditory canal produce a waxy material that serves as a lubricant for the skin, a trap for foreign particles, and a protective barrier against microorganisms. Accumulation of cerumen or deformities of the ear canal may obstruct the canal to sound and can cause ineffective clearance of cerumen. Too little cerumen can cause irritation, inflammation, and infection of the canal.

The eardrum and the ossicular chain are responsible for conducting and amplifying the vibration of sound waves from the external auditory canal to the inner ear through the oval window.

Under normal conditions, the air-containing space of

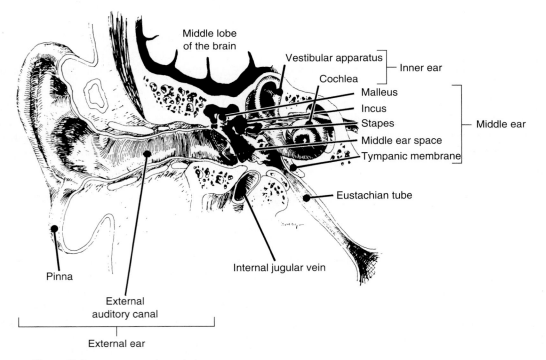

Figure 5-1   Cross section of the ear.

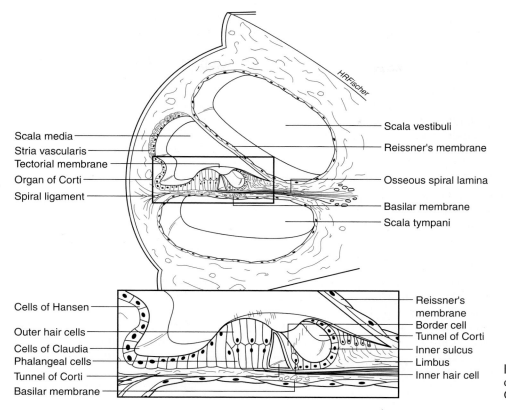

Scala media
Stria vascularis
Tectorial membrane
Organ of Corti
Spiral ligament

Scala vestibuli
Reissner's membrane
Osseous spiral lamina
Basilar membrane
Scala tympani

Cells of Hansen
Outer hair cells
Cells of Claudia
Phalangeal cells
Tunnel of Corti
Basilar membrane

Reissner's membrane
Border cell
Tunnel of Corti
Inner sulcus
Limbus
Inner hair cell

Figure 5-2   Cross section of the cochlea showing the organ of Corti.

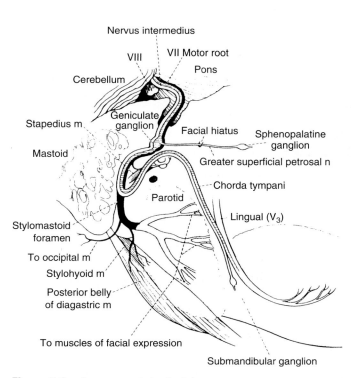

Nervus intermedius
VIII
VII Motor root
Pons
Cerebellum
Geniculate ganglion
Stapedius m
Facial hiatus
Sphenopalatine ganglion
Mastoid
Greater superficial petrosal n
Chorda tympani
Parotid
Lingual (V₃)
Stylomastoid foramen
To occipital m
Stylohyoid m
Posterior belly of diagastric m
To muscles of facial expression
Submandibular ganglion

Figure 5-3   Anatomy of the facial nerve.

the middle ear is periodically inflated when swallowing or chewing; this momentarily opens the eustachian tube, which is normally closed, and allows equalization of negative pressure. The eustachian tube opens by the synergistic action of the tensor veli palatini (innervated by the third division of the fifth cranial nerve) and levator veli palatini (innervated by vagus) muscles. Under these normal conditions, the compliance and resonance of the tympanic membrane and the ossicles are optimal for conduction of sound waves to the stapes footplate. Failure of the middle ear space to remain properly inflated with air may result in the accumulation of secretory fluids (effusion), affecting compliance of the tympanic membrane and the ossicles; this change in compliance may result in a conductive hearing loss.

The inner ear houses three sensory organs (organ of Corti, macula, and crista) that contain hair cell transducers responsible for converting mechanical energy (vibratory, rotational, gravitational) into electrical energy.

Vibratory energy (sound pressure), producing movement of the stapes footplate, causes the propagation of complex waves traveling through the inner ear fluid in the cochlea, which in turn causes the basilar membrane to move up and down. The movement of the basilar membrane with respect to the overlying gelatinous tectorial membrane causes a shearing action, bending the stereocilia at the apical ends of the hair cells. This mechanical deformation triggers electrical energy in the form of nerve impulses emanating from the hair cells. This energy is transmitted to the central nervous system (CNS) through the auditory nerve, ultimately producing the sensation of sound. Each wave has an area of maximum displacement that correlates with the fundamental frequency of the sound that produced it. Hair cells are organized along the basilar membrane so that displacement by waves near the stapes (base of the cochlea) result in high-frequency perception, and waves at the other end (apex) result in low-frequency perception. The basilar membrane is thus said to have a tonotopic organization (Fig. 5-4).

Rotational acceleration of the head (i.e., turning the head) is interpreted by the semicircular canals, whereas linear acceleration (i.e., walking in a straight line) is perceived by the macula of the utricle and saccule. Hair cells are the basic element that transduces the mechanical forces to nerve action potentials in both systems, but their complex organization is different. Energy caused by rotation of the head produces shifts in the fluid of the semicircular canal; these fluid shifts jiggle the gelatinous-like cupulae (within which hair cell cilia are embedded). These jiggles cause a temporary deformation of the cilia, resulting in stimulation of the hair cells (Fig. 5-5). Energy from gravity or changes in linear acceleration produces movement of the utricular stone-like otoconia, resulting in temporary deformation of the cilia-like projections of the hair cells. These mechanical deformations trigger electrical energy in the form of nerve impulses emanating from the hair cells. This energy is transmitted through the supe-

rior and inferior vestibular nerves, ultimately producing the sensation of either rotation or acceleration.

Vestibular input is but one of three systems (i.e., vestibular, ocular, proprioceptive) on which the body depends to maintain orientation in space. Under many circumstances one may be able to maintain relatively normal orientational function without simultaneous input from all three systems; however, denying visual input (eyes closed) or proprioceptive input (weightlessness) to vestibulopathic patients may significantly decrease a person's ability to orient.

Vertigo is an interesting sensory phenomenon associated with the important relation between the input of the left and right vestibular systems into the CNS. If vestibular input is not symmetrical, it will result in discordant output, manifesting as vertigo, which is akin to a sensation of whirling in space. Vertigo is a hallucination of motion when objective motion does not exist. Because of the vestibular-ocular tracts, this fictitious motion produces a number of saccadic ocular tracking motions irrespective of visual input, referred to as nystagmus. This type of asymmetrical input may occur whenever an insult occurs to one rather than both inner ears. However, with time, the vestibular system, unlike the auditory system, is frequently able to compensate for asymmetrical input.

The facial nerve is the motor nerve for muscles of facial expression. When nerve dysfunction exists, paralysis of these muscles occurs; however, depending on the site of the paralyzing lesion, other subtle dysfunction may also

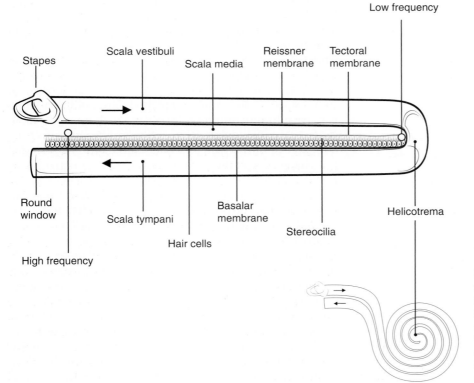

Figure 5-4 Schematic representation of the cochlea unwound. The *arrows* represent the initial fluid shifts as the stapes vibrates. Notice the tonotopic organization of hair cells. High-frequency sounds stimulate the hair cells near the stapes. Low-frequency sounds stimulate hair cells near the apex or helicotrema.

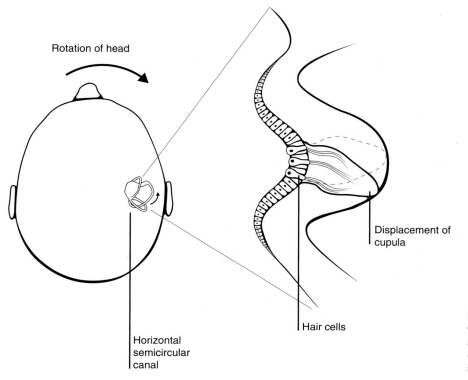

Rotation of head

Displacement of
cupula

Horizontal
semicircular
canal

Hair cells

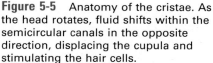

Figure 5-5   Anatomy of the cristae. As the head rotates, fluid shifts within the semicircular canals in the opposite direction, displacing the cupula and stimulating the hair cells.

be present, including loss of lacrimal secretions, contraction of the stapedial muscle, loss of submandibular or nasal secretions or both, loss of sensation in the floor of the mouth, and loss of gustation by the anterior tongue (Fig. 5-6).

If a facial nerve injury is severe, requiring significant regeneration, it is unlikely that normal anatomy will be reduplicated because certain nerve endings may not reinnervate the desired muscles. This aberrant reinnervation may cause very noticeable unintentional simultaneous contraction of multiple facial muscles (synkinesis) and mass movement during facial expression.

Physical Examination

Examination of the ear begins with observation of the auricle. The examiner looks at its shape and the condition of the skin and surrounding area.

The external auditory canal is examined by using an otoscope and the largest speculum that can fit in the ear. Pulling the pinna slightly away from the scalp makes the external canal straight and rigid for easier otoscope manipulation. The external auditory canal is observed for evidence of obstruction, otorrhea, or integumentary abnormality.

Cerumen should be carefully removed to allow adequate examination. A small amount of hard wax in the outer portion of the ear canal is best removed with a wire loop or a curette under direct vision through an otoscope. A large amount of soft wax is best removed by irrigation with warm water or peroxide if there is no perforation of the eardrum. Suctioning may also be used. Wax that is impacted against the tympanic membrane may need to be softened with peroxide drops or other over-the-counter, wax-dissolving agents (e.g., Debrox or Cerumenex) before irrigation or removal is attempted. Occasionally, the patient should be referred to an otolaryngologist for complete removal of the wax with special instruments under a microscope.

The tympanic membrane should be evaluated for deviation from its normal appearance of wax paper–like translucence (Fig. 5-7). In many ears, one can see portions of the ossicular chain (malleus, incus, stapes bones). The eardrum should be evaluated for thickness, opacification, inflammation, and abnormal deposits of materials (e.g., calcium). The presence of any unusually thin spots should be determined. Perforations larger than 1 mm are quite easily seen but are often mistaken for the retraction pocket commonly seen in the ears of patients with chronic dysfunction of the eustachian tube. The eardrum should also be observed for any evidence of middle ear fluid, which may cause a loss of translucency and a speckled light reflex on the eardrum, or may appear as air–fluid levels with bubbles in the middle air space. A pneumatic otoscope with a speculum large enough to completely occlude the ear canal is used to apply negative and positive pressure to the tympanic membrane to determine its freedom of movement, thus evaluating middle ear compliance.

During the course of the history and physical examination, the patient's hearing can be grossly assessed by determining whether the patient is able to understand normal

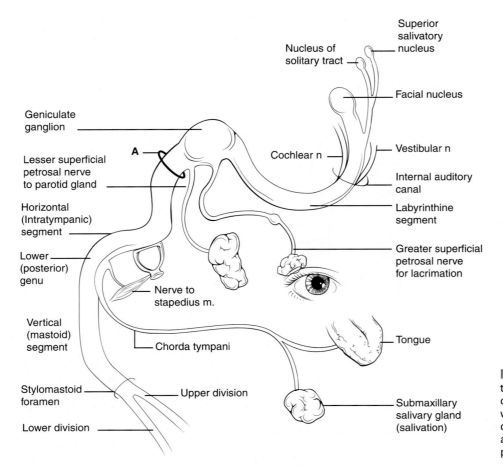

Figure 5-6   Schematic diagram of the facial nerve. Notice how damage to the nerve at site *A* would result in loss of function distal to the lesion, but lacrimation and parotid salivation would be preserved.

conversational speech, which is at 55 decibels (dB) and involves frequencies from 500 to 3,000 Hertz (Hz).

In addition to a standard cranial nerve examination, patients with vestibular complaints should undergo further neurologic examination. The patient is observed for spontaneous or induced nystagmus with position changes. Because disorientation complaints may result from dysfunction of vestibular, ocular, or proprioceptive systems, Romberg testing attempts to "sort out" the cause by removing ocular influence. The Romberg test involves measur-

ing a patient's ability to remain oriented in a standing position with eyes closed. Cerebellar testing (finger to nose, alternating hand test) is also helpful.

Evaluation

Hearing Loss

Although mixed hearing losses exist, the most common hearing losses are fairly pure (i.e., either conductive or

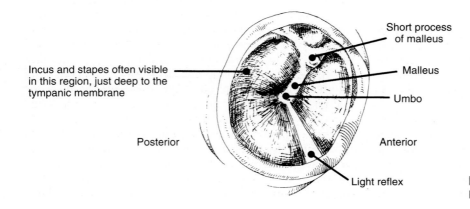

Figure 5-7   The tympanic membrane landmarks.

Table 5-1	Etiologies of Conductive and Sensorineural Hearing Loss

Conductive Hearing Loss	Sensorineural Hearing Loss
External auditory canal obstruction	Cochlear pathology
Cerumen impaction	Presbycusis
Swelling from severe external	Ototoxicity
otitis	Noise-induced hearing loss
Congenital stenosis or atresia	Ménière's disease
Acquired stenosis	Temporal bone trauma
Neoplasm	Meningitis
Middle ear pathology	Viral labyrinthitis
Otitis media	Viral labyrinthitis
Tympanic perforation	Retrocochlear pathology
Unclear etiology	Acoustic neuroma and other
Otosclerosis	inner-ear or skull-base
Ossicular trauma	neoplasms
	Sudden sensorineural hearing
	loss

sensorineural). Making this distinction and determining whether both ears are symmetrically affected are very important in simplifying the differential diagnosis. Table 5-1 categorizes some of the causes of hearing loss as they relate to the inner, middle, or outer ear.

As the term *conductive hearing loss* suggests, patients with this loss have inadequate means of properly conducting sound to the inner ear. This could be produced by any disorder related to the external auditory canal (occlusion), tympanic membrane (large perforation), middle ear space (effusion), or ossicles (disruption). This defect produces a loss of amplification, which may be described as "the volume being turned down too low." The patient with bilateral conductive hearing loss may actually hear better in the presence of background noise, such as at large social gatherings, because people with normal hearing must characteristically "turn up the volume" of their conversation in an effort to overcome the high volume of background noise generated by all of the competing conversations.

In contrast, however, the most common complaint of the patient with bilateral sensorineural hearing loss is difficulty hearing and understanding in large gatherings. Patients with sensorineural hearing loss generally have a distaste for loud music and loud conversation, which add further distortion and discomfort to their already ailing ears. Unilateral hearing loss commonly implies a local cause rather than a diffuse, systemic cause. The clinician must always be concerned about asymmetrical disease in symmetrical organs (i.e., the clinician should wonder if a lesion or neoplasm is responsible).

Tuning fork tests help the clinician differentiate between conductive and sensorineural hearing loss. These tests are most helpful when the hearing loss type is pure (conductive or sensorineural, not mixed) and unilateral. The Weber test is performed with a vibrating 512-Hz tuning fork, placed centrally on the forehead or on the maxil-

lary teeth. The patient is asked whether the sound is heard better in one ear or in the center of the head. If the patient hears the sound better in one ear, either a greater sensorineural hearing loss exists in the contralateral ear or a conductive loss is present in the ipsilateral ear. A conductive loss masks background sounds, resulting in enhanced body and skull sounds. With the Rinne test, the patient is asked to determine whether the tuning fork is heard louder when it is placed on the mastoid bone or when it is held approximately 2 cm from the external canal. A patient with normal hearing or with sensorineural hearing loss will hear the tuning fork better when it is placed adjacent to the ear canal. A patient with a significant conductive loss will hear the tuning fork better when it is placed on the mastoid bone, because air-conducted sounds are masked and skull sounds are enhanced.

Pure tone audiometry qualifies hearing loss according to frequencies, allocating and measuring the amount of loss according to sensorineural and conductive mechanisms. It does not assess speech recognition or discrimination. Pure tone audiometry is performed by presenting a series of variable-intensity tone pips ("beeps") via earphones at six or more frequencies (250, 500, 1,000, 2,000, 4,000, and 8,000 Hz), to which the patient volunteers a response. The threshold is the lowest intensity of stimulus that the patient is able to hear. The zero-dB line on the audiogram is considered normal, and the patient's hearing levels are recorded as dB above or below the zero-dB point along each of the six frequencies.

A hearing threshold of 0 to 20 dB represents normal hearing; 25 to 40 dB, a mild loss; 40 to 70 dB, a moderate loss; 70 to 90 dB, a severe loss; and greater than 90 dB, a profound loss. Sensorineural hearing loss is determined by obtaining bone conduction thresholds. The tone pips ("beeps") are delivered to the cochlea by placing a sound-generating device on the mastoid bone. This, in effect, bypasses the external and middle ear, thus giving a set of bone-conduction scores at each frequency for each ear. Conductive hearing loss thresholds are measured by first delivering the "beeps" through the air via earphones. Sound stimuli delivered in this way must traverse the outer, middle, and inner ear to be heard, thus giving a set of air-conducted scores for each ear. These air-conducted scores are then compared to bone-conducted scores (see above). If the scores match, no conductive hearing loss exists; if the air scores are worse than the bone scores (resulting in an "air–bone gap"), a conductive hearing loss equaling the size of the air–bone gap is present (Fig. 5-8).

The speech reception threshold probably correlates best with one of the most important communication skills: understanding spoken words. This test measures how loud the tester must speak to be understood by the patient. The speech discrimination evaluation, however, requires the patient to discern certain phonetically balanced words from other words (e.g., live, dog, love, girl, bath, dead, boy, die, ball, ride). This ability should be nearly perfect for people with normal hearing and for those with conductive

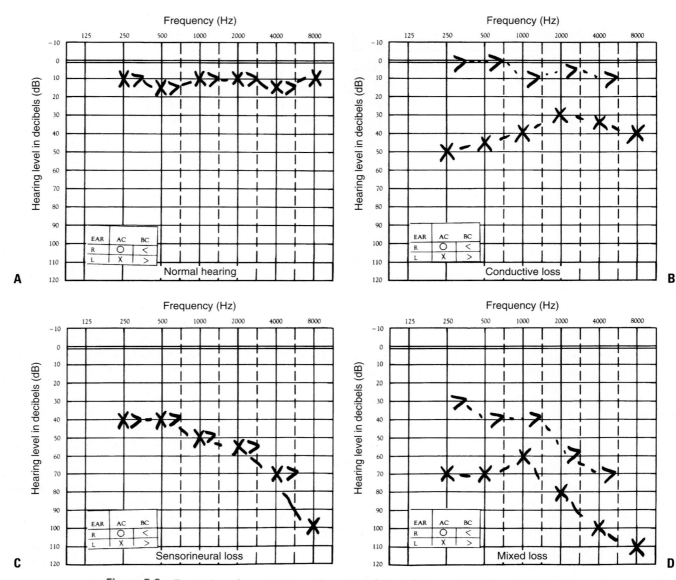

Figure 5-8 Examples of pure-tone audiograms of the left ear only. **A,** Normal hearing (normal air scores = normal bone scores). **B,** Conductive hearing loss (abnormal air scores and normal bone scores, indicating an air–bone gap). **C,** Sensorineural hearing loss (abnormal air scores = abnormal bone scores). **D,** Mixed or combined sensorineural and conductive hearing loss (abnormal air scores are worse than abnormal bone scores, indicating a conductive hearing loss [note air–bone gap] superimposed on a sensorineural hearing loss). Lower limits of normal hearing are about 20 dB.

hearing loss. Pathology of the cochlea, the auditory nerve, or the CNS, however, causes perceptual distortion and thus impairment in speech discrimination.

With electrophysiologic audiometry, the audiologist must interpret an involuntary or reflexive physiologic response. One of the most useful electrophysiologic tests, the **brain stem auditory evoked response (BAER) test,** also known as the **auditory brain stem response (ABR) test,** measures the electroencephalographic responses to sound stimuli. Another useful electrophysiologic test is the **evoked otoacoustic emissions (EOAE) test.** EOAEs are

sounds emitted by the cochlea in response to acoustic stimulation. The hearing of neonates, young children, and patients who are comatose, mentally retarded, or otherwise unreliable is assessed with these techniques, because no volitional response is required.

Tympanometry measures the function of the eardrum with a multichannel probe (containing a speaker, a microphone, and a transducer) that fits into the ear canal. The transducer produces pressure changes from 400 mm H_2O of negative pressure to 200 mm H_2O of positive pressure, while the speaker delivers low-frequency sound. The mi-

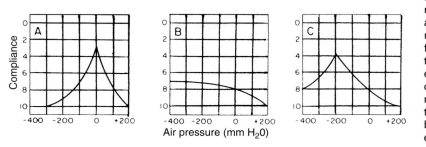

Figure 5-9 Typical patterns obtained with tympanometry. **A,** Peak efficiency occurs with no pressure manipulation. **B,** Often referred to as a flat tympanogram; peak efficiency is not realized at any tympanic position, suggesting fluid in the middle ear (effusion), perforation of the tympanic membrane, or occlusion of the external ear canal. **C,** Peak efficiency occurs only when the position of the tympanic membrane is manipulated outward, suggesting that its resting position is retracted, as would be seen with negative pressure in the middle ear space caused by poor aeration.

crophone senses the amount of sound energy reflected and records it on a tracing. Based on the configuration of the tympanogram, inferences can be made about the function of the middle ear, the presence or absence of fluid, and the presence of a perforation (Fig. 5-9).

Otalgia

Most causes of earache are easy to identify; however, because of the complex sensory innervation of the ear and the temporal bone, pain from many other sources may be referred to the ear and mistaken for ear pathology. In addition to the obvious examination of the ear, the upper aerodigestive tract should be examined because pain at this site is frequently referred to the ear. Queries about exacerbating factors may be helpful. Increased otalgia on chewing, a history of temporomandibular joint (TMJ) trauma, or recent dental work points to the myofascial structures of the TMJ. Tenderness in these areas may be confirmatory in the absence of other physical findings (Table 5-2).

Tinnitus

Tinnitus is "ringing" or some other perceived noise in the ears. It usually occurs in the absence of an objective acoustic stimulus from the outside environment. The very nature of the sound is key to making a diagnosis. Pulsatile tinnitus is usually vascular in origin. Cochlear injury produces a continuous noise that may vary in intensity with background noise or the time of day. Unilateral tinnitus infers pathology of the cochlear end-organ or its nerve, whereas bilateral tinnitus may be from a systemic toxicity or binaural injury. When the onset is acute, other signs of labyrinthine injury (e.g., vertigo, hearing loss, or facial weakness) should be sought. Patients with tinnitus need immediate attention because they may have a pathology that is reversible with early treatment (Table 5-3). Unfortunately, no medications have as yet proved effective in treating tinnitus.

Otorrhea

Drainage from the ear can be of many different consistencies. Thin, watery, yellow-to-clear fluid may be nothing more than bath water mixing with cerumen if the examination reveals normal ear structures. However, when trauma has occurred, a cerebrospinal fluid (CSF) fistula must be considered. A mucoid and purulent discharge from the ear implies infection. Carefully cleaning the ear may reveal a long-standing perforation, an acutely inflamed tympanic membrane and middle ear, or evidence of squamous debris and retraction consistent with otitis media. Bloody discharge may be part of an infectious process, but trauma and neoplasm must also be considered. High-resolution

Table 5-2	Causes of Otalgia
Otogenic	**Nonotogenic**
External ear	Orofacial pain
Otitis externa	Temporomandibular joint disorders
Herpes zoster oticus	Dental pathology
Neoplasm	Parotitis
Middle ear and mastoid	Elongated styloid process (Eagle's
Otitis media	syndrome
Mastoiditis	Visceral
Neoplasm	Pharyngotonsillitis
	Tumors of the hypopharynx, larynx, esophagus

Table 5-3	Disorders Associated with Tinnitus
Continuous	**Pulsatile**
Sensorineural hearing loss	Glomus tympanicum
Ménière's disease (usually unilateral)	Glomus jugulare
Acute noise exposure (e.g., rock concert, explosion)	Dural venous sinus fistula
	Intracerebral aneurysms
Systemic disease (e.g., diabetes, hypertension, thyroid disease)	Arteriovenous malformations
	Atherosclerotic disease
Ototoxicity (e.g., aminoglycosides, cisplatin, salicylates)	Hydrocephalus
Acoustic neuroma (unilateral)	
Viral labyrinthitis	
Bacterial labyrinthitis	

Table 5-4	Basic Differential Diagnosis of Vertigo	
Common	**Unusual**
Disequilibrium of aging	Viral or bacterial labyrinthitis
Vestibular neuronitis	Acoustic neuroma
Benign positional vertigo	Ototoxic or vestibulotoxic drugs
Benign brain stem ischemia	Degenerative neurologic disease
(vasospastic, embolic, and	(e.g., multiple sclerosis)
atherosclerotic)	Systemic disease (e.g., diabetes,
Ménière's disease	hypertension, autoimmune disease,
	thyroid disease)

computed tomography (CT) scans of the temporal bone will provide evidence of bony destruction; however, the usefulness of these scans is limited because the discharge will appear with the same density as soft-tissue defects (e.g., polyp, **cholesteatoma**, tumor).

Vertigo

Dizziness is a common symptom but is usually not otologic in origin. Spinning or whirling vertigo, on the other hand, such as is felt immediately after being spun around or with the nausea of motion sickness, should be distinguished from "light-headedness." Cardiac history, symptoms or findings of orthostatic hypotension, changes in blood pressure medications, or past history of cerebrovascular accident may point to decreased blood flow in the vertebrobasilar system. Complete neurologic examination may point to other CNS findings, especially those of cerebellar pathology. The presentations of these conditions may be identical to those of labyrinthine pathologies (Table 5-4).

Electronystagmography (ENG) takes advantage of the predictable saccadic eye movements (nystagmus) that accompany various types of stimulation of the semicircular canal. Periorbital electrodes are used to precisely sense and record nystagmus; cooling, warming, and head rotation techniques are used to stimulate the semicircular canals. The quantitated nystagmic response can thus be used to measure the integrity of the vestibular system.

Platform posturography alters a patient's visual and proprioceptive feedback to isolate the vestibular system's singular impact on the patient's orientation abilities. In this test, the patient is harnessed inside a chamber that systematically eliminates visual feedback, thus altering the patient's visual surroundings and proprioceptive feedback by eliminating platform stability.

Clinical Presentation, Diagnosis, and Treatment

Congenital Anomalies

During embryologic development, six small hillocks of cartilage (which arise from the first and second branchial arch) eventually fuse to form the pinna. Failure to complete proper embryologic development results in formation of cysts or sinus tracts in the pinna and the preauricular area. If these tracts become recurrently infected, they can be easily resected. More significant anomalies of the first branchial cleft and pouch may lead to marked deformities or absence of the auricle, the external auditory canal, and the middle or inner ear structures. The most important interventions are early audiometric assessment and early placement of hearing aids, preferably within the first year of life. Later, the series of surgical reconstructions of the pinna, the external ear canal, and perhaps the middle ear can begin.

Ear Trauma

Auricular hematoma is caused by a blunt shearing injury that separates the auricular cartilage from the perichondrium, creating a space in which blood and fluid can collect. This collection of fluid eventually forms scar tissue and results in a "cauliflower ear" deformity. This fluid must be evacuated and the skin must be compressed to the cartilage for several days to prevent its reaccumulation.

Frostbite and burns of the ear produce injury that is not fully manifested until days later. It is important to debride eschar conservatively, to keep all exposed cartilage moisturized, to avoid pressure on affected areas, and to control infection topically.

Perforations may develop from previous otitis media. Approximately 90% of traumatic tympanic perforations heal uneventfully. Those that do not heal spontaneously are usually large or have edges curled in such a way that regrowth will not occur. If healing is not evidenced within several months, a tympanoplasty using a temporalis fascia graft is indicated to close the perforation. This procedure is more successful in the absence of recurring otitis media.

Fractures of the base of the skull may traverse the temporal bone and damage the vestibular or auditory mechanisms or both. Classically, two types of fractures are described, depending on location of the fracture in relation to the petrous portion of the temporal bone (Table 5-5): longitudinal and transverse. Longitudinal fractures are far more common, resulting in about 85% of all temporal bone fractures (Fig. 5-10). Physical findings may include hemotympanum, otorrhea containing CSF and blood, hearing loss, and nystagmus. Rarely, a fracture may affect the cochlea or the facial nerve. Balance disturbances and varying degrees of hearing loss may be observed. Ossicular disruptions may need surgical repair. Significant sensorineural hearing loss rarely recovers, but the vestibular system can compensate over a period of months.

Otitis Externa

The skin of the auricle and the external auditory canal is subject to most of the common dermatologic diseases and to some that are unique to the external ear. The most common infectious disease is otitis externa, which can be localized or diffuse. Localized otitis externa (folliculitis

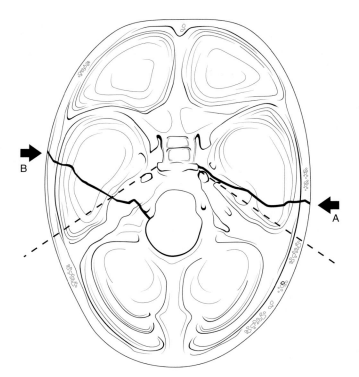

Figure 5-10 Classification of temporal bone fractures. *Dotted lines* represent the axis of the petrous portion of the temporal bone. Fracture **A** depicts a longitudinal fracture, whereas Fracture **B** represents a transverse fracture.

of the external auditory canal) may be caused by trauma (commonly from a fingernail or a hairpin). It produces pain out of proportion to findings on physical examination, which may range from a small red spot to a fluctuant swelling. The patient will complain of extreme pain when the ear is moved or the area is touched. Treatment involves antistaphylococcal antibiotics, drainage, or both.

The term *otitis externa* usually refers to a diffuse process that involves the entire external auditory canal. It is also known as swimmer's ear because moisture remaining in the external canal after swimming or showering may lead to this infection. Trauma to the delicate skin of the canal or exposure to purulent middle ear discharge through a perforation may initiate otitis externa. The most common causative agent is *Pseudomonas*, but *Klebsiella*, *Streptococcus*, and *Staphylococcus* are also frequently implicated. Fungus may appear, but usually as a secondary growth on desquamated epithelium. Findings range from minimal inflammation and tenderness to complete closure of the ear canal, with surrounding cellulitis and adenopathy.

Management involves removing debris from the external auditory canal so that topical ear solutions effective against *Pseudomonas*, *Staphylococcus*, *Candida*, and *Aspergillus* may reach the site of the infection. If the ear canal is so swollen that ear drops cannot be instilled, a small wick is placed into the external auditory canal. With the wick in place, the patient is instructed to use ear drops 2 to 4 times daily for several days. During the course of management, debris should be frequently removed from the patient's ear canal. If there is marked cellulitis or inflammation involving the auricle and the tissues around the ear, systemic antibiotics and steroids are generally effective. Some patients may require hospitalization for treatment with intravenous antibiotics. Pain is a very significant part of the complex of symptoms and narcotic analgesia is often required.

Necrotizing otitis externa, once called malignant otitis externa, is an osteomyelitis of the temporal bone and skull base. The most common offending organism is *Pseudomonas aeruginosa*, but *Proteus* and *Klebsiella* may also be involved. Mortality is high. Patients at risk are those with simple otitis externa who have diabetes or those whose immune system is compromised. The patient develops persistent inflammation of the external auditory canal, persistent pain, and granulation tissue in the ear canal, often with exposed bone and cranial nerve involvement. This infection does not respond to topical therapy. Aggressive treatment with topical and systemic antibiotics over several months is mandatory. Surgical debridement may be helpful in very early cases. To prevent this condition, patients not responding to routine treatment of otitis externa must be referred early to the otolaryngologist.

Foreign bodies in the external ear canal are unfortunately all too common among preschool children. Fortunately, foreign bodies in the ear do not usually represent an emergency unless the object is caustic. However, all

Table 5-5	Classification of Temporal Bone Fractures				
Fracture	**Force of Injury**	**Location of Fracture**	**Examination**	**Hearing Loss**	**Facial Nerve Paralysis**
Longitudinal	Blow to side of head	Parallels the long axis of the petrous bone	Disrupted ear canal skin and tympanic membrane Bloody otorrhea Bruising behind ear (Battle's sign)	Usually conductive	Infrequent (~15%)
Horizontal	Blow to front or back of head	Transects the long axis of the petrous bone	Vertigo common Intact tympanic membrane Hemotympanum	Usually sensorineural May be mixed if hemotympanum present	Common (~50%)

such foreign bodies, whether a soon-to-swell popcorn kernel, a bean, a toy bead, or a trinket, are somewhat difficult to remove. Children will usually allow physicians only one good try; if the attempt is unsuccessful, general anesthesia will almost certainly be required. In the meantime, the use of ear drops containing corticosteroids is prudent.

Otitis Media

Most of the infectious or inflammatory disease processes involving the middle ear space result from dysfunction of the eustachian tube. When the eustachian tube does not open frequently enough to allow equalization between the pressure in the middle ear and that of the atmosphere, a vacuum is created, and oxygen and nitrogen are absorbed into the mucous membranes of the middle ear and the mastoid air cell systems. The consequence is either increased capillary permeability and glandular activity with resultant middle ear effusion, or retraction of the tympanic membrane with possible adherence to the ossicles and the medial wall of the middle ear space. If infectious agents are present, the transudate forms an ideal culture medium, leading to otitis media.

Acute otitis media (AOM) is the most common infection for which antibacterial agents are prescribed for children in the United States. It is defined by a history of acute onset, the presence of middle-ear effusion, and signs and symptoms of middle-ear inflammation. By their second birthday, 75% percent of all children will have had at least three episodes of acute otitis media. The organisms that most commonly cause acute otitis media are *Streptococcus pneumoniae*, *Moraxella catarrhalis*, and *Haemophilus influenzae*. A typical history is onset of pain in one or both ears associated with behavioral changes, including crying, and often occurring in conjunction with an upper respiratory tract infection. Rarely, signs of meningeal irritation are present. Examination shows the eardrum to be red or opaque and possibly bulging, with a loss of normal landmarks secondary to an inflamed and often fluid-filled middle ear. Occasionally, infection results in a rupture of the tympanic membrane before a physician examines the child.

In 2004, the American Academy of Pediatrics (AAP) published updated guidelines for the management of AOM in an attempt to prevent unnecessary use of antibiotics, which can lead to bacterial resistance. If symptoms are not severe or diagnosis is unclear, initial observation only should be performed. The patients should be reevaluated in 48 to 72 hours. If antibiotics are used, then high-dose amoxicillin (90 mg/kg/day) should be used first. Azithromycin, clarithromycin, or erythromycin can be used if a penicillin allergy is present. After therapy is initiated, the pain usually resolves within 3 days and normal eustachian tube function usually returns in 2 weeks. If infection persists after 3 days of antibiotic therapy, then the antibacterial agent should be changed (high-dose amoxicillin–clavulanate). If this fails, a 3-day course of parenteral ceftriaxone should be used. Patients should be followed until the mid-

Table 5-6	Otitis Media: Indications for Urgent Myringotomy
Drainage and Culture	**Culture**
Otitis media with	Immunocompromised patient
Significant sepsis	Neonate
Severe unresponsive otalgia	
Severe unresponsive headache	
Severe unresponsive fever or	
picket fence fever	
Facial paralysis	
Labyrinthitis	
Meningitis	
Acute mastoiditis	

dle ear space is clear, because approximately 10% of children will have persistent effusions for more than 10 to 12 weeks. Some patients might develop recurrent AOM, which is characterized by recurrent episodes of infection despite multiple rounds of antibiotics. Patients who experience six episodes of AOM in a 6-month period are considered candidates for tympanostomy tube placement. This allows direct access to the middle ear space so that topical antibacterial drops may be administered.

Untreated acute otitis media can progress to acute mastoiditis, meningitis, brain abscess, facial nerve paralysis, and labyrinthitis. Drainage was standard therapy in the preantibiotic era; however, tympanocentesis is now infrequently indicated (Table 5-6). The procedure allows the infection to drain as well as material to be obtained for culture.

Otitis media with effusion (OME) is the second most common middle ear disease, with an estimated 2.2 million diagnoses annually in the United States. OME refers to fluid in the middle ear without signs or symptoms of an infection. Tympanometry is useful in its diagnosis. OME may occur spontaneously because of poor eustachian tube function or as an inflammatory response following AOM. The eustachian tubes of children are smaller and more horizontal in orientation than those of adults, thus restricting their ability to open. The function of the eustachian tube is impaired by edema of nasopharyngeal or eustachian tube mucosa caused by infection, allergy, tonsilloadenoidal hypertrophy, nasopharyngeal neoplasm, or cleft palate. Risk factors for OME are listed in Table 5-7.

Table 5-7	Risk Factors for Otitis Media with Effusion

1. Day care
2. Male gender
3. Recent upper respiratory tract infection
4. Bottle feeding
5. Cigarette smoke in the house
6. Increased number of siblings in the home

The AAP also published updated guidelines for the management of OME in 2004. It is a self-limiting disease and initial observation only is recommended unless hearing loss or speech deficit is suspected. Antibiotics, antihistamines, decongestants, and steroids have been shown to have no benefit. Seventy-five to 90% of cases resolve on their own by 3 months. If the eustachian tube does not begin to function, the persistent effusion may create a significant hearing loss. This type of hearing loss can result in language delay and possibly in a learning disability. If fluid persists for more than 3 months despite treatment, myringotomy with placement of middle ear ventilation tubes should be considered. Ventilation tubes allow the middle ear to aerate, reducing the accumulation of fluid and restoring normal conductive hearing. An incision is made in the tympanic membrane and a tube is placed within the incision to maintain this controlled tympanic membrane perforation.

Some patients with chronic dysfunction of the eustachian tube will experience chronic otitis media associated with a nonhealing, chronically inflamed, draining perforation of the tympanic membrane. The middle ear and mastoid mucosa also will be involved and over time may be associated with all of the destructive complications seen in acute otitis media. Treatment is surgical, usually consisting of a combination of tympanoplasty (repair of the ear drum) and mastoidectomy (opening the multiple mastoid air cells into one space).

Cholesteatoma

Cholesteatoma is a skin-lined, keratin-producing middle ear cyst that probably originates from a diseased tympanic membrane. Cholesteatoma tends to develop in a setting of chronic dysfunction of the eustachian tube and chronic negative pressure in the middle ear, resulting in chronic retraction of the tympanic membrane. This retraction produces a cystic, keratin-producing "pocket" of tympanic membrane. These fluid pockets are frequently infected and produce a foul otorrhea. Osteolytic enzymes in the basement membrane of the cholesteatoma produce osteonecrosis. The ossicular chain, the facial nerve, the cochlea, the semicircular canals, and the skull base may be infected and destroyed by this process. A patient with cholesteatoma commonly has chronic and recurrent infections with hearing loss. Facial nerve paralysis, vertigo, or intracranial abscesses may be seen. The pocket of whitish, cheese-like squamous debris inside the cyst may be seen, and the middle ear mucosa is inflamed and often edematous and polypoid, even protruding through a perforation. Surgical excision is necessary and may include a mastoidectomy and removal of the involved ossicles to prevent complications.

Otosclerosis

Otosclerosis is a spontaneous abnormality of the middle ear and occasionally the inner ear. This abnormality is most common in young adults, and it causes an acquired hearing loss. A small focus of spongy vascular bone involves a part or all of the stapes footplate. The result is fixation of the stapes footplate, with a conductive hearing loss. If the cochlea becomes involved, an additional sensorineural hearing loss is produced. Otosclerosis occurs among both men and women, has a genetic predisposition, and may accelerate during pregnancy. A hearing aid may be used to amplify sound for affected patients. Most patients, however, prefer surgical replacement of the fixed stapes footplate by a prosthesis. Infrequent complications include complete loss of hearing in the involved ear or severe postoperative dizziness.

Sensorineural Hearing Loss

Hearing loss affects 1 in 2,000 infants and may be either genetic (usually with a recessive mode of inheritance), developmental (anomalies affecting the temporal bone and the cochleovestibular apparatus), infectious in utero (cytomegalovirus, rubella, syphilis, herpes, toxoplasmosis), or associated with other perinatal factors (meningitis, severe jaundice, prematurity, hypoxia, ototoxic drugs). Early identification is imperative and rehabilitation through language interventions, hearing aids, cochlear implants, or other assistive listening devices may maximize the child's communication skills.

Acquired hearing losses may result from aging, noise exposure, exposure to ototoxicants, and disease processes of the ear and the CNS. Presbycusis, or the hearing loss of aging, results from degeneration of the cochlea. By the age of 80, 75% of people are affected. Exposure to noise in excess of 90 dB, especially if prolonged, may injure the cochlear hair cells, causing a localized loss in the mid- to high-frequency level of 3,000, 4,000, and 6,000 Hz. This loss may be caused by a sudden loud noise, such as a gunshot blast, or by prolonged exposure to industrial or recreational noise, such as factory noise or loud music. Patients should be counseled on the use of noise protection during such activities. Damage to cochlear and vestibular hair cells by toxic levels of aminoglycosides has been well described. Other medications that can cause cochlear dysfunction are cisplatin, vancomycin, loop diuretics, and antimalarial agents. Erythromycin and aspirin can cause a reversible sensorineural hearing loss. Patients will frequently complain of tinnitus and trouble hearing in the presence of background noise. Wearing hearing aids or assistive listening devices and optimizing the listening environment are usually helpful.

Vestibular Pathology

When the vestibular system is disrupted, problems ranging from imbalance to disabling vertigo are produced. As with sensorineural hearing loss, the causes vary.

Vestibular neuritis (previously incorrectly called viral labyrinthitis) is probably a viral inflammation involving the vestibular nerve or the vestibular neuroepithelium. The condition is characterized by the acute onset of severe vertigo, which lasts for a few days and gradually resolves

over several weeks. It may be preceded by a viral upper
respiratory tract condition. Treatment is supportive and
symptomatic, consisting of bed rest and drugs that suppress
vertigo (e.g., meclizine).

Like the cochlea, the vestibular apparatus is subject to
the degenerative process of aging. Patients with such dis-
equilibrium are elderly and somewhat frail; they usually
show evidence of sensorineural hearing loss (presbycusis)
and complain of vertigo induced by changing positions.
These patients should be advised to move carefully and
slowly; some labyrinthine sedation (e.g., meclizine, diazepam) may be prescribed.

Benign positional vertigo is an acute and rather severe
vertigo lasting only a few minutes. The vertigo is reproduced by specific positioning of the head. The condition
is believed to be caused by particulate matter in the endo-
lymph of one of the semicircular canals. The episodes will
subside after several months. Severe persistent disease may
respond to head positioning maneuvers or vestibular destructive procedures.

Ménière's disease, or endolymphatic hydrops, causes
episodic hearing loss, incapacitating vertigo lasting for several hours, tinnitus, and a sensation of aural fullness. This
disease is usually unilateral and is associated with bulging
or rupture of Reissner's membrane (Fig. 5-2) and mixing
of endolymphatic fluid with perilymphatic fluid; this mixture is toxic to vestibular and cochlear hair cells. Medical
treatment consists of a low-salt diet, diuretics, and, under
certain circumstances, allergy therapy. Surgical decompression of the endolymphatic sac or destruction of
the nerves of the inner ear or vestibule is reserved for incapacitating vertiginous symptoms that do not respond to
medical treatment.

Diseases of the Facial Nerve

Pathology in many different locations affects the functioning of the facial nerve because of its long circuitous course
(see Fig. 5-6). In general, the prognosis for recovery of
facial nerve function is good if the paralysis is incomplete
or caused by reversible infection or inflammation. The
prognosis is frequently poor if the paralysis is long-standing
or caused by cancer or trauma of the temporal bone. See
Table 5-8 for a listing of diagnoses.

The most common process producing paralysis is idiopathic or Bell's palsy. Viral infection of the nerve with
herpes simplex is supported by polymerase chain reaction
analysis. The paresis develops in a matter of hours and
may progress to complete paralysis, often with associated
mastoid pain, over a period of several days. Most cases
resolve spontaneously, but treatment with corticosteroids
and acyclovir is recommended. Persistent paralysis warrants imaging studies to rule out the presence of a tumor.

Other infectious or inflammatory diseases known to be
associated with facial paralysis include acute otitis media,
chronic otitis media, herpes zoster oticus, Lyme disease,
HIV infection, sarcoidosis, and Wegener's granulomatosis.
Treatment is generally medical and should be directed at

Table 5-8	Differential Diagnosis of Facial Paralysis
Inflammatory	**Other**
Infection	Tumors
Bell's palsy	Parotid cancer
Acute otitis media	Skull-base cancer
Chronic otitis media	Trauma
Herpes zoster oticus	Temporal bone fracture
Lyme disease	Facial or parotid laceration
Human immune deficiency	Cerebral ischemia
infection	
Inflammation	
Wegener's granulomatosis	
Sarcoidosis	

the underlying disorder. Facial paralysis caused by otitis
media should be treated with wide myringotomy and with
topical and systemic antibiotics.

Supranuclear lesions of the facial nerve, such as are
seen in cerebrovascular ischemia, will frequently spare
dysfunction of the upper facial nerve branches to the forehead because these branches are connected to both
crossed and uncrossed corticobulbar fibers.

Penetrating and blunt injuries involving the side of the
face, the ear, or the temporal bone may affect the facial
nerve. When the main trunk or one of the branches of
the nerve is involved, paralysis of the muscles supplied by
that portion of the nerve may be seen. Transection of the
nerve should be treated by reanastomosis or nerve grafting.

Facial paralysis significantly affects appearance; however, the most serious side effect is an ipsilateral exposure
keratitis caused by inability to close the upper eyelid. If
ignored, this keratitis may lead to corneal scarring and
marked impairment of vision. To protect the eye, the application of artificial tears, ointment, and tape (to keep the
eye closed while sleeping) is recommended. A tarsorrhaphy or the implantation of a gold weight in the upper
eyelid to allow better coverage of the cornea may be required.

Otolologic Neoplasms

Because the skin of the external ear receives as much exposure to ultraviolet light as skin on any other area of the
body, it is subject to the usual ultraviolet-light–induced
skin neoplasms. Actinic keratosis is the most common such
condition. Benign neoplasms unique to the external auditory canal are osteomas and exostoses. Exostoses present
as smooth, hard nodules, usually occurring multiply and
bilaterally. Osteomas are single and unilateral. If either of
these produces marked obstruction or prevents the ear
from cleaning itself naturally, surgical excision is indicated. Of the malignant lesions, squamous cell and basal
cell carcinomas, as well as malignant melanomas, are the

most common. Surgical excision is usually the best treatment, although radiation therapy may also be useful.

Neoplasms of the middle ear and the mastoid are extremely rare. Glomus tympanicum is a very vascular paraganglioma of the middle ear. It is histologically similar to glomus tumors of the carotid body, the vagus, and the jugular bulb. Patients classically complain of unilateral pulsatile tinnitus (Table 5-3) and hearing loss. A reddish tumor mass may be visible beneath an otherwise normal, translucent eardrum. Surgical excision is the best treatment.

Neoplasms of the inner ear are an unusual but important cause of unilateral sensorineural hearing loss. The most common tumor, acoustic neuroma, is a benign intracranial tumor of the eighth cranial nerve. The peripheral tissues in the CNS usually accommodate slow tumor expansion, giving rise to early ear symptoms and late central symptoms. As would be expected with a lesion of the eighth nerve, the hallmark symptom is unilateral sensorineural hearing loss with poor word discrimination, usually accompanied by tinnitus. Late symptoms are severe vertigo, facial nerve paralysis, and ataxia. Magnetic resonance imaging (MRI) is diagnostic, and surgical excision or stereotactic radiosurgery are the treatments of choice.

NOSE AND PARANASAL SINUSES

Anatomy

The external dorsal structures of the nose are formed by a bony and cartilaginous framework covered externally by skin and facial muscles. The upper one third, or bony vault, of the nose consists of the paired nasal bones supported by the frontal process of the maxilla and the nasal process of the frontal bone. The cartilaginous framework consists of the upper lateral cartilages, which are fused to the septal cartilage medially and the lower lateral (alar) cartilages (Fig. 5-11).

The nasal cavity extends from the anterior nares to the posterior choanae and is divided by the nasal septum into two chambers. The nasal valve, located in the anterior nasal cavity, is composed of the inferior turbinate erectile tissue, the septum, and the upper lateral cartilages. This is often the narrowest area of the adult upper airway. Common causes of nasal obstruction occur here, such as a deviated septum or enlarged turbinates due to allergies. The roof of the nose is formed by the cribriform plate of the ethmoid bone. The lateral wall of the nasal cavity is configured by three overhanging scroll-like bones. These turbinates subdivide the lateral nasal wall into a corresponding meatus or opening. Drainage from the nasolacrimal duct passes into the nose through the inferior meatus. The anterior ethmoid, maxillary, and frontal sinuses open into the middle meatus (Fig. 5-12). The region containing the anterior ethmoid sinus and the middle meatus is known as the **osteomeatal complex.** Obstruction here is a common cause for sinus congestion as the maxillary, anterior ethmoid, and frontal sinuses can all be affected. The posterior ethmoid cells drain into the superior meatus, and the sphenoid sinus opens into the sphenoethmoid recess, which is located immediately above and behind the superior turbinate.

Blood supply to the nose arises from both the external and the internal carotid artery systems (Fig. 5-13). The sphenopalatine artery, a branch of the internal maxillary artery from the external carotid, is the primary vessel to the internal nose. It supplies the posteroinferior septum and turbinates. The anterior and posterior ethmoid arteries, branches of the ophthalmic artery from the internal carotid, supply the ethmoid and frontal sinuses, the nasal roof, and the anterosuperior septum and turbinates. Kiesselbach's plexus, a highly vascular area on the anterior septum, receives its blood supply from both the internal and the external carotid artery systems and is the source for a vast majority of nosebleeds. Not unlike the skin, the turbinates contain erectile tissue composed of numerous arteriovenous shunts, referred to as capacitance vessels. Regulation of blood volume in these capacitance vessels in turn regulates nasal lumen and airflow resistance.

Venous drainage from the nose passes through the sphenopalatine, facial, and ethmoid veins. The nose and the sinuses communicate with the orbit and the cavernous sinus through the pterygoid venous plexus of valveless emissary veins and with the anterior cranial fossa via the valveless diploic veins of the posterior frontal sinus wall. The absence of valves in this area is important to remember because simple infections of the face, nose, and sinuses can result in direct hematologic spread to the orbit and CNS. The nose is innervated by the first, fifth, and seventh cranial nerves and by fibers from the sympathetic and parasympathetic systems.

Physiology

Besides serving as the organ of olfaction, the nose is an integral part of the respiratory system. The nose and the sinuses condition the air before it reaches the lungs. The

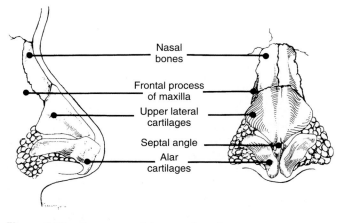

Figure 5-11   Anatomy of the nasal vault.

Nasal bones

Frontal process of maxilla

Upper lateral cartilages

Septal angle

Alar cartilages

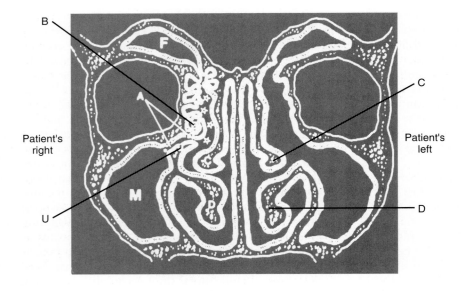

Figure 5-12 The anterior ethmoid sinus–middle meatus region (osteomeatal complex) in the coronal projection. On the patient's right, the middle meatus (*four stars*) receives drainage from the ethmoid bulla (*B*) and other anterior cells. Secretions from the frontal sinus (*F*) must pass through the ethmoidal regions, and maxillary sinus (*M*) secretions must pass through the ostium and the infundibulum (*A*) before reaching the middle meatus. The situation after functional endoscopic ethmoidectomy is shown on the patient's left. The uncinate process (*U*) has been removed, the anterior ethmoid cells opened, and the natural ostium of the maxillary sinus widened. The middle turbinate (*C*) is left intact. Also shown is the inferior turbinate (*D*).

optimal condition of inspired air is a temperature of 94°F, a humidity level of 80%, and a relative freedom from particulate matter. Achieving this condition requires the expenditure of an enormous amount of energy in the physical interaction of the air and the mucosal surfaces of the nose. This interaction disrupts laminar flow, creating large eddy currents in the air stream through the regulation of airflow resistance by the nasal valve. This disturbance ensures increased mixing and contact with respiratory mucosa, facilitating cleansing, humidification, and heating. Any inspired particulate matter is trapped on the mucous blanket overlying the nasal epithelium. The coordinated

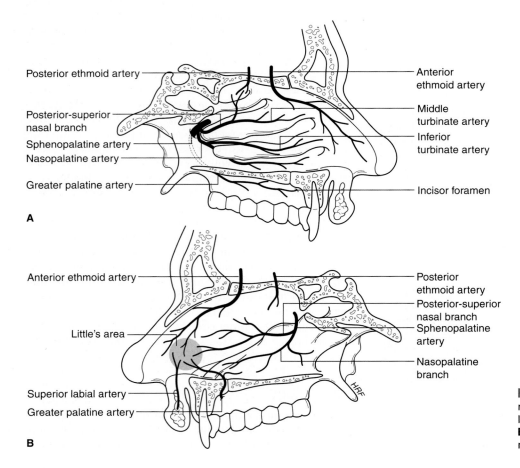

Figure 5-13 Blood supply to the nose. **A,** The arterial supply of the lateral wall of the internal nose. **B,** The arterial supply to the medial wall (septum) of the nose.

movement of the ciliated epithelial cells of the nasal mucosa transports secretions from the nose and the paranasal sinuses to the nasopharynx, where they are swallowed. Chronic contact between mucous membranes, as would occur with intranasal and sinus deformity and edema, disrupts mucociliary clearance, resulting in stasis of secretions with localized inflammation, facial pain and headache, and bacterial colonization.

Physical Examination

Physical examination of the nose begins with both inspection and palpation of the external dorsum. Any asymmetry or collapse (i.e., from trauma) can cause narrowing of the nasal valve with resultant nasal obstruction. Complete inspection of the nasal cavities is difficult without the use of a topical decongestant, a nasal speculum, and a good light, or other specialized instruments. The mucosa of the nasal cavity (septum and inferior and middle turbinates) should be inspected for signs of inflammation, telangiectasias, moisture, drainage, and lesions, including masses or polyps. Obstruction to airflow along the floor of the nose and to sinus mucociliary clearance more superiorly should be noted. Physical examination of the sinuses is also limited to inspection of the sinus ostia and to inspection and palpation of the overlying skin. The application of both flexible and rigid endoscopic instruments allows inspection of these concealed spaces and results in a more precise diagnosis of sinus disease.

Evaluation

Rhinorrhea

Liquid-like drainage from the nose should be classified as unilateral, hemorrhagic, mucoid, or purulent. Patients may have obvious anterior discharge; however, postnasal drip is quite common, producing a variety of symptoms, including dysphagia, asthma exacerbations, and sore throat. Thin, clear-to-white secretions often imply allergic, vasomotor, or viral-induced rhinitis. Unilateral clear drainage may come from a cerebrospinal fistula, warranting collection and analysis of the discharge. Purulent and foul-smelling discharge indicates bacterial infection. The specific site of infection may be the adenoid, the nose, or the sinuses. Nasal examination may demonstrate the discharge, especially in the region of the middle meatus; however, the absence of discharge does not rule out sinusitis. Radiographic imaging, especially coronal CT scans of the sinuses, visualizes areas hidden from endoscopic examination and displays anatomic variation that may predispose the patient to disease. This CT scan optimally evaluates the osteomeatal complex and can be a crucial reference during sinus surgery to safely treat the sinus disease.

Epistaxis

Bleeding from the nose most commonly occurs anteriorly from Kiesselbach's plexus on the nasal septum. Anterior bleeding can be controlled by spraying nasal decongestant spray to the affected side followed by firmly compressing the alar cartilages on both sides of the septum. Posterior epistaxis, more common in older adults, is often associated with arteriosclerotic cardiovascular disease, hypertension, and other systemic disorders; it requires more significant intervention, as explained in the paragraph on management below.

The most common cause of epistaxis is trauma. Bleeding may develop after digital or penetrating injury to the nasal mucosa or as the result of blunt trauma to the nose that produces secondary mucosal laceration. Septal deviations and perforations cause excessive air turbulence and drying and focal inflammation of nasal mucosa, increasing the potential for epistaxis. Acute or allergic rhinitis, especially among children, is another common cause of nasal bleeding. Intranasal foreign bodies, usually seen in pediatric or psychiatric patients, should be suspected if there is unilateral purulent discharge or bleeding. Hereditary hemorrhagic telangiectasia, an autosomal dominant disorder exhibiting arteriovenous malformations of aerodigestive tract mucosa, is characterized by fragility of the vascularity of the nasal mucosa, with recurrent nasal hemorrhage. Epistaxis can be an early symptom of paranasal sinus neoplasm. **Juvenile nasopharyngeal angiofibroma** is a highly vascular, benign tumor of adolescent males, with the classic symptoms of unilateral epistaxis and nasal obstruction. This tumor should always be considered in pubescent males with recurrent unilateral epistaxis.

Epistaxis may also be a sign of systemic disease. Defects in coagulation caused by anticoagulation therapy, blood dyscrasias, lymphoproliferative disorders, and immunodeficiency may cause nasal bleeding. Chronic systemic diseases predisposing patients to epistaxis include nutritional deficiencies, alcoholism, and hereditary hemorrhagic telangiectasia. Recurring or atypical epistaxis warrants a coagulopathy workup.

The initial management of epistaxis focuses on control of acute blood loss and airway relief if necessary. If the site of bleeding can be identified, it is cauterized electrically or chemically with silver nitrate. If the site cannot be identified, an anterior nasal pack is placed. Figure 5-14 demonstrates a classic anterior gauze pack; however, placement of expanding nasal tampons, sponges, or use of bioabsorbable hemostatic material may suffice for minor anterior nosebleeds. If a well-placed anterior pack fails to control bleeding (often demonstrated by continued bleeding into the pharynx) a posterior pack may be required. Posterior bleeding is often more profuse than anterior. A posterior pack seals the choanae and provides a bolster against which anterior packing can be placed to tamponade posterior nasal vessels. Foley catheters or gauze packing is seated in the nasopharynx, against the choanae with anterior traction, while a formal anterior pack is placed. Several manufactured posterior nasal pack balloons, which are easier to place and very effective, are available. Patients requiring posterior nasal packing need to be hospitalized so that they may be monitored for further bleeding, hypoxia caused

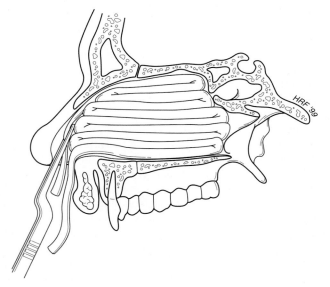

Figure 5-14 Formal anterior packing of the nose requires introduction of a continuous $\frac{1}{2}$-inch, ointment-coated, layered gauze to completely fill the nasal cavity.

by nasal reflexes, aspiration of blood, and for sedation if necessary. Further, these patients will require humidified oxygen, prophylactic antibiotics, narcotic analgesia, and bed rest.

If anterior and posterior packs fail to control bleeding, the arterial supply to the bleeding portion of the nose must be disrupted. The profound collateral blood supply of the nasal cavity demands ligation or embolization close to the bleeding site. Ligation of the anterior and posterior ethmoid arteries is indicated for superior epistaxis, whereas ligation or angiographic embolization of the internal maxillary artery is performed for posterior bleeding.

Nasal Congestion and Obstruction

Nasal pathologies associated with congestion, obstruction, stuffiness, or inability to clear, blow, or breathe through the nose are usually associated with obstruction along the floor of the nasal cavity. Shelf-like spurs along the base of the septum, deviation of the entire septum, and enlarged inferior turbinates or nasal masses are usually responsible. The turbinate swelling may be due to inflammatory pathology such as viral, bacterial, allergic, or vasomotor rhinitis. All intranasal masses deserve close attention to rule out neoplasm. Other entities in the differential diagnosis include nasal polyps, pyogenic granuloma, and hypertrophic or polypoid turbinates. Polyps are rarely unilateral; thus, unilateral polyps, especially in the presence of bleeding, increase the suspicion that the polyps represent neoplasm. Polypoid sinusitis is rare among children and should prompt a workup to rule out cystic fibrosis and immunodeficiency.

Clinical Presentation, Diagnosis, and Treatment

Acute Viral Rhinitis

Acute viral rhinitis, or the common cold, is the most common infectious disease of human beings and is most prevalent among children younger than 5 years of age. The viral infection produces desquamation of ciliated epithelial cells. Symptoms, which vary significantly in severity, include nasal stuffiness, rhinorrhea, sneezing, and airway obstruction. There may be associated cough, headache, temperature elevation, sore throat, and generalized malaise. Mucopurulent drainage replaces the initial mucoid secretions, and resident flora may cause secondary bacterial infection. The disorder is self-limited; regeneration of epithelium occurs by approximately the day 14, but return of ciliary function and relief of rhinitis symptoms may lag for several weeks.

Bacterial Rhinitis

Acute bacterial rhinitis is most commonly seen among children, but adults may also develop the condition after nasal trauma, viral upper respiratory tract infection, or surgery. The clinical presentation of acute bacterial rhinitis may be identical to that of the common cold. Causative organisms include *S. pneumoniae*, *H. influenzae*, and *Staphylococcus aureus*. Clinical signs that distinguish bacterial rhinitis from acute sinusitis may be subtle, and both conditions may occur in a patient whose defenses have been compromised by an intercurrent viral inflammatory process. An adherent gray membrane that bleeds on attempted removal may be found. Treatment with oral antibiotics may shorten the course of the disease.

Chronic bacterial inflammation of the nasal cavity is relatively uncommon, and the initial clinical manifestations of congestion, obstruction, and drainage are nonspecific. If these symptoms persist despite standard medical treatment, culture and biopsy should be considered to rule out infectious causes, such as tuberculosis, syphilis, rhinoscleroma (*Klebsiella rhinoscleromatis*), and leprosy. The clinician should also consider autoimmune diseases (e.g., Wegener's granulomatosis, lupus) and lymphoproliferative disorders (e.g., polymorphic reticulosis). Children with an indolent history of unilateral purulent nasal discharge with or without blood may be harboring a nasal foreign body.

Allergic Rhinitis

Allergic rhinitis is the most common allergic disease, affecting 20% of the population. It is a disease of the immune system, mediated by immunoglobulin E (IgE). Allergic rhinitis is caused by hypersensitivity to inhaled particulates (e.g., grass, ragweed, and tree pollens; animal dander; dust; mold spores). The disease most commonly affects children and young adults and is often associated with reactive lower respiratory tract disease. A positive family history is found in 50% of patients. Symptoms, which may be seasonal or perennial, include rhinorrhea, nasal obstruction, sneezing, and pruritus. Although pale-bluish, edematous mucosa is suggestive of the disease, no rhinoscopic findings are unique to allergic rhinitis. The results of skin tests, accomplished by injecting small amounts of extracts prepared from the culprit allergens, are usually positive, and elevated allergen-specific serum IgE levels are usually found.

Medical management begins with the identification and avoidance of offending allergens. If this measure fails to control symptoms adequately, pharmacotherapy with antihistamines, decongestants, and topical corticosteroid nasal sprays should be tried. Topical cromolyn sodium provides symptomatic relief by preventing the degranulation of mast cells.

Allergen immunotherapy should be considered to desensitize allergic patients whose symptoms are not controlled adequately with medication and avoidance measures. Immunotherapy is usually accomplished by injecting the patient with progressively larger amounts of allergenic extract, which stimulates T-suppressor cell regulation of IgE synthesis. This treatment is effective only for disease caused by IgE mechanisms and must usually be continued for several years.

Hormonal Rhinitis

Hormonal rhinitis (rhinitis of pregnancy) most commonly occurs in association with rising endogenous estrogen levels during pregnancy. Estrogens, which cause vascular engorgement of the nose, cause the nasal congestion and obstruction occurring in association with the immediate premenstrual period and with the use of oral contraceptives. Hormonal rhinitis may also be seen in hypothyroidism and is caused by extracellular edema.

Rhinitis Medicamentosa

Rhinitis medicamentosa is a drug-induced nasal inflammation, most commonly caused by the abuse of decongestant nasal sprays. Chronic use of these medications causes rebound congestion sooner and sooner after each use, because the chronic vascular embarrassment eventually forces the abuser to spray more and more frequently to counteract this rebound congestion. Although marked erythema of the mucosa may be seen, physical findings vary. *Management requires total withdrawal of topical decongestants and treatment of the underlying nasal disease that led to the use of intranasal drugs.* Oral steroids, steroid nasal sprays, and systemic decongestants help minimize withdrawal symptoms.

Mucociliary Dysfunction and Nasal Polyposis

The obstruction, congestion, and rhinorrhea so familiar to chronic sinus sufferers may be the result of mucociliary dysfunction, nasal polyposis, or both. Mucociliary dysfunction is a presently ill defined but probably a genetically related group of disorders that share the unfortunate char-

acteristic of dysfunctional sinonasal mucociliary transport. Kartagener's syndrome (immotile cilia syndrome) is a member of this group. Chronic smoke inhalation, viral rhinitis, chronic inflammatory disease, and trauma are some causes of acquired mucociliary dysfunction.

Nasal polyps (sinonasal polyposis), another example of the mucociliary dysfunction entities, are characteristically bilateral, multiple, translucent masses that arise from the osteomeatal complex and extend into the nose. Although the cause of polyps is not well understood, multiple factors are probably implicated, including chronic mucosal inflammation, injury, and obstruction. Nasal polyps are seen in the presence of reactive airway disease and asthma, aspirin hypersensitivity, cystic fibrosis, and chronic ethmoidal sinusitis. Initial management of nasal polyps can include both topical steroids and a short course of systemic steroids. Surgical excision of the polyps is reserved for those patients for whom steroids are contraindicated or ineffective in restoring adequate nasal airway. Recurrence is frequent; ethmoidectomy and the use of intranasal topical steroid sprays may help prolong time to recurrence of polyps.

Nasal and Septal Deformity

The nasal bones are the most frequently fractured bones in the body. In addition to causing bony injury, nasal trauma may result in displacement of the septum or the lateral cartilages. Clinical findings of nasal fracture include edema, ecchymosis, epistaxis, abnormal mobility, crepitus, dorsal asymmetry, or palpable bony deformity. The most frequent deformity is depression of one nasal bone and outward displacement of the contralateral bone, and it usually occurs after a lateral blow. Direct frontal blows may result in flattening and widening of the nasal dorsum. If the injury is severe, forces can be transmitted posteriorly to involve the ethmoid sinus, the medial orbital walls, and the cribriform plate, with resultant CSF rhinorrhea, hypertelorism (secondary to disruption of medial canthal tendons), and anosmia.

Evaluation of a patient with suspected nasal fracture must include inspection of the septum for hematoma. Septal hematoma is caused by the accumulation of blood between the cartilage and the overlying mucoperichondrium, effectively separating this cartilage from its blood supply. *Prompt drainage is required to prevent formation of an abscess and resorption of cartilage, which produces a saddle nose deformity.* Nondisplaced fractures of the nasal bones do not require reduction. Minimal deviations of the bony dorsum, with no appreciable septal displacement, are managed with closed reduction. More complex injuries and those associated with septal displacement require open reduction with repositioning of the septum to achieve satisfactory functional and cosmetic results.

Septal deviations are traumatic or congenital. Septal deviation may cause high-velocity, excessively turbulent airflow or chronic contact with the lateral nasal wall producing nasal obstruction, snoring, sleep apnea, epistaxis, facial pain, headache, or sinusitis. Intranasal septoplasty will correct the deformity.

Choanal Atresia

Persistence of the nasobuccal membrane during gestation results in incomplete opening of the posterior nasal cavity or choanae. Resultant choanal atresia may be unilateral or bilateral. Because the newborn is an obligate nasal breather, bilateral **choanal atresia** is a medical emergency. Diagnosis is suspected when a newborn's initial feedings result in progressive obstruction, cyanosis, choking, and aspiration. *The airway obstruction is temporarily relieved by crying, since that is the only time the neonate inhales through the mouth.* An inability to pass a small catheter through the nose and into the nasopharynx suggests this diagnosis. Immediate treatment includes stenting with an oral airway or endotracheal intubation. The infant should also be evaluated for other craniofacial and upper aerodigestive anomalies (e.g., cleft palate, subglottic stenosis, craniofacial synostosis, tracheoesophageal fistula) because these anomalies often cluster together. Surgical opening of the choanae with prolonged stenting is required for correction.

Acute Sinusitis

Acute sinusitis most frequently develops as a complication of a viral upper respiratory tract infection (i.e., the common cold). The symptoms of periorbital tenderness, facial pain, headache, fever, and purulent nasal discharge usually indicate involvement of the sinuses. Acute sinusitis is caused by ostial closure as the result of inflammatory edema from viral upper respiratory tract infection or allergies. The resultant stasis of secretions leads to infection with bacteria. Common causative organisms in acute sinusitis are *S. pneumoniae*, *H. influenzae*, and *Moraxella catarrhalis*. The diagnosis is usually established based on clinical findings of mucopurulent nasal drainage, inflamed turbinates, pain over the anterior face, and fever.

Medical therapy is begun empirically in the uncomplicated case. A 7- to 14-day course of amoxicillin–clavulanate, cefprozil, cefuroxime, clarithromycin, or loracarbef and a short course of topical decongestants are recommended. Supportive measures include systemic decongestants, saline nasal sprays, expectorants, humidification, warm compresses, and analgesics.

Surgical treatment is indicated for acute sinusitis if the response to adequate medical therapy is poor or in the presence of a high risk for extranasal complications of sinusitis, such as orbital infection, meningitis, intracranial sinus thrombosis, and facial cellulitis. The maxillary sinus is aspirated and irrigated through a trocar that is punctured into the sinus. Aspiration and drainage of the frontal sinus is performed through an incision in the medial supraorbital region. Ethmoidal drainage can usually be accomplished through an intranasal approach.

Chronic Sinusitis

Chronic sinusitis is one of the most common health care complaints in the United States. It results when mucosal contact disrupts mucociliary clearance or forces closure of the sinus ostium, as shown in Figure 5-15. The resulting accumulation of secretions may cause chronic inflammation, ciliary injury, hyperplasia of seromucinous glands, and increasingly viscous mucus. Sinus hypoventilation interferes with local defense mechanisms and may lead to anaerobic infection. The region of the anterior ethmoid sinus and middle meatus (osteomeatal complex) is the site of 90% of inflammatory sinus disease. Because both the maxillary and the frontal sinus ostia open into the osteomeatal complex, these sinuses may be secondarily inflamed by disease in the anterior ethmoid sinuses.

Although the symptoms of chronic sinus disease vary, most patients note a sensation of obstruction, facial pressure, or pain. The pain is often referred to areas supplied by the ophthalmic or maxillary division of the trigeminal nerve and is characterized as dull, deep, and nonpulsatile.

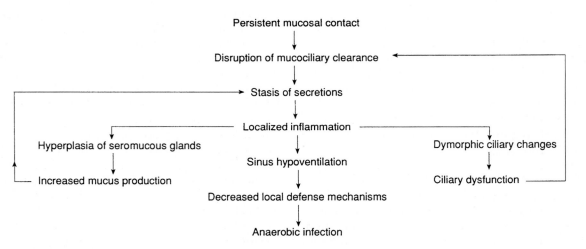

Figure 5-15 Pathophysiology of chronic sinusitis.

The clinical picture in chronic sinus disease may be dominated by nonspecific symptoms such as congestion, discharge, headache, aural pressure, sore throat, cough, generalized fatigue, and dizziness. Causes include ciliary dysfunction, immune deficiency, and nasal allergy. Structural variations that interfere with ventilation or mucociliary clearance in the osteomeatal complex also will produce chronic sinus disease.

The goals of medical therapy are to treat infection, to improve mucociliary clearance, and to maintain patency of sinus ostia. Antimicrobial treatment of chronic sinusitis is indicated in the presence of coexistent acute inflammation and for patients who have not received a prolonged course of a β-lactamase–resistant antibiotic. Topical intranasal steroid sprays are important adjuncts to antibiotic therapy because of their anti-inflammatory effect, which helps restore ostial patency and relieves chronic symptoms. Saline nasal sprays, expectorants, smoking cessation, and increased fluid intake enhance mucociliary clearance by reducing the viscosity of mucus.

Surgical treatment of chronic sinus disease focuses on the pivotal role of the osteomeatal complex in the pathophysiology of disease. When a rigid endoscope is used for improved visualization, the important ostia in the anterior ethmoid region are opened to establish normal ventilation and mucociliary clearance (Fig. 5-12). By restoring the normal physiologic function of the osteomeatal complex, ethmoidectomy may allow the clearance of secondary disease in the frontal or maxillary sinuses.

Nasal and Sinus Mycotic Infections

Fungal infections involving the nose and paranasal sinuses are usually caused by the opportunistic organisms *Phycomycetes (Mucor, Rhizopus)* and *Aspergillus*. These normally innocuous organisms produce fulminant, invasive, frequently lethal disease among immunocompromised patients. One should maintain a high clinical suspicion in this subset of patients because this disease can invade rapidly to involve the orbit or CNS. Characteristic clinical signs are nasal pain, bloody nasal discharge, and black, necrotic turbinates. Diagnosis depends on histologic identification of invasive fungus in biopsy specimens; nasal smears are inadequate for diagnosis. Treatment requires radical surgical debridement of all involved tissues and therapy with high-dose antifungal therapy.

Nasal and Sinus Neoplasms

Benign neoplasms of the sinonasal tract are treated with simple excision, in most cases for cure. Squamous papilloma is a wart-like benign neoplasm occurring at the mucocutaneous junction of the nasal vestibule. Osteoma is the most common tumor involving the paranasal sinuses. It arises in the frontoethmoid region and is often an incidental finding of sinus radiographs. If the osteoma is asymptomatic, annual radiographs are sufficient to track its growth. Progressively growing osteomas are removed surgically. Although histologically benign, inverting papillomas are locally invasive, and 10% to 15% may have foci of squamous cell carcinoma. For this reason, wide local excision is preferred. Juvenile nasopharyngeal angiofibroma arises in the pterygomaxillary fossa and presents as a unilateral nasal mass among adolescent boys, causing epistaxis and nasal obstruction. Diagnosis is clinical and radiographic because hemorrhage from biopsy may be hazardous. Hemorrhage after surgical excision is reduced by preoperative embolization.

Malignant neoplasms of the nose and sinus represent fewer than 1% of cancers. Bony destruction shown by CT scan is highly suggestive of malignancy; MRI scan distinguishes secondary inflammatory sinus disease from primary malignancy. Diagnosis depends on biopsy and histologic study. Epithelial neoplasms, such as squamous cell carcinoma, adenocarcinoma, and salivary malignancies, are predominant in this rare group of tumors and are optimally treated with wide local excision combined with irradiation. The structures of the orbit, maxilla, and anterior fossa will be affected to some extent by the treatment of these lesions. Local recurrence is the most common cause of treatment failure. Olfactory neuroblastoma (esthesioneuroblastoma) metastasizes frequently and responds best to chemotherapy, surgery, and radiation therapy. Rhabdomyosarcoma, a tumor of striated muscle, is the most common intranasal cancer among children. Advances in chemotherapy and radiation therapy techniques have reduced the role of surgery to a diagnostic procedure in most cases.

THE ORAL CAVITY AND PHARYNX

Anatomy

The oral cavity consists of the space posterior to the lips and anterior to the tonsils and soft palate (Fig. 5-16). The vestibule is a space bounded by the lips anteriorly and by the cheeks, the gingiva, and the teeth posteriorly. The oral cavity is bounded anteriorly and laterally by the alveolar arches, superiorly by the hard and soft palates, and inferiorly by the tongue. The tongue is the predominant organ of the mouth and plays an integral role in chewing and swallowing food. It is an essential organ of speech because its complex movements determine articulation. Its movements are controlled by paired extrinsic and intrinsic muscles, all of which are innervated by the hypoglossal nerve. Sensory innervation is supplied by both special visceral and general somatic nerves. The sensation of taste is transmitted from the anterior two thirds of the tongue by the lingual nerve to the chorda tympani branch of the facial nerve. The lingual branch of the glossopharyngeal nerve carries special visceral afferent nerves from the posterior one third of the tongue. General sensation is through branches of the fifth, ninth, and tenth cranial nerves.

Saliva is produced by a set of six paired major glands and by more than 100 minor salivary glands. Most saliva is produced in parotid, submandibular, and sublingual

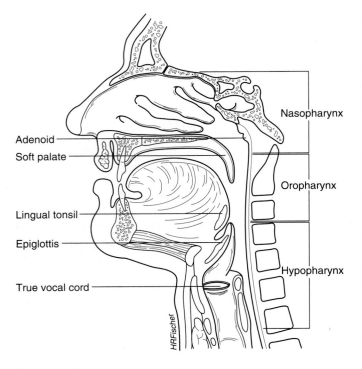

Figure 5-16   Sagittal view of the pharynx.

major salivary glands and flows through ducts into the oral cavity. The minor salivary glands empty directly into the oral cavity and are located in the palate, the lips, the tongue, the tonsils, and the buccal mucosa. The oral cavity ends at the fauces, the archway composed of the posterior soft palate and the glossal palatine folds.

The pharynx lies posterior to the nasal cavity, the mouth, and the larynx (Fig. 5-16). The three major muscles of the pharynx are the superior, middle, and inferior constrictor muscles, which play important roles in the process of swallowing. The nasopharynx lies above the level of the soft palate and communicates with the nasal cavity through the choanae. Opening into the lateral walls of the nasopharynx are the eustachian tubes, which allow aeration of the middle ear through the opening action of the tensor veli palatini muscles. On the posterior wall lies the adenoidal tissue.

The oropharynx extends from the level of the hyoid bone to the soft palate. It opens anteriorly into the oral cavity and contains the palatine tonsils laterally. The hypopharynx reaches from the hyoid bone to the lower border of the cricoid cartilage, where it narrows to become continuous with the esophagus. It communicates anteriorly with the larynx. Immediately lateral to the larynx are mucosal recesses called the pyriform sinuses that lead inferiorly around the larynx to the esophageal introitus.

Physiology

The oral cavity and pharynx play important roles in breathing, mastication, swallowing, and articulation of speech.

Each of these functions requires motor and sensory information for optimal performance.

Swallowing is divided into four phases. The first is the preparatory phase, in which a food bolus is crushed, macerated, and mixed with saliva. This preparation ensures an optimal consistency for passage to the stomach. In the second phase, voluntary control of the tongue sweeps the bolus posteriorly against the soft palate into the oropharynx. When the bolus traverses the fauces, the third phase, which is controlled involuntarily, begins. The larynx elevates, opening the pyriform sinuses. The epiglottis moves over the larynx, acting as a keel to direct food into the pyriform sinuses. The pharyngeal constrictors function as the soft palate elevates to seal the nose from the oral cavity. These movements drive the bolus to the esophageal introitus, which opens by relaxing the cricopharyngeal muscle. In the fourth phase, the esophagus drives the bolus to the stomach with stripping peristaltic waves. Dyscoordination, lack of sensory feedback, or other anatomic derangement will lead to dysphagia, aspiration, or both.

The tongue, palate, and lips are key structures in shaping the sounds produced in the larynx into intelligible speech. Anatomic or neurologic dysfunction of these organs produces dysarthria.

Physical Examination

Physical examination of the oral cavity and pharynx is facilitated by ample lighting and the use of tongue blades for retraction of the cheeks and tongue. Congenital, inflammatory, or neoplastic abnormalities should be sought. Complete inspection includes full examination of the buccal mucosal recesses, the palate, the floor of mouth, and the dental alveolar structures. The standard instruction, "Open your mouth and say ahh," is always inadequate for a comprehensive examination, but does allow evaluation for asymmetrical palatal elevation, which could indicate cranial nerve weakness. Most areas of the pharynx can be inspected with direct vision, mirrors, or fiberoptic endoscopes. Digital palpation of the oral cavity is mandatory because many lesions may be difficult or impossible to visualize. Lesions of the oral cavity and the oropharynx may be submucosal or may have a surface that blends into the irregular normal surface of the tongue or tonsil. Palpation of the induration they produce will aid in their detection.

Evaluation

Sore Throat

Chronicity, concurrent systemic symptoms, patient age, and physical examination will help narrow the wide differential diagnosis. Sore throat for less than a week implies infection, whereas neoplasms usually cause symptoms for much longer periods. The presence of fever and malaise suggests infection, and weight loss over the months before treatment is sought raises the possibility of malignancy.

Careful inspection and palpation of the entire oral cavity and pharynx may reveal a lesion. The innervation of the pharynx is variable and it is often difficult for the patient to localize pain. Reproducing the patient's pain by palpation locates the site of pathology.

Snoring and Sleep Disturbance

Patients with disordered sleep may present with chronic fatigue, daytime somnolence, or right-sided heart failure. Snoring occurs more commonly as a person ages and is not pathologic in the adult. Children should not snore. More importantly, the physician must elicit any history of apnea (i.e., cessation of breathing) during sleep. Complete examination of the upper airway is mandatory. Any significant obstruction is exacerbated during sleep, when the resting tone of the upper airway is reduced.

Dysphagia

Patients with trouble swallowing describe many different sensations. It is crucial to determine whether the dysphagia represents a mechanical obstruction or a neurologic coordination problem. Dysphagia for solids only, or a progressive dysphagia that began with solids and progresses to include liquids, implies mechanical blockage. Chronic odynophagia (painful swallowing) associated with this type of dysphagia indicates a possible malignancy. Patients with this condition require laryngoscopy and esophagoscopy for evaluation and possible biopsy. Transnasal esophagoscopy is a new visualization technique that allows evaluation of the esophagus and stomach in clinic without the need for general anesthesia or sedation. Barium swallow also provides useful anatomic information about larger lesions. Patients may describe choking, especially with liquids, representing a loss of bolus control present in neurologic problems (central as well as peripheral). The modified barium swallow will define the functional movement of the upper aerodigestive tract in swallowing. Some patients may have little difficulty swallowing, yet may complain of having "something stuck" in their throats. Physical examination of these patients often reveals no significant findings; in this case, other causes of pharyngeal irritation, such as gastroesophageal reflux, postnasal drip, and inhaled irritants, must be sought. Treating these conditions may help relieve the symptom. Undiagnosed, long-standing dysphagia requires at least a barium swallow to rule out significant pathology.

Clinical Presentation, Diagnosis, and Treatment

Acute and Chronic Pharyngitis or Stomatitis

Inflammatory diseases of the oral cavity and the pharynx are common and are frequently viral in origin. Viral upper respiratory tract infections may produce lesions of the pharynx, the oral cavity, or both. These lesions range from diffuse inflammation to vesicular eruptions. Various viruses, including parainfluenza, adenovirus, influenza, and Epstein-Barr, have been identified in pharyngotonsillitis. The Epstein-Barr virus has been identified as the cause of mononucleosis, and systemic involvement may also include the liver and the spleen. Occasionally, aseptic meningitis also occurs. Viral pharyngitis or stomatitis is self-limiting and requires only symptomatic treatment. Herpes virus type 1 may cause a painful, recurring, blistering infection that responds to early antiviral therapy. Aphthous ulceration is common in the oral cavity. Aphthous ulcers are single or multiple, shallow, painful ulcers presenting without other disease. When these lesions are recurrent or severe, topical steroids may shorten the course of the disease.

Inflammation of the oral cavity and pharynx can also occur with the ingestion of caustic materials, such as acid or alkali. Alkaline ingestion causes liquefaction necrosis, which usually results in more severe damage to the esophagus, whereas acidic ingestion causes a coagulation necrosis. It is important to remember that the severity of external and oropharyngeal damage may not correlate with the extent of esophageal or gastric injury. A seemingly benign oral examination may mask a more severe distal injury. If severe, the resulting mucosal necrosis can result in pharyngeal or esophageal perforation and airway obstruction caused by mucosal edema. Long-term strictures can require years of dilation or significant reconstructive surgery.

The most common fungal infection of the oral cavity is moniliasis or thrush, caused by *Candida albicans*. This infection is common in the neonate or in the adult during or following a course of systemic antibiotics. It is also seen in patients with a compromised immune system. Thrush responds to topical therapy with agents such as miconazole or nystatin, although more severe or recalcitrant infections may require systemic antifungal agents (e.g., ketoconazole or fluconazole).

Streptococcal pharyngitis occurs more commonly in patients older than 2 years of age. The infection is caused by α-hemolytic streptococcus, which can be cultured from the exudate of the tonsils and the pharynx. It is characterized by fever, malaise, cervical adenopathy, and exudative tonsillitis. Penicillin, administered intramuscularly or orally, provides adequate treatment against the organism. However, if the infection recurs frequently, removal of the tonsils is necessary to eradicate the disease.

Bacterial infections of the tonsils can be caused by various organisms, including anaerobes. Patients whose infections do not respond to penicillin may have resistant bacteria and may require a different antibiotic. Chronic or repeated acute bacterial tonsillitis may require tonsillectomy. Occasionally, the tonsillitis spreads to the peritonsillar region, resulting in peritonsillar abscess, peritonsillitis, or necrotizing tonsillitis. In most cases, these infections respond to systemic antibiotics, but peritonsillar abscess usually requires aspiration or surgical drainage. Peritonsillar abscess is characterized by asymmetry of the tonsils and swelling of the soft palate, resulting in uvular deviation away from the affected side. Patients often complain of inability to swallow and speak with a muffled tone referred to as "hot potato voice."

Adenoidal tissue can also be infected, producing recurrent purulent nasal discharge and obstruction of the nose. If the obstruction does not respond to antibiotic therapy or is recurrent, adenoidectomy is indicated. Young patients with recurrent tonsillitis have infection of the adenoidal tissue as well. For this reason, children usually undergo simultaneous tonsillectomy and adenoidectomy. Because the adenoid may contribute to recurrent otitis media, adenoidectomy will decrease recurring otitis in some cases. Table 5-9 summarizes current indications for tonsillectomy.

Congenital Anomalies

The more common congenital disorders of the oral cavity include ankyloglossia, in which the tongue is bound to the mandible because of a shortened frenulum; cleft lip, cleft palate, or both; supernumerary teeth; micrognathia; cysts of the alveolar ridge or palate; lingual thyroid; and hemangiomata. If the lesions neither obstruct the airway nor interfere with swallowing, most congenital defects can be corrected surgically when the child is older.

In addition to the esthetic consequences, cleft lip also impairs the child's ability to form an oral seal for suckling. Surgical correction is begun during the first months of life. The rule of 10s is loosely applied to timing a cleft lip repair (when the child is >10 weeks old, weighs >10 lb, and has Hgb >10.) Children with cleft palates due to the inability to constrict the velopharynx have no means of separating oral from nasal airflow or of controlling oral contents or pressure (i.e., velopharyngeal incompetence). They are incapable of normal speech articulation, and they often experience reflux of foods into the nasal cavity when eating. In addition, they have decreased swallowing pressures, preventing them from propelling boluses of food posteriorly and inferiorly. Further, patients with clefts involving the soft palate routinely have chronic middle ear effusions because the palatal musculature is reoriented, causing impaired opening of the eustachian tube. Cleft palate closure is performed before 2 years of age to allow for more normal speech development. Ventilation tubes are usually inserted into the tympanic membranes to treat recurrent otitis media with effusion. (Cleft lip and cleft palate are further discussed in Chapter 3.)

Children with Pierre Robin syndrome (characterized by mandibular hypoplasia, glossoptosis or ptotic tongue, and cleft palate) are at risk for airway obstruction caused by posterior displacement of the tongue. Infants with this problem have no mandibular support for the tongue and experience choking and aspiration during feeding. Special bottles, surgical fixation of the tongue, and tracheostomy may be necessary to treat more severe cases.

Obstructive Sleep Apnea and Snoring

Obstructive sleep apnea, characterized by recurring periods of apnea during sleep and associated with respiratory efforts, is caused by a central loss of muscle tone, causing the upper airway to collapse during the negative pressure of inspiratory flow. During periods of sleep apnea, the respiratory pattern is disrupted and oxygen saturation drops. Although many treatments aim at reducing anatomic airway obstruction, this obstruction occurs only during sleep.

Obstructive sleep apnea is most common in obese adults, especially those with nasal airway obstruction. In children, body habitus is usually normal and hypertrophied adenoids and tonsils are present. Neuromuscular diseases and craniofacial anomalies may also lead to the condition. Snoring at night and mouth breathing are common characteristics of patients with this condition. Long-term systemic problems include cor pulmonale (right-sided heart failure secondary to chronic upper airway obstruction and pulmonary hypertension) and growth retardation. Polysomnography (sleep study) monitors electroencephalography, respiratory efforts, heart rate, and oxygen saturation during sleep. Clinical diagnosis is usually correct, but confirmation with polysomnography determines whether the condition warrants treatment. The treatment of adult sleep apnea is continuous positive airway pressure (CPAP) during sleep. For obese patients, weight loss to ideal body weight is frequently curative. For patients who cannot lose weight or tolerate CPAP, modification of the upper airway with septoplasty, turbinate reduction, tonsillectomy, or soft palate reduction (uvulopalatopharyngoplasty) is frequently helpful. Other surgical procedures, such as tongue reduction, hyoid advancement, and mandibular advancement, may be helpful in selected cases. In severe cases, tracheostomy will bypass the obstructed airway, relieving the condition in most cases. Children are frequently cured by simple tonsillectomy and adenoidectomy.

Neoplasms

Benign neoplasms of the oral cavity and pharynx are frequently diagnosed by biopsy. Of malignant neoplasms in

Table 5-9	Indications for Tonsillectomy	
Infectious	**Other**	
Tonsillitis	Upper airway obstruction	
Recurrent acute tonsillitis	Symptomatic	
6 episodes in 1 yr	Obstructive sleep apnea	
3–5 episodes/yr in 2 yr	Suspected malignancy	
3 episodes/yr for <3 yr		
Chronic tonsillitis		
Peritonsillar abscess		
Recurrent peritonsillar abscess		
Peritonsillar abscess when general		
anesthesia is required for		
incision and drainage of first		
abscess		

this region, 90% are squamous cell carcinomas. Like all head and neck carcinomas, they are strongly related to tobacco and alcohol use. These carcinomas may bleed or cause pain. New lesions are staged according to the system proposed by the American Joint Committee on Cancer, taking into consideration tumor size and location, cervical nodal involvement, and metastasis. Patients whose tumors are small, with neither nodal involvement nor evidence of metastasis, have a much greater survival rate than those with evidence of tumor spread.

Squamous cell carcinoma of the lip, a cross between cutaneous and oral cavity squamous cell carcinoma, is associated with sun exposure and tobacco use. Lip cancers have a better prognosis than oral cavity tumors but are more aggressive than similar cutaneous squamous cell carcinomas. Carcinomas of the oral cavity usually occur on the floor of the mouth and on the mobile tongue. They may present as enlarging masses or infiltrating ulcers. Neoplasms of the tonsillar area, the retromolar trigone, or the base of the tongue may cause hemoptysis, dysphagia, dysarthria, trismus (inability to open the mouth due to pterygoid muscle spasm), odynophagia, or referred otalgia. Patients with nasopharyngeal cancer may be seen with middle ear effusion caused by mechanical obstruction of the eustachian tube. Any adult with a unilateral serous otitis should be evaluated for a nasopharyngeal tumor. These cancers, which are frequently asymptomatic, are often discovered during the workup of metastatic cervical lymph nodes.

Malignant neoplasms of the oral cavity and pharynx are treated by radiation therapy, surgery, chemotherapy, or some combination of these treatments. Small, superficial lesions without nodal metastasis can be treated with either surgery or radiation therapy alone. Unfortunately, most cases of squamous cell carcinoma of the oral cavity and pharynx are associated with high rates of occult nodal metastasis, requiring surgical excision or radiation treatment of the lymph nodes that drain the region of the primary cancer. Larger primary tumors and those associated with cervical adenopathy usually require a combination of surgery and radiation therapy. Results of recent studies on the effect of chemotherapy used concurrently with radiation therapy in the pharynx are encouraging. Many patients show equivalent survival rates to those treated with surgery and postoperative radiation therapy. Therefore, specific treatment schemes are tailored to the individual patient's medical and psychosocial needs.

The oral cavity and the pharynx are functionally impaired after surgery or radiation therapy. Patients with this type of impairment require a large team of physicians and therapists for rehabilitation. The techniques of surgical reconstruction and irradiation continue to advance; the goal is to minimize the morbidity associated with treatment. Oral and facial prostheses also play a valuable role in rehabilitating the patient with speech, swallowing, and cosmetic defects.

THE LARYNX

Anatomy

The larynx occupies the central compartment of the neck and has muscular attachments to the tongue, mandible, skull base, sternum, and clavicles. The laryngeal framework consists of nine cartilage structures. There are three single cartilage structures (epiglottis, thyroid, and cricoid) and three paired cartilage structures (arytenoids, corniculate, and cuneiform) (Fig. 5-17). The epiglottis is an anterior leaf-like structure overlying the laryngeal inlet. The

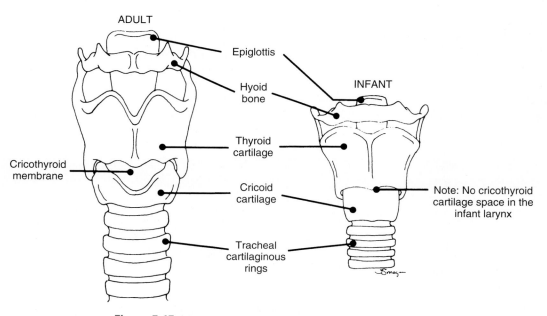

Figure 5-17   Laryngeal framework of the adult and infant.

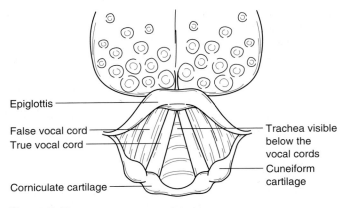

Epiglottis

False vocal cord
True vocal cord

Trachea visible
below the
vocal cords

Cuneiform
cartilage

Corniculate cartilage

Figure 5-18   Superior view of the larynx.

shield-shaped thyroid cartilage (i.e., Adam's apple) contains the anterior origin of the vocal ligaments and is readily palpated in the adult neck. The cricoid cartilage, the only complete cartilaginous ring in the larynx, is shaped like a signet ring. It lies below the thyroid cartilage and is attached posteriorly to the cricothyroid joint, laterally to the cricothyroideus muscle, and anteriorly to the cricothyroid membrane. The paired arytenoid cartilages have a three-sided pyramidal shape and articulate with the cricoid inferiorly. They lie immediately below two small cartilages, the cuneiform and corniculate cartilages (Fig. 5-18). Laterally, several intrinsic laryngeal muscles insert at the muscular process of the arytenoid. The vocal process arises medially and attaches to the vocal ligament and the vocalis muscle. Medial movement of the vocal processes adducts the vocal cords, closing the airway at the glottic opening.

The muscles of the larynx are classified as extrinsic or intrinsic. The extrinsic muscles elevate and depress the larynx as a unit, whereas the intrinsic muscles move the vocal cords. The posterior cricoarytenoid muscle rotates the arytenoid laterally, abducting (opening) the vocal cords for respiration. The remainder of the intrinsic muscles adduct (close) the vocal cords for phonation, coughing, and swallowing. The vocal cords have a unique and complex structure that facilitates their vibration during phonation. The vocalis muscle is lined by three connective tissue layers and a layer of squamous epithelium.

The nerve supply to the larynx derives from two branches of the vagus nerve: the superior laryngeal nerve, which provides sensory function and innervates the cricothyroid muscle, and the recurrent laryngeal nerve, which supplies motor functions to all remaining intrinsic muscles. Table 5-10 lists all the intrinsic muscles of the larynx as well as their innervation and action. The superior laryngeal nerve enters the larynx through the lateral thyrohyoid membrane. The recurrent laryngeal nerve leaves the vagus and courses around the aortic arch on the left and the subclavian artery on the right. It then ascends near the tracheoesophageal groove, branching to innervate the larynx. The left recurrent laryngeal nerve has a longer course in the chest and thus is more susceptible to injury.

The laryngeal lymphatic drainage is site dependent. The larynx is formed embryologically at the fusion of the respiratory diverticulum and the gut tube. The supraglottic larynx has a rich bilateral lymphatic drainage to the deep jugular lymph nodes. The glottic and subglottic larynx has sparse lymphatics, which drain to the pretracheal and paratracheal lymph nodes.

Physiology

The primary functions of the larynx are respiration, airway protection, and phonation. During normal respiration, the glottis opens widely, before the descent of the diaphragm. During deglutition, the larynx acts as a valve by carrying out a complex, intricately timed series of events to close the airway, thus preventing aspiration. Before the food bolus reaches the larynx, the extrinsic muscles of the larynx elevate it. This movement opens the pyriform sinuses widely, and the epiglottis covers the larynx to divert the bolus laterally into the pyriform sinuses. The false and true cords also adduct to close off the airway.

Voice is produced by the movement of air through an adducted glottis. This air movement through the narrowed, tense glottis produces a repeating wave of the vocal folds. Fine adjustments of the vocal fold tension and intrathoracic air pressure will then define both the frequency of this motion and the volume of the sound generated. This mechanism produces the rudiments of voice; however, the complex sounds of speech require the resonance of the pharyngeal, oral, and nasal cavities. Articulation of

Table 5-10	**Intrinsic Muscles of the Larynx**				
	Cricothyroid	**Lateral Cricoarytenoid**	**Posterior Cricoarytenoid**	**Thyroarytenoid**	**Interarytenoid**
Innervation	SLN	RLN	RLN	RLN	RLN (has bilateral innervation)
Effect on vocal cords	Lengthen and tighten cords for higher voice production	Adducts vocal cords	Abducts vocal cords	Thickens and adducts vocal cords for stronger voice production	Adducts the vocal cords

RLN, recurrent laryngeal nerve; SLN, superior laryngeal nerve.

speech occurs when the voice is modified continuously by the musculature that shapes these three cavities.

Physical Examination

Special equipment is required for physical examination of the larynx and the hypopharynx. Indirect laryngoscopy, which provides good visualization, requires the use of a head light or head mirror, a laryngeal mirror, a mirror warmer, gloves, and a gauze sponge. The patient should be sitting in an upright position facing the examiner. The patient is asked to open the mouth and protrude the tongue. The examiner gently holds the tongue out with a gauze sponge in the left hand, permitting visualization of the oropharynx. The laryngeal mirror is warmed to prevent fogging but should not be too hot; proper temperature can be determined by touching the mirror to the back of the examiner's hand before introducing it into the patient's mouth. The mirror is placed against the soft palate, and the head-mounted light source is directed on the mirror. The base of the tongue, the epiglottis, and the larynx and pyriform sinuses should be visualized. The patient is asked to repeat the sound "eee" and then to take a deep breath, which allows visualization of the vocal cords in both adduction and abduction. For patients with a sensitive gag reflex, topical spray anesthetic can be applied to the posterior pharynx. A flexible fiberoptic laryngoscope also allows visualization of the hypopharynx and the larynx; after the nose has been anesthetized, the scope is passed through the nose and over the soft palate.

Evaluation

In all complaints related to the larynx and the hypopharyngeal area, certain elements of history are critical. Basic features, such as duration of the complaint and exacerbating and relieving characteristics, are helpful in narrowing the differential diagnosis. Systemic signs of infection help confirm the presence of an inflammatory process, such as laryngitis or epiglottitis. Weight loss raises the suspicion of malignancy. Further, in a patient with odynophagia or dysphagia, weight loss will better define the degree of morbidity caused by the symptom. In the adult population, neoplastic disease must be considered; thus, knowledge of risk factors such as tobacco use, alcohol use, and toxic exposure (e.g., to carcinogenic chemicals) is key.

Hoarseness

Hoarseness is related to the disruption of the normal mechanisms of voice production. The characteristics of the vocal change help distinguish motor disturbances from dysfunction of the vocal fold vibratory characteristics. Breathiness of the voice indicates incomplete adduction of the cords, which can be caused by denervation of the larynx, functional disorders, or senile atrophy of the vocalis muscle. Strained or strangled vocal characteristics imply spasticity of movement. A muffled quality ("hot potato voice") is present in patients with mass lesions or inflammatory conditions above the true vocal cords.

The patient with a roughened vocal quality has pathology of the vocal fold. Inflammatory conditions are more likely to improve and deteriorate repeatedly over time. Neoplastic voice disturbance is usually progressive; however, patients with neoplasms may have elements of a concurrent inflammatory process. The larynx of a patient with hoarseness that does not resolve over a 1-month period should be carefully visualized.

Chronic Cough

The patient with chronic cough can be very challenging to treat because the diagnosis is frequently difficult to confirm. Pulmonary causes, including bronchospastic disease without wheezing, must be carefully eliminated. Cough that occurs immediately after eating is usually the result of aspiration. Patients may also note feeling "strangled" when swallowing; this symptom occurs more commonly with liquids. The larynx is frequently irritated by a number of factors, such as postnasal drip produced by sinusitis, allergic rhinitis, and vasomotor rhinitis producing a chronic cough. Gastroesophageal reflux may cause inflammatory changes of the vocal folds, inducing cough. Children or adults with gastroesophageal reflux may develop pneumonitis when gastric secretions are aspirated, although this condition is uncommon. Drugs such as angiotensin-converting enzyme inhibitors may cause a mild edematous process of the vocal fold, inducing cough. Unfortunately, the continuous trauma of chronic cough usually induces mild edema or erythema of the larynx, leaving the physician to answer the "Which came first?" question.

Hemoptysis

Although the classic teaching is that hemoptysis is caused by lung pathology, the condition may also indicate a bleeding lesion elsewhere in the upper aerodigestive tract. The physician cannot rule out the possibility of aspiration of blood from an upper aerodigestive source such as a posterior nasal bleed.

Stridor

Stridor is a high-pitched noise audible without a stethoscope that is a result of turbulent airflow through a narrowed portion of the airway. It represents significant obstruction of the airway and demands diagnosis. It can be characterized as inspiratory, expiratory, or biphasic (occurring during both inspiration and expiration). One can often determine the location of stenosis just by the nature of the stridor (Fig. 5-19). In general, narrowing of the airway above the level of the vocal cords results in inspiratory stridor. Stenosis at the level of the vocal cords or in the extrathoracic trachea causes biphasic stridor, and narrowing or partial obstruction of the intrathoracic trachea results in expiratory stridor. The latter is often mistaken for asthma, and patients may be improperly diagnosed and treated for some time. Patients who are not responding to

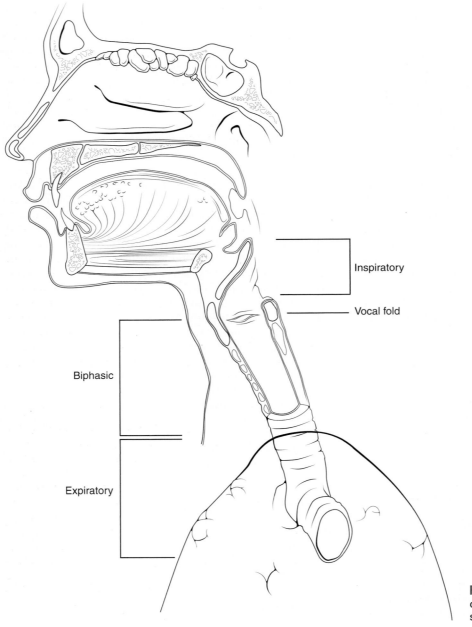

Figure 5-19 Location of airway obstruction with respect to type of stridor.

asthma medications should be evaluated for possible other causes of airway narrowing.

In the infant, laryngomalacia, subglottic stenosis, laryngeal webs, and benign neoplasms are the most likely diagnoses; laryngoscopy or bronchoscopy is required for evaluation. Associated systemic illness in a child implies laryngotracheobronchitis or tracheitis and epiglottitis. In the adult, these illnesses are less commonly associated with stridor and airway compromise because of the increased size of the adult glottis and its ability to tolerate the associated edema. In stridorous adults, neoplasm is more frequently diagnosed. Table 5-11 lists common causes of stridor in adults and children.

Odynophagia and Dysphagia

Patients with difficulty swallowing describe an inability to pass food, pain with swallowing, or the sensation of something caught in the throat. The physician must first identify the consistency of the food that causes symptoms. Neuromuscular disorders will first affect the ability to swallow liquids, but will eventually affect swallowing of foods of all consistencies. Difficulty in passing solid foods implies a mechanical obstruction, such as stricture, neoplasm, or diverticulum. An adult with chronic pain on swallowing requires careful evaluation to rule out malignancy. Unfortunately, superficial lesions can be quite painful and may

Table 5-11	Common Causes of Stridor	
Inspiratory	**Pediatric**	**Adult**
Inspiratory	Laryngomalacia	Neoplasm
	Epiglottitis	Angioedema
	Foreign body	Trauma to larynx
Biphasic	Croup	Vocal cord neoplasm
	Vocal cord web	Vocal cord paralysis
	Vocal cord paralysis	Laryngeal trauma
	Tracheomalacia	Subglottic stenosis
	Subglottic hemangioma	
	Vascular rings or slings	
Expiratory	Foreign body (tracheal or bronchus)	Tracheal neoplasm
	Asthma	Bronchial neoplasm
	Broncheomalacia	Foreign body

escape radiologic assessment. Patients with risk factors for malignancies who have chronic unexplained odynophagia must undergo complete assessment of the upper aerodigestive tract. The sensation of something caught in the throat is quite common and is frequently associated with no other demonstrable pathology. History of swallowing a rough food that may have scratched the throat may be helpful. Symptoms that persist for more than 1 month should be further evaluated.

Clinical Presentation, Diagnosis, and Treatment

Pediatric Structural Pathology

Laryngomalacia is the most common cause of stridor among infants, accounting for 60% of all cases. The supraglottic structures prolapse into the airway, producing inspiratory stridor. The condition is present at birth; most children will be seen during the first 2 months of life. The stridor worsens when the child is in the supine position but rarely results in severe distress. Diagnosis is permitted by flexible laryngoscopy, which demonstrates the airway collapse during spontaneous ventilation. Rigid laryngoscopy under general anesthesia will also demonstrate severe cases of malacia. The symptoms are usually self-limiting, with spontaneous recovery by the second year of life. Parents should be reassured but should also be advised to avoid keeping the baby in the supine position, especially during sleep. In the rare severe case, resecting redundant supraglottic tissue can be beneficial. This procedure, called a supraglottoplasty, is generally reserved for patients with worrisome apnea spells or failure to thrive.

Tracheomalacia is seen as expiratory or biphasic stridor caused by collapse of the trachea in the anterior-posterior direction. The cartilage is often abnormally shaped and soft. Spontaneous resolution can usually be expected by the time the child reaches the age of 18 months. Occasionally, surgical treatment (e.g., trachelopexy) is required.

In the infant, the subglottic airway is the narrowest region of the upper airway. Stenosis of this region can occur congenitally but more commonly results from local trauma, such as prolonged intubation. If severe, this condition causes biphasic stridor. In most cases, children with mild stenosis are seen with stridor during upper respiratory tract infections or after intubation. Even the slightest circumferential narrowing of the airway results in significant reduction of the total area. The narrowed subglottis becomes critical with additional airway edema, and the child develops stridor or recurrent **croup.** These exacerbations usually respond to conservative measures, such as nebulized racemic epinephrine and systemic corticosteroids. The problem often resolves as the infant grows because the stenotic segment grows along with the rest of the larynx. If severe, the stenosis can be corrected by surgically incising and stenting the cricoid cartilage ("cricoid split").

Vocal cord webs are usually membranous and usually involve the anterior true cords. Congenital webs are formed when normal embryonic laryngeal recanalization fails to occur. More commonly, they result from trauma and subsequent scarring of the anterior commissure. They may cause hoarseness or stridor, depending on their extent. The recommended treatment is endoscopic laser excision. Rarely, an open surgical repair is required, which consists of splitting the thyroid cartilage anteriorly.

Blunt and Penetrating Trauma of the Larynx

Laryngeal injuries are immediately life threatening because they may cause airway obstruction. The airway must be carefully assessed; if it is compromised, it should be secured by tracheotomy. A fractured larynx can lead to false passage on attempted oral or cricothyroid intubation. Diagnosis of these injuries is facilitated by laryngeal examination. Findings such as neck tenderness, voice change, the presence of subcutaneous emphysema, glottic mucosal disruption, or hematoma indicate possible laryngeal fracture. Blunt injuries causing fracture may escape detection if the patient is intubated for other reasons; the fracture may be discovered when attempts to extubate are unsuccessful. Penetrating injuries are readily apparent and usually require surgical repair.

Tracheal and Subglottic Stenosis

Trauma to the trachea can also occur from internal injury, the most common of which is prolonged intubation. The pressure of the endotracheal tube cuff can cause local ischemia and subsequent mucosal damage. If perichondritis and chondritis follow, significant scarring may occur. Occasionally, the cartilage is damaged, leaving a malacic segment that collapses on inspiration. A tracheostomy may also cause tracheal narrowing. These conditions may occur days to months after extubation as the scar continues to contract. Treatment with sleeve resection of the trachea is usually necessary. Occasionally, endoscopic laser excisions and dilations can be curative if the stenotic segment is less than 1 cm in length. Oftentimes these areas become restenotic, requiring multiple endoscopic procedures. Recently, the topical application of mitomycin C to a freshly dilated segment has shown promise in preventing recurrent stenosis. Mitomycin C is a chemotherapeutic agent that prevents proliferation of fibroblasts (cells essential for scar formation).

Inflammatory Conditions

Patients of all age-groups can suffer inflammatory processes of the larynx, usually causing hoarseness. Infectious conditions may cause odynophagia and systemic symptoms. The larynx of a child is substantially smaller than that of an adult, and the swelling caused by laryngeal infections can produce life-threatening airway compromise.

Epiglottitis

Epiglottitis is a potentially lethal inflammation of the supraglottis, usually caused by the bacteria *H. influenzae.* The incidence of epiglottitis has decreased substantially with the introduction of the *H. influenzae* vaccine. The condition occurs most commonly among children 3 to 6 years of age, but may also occur well into adulthood. The child is seen with a sudden onset of fever and stridor. Physical examination reveals a child in moderate to severe distress sitting upright with the head hyperextended to straighten the upper airway in an effort to facilitate air exchange. The child may be drooling and may also have severe odynophagia. A tongue blade must not be used to examine the child's throat because this may produce severe laryngospasm and loss of the airway. The child should be kept calm; if the child's condition permits, a portable lateral neck radiograph should be made to look for loss or blunting of the usual sharp borders and thin contour of the epiglottis.

If epiglottitis is considered, the child is taken to the operating room for anesthesia, direct laryngoscopy, and oral intubation. A nasotracheal tube is often inserted later because it is more stable and less likely to become displaced. In addition to an experienced anesthesiologist, an otolaryngologist or pediatric surgeon should be in attendance in the event that intubation cannot be carried out and bronchoscopy, tracheostomy, or both become necessary. Once the airway is established, cultures are taken and treatment with intravenous antibiotics effective against *H. influenzae* are instituted. From the operating room, the child is taken to the intensive care unit, where the nasotracheal (preferable) or orotracheal tube is kept secure. The edema usually resolves rapidly and the child can be extubated within 72 hours.

Croup

Laryngotracheobronchitis, frequently referred to as croup, most commonly affects children 2 years of age or younger. It is viral in origin and generally affects the subglottic larynx, although it may extend the length of the trachea. The child is seen with symptoms of an upper respiratory tract infection of a few days' duration. Over a period of several hours, the child develops a barking cough as the primary symptom. Fever is usually low grade or absent. Physical examination reveals an irritable infant with mild stridor and barking cough. A lateral neck film reveals a normal epiglottis but a narrowed subglottic air column. Treatment is based on severity of symptoms. In mild cases, humidified air alone suffices. In moderate cases, racemic epinephrine treatments may be required in the emergency room. In severe cases, the child may require hospitalization, with frequent racemic epinephrine treatments and intravenous or aerosol administration of steroids to decrease inflammation. Rarely, the airway distress is so severe that endotracheal intubation is required to secure the airway. The edema from croup resolves more slowly than that from epiglottitis, often requiring 5 to 7 days for full resolution. Because several viruses cause croup, recurrences are common. Rarely, bacterial tracheitis is seen and is associated with a more virulent course, requiring intubation and therapeutic bronchoscopy. For a comparison of presentation and treatment of epiglottitis and croup, see Table 5-12.

Laryngitis

The most common inflammatory condition of the larynx among adults is acute laryngitis. It is usually viral in origin, causing hoarseness and symptoms of upper respiratory tract infection. Examination of the vocal cords reveals edema and erythema. The disease usually resolves spontaneously, but improvement can be expedited with humidification and voice rest. It should be emphasized that an adult with hoarseness that persists for more than 1 month should undergo examination of the vocal cords.

Chronic laryngitis is precipitated by chronic irritation of the larynx, usually resulting in painless dysphonia. The vocal cords are erythematous, with some degree of edema. In some cases, the edema becomes quite pronounced and is described as polypoid degeneration; occasionally, classic polyps form and should be excised. The treatment is removal of the irritating condition, which is usually an inhaled irritant (e.g., tobacco smoke, an allergen, or some noxious compound). Gastroesophageal reflux and postnasal drainage of inflammatory mucus may also lead to chronic laryngitis.

Vocal Cord Paralysis

Simple unilateral vocal cord paralysis usually causes a weak, breathy voice and sometimes aspiration. The patient will commonly relate coughing when swallowing thin liquids. The cause is frequently denervation. The recurrent laryngeal nerve can be traumatized or iatrogenically injured during carotid, thyroid, or thoracic surgical procedures. Central lesions, such as brain stem stroke, amyotrophic lateral sclerosis, and multiple sclerosis, will usually have other neurologic manifestations. Tumor at the base of skull or within the lung, thyroid, esophagus, hypopharynx, or larynx may disrupt the innervation of a vocal cord if it extends to involve the nerve. Unilateral vocal cord paralysis can be a congenital defect, usually caused by

Table 5-12	Symptoms and Treatment of Epiglottitis versus Croup	
	Epiglottitis	**Croup**
Definition	Inflammation of the supraglottis	Laryngotracheobronchitis
Etiopathology	Bacteria: *Haemophilus influenzae* type B	Viral (several: parainfluenza virus type 1, RSV, influenza A and B, adeno-, entero-, rhino-, and measles viruses)
Age	Most common among children 3–6 yr of age but may also occur well into adulthood	Most commonly affects children 2 yr of age or younger
Onset	Acute and fulminating	Less fulminant in onset
Presentation	Fever	Fever low grade or absent
Symptoms	Stridor	Mild stridor
		Symptoms of an upper respiratory tract infection of a few days
Physical examination	Child in moderate to severe distress, sitting upright with the head hyperextended to straighten the upper airway in an effort to facilitate air exchange	Irritable infant
	Odynophagia	
Key word	Drooling	Barking cough
Investigation (lateral neck film)	Loss or blunting of the usual sharp borders and thin contour of the epiglottis	Normal epiglottis but a narrowed subglottic air column (subepiglottic narrowing)
	Thumb-printing sign	Steeple sign
Treatment	(A) IV antibiotic effective against *H. influenzae*, β-lactamase–resistant antibiotic, ampicillin, third-generation cephalosporin, chloramphenicol	(A) *Mild:* Humidified air
	(B) The child is taken to the OR for anesthesia, direct	(B) *Moderate:* Racemic epinephrine in the ER
		(C) *Severe:* Hospitalization with frequent racemic epinephrine and IV or aerosol administration of steroids
		(D) Very severe: endotracheal intubation
Afterward	Edema resolves rapidly in 72 hr	The edema resolves more slowly, often requiring 5–7 days
Recurrence	Uncommon	Common

Table courtesy of Mohammed I. Ahmed, MBBS, MS (Surgery).

trauma resulting from stretching the recurrent laryngeal nerve during pregnancy or delivery. Often, the workup will reveal no cause (i.e., idiopathic vocal cord paralysis). Idiopathic vocal cord paralysis is probably similar to other cranial nerve neuropathies and may reverse itself without treatment. If after 6 to 12 months no function returns and the patient has an uncompensated paralysis, the paralyzed vocal cord can be medialized. This procedure allows the mobile contralateral vocal cord to approximate the paralyzed cord, producing voice and protecting the airway (Fig. 5-20). Endoscopic injection techniques and external approaches can be used to perform this medialization.

Bilateral vocal cord paralysis is quite uncommon and may be caused by central and systemic pathology. Adults with this condition will have a near-normal voice and marked biphasic stridor. Both vocal cords can be paralyzed at birth because of a brain stem lesion, such as Arnold-Chiari malformation. Initial treatment for airway distress is intubation. Tracheotomy is usually performed in cases with airway distress. Tracheotomy preserves the normal voice and provides an adequate airway. Frequently, patients find the secretions and management associated with a long-term tracheostomy unsatisfactory. In those cases, vocal cord lateralization procedures, unilateral arytenoidectomy, or unilateral vocal cordotomy can be performed. These procedures will compromise the voice as they enlarge the laryngeal airway. Reinnervation procedures have been reported but are generally unsuccessful.

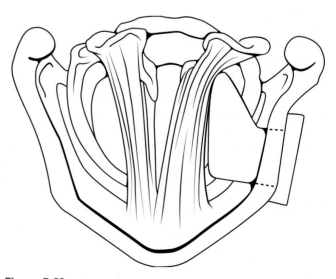

Figure 5-20   Coronal section of the larynx at the level of the vocal cords. An implant has been surgically placed on the left inside of the thyroid cartilage to medialize the left vocal cord.

Chronic Lesions of the Vocal Folds

Vocal cord nodules are a common cause of chronic hoarseness and occur in children and adults. They are usually the result of localized chronic inflammation from improper vocal use and vocal abuse. Also known as "singer's nodules," they may occur among vocalists, especially those without voice training. Examination reveals symmetrical white nodules at the junction of the anterior and middle third of the true vocal cords. Correcting the patterns of voice use and abuse will in many cases enable spontaneous clearing of nodules; however, many patients will require endoscopic excision. Without speech or voice therapy, the nodules will probably recur.

Granuloma formation can occur at the posterior true vocal cords as a result of trauma, usually in the presence of gastroesophageal reflux. Granuloma formation is frequently associated with endotracheal intubation or repeated vocal trauma, such as throat clearing and chronic cough. The condition will frequently respond to aggressive treatment of the gastroesophageal reflux, antibiotics, and a short course of corticosteroids. Lesions that do not respond to the above measures can be treated by injection of botulinum toxin (Botox) into the laryngeal adductors (thyroarytenoid and lateral cricothyroid muscles). Botox provides neuromuscular paralysis by preventing the release of presynaptic acetylcholine. This results in less forceful adduction of the vocal cords, which allows the granuloma to resolve and the area to heal. In rare instances, granulomas are removed surgically because they cause airway obstruction, or to rule out malignancy.

Benign Neoplasms of the Larynx

The most common benign tumor in children is the squamous papilloma, which can also involve the trachea and the bronchi. The papilloma is an epithelial lesion of connective tissue covered by squamous epithelium that may be keratinized. Papillomas are believed to be caused by viruses and to be influenced by hormonal changes, as evidenced by their tendency to remit spontaneously around the time of puberty. Papillomas usually involve the anterior portions of the vocal cords but can also involve the false cords superiorly and the immediate subglottic area. In children, onset usually occurs before the age of 5 years, and the condition can persist until late adolescence. Papillomas arising in adults are not as aggressive. Papillomas spread by manipulation and can seed up and down the respiratory tract.

Treatment is endoscopic laser ablation of the papilloma. Radiation therapy is not helpful. Systemic therapies, such as α interferon, ribavirin, acyclovir, and indole 3, are currently under investigation for more severe cases. It is difficult to determine the best treatment because the natural history of this disease involves waxing and waning of severity.

Subglottic and tracheal **hemangiomas** are vascular lesions seen during the first year of life in association with stridor. Like hemangiomas of the skin, they usually regress by 4 years of age; thus, a conservative approach is warranted. If these lesions cannot be managed with endoscopic laser excision, tracheotomy may be necessary. Steroids have been used with varying degrees of success.

Malignant Neoplasms of the Larynx

The most common laryngeal malignancy is squamous cell carcinoma; all other malignancies combined make up less than 5% of laryngeal malignancy. In most populations, the incidence of laryngeal malignancy is 10% that of lung cancer. Tobacco smoking and alcohol are strong risk factors. The peak incidence is in the sixth and seventh decades of life; men are affected more commonly than women.

A diagnosis of carcinoma of the larynx requires a biopsy of the lesion or an obvious lymph node metastasis. In addition to indirect mirror and fiberoptic examination of the larynx, direct operative laryngoscopy best delineates the mucosal involvement. CT or MRI scans can demonstrate depth of invasion and lymph adenopathy. New lesions found in the larynx are then staged according to the system proposed by the American Joint Committee on Cancer, accounting for tumor size and location, cervical nodal involvement, and metastasis. Patients whose tumors are small, with no nodal involvement and no evidence of metastasis, have a much greater survival rate than those with evidence of tumor spread.

Primary treatment methods are surgery and radiation therapy. Chemotherapy given in conjunction with radiation therapy improves the survival rates for many stages of larynx cancer and obviates the need for surgery in some cases. For end-stage malignancies, chemotherapy has been used palliatively with very limited success. To determine the therapeutic modality, the size and location of the tumor, the presence or absence of cervical nodes, and the patient's own desires and physical status are taken into account.

The surgery for laryngeal carcinoma is dictated by the primary tumor and the patient's premorbid conditions. Endoscopic excision or partial laryngectomy is used with good success for small tumors. These procedures preserve function; however, more extensive resections of the vocal folds will disturb the quality of the voice. Partial laryngectomy, especially supraglottic laryngectomy, may allow for intermittent aspiration. Total laryngectomy is reserved for larger lesions and for smaller lesions in patients with marginal pulmonary lung function who could not tolerate aspiration. This completely disconnects the airway from the alimentary tract. The trachea is matured as a stoma to the skin at the base of the neck above the sternal notch. Once laryngectomy has been performed, the patient is able to produce good, intelligible speech by using an electrolarynx or by using the esophagus and the neopharynx to produce a vibratory noise. Prosthetic valves are often placed into the tracheostoma connecting to the esophagus, allowing the patient to produce a vibratory sound. The articulating mechanisms of the pharynx, nose, and mouth then shape the sound into audible speech.

Radiation therapy can be delivered to the larynx alone with little morbidity. Small tumors are usually treated with radiation therapy, particularly when they involve the true vocal cords. For small superficial cancers of the larynx with no cervical node involvement, either surgery or radiation therapy will produce a 3-year survival rate of greater than 90%. Tumors of the supraglottic larynx are associated with a high rate of lymph node metastasis, and even small lesions without palpable adenopathy will necessitate treatment of the neck. Patients treated with radiation for supraglottic cancers must have a much larger proportion of the neck treated than those with glottic cancers. Therefore, the morbidity rates associated with irradiation increase. Surgical treatment is used for patients whose disease recurs or does not respond to therapy.

As is true for other squamous cell carcinomas of the head and neck, the presence of cervical adenopathy is an indicator of a much poorer prognosis, reducing the predicted 5-year survival rate by as much as 70%. These advanced-stage lesions are frequently treated with a combination of irradiation and surgery.

Surgery has been the standard of care for many years with good success. Over the past 10 years, many of these patients have received chemotherapy with radiation to improve the response of their laryngeal tumors to radiation. This combination of treatments allows cure without laryngectomy in about two thirds of patients. However, the survival rates are inferior to those associated with surgery unless all patients whose disease recurs or does not respond to this combination are treated with surgery. Such treatment requires a cooperative patient and close follow-up by a surgeon familiar with the appearance of recurrent cancer of the larynx.

THE NECK AND SALIVARY GLANDS

Anatomy

A significant portion of any gross anatomy course is spent covering the complex structures of the neck. The neck serves two basic functions. It is a portal through which a vast array of visceral and neurovascular structures traverse, and it also serves as the fifth limb, allowing movement of the head. The musculature connects the cervical vertebrae to move the head and to elevate the ribs and the shoulder girdle. The sternocleidomastoid muscle divides the neck into two triangles. The anterior triangle of the neck is bounded medially by the midline of the neck, superiorly by the angle of the mandible, posteriorly by the sternocleidomastoid muscle, and inferiorly by the clavicle. The posterior triangle is bounded medially by the sternocleidomastoid muscle, superiorly by the mastoid tip and the superior nuchal line, posteriorly by the trapezius muscle, and inferiorly by the clavicle. Normal structures in the anterior triangle that can be seen or palpated include the sternocleidomastoid muscle, the hyoid bone, the larynx, the trachea, the thyroid gland, the parotid gland, and the submandibular gland. Deep to the sternocleidomastoid muscle in the anterior triangle lies the carotid sheath, which contains the common, external, and internal carotid arteries; the internal jugular vein; the vagus nerve; the sympathetic chain; and the deep jugular lymph nodes. The lymphatics drain the mucosal surfaces of the upper aerodigestive tract (Fig. 5-21). This leads to a somewhat predictable spread of infection or tumor into the cervical lymphatics.

Four distinct layers of cervical fascia envelop the contents of the neck. Deep to the skin is an external layer of fascia. The platysma muscle lies just below this external layer. Immediately below the platysma is the investing layer of the deep cervical fascia, which splits to envelop the sternocleidomastoid and strap muscles. The middle layer of deep fascia envelops the thyroid, pharynx, larynx, and trachea as the visceral fascia. Laterally, the middle layer forms the carotid sheath. The deepest layer is the prevertebral fascia, enveloping the paraspinous musculature of the neck.

The major salivary glands are the parotid, the submandibular, and the sublingual glands (Fig. 5-22). These paired glands are located outside the mucosa of the oral cavity, to which they are connected by ducts. The minor

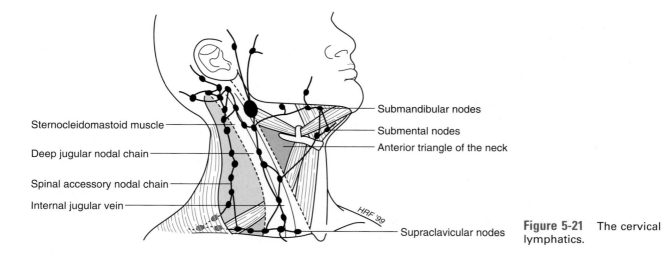

Sternocleidomastoid muscle

Deep jugular nodal chain

Spinal accessory nodal chain

Internal jugular vein

Submandibular nodes

Submental nodes

Anterior triangle of the neck

Supraclavicular nodes

HRF '99

Figure 5-21   The cervical lymphatics.

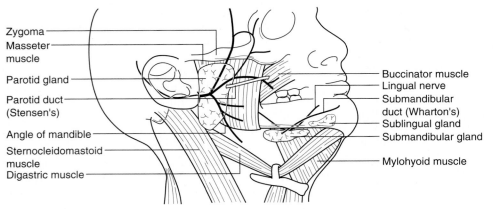

Zygoma
Masseter muscle
Parotid gland
Parotid duct (Stensen's)
Angle of mandible
Sternocleidomastoid muscle
Digastric muscle

Buccinator muscle
Lingual nerve
Submandibular duct (Wharton's)
Sublingual gland
Submandibular gland
Mylohyoid muscle

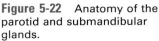

Figure 5-22 Anatomy of the parotid and submandibular glands.

salivary glands are scattered throughout the oral cavity and the oropharynx. They lie just deep to the mucosa and connect with the oral cavity and the pharynx by way of rudimentary ducts.

The parotid gland is the largest. It lies anterior to the ear, overlying the masseter muscle, and has a tail portion that extends inferiorly to the mandibular angle and posteriorly below the mastoid tip. Its duct (Stensen's) arises anteriorly approximately 1 cm below the zygoma. It traverses the masseter muscle and terminates orally in an ampulla opposite the upper second molar tooth. The most important of the multiple nerves associated with the parotid gland is the facial nerve, which exits the mastoid bone through the stylomastoid foramen and passes through the center of the gland, where it branches into the cervical, marginal mandibular, buccal, zygomatic, and temporal motor nerves. The secretomotor supply to the gland is parasympathetic via the ninth cranial nerve from the inferior salivatory nucleus in the brain stem.

The submandibular gland lies in a concavity inferior to the mandible, between the anterior and posterior bellies of the digastric muscle. Its duct (Wharton's) runs anteriorly from the gland between the mylohyoid and hyoglossus muscles. It ends in an ampulla near the lingual frenulum. The parasympathetic secretomotor nerve supply is derived from the superior salivatory nucleus by way of the chorda tympani and the lingual nerve.

The sublingual gland, the smallest of the major glands, lies directly under the oral mucosa, forming a ridge next to the tongue. The gland empties directly into the floor of the mouth through several ducts on its superior surface. It lies close to the superior part of the submandibular gland and minor sublingual ducts may enter the submandibular gland. The secretomotor nerve supply is the same as that of the submandibular gland.

Physiology

The salivary glands produce approximately 500 mL of saliva per day, of which 90% is secreted by the parotid and submandibular glands. Saliva acts both as a lubricant and as a protective agent throughout the upper aerodigestive tract. It promotes clearing of debris and bacteria, sweeping these contaminants into the lower gastrointestinal tract. It also helps maintain oral and dental hygiene and indirectly aids in body hydration. The main digestive enzyme of saliva is β-amylase, which is important for the enzymatic breakdown of starch.

Physical Examination

The physical examination must be performed in a systematic way to avoid omitting a structure. Visual inspection for lesions and scars on the skin and for signs of muscular atrophy or deformity must always precede palpation. Then, the parotid gland should be palpated. To allow complete assessment of the submandibular triangle, a gloved finger should first be inserted into the floor of the mouth, allowing bimanual palpation. Otherwise, the contents of the submandibular triangle will elevate on palpation. The anterior triangle should be palpated to assess the cervical lymphatics and anterior airway cartilages. Then the posterior triangle should be palpated for masses. The thyroid gland should be palpated anteriorly by insinuating the fingers between the trachea and the sternocleidomastoid muscle. Having the patient swallow will cause the gland to move under the palpating fingers, facilitating the detection of nodules.

Evaluation

Patients with a neck mass present a diagnostic challenge because the differential diagnosis is quite lengthy. In broad categories, these lesions are traumatic, congenital, inflammatory, or neoplastic. The temporal history of the lesion, associated pain, systemic manifestations of disease, and other symptoms of aerodigestive pathology are quite important. Past medical history and patient demographics complete the information required to shape the differential diagnosis. The location of the lesion is also important. The tail of the parotid and the submandibular gland are frequently confused with adenopathy. Certain bony protuberances, such as the angle of the jaw and the transverse process of C-1, can be mistaken for neck masses. The physician should carefully feel for the characteristics of the lesion. If it is pulsatile, is there a symmetrical mass on the contralateral side (does it represent a prominent carotid bulb)? Is there a thrill or bruit, as in a vascular tumor? Is the mass discrete or infiltrating? Are there other masses?

Nontender Neck Mass

In an adult older than 40 years of age, a nontender neck mass indicates neoplasm until proven otherwise. Squamous cell carcinoma commonly metastasizes to the cervical lymph nodes from the upper aerodigestive tract. Distant metastasis from lung cancer or the abdomen may occur in the supraclavicular fossae. Thyroid carcinoma may also metastasize to the cervical lymph nodes without obviously palpable pathology in the thyroid gland. A careful examination of the head and neck should be performed. If a primary site is identified, a biopsy of the primary tumor should be performed. If no primary site can be found, a fine-needle biopsy performed properly and read by a skilled cytopathologist is quite accurate in providing a diagnosis. An open biopsy of a neck mass is performed only as a "last resort," because it may compromise future treatment. Therefore, it is to be done only after repeated fine-needle aspiration is nondiagnostic and examination of the upper aerodigestive tract under anesthesia (including ipsilateral tonsillectomy and biopsies of the nasopharynx and base of tongue) fails to discover a primary site of malignancy. CT scans and MRI provide detailed information about nonpalpable pathology; these imaging methods also allow good visualization of the nasopharynx, which can be difficult to assess fully.

In the adolescent and young adult, cancer is a less common diagnosis. A compliant patient with a mass smaller than 3 cm in size may be followed. Reactive lymph nodes do not always return to normal size. Certain infectious conditions may produce nontender adenopathy. A history of exposure to tuberculosis, human immunodeficiency virus (HIV), and animal bites and scratches may be helpful. Larger and solid lesions that enlarge over time raise the suspicion of lymphoma and demand fine-needle aspiration. Fine-needle aspiration is diagnostic and can provide tissue for flow cytometry to aid in defining the subtype of lymphoma. Occasionally, a lymphoma may depend on histologic architecture, making open biopsy necessary. Cystic congenital lesions are seen most commonly among patients in this age-group. Because of the thick fascial layers of the neck, differentiating cysts from solid lesions can be difficult. Ultrasound and CT or fine-needle aspiration will help to make the diagnosis.

Tender Neck Mass

Inflammatory processes are usually more recent in onset and shorter in duration; they may be accompanied by fever and symptoms related to an upper respiratory tract infection, such as sore throat or congestion. Tender adenopathy that is not responsive to antibiotics may imply granulomatous infections, which may be identified through fine-

needle cytopathology and culture. Useful laboratory tests include a complete blood cell count with differential, an erythrocyte sedimentation rate, and a serum test as appropriate for mononucleosis, cat scratch disease, and HIV.

Clinical Presentation, Diagnosis, and Treatment

Acute and Chronic Sialadenitis

Inflammatory diseases of the salivary glands include mumps, acute suppurative **sialadenitis,** parotid abscess, chronic sialadenitis, and Sjögren's syndrome. Acute sialadenitis is a bacterial infection most frequently involving the submandibular gland. Adults are more commonly affected. Debilitated and dehydrated patients are particularly susceptible. The gland becomes hard and tender, and purulent discharge can be seen from the duct, producing a bad taste in the patient's mouth. Causative organisms include S. *aureus*, S. *pneumoniae*, and hemolytic streptococcus. Treatment includes hydration and appropriate antibiotics targeting Gram-positive organisms. Abscesses of the salivary glands are treated by incision and drainage.

Chronic sialadenitis is characterized by recurrent tender enlargements of the glands and is frequently associated with strictures or calculi involving the ductal system. These conditions can be treated with ductal dilation, removal of stones, or sialodochoplasty (reconstruction of the duct). Treatment of chronic sialadenitis is usually conservative, including sialagogues (saliva stimulants, such as sour candy), massage, and antibiotics. When conservative measures are unsuccessful, superficial parotidectomy or excision of the submandibular gland may be the most appropriate means of treatment.

Sjögren's syndrome is an autoimmune disease of the salivary glands and includes xerostomia, keratoconjunctivitis sicca, and connective tissue disorders. The cause of the syndrome is unknown, but most patients exhibit hypergammaglobulinemia with elevated IgG fraction. Rheumatoid arthritis is a common characteristic of the syndrome, and antinuclear antibodies are present in 50% of the cases, with or without clinical arthritis. Treatment of head and neck symptoms includes local measures to counteract xerostomia and conjunctivitis. If the salivary glands are infected, antibiotic therapy is also recommended. Patients with this syndrome should be observed for increasing size of the glands because they are at higher risk for salivary lymphoma.

Benign Neoplasms of the Salivary Glands

Tumors of the salivary glands account for approximately 1% of all head and neck tumors, and 85% of them arise from the parotid gland. Of these, 75% are benign; in comparison, 50% of submandibular gland tumors and 30% of minor salivary gland tumors are benign. Diagnostic procedures for tumors of the salivary glands include fine-needle aspiration, sialography, scintillation scanning, CT scanning, and magnetic resonance imaging. The introduction of CT scanning and MRI over the past 15 years and the increased use of fine-needle aspiration for tumor information have resulted in a dramatic decrease in the use of other diagnostic techniques.

Benign tumors usually display painless, slow growth and tumor mobility; they may occasionally cause secondary fibrosis or inflammation. Because of secondary infection or cystic degeneration, pain may be present but is not common. Minor salivary gland tumors usually occur on the palate but may occur anywhere in the upper aerodigestive tract. They are firm, nontender, mucosally covered masses.

Approximately 80% of benign tumors are mixed tumors or pleomorphic adenomas, which tend to occur in the third and fourth decades of life. Warthin's tumor occurs 8% of the time, primarily in the tail of the parotid gland and principally among male smokers. Treatment of these benign tumors consists of total removal of the submandibular gland or minor salivary gland, or removal of the appropriate portion of the parotid gland, preserving the facial nerve.

The most common benign parotid gland tumor among children is the hemangioma, which usually resolves spontaneously. Surgery should be reserved for rapidly growing tumors or those that do not resolve by the time the patient has reached 2 or 3 years of age.

Parotid cysts occur frequently among patients with acquired immunodeficiency syndrome (AIDS). These cysts may respond to laser treatment or low doses of radiation. Surgical excision is reserved for symptomatic cysts for which other treatment methods have failed.

Malignant Neoplasms of the Salivary Glands

Malignant lesions of the salivary glands share many of the characteristics of their benign counterparts. However, certain signs and symptoms indicate malignancy: rapid growth, large size, fixation of the tumor to the overlying skin, facial nerve dysfunction, and cervical node enlargement. Children tend to have a higher rate of malignancy with salivary gland tumors.

Fine-needle aspiration allows diagnosis of malignancy in 85% to 95% of cases. Open or partial biopsy is performed only when mucosal or skin involvement is noted. Minor salivary gland biopsy may be performed if the tumor is not accessible by fine-needle aspiration. Biopsies of small tumors of the submandibular gland are best performed by removal of the gland. New lesions found in the salivary glands are staged according to the tumor node metastasis system, described earlier, proposed by the American Joint Committee on Cancer.

The most common malignancy of the major salivary glands is mucoepidermoid carcinoma, followed by adenoid cystic carcinoma and acinic cell carcinoma. Each of these tumors shows a wide spectrum of biologic behavior. They are histopathologically classified into low- and high-grade tumors. Low-grade cancers usually have a favorable prognosis, grow locally, and metastasize to upper neck nodes infrequently and late in the course of the disease. High-grade cancers commonly metastasize to the neck nodes and lungs. Adenoid cystic carcinoma, the most common malignancy in all but the parotid gland, tends to invade lymphatics and nerves. This tumor is characterized by late distant metastasis; the 10- to 20-year survival rate is poor. Other malignant tumors of the salivary glands include adenocarcinoma and squamous cell carcinoma. The primary treatment of malignancies of the salivary glands is removal of the tumor and the involved lymph nodes, followed by radiotherapy. If possible, the facial nerve should be spared in this resection. If there is preoperative facial nerve paralysis, or obvious nerve involvement with tumor, the nerve should be sacrificed to provide adequate tumor resection. Numerous plastic surgery techniques are available to reanimate the paralyzed face, if needed.

Cervical Adenitis

Most inflammatory neck masses are inflamed lymph nodes, especially in children. Nearly every person has lymphadenitis at some point in life, most commonly during childhood; the disease may be bacterial, viral, or granulomatous. In children, concurrent viral upper respiratory tract illness is associated with swollen tender adenopathy.

Frequently, staphylococcal and streptococcal bacteria species infect the cervical nodes, requiring treatment with appropriate antibiotics. The source of initial infection is frequently the adenotonsillar tissues; however, bacterial adenitis may appear without obvious initiating sources. Posterior cervical nodes may be enlarged as the result of scalp lesions, such as those associated with head lice, or other cutaneous infections. The treatment is appropriate oral antibiotic therapy, with resolution expected in days to weeks.

Occasionally, lymphadenitis may become suppurative, particularly in infants and children. In children, a trial of intravenous antibiotics is often curative. If the suppuration becomes more superficial or fails to improve within 24 to 48 hours of antibiotic therapy, incision and drainage are appropriate. Rarely, the suppurative adenitis involves one or more of the deep jugular lymph nodes; in these cases, patients are toxic with fever and leukocytosis, and they exhibit diffuse erythema and swelling of the lateral neck with a brawny edema. Fluctuance is not present in most cases because of the deep location of the purulence. In the adult, deep neck infections frequently result from dental pathology. CT scanning is of great benefit in diagnosing the extent of the deep neck abscess. In children, the CT scan can be misleading, indicating abscess where there is only phlegmon. Because these nodes and resultant abscesses are within the carotid sheath, careful incision and drainage through a lateral neck incision are indicated. If these potentially dangerous, deep neck abscesses are not drained adequately, the infection may tract along tissue planes into the mediastinum, with a significant additional morbidity and risk of mortality.

Granulomatous Cervical Adenitis

Cat scratch fever is a bacterial granulomatous adenitis, often occurring after exposure to or a scratch from a cat or a dog. Usually, the lymph node on the ipsilateral side of the scratch becomes enlarged and tender. Initial systemic symptoms include low-grade fever, malaise, and myalgia. The adenopathy may resolve spontaneously over months, and management is usually supportive. Antibiotics for Gram-negative infections may shorten the clinical course. If suppuration occurs, needle aspiration and, rarely, excision of the node or nodes are indicated.

Mycobacteria produce a granulomatous adenitis, usually without systemic symptoms. The majority of mycobacterial cervical infections in adults are caused by *Mycobacterium tuberculosis*. Cases involving atypical organisms, most commonly *Mycobacterium avium-intracellulare*, occur more frequently in children and are more common than tuberculous cervical adenitis. Affected patients may have a weakly positive tuberculin skin test. They often present with a nontender fluctuant mass, usually around the parotid or submandibular glands. The overlying skin develops a violaceous hue, and, if left alone, the mass will often progress to rupture and drainage. These highly resistant organisms are best treated with surgical excision of the involved nodes. Antibiotic therapy is reserved for recurrent disease or for disease that can only be partially excised to prevent development of a chronic draining fistula. Tuberculous cervical adenitis, historically known as scrofula, is best treated with antibiotic therapy. Surgery is helpful in making the diagnosis if culture material is unobtainable through needle biopsy. Curiously, most patients exhibit no evidence of pulmonary tubercular infection.

Benign Cervical Cysts

Thyroglossal duct cysts occur as soft, painless, persistent midline neck masses and are formed during the first or second decade of life (Fig. 5-23). Physical examination shows that the cyst elevates on swallowing or on protruding the tongue; this occurs because the cyst or tract is tethered to the hyoid bone. The thyroid develops embryologically at the tuberculum impar at the base of the tongue and descends through the neck to its final location, creating a thyroglossal tract of tissue. Thyroglossal duct cysts are caused by failure of this cyst to obliterate. Excision is usually performed because these cysts may enlarge, become infected, or undergo malignant degeneration. Surgical excision should include the cyst and the complete tract, thus necessitating excision of the midportion of the hyoid. Before the cyst is excised, the normal position and function of the thyroid gland should be carefully documented. On rare occasions, the cyst may contain the only functioning thyroid tissue.

Branchial cleft anomalies arise from a failure of the embryologic cervical sinus of His to obliterate during fetal development. Branchial anomalies can involve the first through fourth arches but most commonly involve the second branchial arch. They usually present as persistent, painless (unless infected) cysts just anterior to the middle third of the sternocleidomastoid muscle. They may also be seen as sinuses or fistulae. These cysts may occur in a patient of any age; however, fistulae and sinuses usually occur during infancy, and cysts commonly occur during the second and third decades of life. A second branchial arch anomaly classically courses superiorly between the internal and external carotid arteries, superior to the hypoglossal nerve. The tract of the second branchial cleft begins in the central cleft of the pharyngeal tonsil and courses above the hypoglossal nerve between the internal and external carotid arteries, and out to the skin of the lower third of the neck, anterior to the sternocleidomastoid muscle. These masses or tracts are subject to recurrent infection, usually in conjunction with an upper respiratory tract infection. Surgical excision of the cyst, the fistula tract, or both is recommended during a quiescent period. See Table 5-13 for a comparison of thyroglossal duct cysts and branchial cleft cysts.

Dermoid cysts, like thyroglossal duct cysts, are soft, painless, persistent midline neck masses occurring during the first or second decade of life. Unlike thyroglossal duct cysts, however, they do not elevate with swallowing because they are not attached to the hyoid bone. Pathophysiologically, they are developmental anomalies involving pluripotential embryonal cells that become isolated and subsequently undergo disorganized growth. They are composed of ectoderm and mesoderm and often contain hair follicles, sweat glands, and sebaceous glands. The treatment of choice is complete surgical excision.

Lymphangioma and Hemangioma

Lymphangioma and hemangioma are pathologically similar; **hemangiomas** contain blood-filled channels, and **lymphangiomas** contain lymph-filled channels. These lesions are classified as capillary, cavernous, or mixed.

Cystic hygromas are soft, painless, often very large mul-

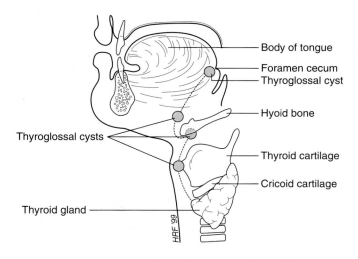

Figure 5-23   Localization of thyroglossal duct cysts.

Labels: Body of tongue, Foramen cecum, Thyroglossal cyst, Hyoid bone, Thyroglossal cysts, Thyroid cartilage, Cricoid cartilage, Thyroid gland

Table 5-13	Thyroglossal Duct Anomalies versus Branchial Cleft Anomalies	
	Thyroglossal Duct Anomalies	**Branchial Cleft Anomalies**
Presentation	Cysts/sinuses/fistulae	Cysts/sinuses/fistulae/cartilaginous rests
Age	Most present in childhood or in early adult life	Commonly present in young adults
Histology	Usually lined by stratified squamous epithelium or pseudostratified columnar epithelium with mucus-secreting glands	Lined by squamous or columnar epithelium and often have lymphoid tissue
Anatomic location	Almost always in the midline, from the tongue base to the thyroid isthmus; when adjacent to the thyroid cartilage, may lie slightly to one side of the midline	Lateral along the anterior border of the sternocleidomastoid, anywhere from the angle of the mandible to the clavicle
Physical	Cyst not only moves upwards on swallowing, but also on protrusion of the tongue, as it is attached by the tract remnant to the foramen cecum	Not so
Clinical	Cyst does not have a sinus opening to the skin unless infection has resulted in spontaneous drainage or an incomplete excision or incision and drainage procedure has previously been performed	Sinuses present as cutaneous openings marked by skin tags or subcutaneous cartilaginous remnants
	Discharges mucus	Nonpurulent drainage (before infection) cysts contain a yellow fluid, which on microscopy is rich in cholesterol, hence they do not transilluminate
Origin	Thyroglossal fistula is never congenital; it follows infection or inadequate removal of a thyroglossal cyst	Congenital
	Characteristically the cutaneous opening of a thyroglossal fistula is drawn upwards on protrusion of the tongue	Not so
Risk	Infection	Infection
	Malignant potential of the dysgenetic thyroid tissue	
Treatment	Sistrunk's operation	McFee step-ladder technique
Differential diagnosis	Dermoid inclusion cyst	Pathologic lymph nodes
	Pathologic lymph nodes	
	Cervical thymic cysts	
	Bronchogenic cysts	
	Ectopic thyroid tissue	

Table courtesy of Mohammed I. Ahmed, MBBS, MS (Surgery).

tiloculated masses that are usually evident at birth or occur during the first year or two of life. These masses are cavernous lymphatic malformations that can occur anywhere in the body but are most common in the posterior triangle of the neck. They often enlarge during upper respiratory tract infections. When allowed to enlarge massively, they may compress the larynx, the trachea, or the esophagus. These masses are unencapsulated arcades of disorganized, thinly lined, fluid-filled spaces that often surround vital nerves and blood vessels, making excision difficult. Before the lesions are excised, MRI scanning should be performed to delineate their extent and to rule out thoracic involvement. Complete surgical excision, although desirable, should not sacrifice important structures. With large hygromas, multiple excisions are likely to be necessary over the course of the first several years of life.

Congenital hemangiomas, usually easily diagnosed, are developmental abnormalities present at birth. They appear as bluish masses in the oral cavity, the pharynx, the parotid gland, or the neck, and they generally increase in size when the infant cries or strains. Because most hemangiomas regress spontaneously by the time the patient reaches 5 years of age, a conservative approach is warranted. Laser surgery or excision may be beneficial when hemangiomas do not resolve. Steroids have also been used with varying

degrees of success. Cutaneous hemangiomas of the head and neck are sometimes associated with hemangiomas of the airway, particularly of the subglottis. This diagnosis should always be considered in an infant with breathing difficulties and known facial hemangioma. Subglottic hemangioma can often be treated with a carbon dioxide laser.

Other Benign Neoplasms

Typically, benign neoplasms are slow-growing, nontender neck masses that are often present for a number of years. Lipomas are common asymptomatic soft masses located in the subcutaneous tissues or the deeper spaces of the neck; they are usually quite characteristic on physical examination. Lesions that enlarge or that are troublesome to the patient are excised. Neurogenic tumors consist primarily of schwannomas and neurofibromas. They arise from the peripheral nerve sheath of cranial nerves (e.g., the vagus or glossopharyngeal nerve) or from the cervical sympathetic chain. They usually occur as solitary lesions in the neck. Of the two neurogenic tumors, schwannomas are the more clinically benign. Because the individual nerve axons drape around the tumor, nerve-sparing excision should always be attempted. Neurofibromas are more difficult to treat because nerve fibers pass through the tumor rather than around it. Removing the tumor thus requires sacrificing the involved nerve. Patients with multiple neurofibromas should be suspected of having neurofibromatosis (von Recklinghausen's disease).

Malignant Tumors

Malignant lymphomas are the most common neoplastic neck mass among children and young adults, accounting for more than 50% of cases. The masses may be bilateral, are usually nontender, and enlarge progressively. Other signs and symptoms of lymphoma include hepatosplenomegaly, abnormal chest radiograph with hilar adenopathy, and weight loss. Lymphomas are classified as Hodgkin's or non-Hodgkin's. The nodular sclerosing histologic type of Hodgkin's disease is the most common and is often localized to the cervical and upper mediastinal lymph nodes. Pathologic confirmation is mandatory, and this is usually the only role played by surgery in treating this condition. Treatment generally consists of chemotherapy, irradiation, or both. For a complete discussion of lymphoma, see Chapter 25 in Lawrence's *Essentials of General Surgery*, 4th ed.

Rhabdomyosarcoma, usually the embryonal form, is the most common solid primary tumor of the neck in children. This lesion was once considered universally fatal, but the combined treatment of surgery, radiation, and chemotherapy has significantly improved survival rates.

Squamous cell carcinoma is the type of cancer that most commonly metastasizes to the neck; the primary site is usually in the upper aerodigestive tract. The mucosa of the upper aerodigestive tract should be carefully examined during a search for the primary tumor site. A chest radiograph should be obtained to check for lung metastasis and rule out the lung as a primary tumor site, particularly for supraclavicular masses. A CT scan or MRI can help determine the extent of large masses and their relation to the base of the skull, the prevertebral fasciae, and the carotid artery. Recently, positron emission tomography (PET) scanning has become popular for evaluating tumor extent and metastasis and even for identifying unknown primary site location. PET scanning utilizes a radiolabeled glucose molecule that is injected into the patient. The glucose is "taken up" by rapidly dividing cells (i.e., malignancies), therefore concentrating the radio isotope so that it can be identified on scanning. Fine-needle aspiration can often be used as part of the early evaluation to confirm the cytology. Open biopsy is not performed unless either the workup for a primary lesion or multiple attempts at fine-needle aspiration are unsuccessful. Treatment for the primary tumor site generally consists of irradiation, surgery, or both, depending on the site and size; neck dissection is performed to remove the nodal contents of the anterior and posterior triangles of the ipsilateral neck. For 5% to 10% of patients with metastatic squamous cell cancer of the neck, no primary tumor can be identified by examination or endoscopy. Treatment for these patients consists of radical neck dissection with possible irradiation treatment of the most likely primary tumor site. For 30% of these patients, the primary tumor will manifest itself within 2 years, making regular follow-up imperative.

Cancer metastatic to the neck from more distant sites—such as the lung, kidney, or gut—is usually treated with radiotherapy or chemotherapy. Melanoma metastatic to the neck will usually require neck dissection. Adjuvant postoperative radiotherapy for cervical melanoma metastasis is currently under study and may help to prevent regional recurrence of the disease. Metastatic thyroid cancer first may be seen as a nodal metastasis. The treatment is excision with total thyroidectomy. See Chapter 21 in Lawrence's *Essentials of General Surgery*, 4th ed, for a discussion of thyroid malignancy.

The Surgical Airway

The indications for a surgical airway are listed in Table 5-14. In most instances, a tracheotomy is performed in a controlled, planned procedure.

Cricothyrotomy

In cases of acute airway obstruction when attempted orotracheal intubation fails, the fastest, safest surgical airway is a **cricothyrotomy**. The technique involves making a vertical skin incision directly over the cricothyroid membrane. The incision can be spread horizontally, and the landmarks of the cricoid and cricothyroid membrane are palpated through the incision. The cricothyroid membrane is incised horizontally, opening the airway to allow the insertion of an available endotracheal tube. In young children, this is not possible, and the airway is best entered between the cricoid and the first tracheal ring (Fig. 5-17). Because there is a higher incidence of subglottic stenosis associated with cricothyrotomy, conversion to a tracheostomy is prudent if the airway is needed longer than a few days. See Lawrence's *Essentials of General Surgery*, 4th ed, Trauma chapter (especially Figs. 10-6 and 10-10) for further information.

Tracheotomy

Tracheotomy is the act of cutting the trachea to create an airway that bypasses the upper aerodigestive tract. The hole connecting the trachea to the skin is known as a tracheostomy. The procedure can be performed under local or

Table 5-14	Indications for Tracheotomy

Bypass upper airway obstruction
Expect prolonged ventilatory dependence (usually over 2 weeks)
Allow direct access for irrigation and suctioning of the airway (pulmonary toilet)
Prevent chronic aspiration
Decrease the dead space to overcome in patients with poor ventilatory effort or CNS depression

general anesthesia. A horizontal skin incision is made two fingerbreadths above the sternal notch and carried down through the subcutaneous tissue. The strap muscles are identified and spread apart in the midline, exposing the pretracheal fascia. Frequently, the thyroid isthmus overlies the trachea and must be retracted or divided. A tracheal hook is placed under the cricoid to elevate and expose the tracheal rings. A hole is created in the tracheal cartilage usually between the second and fourth tracheal rings. Stay sutures are placed in the tracheal cartilages to facilitate reinsertion of the tracheotomy tube accidentally displaced. In the intubated patient, this procedure can be performed percutaneously. A similar skin incision is made, and the trachea palpated within the incision. A needle is used to enter the trachea, and serial dilations of the tracheotomy site are performed over a wire and plastic stent.

After the tracheotomy is created, a tracheotomy tube is inserted, breath sounds are checked to ensure proper placement. The tube is sutured in and secured with circumferential ties around the neck. Because the patient with a tracheostomy tube has lost the access between the lower and upper airway, the nasal functions of warming and humidifying air are lost. Humidified air and frequent suctioning are important, especially in the early postoperative period, to keep the secretions from drying and plugging the airway. Potential early complications of tracheostomy are bleeding, mucous plugging, pneumothorax, accidental decannulation, false passage into the mediastinum, and cardiac arrest. Late complications include granulation tissue formation with bleeding and airway obstruction, persistent tracheocutaneous fistula following decannulation, tracheal stenosis, tracheoinnominate fistula, and tracheoesophageal fistula.

SUGGESTED READINGS

American Academy of Family Physicians, American Academy of Otolaryngology–Head and Neck Surgery, and American Academy of Pediatrics. Subcommittee on Otitis Media with Effusion. Otitis media with effusion. *Pediatrics* 2004;113:1312–1429.

American Academy of Pediatrics. Subcommittee on Management of Acute Otitis Media. Diagnosis and management of acute otitis media. *Pediatrics* 2004;113:1451–1465.

Benninger MS, Ferguson BJ, Hadley JA, et al. Adult chronic rhinosinusitis: definitions, diagnosis, epidemiology, and pathophysiology. *Otolaryngol Head Neck Surg* 2003;129(3 suppl)1:S1–S32.

Forastiere AA, Ang K, Brizel D, et al. Head and neck cancers. *J Nat Compr Canc Netw* 2005;3:316–391.

Forastiere AA, Goepfert H, Maor M, et al. Concurrent chemotherapy and radiotherapy for organ preservation in advanced laryngeal cancer. *N Engl J Med* 2003;249:2091–2098.

Ford C. Evaluation and management of laryngopharyngeal reflux. *JAMA* 2005;294:1534–1540.

Lawrence PF. *Essentials of General Surgery*, 4th ed. Philadelphia: Lippincott Williams & Wilkins; 2006.

Postma GN, Cohen JT, Belafsky PC, et al. Transnasal esophagoscopy: revisited. *Laryngoscope* 2005;115:321–323.

Shah JP, Lydiatt W. Treatment of cancer of the head and neck. *CA Canc J Clin* 1995;45:352–368.

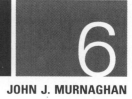

6

JOHN J. MURNAGHAN

Orthopedic Surgery: Diseases of the Musculoskeletal System

231

20 List and discuss common causes of low back pain and cervical pain.
21 Describe the signs and symptoms of lumbar or cervical disc herniation, and outline the diagnostic workup for these conditions.
22 Define osteoporosis and osteomalacia and list the common etiologies of each.
23 Discuss the pathophysiology, symptoms, and laboratory and radiographic findings of hyperparathyroidism and Paget's disease.

24 List the common primary and secondary malignant neoplasms of bone.
25 Outline the diagnostic workup for a patient with a suspected primary or secondary malignant neoplasm of bone.
26 Describe the basic components of gait, and discuss common gait abnormalities in relation to mechanical or neurologic disorders.

The musculoskeletal system is composed of connective tissue of mesodermal origin. Bones, joints, muscles, tendons, ligaments, and aponeurotic fascia constitute 70% of total body mass. Although disorders of the musculoskeletal system do not usually affect longevity, they frequently interfere with the quality of life. Musculoskeletal problems are the second most frequent cause of visits to a physician and are second in the consumption of health care dollars. Forty percent of emergency room visits are related to musculoskeletal problems. It is estimated that osteoporosis affects more than 20 million postmenopausal women and that associated hip fractures occupy almost 20% of surgical hospital beds. Back pain is the most common cause of time lost from work and disability in patients younger than 45 years of age. The annual cost of treatment and compensation for back conditions is greater than 14 billion dollars. Based on these statistics, it is clear that a working understanding of the musculoskeletal system is necessary to all physicians, especially those who practice primary care.

TRAUMA

Fractures, Subluxations, and Dislocations

A fracture is a break or loss of structural continuity in a bone. In a subluxation, the normally apposing joint surfaces are partially out of contact (Fig. 6-1A). In a dislocation, those surfaces are completely out of contact (see Fig. 6-1B). Joint subluxation may be a transient phenomenon in which the joint surfaces approach dislocation but reduces themselves.

Fractures

Description

Knowledge of the accepted fracture nomenclature allows for communication between medical colleagues and may affect decision making. Therefore, it is essential to describe fractures in a precise and detailed manner. Fractures are described according to type, site, pattern, and degree of displacement. In children, growth plate fractures are described according to the Salter-Harris classification of growth plate injuries (discussed below).

Type. Fractures are either open or closed. A fracture is open when there is a break in the surrounding skin or mucosa that allows the fracture to communicate with the external environment. Although most open fractures are obvious to cursory inspection, others, such as pelvic fractures, may communicate with the rectum or vagina and are discovered only in the course of a thorough physical examination. All open fractures are by definition contaminated and require emergency treatment to prevent infection. A fracture is closed when the skin or overlying mucosa is intact.

Fractures usually are the result of a single forceful impact. However, repeated submaximal stress can produce microscopic fractures, which, if not allowed to heal, will coalesce into a stress fracture (discussed below). Stress fractures are frequently seen in army recruits or in insufficiently conditioned patients who participate in vigorous athletic training routines. A fracture produced by minimal trauma through abnormal bone is termed a pathologic fracture. Pathologic fractures occur in bone that is weakened by metabolic bone diseases (e.g., osteoporosis) or in bone harboring primary or metastatic tumors.

Site. When describing the location of a fracture, the bone affected is identified, as well as the specific site involved; such as the proximal or distal epiphysis, metaphysis, or diaphysis (Fig. 6-2). A fracture in the epiphyseal region suggests intra-articular fracture extension that would violate the joint surface and could result in traumatic arthritis. By convention, the diaphysis of a long bone is described in thirds: proximal, middle, or distal (Fig. 6-2). Fracture location has implications for healing. Fractures of metaphyseal or cancellous (spongy) bone with a rich blood supply and high bone turnover rates usually heal quite rapidly. In contrast, cortical, diaphyseal bone heals more slowly. Diaphyseal fractures, therefore, require lengthier periods of stress protection by immobilization or protection from weight bearing.

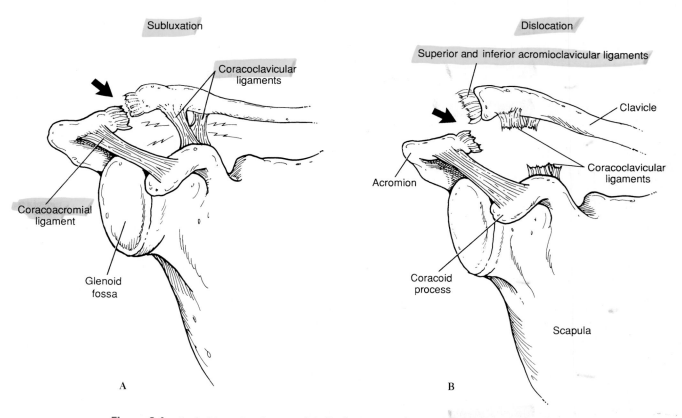

Figure 6-1 **A,** Subluxation is a partial displacement of apposing joint surfaces. This phenomenon may be transient and reduce itself. **B,** Dislocation is complete displacement of apposing joint surfaces. A reduction maneuver is often needed to restore joint alignment. (Modified from Rockwood C, Green D. *Fractures in Adults,* 3rd ed. Philadelphia: JB Lippincott; 1982:1193.)

Pattern. The fracture pattern suggests the type and amount of kinetic energy imparted to the bone. A transverse fracture (Fig. 6-3A) is a low-energy injury, usually the result of either a direct blow to a long bone or a ligament avulsion. A "nightstick" fracture is a transverse fracture of the ulna that occurs when the forearm is used to fend off a blow. Stress and pathologic fractures usually have a transverse pattern. Spiral or oblique fractures (see Fig. 6-3B,C) result from a rotatory, twisting injury. These fractures have a tendency to displace and shorten after reduction and immobilization. A fracture with more than two fragments is termed comminuted or multifragmented. The middle fragment may be triangular and is called a butterfly fragment (Fig. 6-4A); when cylindrical in configuration, it is described as segmental (Fig. 6-4B). Comminuted fractures occur as a result of larger forces and imply greater degrees of damage to the intramedullary blood supply to the bone and surrounding soft tissues, which may compromise the healing of one or both fracture sites. An impacted fracture (Fig. 6-5A; also see Fig. 6-15) is commonly seen in metaphyseal bone, such as with femoral neck, distal radius, or tibial plateau fractures. These are low-energy injuries in which two bone fragments are jammed together. A compression fracture signifies that trabecular or cancellous bone is crushed; it often occurs in vertebral bodies (Fig. 6-5B). Although most bone fractures are complete, an incomplete buckling of only one cortex is seen in children and is known as a greenstick fracture (Fig. 6-6).

Displacement. Fractured bone fragments may be displaced by the force of an injury, gravity, or muscle pull. Displacement is described in terms of anterior-posterior (AP), medial-lateral, and length (either shortening or distraction).

Displacement is described in both the mediolateral (coronal) and the anteroposterior (sagittal) planes. The position of the distal fragment is always named relative to the proximal fragment. This naming convention is helpful, because most fractures are aligned by reducing the displaced distal fragment to the proximal one. Fracture displacement is customarily quantified as a percentage (Fig. 6-7). This description can be misleading because 50% posterior (Fig. 6-7B) and 50% lateral displacement (Fig. 6-7A), may, when viewed in three dimensions, represent only 25% bone apposition (Fig. 6-7C). Angulation is the relationship between the long axis of the distal fragment

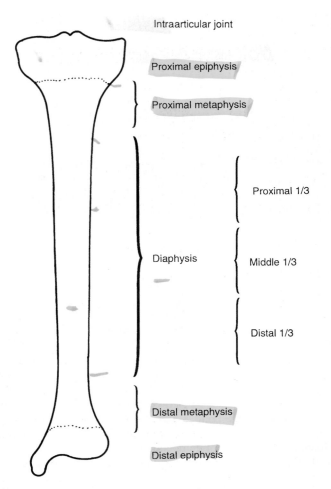

Intraarticular joint

Proximal epiphysis

Proximal metaphysis

Diaphysis

Proximal 1/3

Middle 1/3

Distal 1/3

Distal metaphysis

Distal epiphysis

Figure 6-2   Anatomic regions of a long tubular bone.

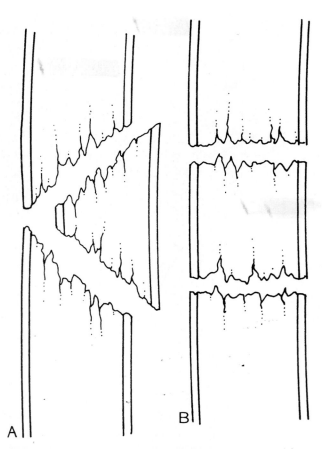

Figure 6-4   Comminuted fractures. **A,** Triangular butterfly fragment. **B,** Cylindrical segmental fracture.

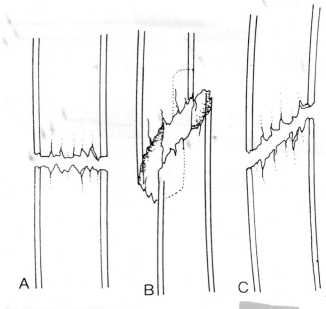

Figure 6-3   Common fracture patterns. **A,** Transverse fracture. **B,** Spiral fracture. **C,** Oblique fracture.

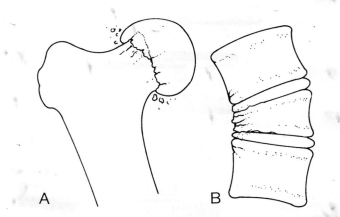

Figure 6-5   **A,** Impacted femoral neck fracture. **B,** Anterior compression fracture of vertebral body.

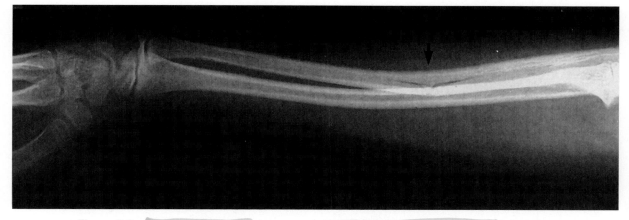

Figure 6-6 Greenstick fracture of the ulna in which only one cortex is broken (*arrow*) and the bone is bowed with its apex anterior. The fracture must be completed (the other cortex broken) to prevent angular deformity. Greenstick fractures typically occur in children whose bones are more plastic and less brittle than those of adults.

to the long axis of the proximal fragment. It may be described by one of two conventions. In the first convention, the direction to which the distal fragment is inclined is identified (Fig. 6-8). In the second convention, the location of the fracture angle apex is described. Reference to either the distal fragment or apical angulation should be mentioned in reports of fracture alignment. For example, in Figure 6-8, the distal fragment is inclined in the posterior and lateral directions, or the fracture apex is angled anteromedially.

The terms **varus** and **valgus** are also used in the descriptions of fractures and postural deformity. These terms refer to the direction of an angular deformity in relation to the midline of the body. If the deformity apex is pointed away from the midline (Fig. 6-9A), the term varus is used. If the deformity apex is directed toward the midline (Fig. 6-9B), it is called valgus. Thus, bowlegs in which the deformity apex at the knee (genu) is away from the midline are called **genu varum**, whereas knock-knees are called **genu valgum.**

Fracture apposition, angulation, and shortening are quantified in percentage, degrees, and centimeters, respectively, from radiographs. Rotation describes angular shifts around the long axis of the bone. It is best judged clinically. Rotational deformity is expressed by identifying the posi-

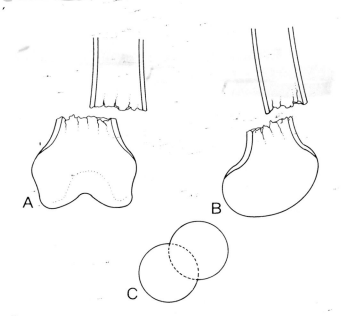

Figure 6-7 Fracture displacement. **A,** The anterior-posterior (*AP*) view shows approximately 50% lateral displacement of the distal fragment. **B,** The lateral view shows 50% posterior displacement of the distal femur. **C,** Additively in three dimensions, the amount of bone apposition is approximately 25%, an amount that is underestimated by either view (**A** or **B**) in isolation.

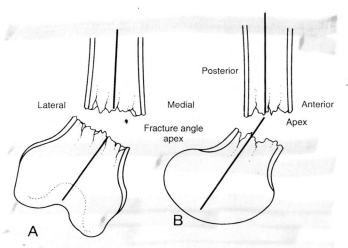

Figure 6-8 **A,** On the anterior-posterior view (coronal plane), the distal fragment is angulated laterally and the fracture angle apex is medial. **B,** On the lateral view (sagittal plane), the distal fragment is angulated posteriorly and the angle apex is anterior.

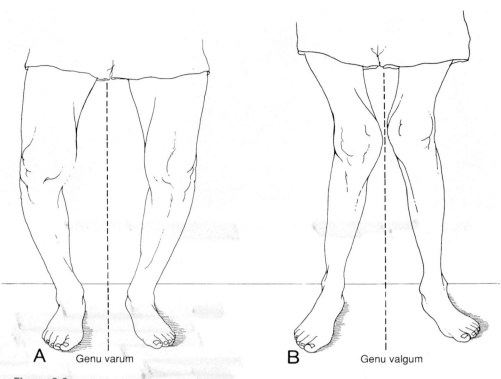

A   Genu varum

B   Genu valgum

Figure 6-9   The terms varus and valgus refer to the relation of a deformity to the midline of the body. **A,** Genu varum, or bowlegs, occurs when the deformity apex is pointing away from the midline. **B,** Genu valgum, or knock-knees, occurs when the deformity apex is directed toward the midline; it is called valgus. In knock-knees, the knee resembles the letter L, which is a helpful mnemonic in distinguishing between these confusing terms. (Modified from American Orthopaedic Association. *Manual of Orthopaedic Surgery,* 6th ed. Park Ridge, IL: American Orthopaedic Association; 1985.)

tion of the distal fragment as it relates to the proximal one. For example, if the foot is twisted outward, the fracture is externally rotated.

The Salter-Harris Classification of Growth Plate Fractures. In children, the growth plate (physis) is a zone of cartilage situated between the epiphysis and the metaphysis of long bones. Cartilage is weaker than bone and thus it is a common site of fracture. The Salter-Harris classification of growth plate injuries is descriptive, is generally recognized, and has important prognostic implications (Fig. 6-10).

The Salter-Harris type I fracture is a separation of the epiphysis from the metaphysis (Fig. 6-10). If the periosteum is not torn, the fracture remains undisplaced. In this injury, there is tenderness over the growth plate. The Salter-Harris type II fracture passes through the growth plate and exits through the metaphysis. This fracture is due to a bending movement that tears periosteum on the side opposite the triangular metaphyseal fragment. In a Salter-Harris type III injury, the fracture extends from the growth plate through the epiphysis to enter the joint. This fracture is intra-articular and requires a perfect reduction to avoid arthritic sequelae. The Salter-Harris type IV frac-

ture line extends from the metaphysis through the growth plate cartilage into the epiphysis. This fracture pattern is also intra-articular. These fractures must be operatively fixed to prevent nonunion and joint surface incongruity. Salter-Harris types III and IV fractures have the highest incidence of growth disturbance if not properly managed. A Salter-Harris type V fracture involves a crushing of the epiphyseal growth plate. These fractures may appear innocuous on radiographs and therefore are difficult to identify prospectively. The type V injury causes a bony bar to replace the growth plate, which will result in asymmetrical, angular growth.

Growth plate injuries, no matter how trivial, have the potential to cause growth disturbance of the involved long bone. The larger Salter-Harris numbers represent greater degrees of injury to the growth plate. Consequently, the type IV fracture has a poorer prognosis and higher incidence of growth disturbance than the type I injury. The possibility of a growth disturbance requires that all growth plate fractures be followed radiographically for at least 1 year after injury.

Evaluation of Patients with Musculoskeletal Trauma

The patient usually has a history of injury, although in pathologic fractures the injury may be minimal. In chil-

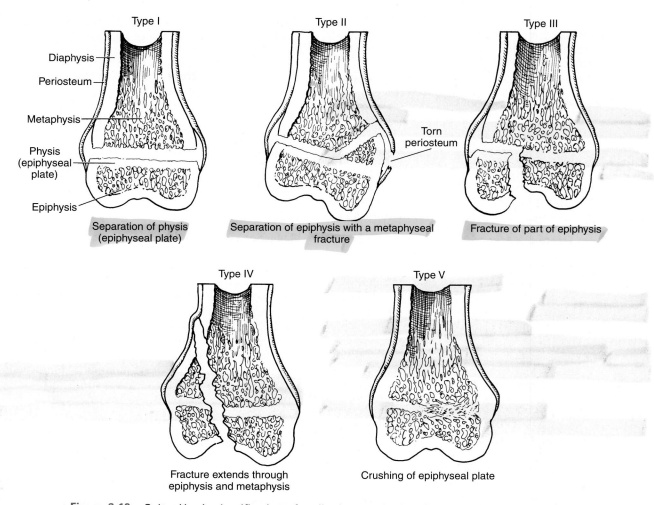

Figure 6-10   Salter-Harris classification of pediatric growth plate fractures. The greater the classification number, the more violent is the injury to the epiphyseal plate and the greater the risk of long bone growth and healing problems. (Reprinted with permission from Rang MC. *Children's Fractures,* 2nd ed. Philadelphia: JB Lippincott; 1983.)

dren, either a limp or the refusal to use an extremity suggests a possible fracture. Symptoms of musculoskeletal injury include pain, swelling, and deformity. Bony tenderness, crepitus, or deformity strongly suggests a fracture. The examiner should inspect the extremity circumferentially for small puncture wounds. Vascular integrity (pulses, capillary return) and neurologic status (sensory, motor, and reflex functions) must be assessed and documented. Active motion of articulations distal to the fracture site implies an element of soft tissue integrity and neurologic function. The two most important clinical features of the fracture (whether it is open or not and whether the neurovascular status is compromised) are determined by clinical examination before x-ray films are obtained.

A complete radiologic evaluation includes the following:

1 Two views of the affected bone or joint at right angles to each other must be taken. Because fractures occur in three dimensions, a single radiographic view will not permit an accurate description (i.e., displacement and angulation) of the injury (Fig. 6-7). Two views taken perpendicular to each other, usually an AP and a lateral view meet these requirements.

2 The joint above and the joint below the injured area must be visualized. It is not uncommon for a knee injury or hip fracture to be associated with a fracture of the femoral shaft.

3 Known injury associations warrant special radiographic examination. Cervical spine radiographs are mandatory in all patients with facial and head injuries; hip dislocations are associated with injuries to the knee. Fractures of the axial skeleton (spine and pelvis) occur with injuries to the thoracic, abdominal, or pelvic viscera, as well as neural structures.

4 If a fracture is not evident radiographically but is suspected clinically (e.g., scaphoid fracture), the patient will not be harmed if the extremity is immobilized

and reassessed. Repeated radiographs, stress views, or other imaging techniques — such as polytomography, bone scan, computed tomography (CT), or magnetic resonance imaging (MRI) — may be needed to establish the diagnosis.

Trauma patients with long bone fractures are prone to fat embolism. Clinical examination should watch for petechiae in conjunction with alteration of mental status. Patients are often dyspneic and have low oxygen saturation. Chest x-ray films reveal diffuse opacification without focal findings. Fat embolism syndrome is a clinical diagnosis because there is no specific laboratory finding. Treatment is supportive and in severe cases may require intubation and positive pressure ventilation with up to 100% O_2.

Principles of Fracture Management

A patient with a fracture should be managed as a traumatized patient (see Chapter 10 in Lawrence's *Essentials of General Surgery*, 4th ed.). Life-threatening conditions are always treated first. It is essential to check the integrity of neural and vascular structures distal to any fracture site. All musculoskeletal injuries must be splinted in the field. Splints are to remain in place whenever the patient is transported. Splinting prevents fracture motion, thus minimizing further damage to the surrounding soft tissues (nerves, blood vessels, and muscle; shown in Fig. 6-16), limits blood loss, and decreases the pain of injury. Proper splinting requires that the joint above and the one below the fracture site be immobilized. Similarly, with a dislocation, the bone above and the bone below the joint should be splinted.

All open fractures are considered contaminated with bacteria. Treatment is aimed at preventing subsequent infection. After the extremity has been splinted, a culture is taken from the wound and the wound is covered with a sterile dressing. Tetanus prophylaxis is administered if necessary (see Chapter 3) and antibiotic treatment initiated. Intravenous first-generation cephalosporin is used for mildly contaminated wounds. Extensive open wounds or those that occurred in barnyards should receive an aminoglycoside and metronidazole (Flagyl) in addition. The patient is prepared for surgery, preferably under general anesthesia. A 1-mm margin of devitalized skin is excised, with care being taken not to sacrifice viable skin. The wound is extended as needed to expose the bone ends and debride all foreign material and necrotic tissue. The wound is irrigated with copious amounts of normal saline ($\geq$6 L). Only after thorough irrigation and surgical debridement is an open fracture reduced and immobilized. The wound is reexplored 48 to 72 hours later for debridement of tissue that was marginally viable at first surgery and has subsequently necrosed. Delayed wound closure or the need for special soft tissue coverage techniques (e.g., a myocutaneous or a free microvascular flap) are planned at the "second look" procedure (see Chapter 3).

Fracture management requires knowledge of the stages of fracture healing (Table 6-1). The two principles of fracture care are obtaining a reduction and maintaining the reduction.

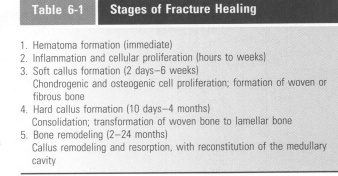

Table 6-1	Stages of Fracture Healing

1. Hematoma formation (immediate)
2. Inflammation and cellular proliferation (hours to weeks)
3. Soft callus formation (2 days–6 weeks)
   Chondrogenic and osteogenic cell proliferation; formation of woven or fibrous bone
4. Hard callus formation (10 days–4 months)
   Consolidation; transformation of woven bone to lamellar bone
5. Bone remodeling (2–24 months)
   Callus remodeling and resorption, with reconstitution of the medullary cavity

Reduction. Fracture deformity is reduced to restore bone apposition and alignment. Reduction can be achieved by closed or open methods. Closed reduction involves the manipulation of the fracture into a functional position. Generally, in a closed reduction, traction is applied to the distal segment to separate the impacted fragments. Force is applied to realign the bone fragments. When closed reduction has been unsuccessful, an open reduction may be required. The fracture is surgically exposed, and bone fragments are manipulated directly. Open reduction is indicated when closed reduction methods fail or with intra-articular fractures in which the joint surface must be perfectly restored to prevent the development of post-traumatic arthritis.

Maintenance of Reduction. Once the fracture has been reduced, alignment must be maintained until the process of bone healing is completed. Maintaining alignment requires some form of fracture immobilization, which may include casting, traction, functional bracing, and internal or external fixation. The type of immobilization employed depends on fracture stability or its propensity for displacement. A circumferential plaster or fiberglass cast is the traditional method of immobilization. A cast protects and maintains fracture alignment until healing occurs. Early clinical and radiographic follow up is necessary to ensure that fracture reduction is not lost as swelling diminishes.

Continuous traction applied through the skin, the skeleton, or by gravity is a technique that can both effect and maintain reduction. With skin traction, a foam rubber boot or sleeve is wrapped directly against the skin and traction is applied via friction of the foam–skin interface. The risk of skin breakdown limits the amount of traction that can be used to no more than 7 lb. Therefore, skin traction is useful in small children or to temporarily splint an adult with a hip fracture before surgery. Skeletal traction requires that a pin be inserted through bone distal to the fracture site. Large **distraction** forces can then be applied directly to the bone and can overcome the contractile forces of large muscles in patients with pelvic, femoral, or tibial fractures (Fig. 6-11). A common site for skeletal traction pin placement is the proximal tibia (occasionally, the distal femur or calcaneus); in the upper extremity the pin placement site is often through the olecranon process

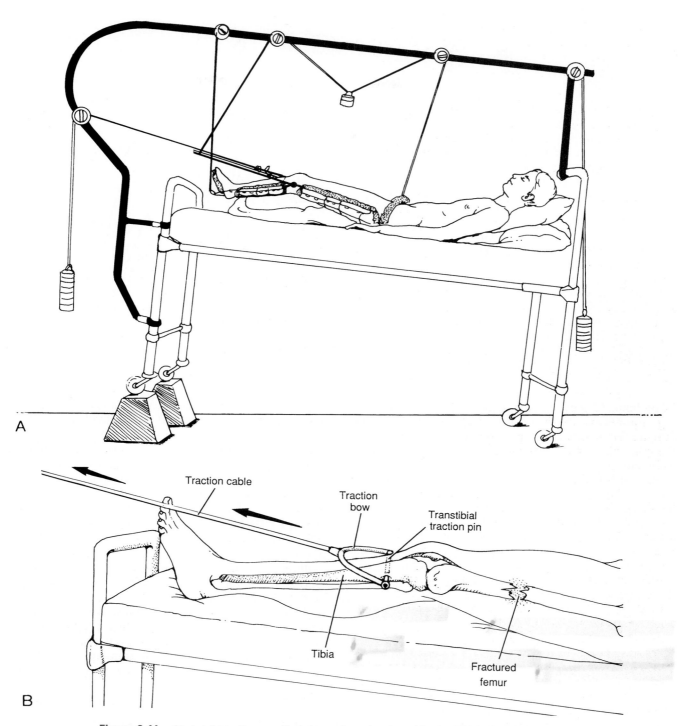

A

B

Traction cable

Traction bow

Transtibial traction pin

Tibia

Fractured femur

Figure 6-11   Skeletal traction applied through a pin placed in the tibia is useful for treating femur or pelvic fractures. The leg is supported in a suspension apparatus, and the foot of the bed is raised to permit body weight and gravity to act as countertraction.

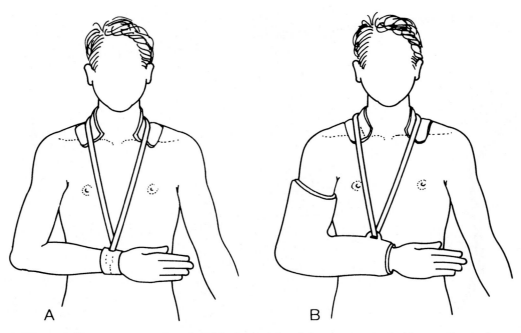

Figure 6-12 Gravity traction. **A,** With the weight of the arm supported by a collar and cuff. **B,** With a hanging cast.

of the ulna. Gravity acting through a dependent extremity can also act as a traction force. In humeral fractures, the weight of the distal arm applies traction if the body is kept upright (Fig. 6-12A). Application of a forearm cast can augment this type of traction (Fig. 6-12B).

Several complications are associated with casts and traction. Circumferential bandages may cause circulatory impairment in acutely traumatized limbs in which further swelling is expected. A cast or dressing that is too tight must be completely released to the level of skin. Excessive traction can cause nonunion and peripheral nerve injury. Ulcerative skin problems may occur with both skin and skeletal traction. Skeletal traction causes frictional shearing forces between the patient's sacrum and the bed, which can result in a sacral decubitus ulcer. A poorly applied cast can cause a pressure ulcer over an inadequately padded bony prominence or a displaced bone end. Joint stiffness and muscle atrophy are common problems after prolonged immobilization.

Functional braces allow for early joint motion while maintaining fracture alignment through a compressive hydraulic effect on the soft tissues. Conversion from a cast or splint to a functional brace after early evidence of fracture healing hastens both healing and rehabilitation.

Internal fixation devices include pins, screws, plates (Fig. 6-13), circumferential wires or bands, and intramedullary rods (see Fig. 6-19). Indications for internal fixation are listed in Table 6-2. Metallic fracture fixation implants may appear sturdy on radiographs. However, like a cast, they simply position the fracture until healing is complete. Fracture fixation hardware should be considered an internal splint that must respect the biology of fracture healing.

The mere presence of an internal fixation device does not guarantee fracture healing. If the fracture does not unite, repetitive (cyclic) loading of a fracture implant will ultimately lead to its loosening or to metal fatigue and breakage. Whenever internal fixation is employed, there is a race between fracture healing and implant failure. Although internal fixation enhances early patient mobility, it has a number of potential complications. Internal fixation requires a surgical exposure that itself can devitalize tissue and adds to the risk of infection and nonunion. A second surgical procedure may be needed if the implant is to be removed. Finally, after hardware removal, the bone can refracture through screw holes, especially when they are in cortical, diaphyseal bone.

External fixation is a minimally invasive method of maintaining fracture alignment. Threaded pins are placed into the bone above and below the fracture site and are attached to an external frame to immobilize the fracture (Fig. 6-14). It functions as a portable traction device. Indications for external fixation are listed in Table 6-3. Complications include pin track infection and delayed union.

Rehabilitation of Function. Rehabilitation planning begins with the initial phases of fracture management. To avoid joint stiffness common to periarticular and intra-articular fractures, the limb is immobilized in a position of maximum function. Isometric exercises of immobilized muscles are started to avoid excessive atrophy. Range-of-motion exercises for adjacent joints that are not immobilized are encouraged from the onset of care. After a cast or brace is removed, active range-of-motion and resistive muscle strengthening exercises are initiated.

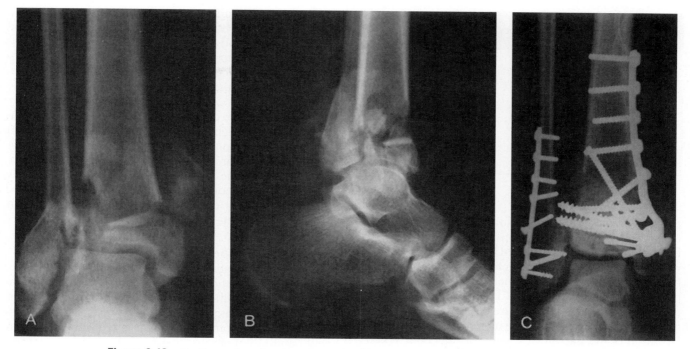

Figure 6-13 Radiographs of a comminuted ankle fracture. **A,** Anterior-posterior radiograph. **B,** Lateral radiograph. **C,** Intra-articular fracture treated with a complex array of internal fixation plates and screws.

The speed of rehabilitation depends on the rate and quality of fracture healing. Exuberant rehabilitative activities or exercises may result in delayed healing, implant failure, and loss of reduction. A rational rehabilitation plan incorporates those factors that influence the speed and success of fracture healing. These factors include the amount of energy imparted to the bone during injury (open, multifragmented, and displaced fractures heal slowly), the type of bone involved (cancellous or cortical), the integrity of the soft tissue envelope, and the patient's general health and age (children heal more rapidly than adults).

Bone healing is evaluated clinically and radiologically. Clinically, healing is evident when the fracture is no longer tender to palpation or stress. Radiographically, healing is evident when distinct bony trabeculae are seen crossing the fracture site on radiographic images.

Complications of Fracture Healing

Local Complications
Local complications of fracture healing include infection, delayed union, nonunion, malunion, avascular necrosis, and, in children, growth disturbances. Fractures that are open, either from injury or surgical intervention, have a higher incidence of infection than closed fractures. Delayed union is characterized by fracture healing that ap-

Table 6-2	Indications for Internal Fixation of a Fracture

Failure of nonoperative reduction methods
Anatomic reduction of intra-articular fractures
Fractures not amenable to traction or cast immobilization (e.g., femoral neck fractures, intertrochanteric fractures in the elderly)
Pathologic fractures
Multiple fractures in the same extremity or same patient
Fractures in paraplegics (to assist nursing care)

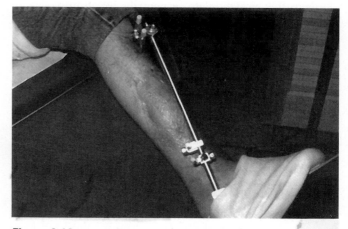

Figure 6-14 Severely comminuted open tibia fracture treated with an external fixator. This form of fixation immobilizes the fracture while permitting access to the wound for observation and care.

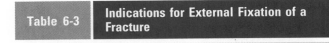

Table 6-3	Indications for External Fixation of a Fracture

Open, unstable fractures (to allow access to and care of the wound and to avoid the use of internal fixation devices in contaminated wounds)
Infected fractures
Unstable pelvic fractures
Severely comminuted or unstable fractures not amenable to internal fixation
Fractures involving bone loss in which bone length must be maintained until a bone graft can be performed

pears to be taking place, but slower than the usual. Non-union is characterized by incomplete and nonprogressive fracture healing. The nonunited fracture gap may be filled with fibrous tissue or, if subjected to significant motion, may form a synovial membrane with joint fluid called a pseudarthrosis (a "false joint"). Delayed unions and non-unions are caused by fracture separation, soft tissue interposition, excessive fracture motion, inadequate vascularization of the fracture segments, or infection. When a fracture heals with a deformity that causes cosmetic or functional impairment, it is called a malunion. Malunited fractures can be shortened, angulated, or rotated. A corrective osteotomy may be required to regain alignment and function.

Avascular necrosis occurs when the blood supply to a bone is injured by the traumatic event (see Bone Necrosis later in this chapter). Bones that are extensively covered by articular cartilage and have a minimal muscular envelope are particularly vulnerable to osteonecrosis (e.g., the femoral head, the scaphoid, or the talus).

Growth disturbance is a fracture complication specific to children. The epiphyseal plate is composed of cartilage and is the site of longitudinal growth in bones. Because cartilage is weaker than bone, the growth plate is often involved in pediatric fractures. Fractures in children may damage the growth plate, especially by compressive or shearing mechanisms. When the entire growth plate is damaged, growth will cease and the affected limb will be shorter than the unaffected limb by the end of growth. If only part of the epiphyseal plate is damaged, the bone may grow asymmetrically and cause an angular deformity. A growth plate injury can be detected only by serial radiographs. Most growth plate problems can be identified by radiographs taken at the 1-year anniversary of the injury, a date that parents should mark down so they are reminded to present for follow-up radiographs. Lower limb shortening of less than 1 cm is well tolerated; shortening between 1 and 2 cm can be managed by a shoe lift. A leg length discrepancy of more than 2 cm can be corrected by fusion of the opposite growth plate, a procedure known as epiphysiodesis. The timing of this procedure is calculated from growth tables. Angular deformity from a partial growth plate arrest is managed surgically and is best handled when diagnosed early.

Post-traumatic arthritis is a complication of displaced intra-articular fractures. Articular cartilage has no blood supply and depends on synovial fluid for nourishment. When injured, articular cartilage has minimal healing potential. If intra-articular fractures are not anatomically reduced, the irregular surface may cause rapid arthritic change.

Arthritis can also develop indirectly from a severe angular deformity. Weight-bearing forces can be concentrated in the part of the joint causing abnormal stress concentration and joint wear. Depending on the magnitude of injury, post-traumatic arthritis can occur rapidly or slowly over a decade or more. Patients who have had a traumatic hip dislocation, for example, usually have hip arthritis in 10 to 20 years later.

Systemic Complications

Systemic complications are unusual following a fracture. Systemic complications usually result from trauma in general and not from the fracture itself. These complications include shock, sepsis, tetanus (in open injuries), gas gangrene, venous thrombosis, and fat embolism. The emergent stabilization of spine, pelvic, and long bone fractures is necessary to minimize blood loss and to allow a patient to sit upright and receive proper pulmonary physiotherapy. Accomplishing this can significantly decrease the incidence of respiratory insufficiency in multisystem trauma patients.

Joint Subluxation and Dislocation

Diagnosis and Evaluation

Subluxation of a joint is usually a transient phenomenon, when articular surfaces of a joint become partially separated. When a joint is dislocated, the articular surfaces of a joint are no longer in contact with each other. The patient is reluctant to move it. The limb may be held in a typical posture (e.g., when a hip is posteriorly dislocated, the thigh is held in flexion, adduction, and internal rotation). Neurovascular structures, in close proximity to joints, can be injured with dislocations, especially in older patients whose arteries may be thickened by atherosclerotic plaque. Not all vascular injuries are acute occlusive phenomena. An intimal tear of the artery may slowly cause thrombus formation, delaying the presentation of vascular compromise. Therefore, serial neurovascular evaluations are essential after the reduction of a dislocated joint. Asymmetry in pulses, which is detected by palpation or Doppler ultrasonography, warrants further vascular workup, especially in young patients who have had little stimulus to develop collateral circulation.

Radiographs of the involved joint are obtained in the dislocated posture. This radiograph demonstrates the pathology and allows the treating physician to infer which specific ligamentous structures are damaged. Like a fracture, a dislocation can be described as open or closed and according to the position of the distal fragment relative to the proximal fragment. If radiographic assessment will be delayed and if skin is compromised (e.g., ankle fracture or dislocation) or if neurovascular integrity is in question (e.g., knee dislocations), then reduction should be attempted immediately.

Treatment

Dislocations are usually realigned by traction along the normal axis of the extremity. Occasionally, bone or soft tissue may be interposed between joint surfaces and will require a surgical (open) reduction. Postreduction radiographs must be taken to ensure the adequacy of reduction and rule out an associated fracture.

Common Musculoskeletal Injuries

Upper Extremity

Carpal Scaphoid Fracture. The scaphoid is the bone most frequently fractured of the carpal bones. A fracture through the waist of the scaphoid usually occurs after a fall on the outstretched hand, with the wrist positioned in dorsiflexion and radial deviation. If a fracture is suspected from the mechanism of injury and tenderness in the anatomic snuff box, the patient should be treated as if there were a fracture (even if radiographic views do not indicate a fracture). A bone scan, CT scan, or follow-up radiographs at 7 to 14 days will confirm or disprove the diagnosis. The scaphoid bone is extensively covered by hyaline cartilage and has limited soft tissue attachments and blood supply. Complications of avascular necrosis, delayed union, and nonunion are increased by failure to treat a scaphoid fracture initially. Undisplaced fractures are treated in a thumb spica cast (a forearm cast extended to incorporate the thumb in the pinch position). Displaced scaphoid fractures are treated by open reduction and internal fixation.

Distal Radius Fracture. A distal radius fracture is also caused by falling on an outstretched hand. When this injury causes a transverse fracture of the distal radius just proximal to the wrist it is referred to as a Colles fracture. It is a common fracture in elderly, osteoporotic patients. Radiographically, dorsal comminution can be noted, and the distal fragment is impacted and shortened with apex palmar angulation (Fig. 6-15). The ulnar styloid is often fractured.

Reduction is obtained by longitudinal traction applied to the hand, disimpacting the fracture. The wrist and distal fragment are manipulated into flexion and ulnar deviation to correct the dorsal and radial displacement. After reduction, a splint is applied from the elbow to the palm. A repeat radiograph should be taken following reduction at approximately 10 days to assess whether the reduction has been maintained. If it has not, a repeat manipulation or external fixation is required. The deformity tends to recur because of dorsal cortical comminution. Occasionally, a Kirschner wire, or K-wire, is inserted percutaneously to prevent loss of fracture alignment.

The median nerve is in close proximity to the volar aspect of the wrist. Its function must be documented be-

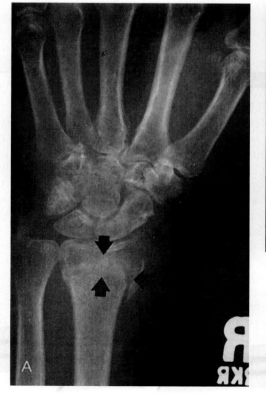
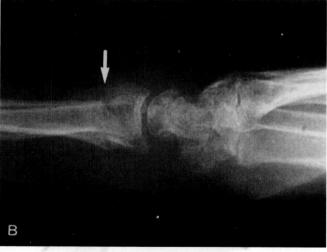

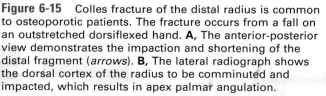

Figure 6-15 Colles fracture of the distal radius is common to osteoporotic patients. The fracture occurs from a fall on an outstretched dorsiflexed hand. **A,** The anterior-posterior view demonstrates the impaction and shortening of the distal fragment (*arrows*). **B,** The lateral radiograph shows the dorsal cortex of the radius to be comminuted and impacted, which results in apex palmar angulation.

fore and after fracture manipulation. The shoulder–hand syndrome is a common complication of a Colles' fracture in the elderly. In this syndrome, shoulder and finger stiffness results from disuse during the treatment period. Patients are encouraged to exercise the shoulder and fingers during the early phases of fracture healing.

Olecranon Fracture. An olecranon fracture is usually caused by a fall in which there is a direct blow to the point of the elbow. The fracture is displaced by contraction of the triceps muscle. Thus, there is loss of active elbow extension. The fracture also involves the elbow joint surface. Any displacement of the fracture fragments requires an open reduction to restore the articular surface and triceps integrity.

Pulled Elbow. This is a painful condition that affects young children aged 1 to 4 years. It occurs frequently when the child has been pulled forcibly by the hand. The child tends to hold the elbow slightly flexed and avoids moving it. The pain is believed to be due to impingement of the annular ligament of the radial neck. Treatment is to flex the elbow slightly and supinate the child's hand. This repositions the annular ligament around the radial neck and relieves the symptoms.

Supracondylar Humerus Fracture. A supracondylar humerus fracture is commonly seen in children 5 to 10 years of age. It occurs from a fall on an outstretched hand with the elbow extended. The distal fragment is usually displaced posteriorly. It can cause significant neurovascular complications by entrapping the brachial artery and the median and radial nerves, either at injury or during reduction (Fig. 6-16). This fracture is a frequent cause of a forearm **compartment syndrome** because of ischemia (Volkmann's ischemic contracture). It must be treated with great care and vigilance. Usual management of displaced fractures is with prompt reduction and percutaneous pin fixation in the operating room.

A forearm compartment syndrome can be caused by kinking of the brachial artery at the site of the supracondylar fracture. If the flow of blood with the delivery of oxygen and removal of metabolic waste from the muscles is not restored, severe and even permanent muscle injury can occur. If muscle is ischemic at normal body temperature for more than 2 hours, there is some permanent muscle damage. If the warm ischemia time exceeds 8 hours, then the muscle is likely dead and revascularizing the limb can lead to systemic complications from hyperkalemia and release of myoglobin. The flexor compartment of the forearm is completely dependent on the blood supply from the brachial artery. If the muscles die, the fibers contract and leave a nonfunctional hand due to fingers and thumb that are flexed into the palm. There is no effective tendon transfer to restore hand and wrist function when the entire flexor compartment has stiffened and scarred.

Shoulder Dislocation. The shoulder is the most frequently dislocated joint in the body. In more than 90% of trau-

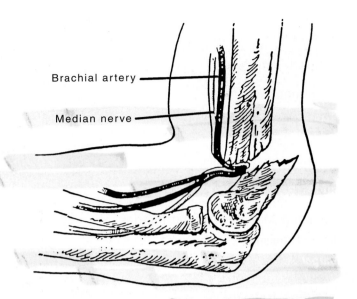

Figure 6-16 The dangerous supracondylar distal humerus fracture may entrap the brachial artery and the median and radial nerves. This fracture is associated with forearm compartment syndrome and warrants cautious and frequent neurovascular monitoring. (Reprinted with permission from American Academy of Orthopaedic Surgeons. *Athletic Training and Sports Medicine,* 2nd ed. Park Ridge, IL: American Academy of Orthopaedic Surgeons; 1991:277.)

matic dislocations, the humeral head is anterior to the scapular glenoid fossa (Fig. 6-17A). The axillary nerve and artery can be endangered by this injury. The integrity of the axillary nerve should be documented by testing sensation over the deltoid patch and motor function of the deltoid muscle before and after reduction of the shoulder dislocation. An anterior shoulder dislocation occurs with forced external rotation of the abducted arm. This type of injury may be caused by an arm tackle in football or by blocking a basketball shot.

Reduction can be achieved by gradual shoulder abduction while longitudinal traction is placed on the arm and countertraction is placed through the axilla with a sheet (Fig. 6-17B). Sedation and muscle relaxation facilitate the manipulation.

Posterior shoulder dislocations, although rare, are often missed because of improper interpretation of the AP radiograph, which appears to show the humeral head aligned with the glenoid. An axillary view shows the humeral head to lie posterior to the glenoid, which should reinforce the principle that two radiographs taken in perpendicular planes are needed for proper radiographic evaluation of any bony structure. Clinically, the arm is held internally rotated and cannot be externally rotated beyond the neutral position. A posterior dislocation should be considered in all patients with shoulder symptoms after an electrocution or a seizure due to epilepsy, alcohol withdrawal, electroconvulsive therapy, or electrocution.

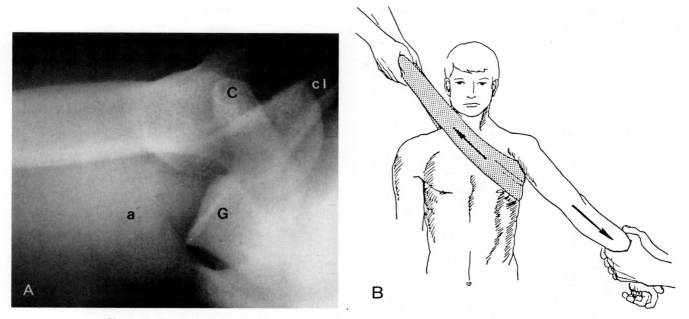

Figure 6-17   **A,** Axillary lateral radiograph of an anterior shoulder dislocation. The humeral head lies out of the glenoid fossa (*G*). The coracoid process (*C*) is an anterior scapular structure and orients the film. **B,** Closed reduction of an anterior shoulder dislocation via traction countertraction. *a,* acromion; *cl,* clavicle. (Reprinted with permission from Rockwood C, Green D. *Fractures in Adults,* 3rd ed. Philadelphia: JB Lippincott; 1982:1092.)

Lower Extremity

Hip Fractures. Low-energy hip fractures are common in elderly, osteoporotic patients. They account for about 33% of admissions to large orthopedic centers. The common types are femoral neck (Fig. 6-5A) and intertrochanteric hip fractures (Fig. 6-18). In both fractures, the affected limb is externally rotated and shortened. The patient cannot bear weight and slight amounts of hip motion cause pain.

The blood supply to the femoral head comes from vessels that run along the posterior femoral neck. These vessels can be damaged by a femoral neck fracture. If the femoral head is rendered avascular, the bone cells die. When dead bone is subjected to repetitive weight-bearing loads, it will collapse and fragment. Femoral neck fractures have a higher incidence of nonunion because the fracture is within the hip joint (intracapsular), with a thin periosteum and no muscle envelope. Femoral neck fractures are either reduced and surgically fixed or, because of attendant complications, replaced with a metal hemiarthroplasty. An intertrochanteric hip fracture occurs outside the hip joint (extracapsular). There is a good blood supply, and the fracture usually heals (Fig. 6-18A). Intertrochanteric fractures are reduced under radiographic guidance and fixed with a sliding screw and sideplate device (Fig. 6-18B). Surgical treatment allows for early patient mobilization and decreases problems related to prolonged bed confinement (e.g., pneumonia, thrombophlebitis, decubitus ulcers).

Femoral Shaft Fractures. The femoral shaft is the strongest bone in the body. In young patients, femur fractures require high-energy trauma and are incurred by motor vehicle accidents and falls from heights. Blood loss may be considerable. In a closed fracture, 1 to 3 units of blood may be lost into the thigh and the patient may present in hypovolemic shock. Other sources of hypovolemia (e.g., such as intra-abdominal and intrathoracic injuries or pelvic fractures) must be excluded. In all patients with a fractured femur, the pelvis and hip must be assessed radiologically to rule out associated fractures or dislocations. Knee stability should be evaluated.

Closed, interlocked intramedullary nailing is the preferred treatment (Fig. 6-19). Because the nail can be locked proximally and distally, the fracture can be rendered quite stable and allow early ambulation. This approach prevents the lengthy periods of bed rest required with skeletal traction (Fig. 6-11) and minimizes the risks of venous thrombosis, knee stiffness, quadriceps contracture, muscle atrophy, and disuse osteoporosis.

Hip Dislocation. Hip dislocation often occurs in motor vehicle accidents when the knee strikes the dashboard. Seated posture places the hip in adduction and 90 degrees of flexion. The longitudinal load of unrestrained dashboard impact drives the hip posteriorly out of the acetabular socket and may stretch the sciatic nerve. All patients with posterior hip dislocations should be assessed for a foot

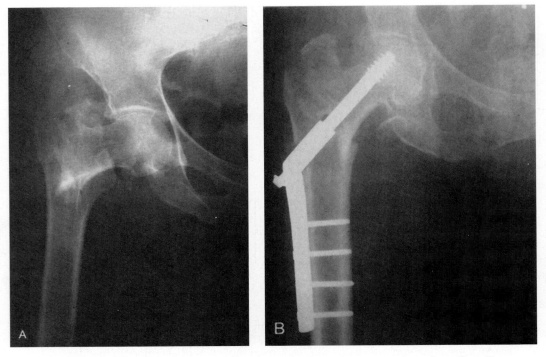

Figure 6-18   **A,** Intertrochanteric hip fracture. The bone is osteopenic and rarefied. **B,** This fracture has been reduced and internally fixed with a screw and sideplate device. This type of fixation will permit early patient mobilization.

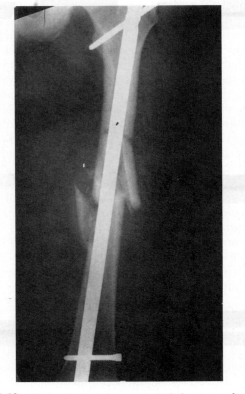

Figure 6-19   Comminuted femoral shaft fracture after internal fixation with an interlocked intramedullary nail.

drop. The hip should be reduced urgently and associated fractures repaired to restore stability of the hip joint. Delays in treatment beyond 8 to 12 hours from injury can increase the risks for avascular necrosis of the femoral head and post-traumatic arthritis of the hip.

Tibia and Fibular Shaft Fracture.   Shaft fractures of the tibia and fibula occur nine times more often than femoral shaft fractures. Almost 33% of the tibial surface is subcutaneous. For this reason, tibia fractures are often open and contaminated. The limited blood supply to the tibia causes fractures of this bone to have delayed union and nonunion. Tibia fractures are at risk for compartment syndrome (discussed later), which requires attentive observation and early diagnosis. The key clinical sign in a conscious patient is pain that is out of proportion to the injury. Complications associated with tibia fracture management are the most frequent cause of trauma-related orthopedic malpractice suits.

Closed reduction and above-the-knee cast immobilization are the standard treatment for uncomplicated closed fractures of the tibia and fibula. Open reduction and internal fixation are considered only when an acceptable reduction cannot be achieved by closed means or the reduction cannot be maintained by a plaster cast. External fixation (Fig. 6-14) is frequently used in managing open fractures of the tibia: stability and alignment of the fracture fragments are maintained while allowing access to treat the soft tissue wound. Current trends are toward adequate surgical debridement at the time of injury followed by internal fixation. The implant of choice is a reamed intramedullary nail.

Ankle Injuries. Ankle injuries are common in young, athletic individuals and may involve both ligamentous and bony structures. The ankle is a mortise and tenon joint. The three-sided mortise is composed of the tibial malleolus, the tibial plafond (ceiling), and the fibular malleolus. The talus represents the tenon. The mechanism of injury can be inferred from the plane of the fracture line (Fig. 6-20). A transverse fracture line occurs from a tensile or "pulling off" force. Thus, when the medial malleolus fracture is transverse, it suggests an abduction (eversion or pronation) force of the foot on the leg (Fig. 6-20B and 6-20C). If the lateral malleolus fracture is transverse, the force applied to the foot is adduction (inversion or supination; Fig. 6-20A). A spiral fracture configuration implies a rotatory force. A coronal plane spiral fracture is a common lateral malleolar fracture pattern and is seen when the foot is externally rotated on the leg and body (Fig. 6-20C). Bimalleolar ankle fractures are common. When a posterior tibial fragment is seen on the lateral radiograph, it is called a trimalleolar fracture and results from vertical loading of the plantar flexed ankle (Fig. 6-20D).

Because ankle fractures are intra-articular, anatomic restoration of the joint congruity is an essential treatment principle. One millimeter of ankle displacement can reduce joint surface contact by 40%. Anatomic open reduction with internal fixation is the ideal treatment for displaced ankle fractures.

Spinal and Pelvic Fractures

Spinal and pelvic fractures in young people result from high-velocity trauma and are associated with intrathoracic, intra-abdominal, and extremity injuries. In the elderly, spine fractures may occur after minimal trauma in bone that is weakened by osteoporosis or tumor.

Spinal Fractures. Spinal stability is the critical concept in the treatment of spinal fractures. The spine is unstable if unprotected movement causes fracture displacement that can compromise the integrity of neural structures. In all cases of suspected spinal injury, a complete and detailed baseline neurologic assessment should be performed and documented as soon as the patient's condition permits. In unconscious patients or in those with any injuries above the level of the clavicle (facial), the cervical spine is presumed to be injured until proven otherwise (see Chapter 10 in Lawrence's *Essentials of General Surgery*, 4th edition). Patients with minor wedge compression fractures (Fig. 6-5B) of the lower thoracic or lumbar spine often develop an ileus from retroperitoneal bleeding and should not be fed enterally until the ileus has resolved. If paraplegia results from a catastrophic spinal column injury, the signs of other injuries are masked by the lack of sensation. A systematic and thorough examination of all vital structures must therefore be carried out in patients with paraplegic. The patient with suspected spine trauma is properly splinted at the site of injury in a cervical collar with the head secured by taped sandbags. The thorax, abdomen, and extremities are strapped to a spine board. Consultation

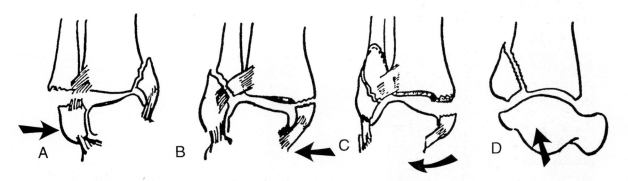

Figure 6-20 Ankle fractures. The basic mechanism of injury can be identified by the characteristic fracture patterns. A transverse fracture line implies that tensile, avulsive force was applied to the bone and is usually the first fracture to occur in the injury pattern. **A,** Adduction (inversion), in which the lateral malleolus is pulled off transversely and the medial malleolus is pushed off obliquely by the talus. **B,** Pure abduction (eversion) in which the medial malleolus is pulled off transversely, the fibula pushed off obliquely by the talus. The lateral malleolus is fractured in the sagittal plane. In some cases, the fibula is fractured above the joint line, indicating a tear in the interosseous membrane. **C,** Abduction (eversion) and external rotation (common), in which the medial malleolus is pulled off transversely while the lateral malleolus is obliquely fractured by the talus as it externally rotates and abuts the fibula. The fibular fracture is in the coronal plane. **D,** Vertical load, in which the posterior malleolus, seen best on a lateral x-ray film, can be fractured by a vertical compression load as the talus impacts the posterior tibia. The addition of this fracture fragment to any of the above constitutes a trimalleolar fracture. (Reprinted with permission from Rockwood C, Green D. *Fractures in Adults,* 3rd ed. Philadelphia: JB Lippincott; 1982.)

with a neurosurgeon or an orthopedic surgeon is indicated if the physician has any doubt about the stability of the spine injury.

Pelvic Fractures. The pelvis transfers body weight through the sacroiliac joints and acetabula in stance and through the ischial tuberosities in seated postures. The pelvis also protects the lower abdominal and genitourinary tracts. The pelvis houses the extensive vascular arborizations of the iliac vessels and the lumbosacral plexus of nerves. Pelvic fractures usually occur after high-velocity blunt trauma and can be associated with massive blood loss and multiorgan system injuries (Fig. 6-21). Therefore, in a hemodynamically unstable patient, emergency pelvic stabilization with external fixation is considered essential to the trauma resuscitation. The two goals of acute pelvic fracture surgery are to stop bleeding and permit sitting stability to facilitate pulmonary physiotherapy.

Almost one in five pelvic fractures has a concomitant bladder or urethral injury in males. When blood is seen at the external urethral meatus or when the patient cannot pass urine, a retrograde urethrogram is obtained to evaluate the integrity of the urethra before an indwelling catheter is placed. With hematuria, an intravenous pyelogram is performed to show renal function. If blood is detected in the rectum or vagina, the pelvic fracture may be open. Open pelvic fractures are treated with a diverting colostomy after debridement and external fixation to prevent ongoing fecal soilage of the fracture.

Traumatic Amputations and Replantation

With the advent of microsurgical techniques, completely severed digits and limbs can be surgically reattached. Limb replantation is most successful if the part is amputated cleanly with a minimum of crushed tissue. Children enjoy better nerve regeneration than adults and are ideal candidates for replantation. A general rule applies to replantation: Because muscle tissue is sensitive to ischemic injury, the greater the amount of muscle attached to the amputated part, the poorer is the prognosis for its function after replantation.

The best amputation levels for replantation in adults are the thumb, multiple digits, and the wrist or metacarpal level of the hand. In children, amputations at any level have a good chance for successful replantation. Contraindications to replantation include amputations with large crush or avulsive components; body parts that have been amputated at multiple levels; individual digit amputations (other than the thumb), especially proximal to the middle phalanx; and amputation in older patients who have concurrent disease or mental instability.

An amputated part may remain viable for approximately 6 hours of warm (36°C) ischemia. Cooling decreases tissue metabolism and increases the duration of viability. Amputated tissues can tolerate up to 16 hours of cold (10°C) ischemia. Thus, preparation of a severed part for transportation should include cleansing of superficial contamination, wrapping in moist gauze, and placement in an airtight plastic bag that is then immersed in ice water. Dry ice is never used because it causes frostbite and further tissue damage.

Of digital replants, 85% remain viable. Joint motion is usually about 50% of normal and two-point sensory discrimination is protective (>10 mm) in half of adults while being almost normal (>5 mm) in children. All digits are cold intolerant for a period of at least 2 years and 80% of epiphyses will continue to grow after replantation.

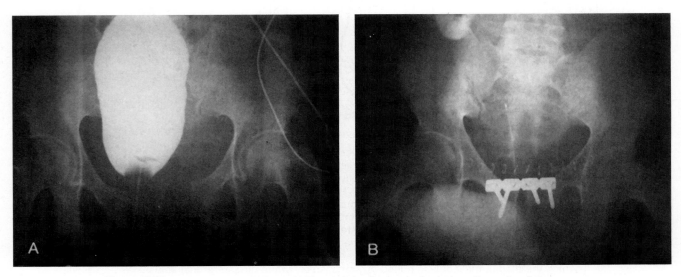

Figure 6-21   A, Anterior-posterior (AP) pelvis radiograph depicting diastasis of the symphysis pubis. The retrograde cystogram demonstrates bladder compression from a large pelvic hematoma. This type of pelvic injury can cause massive amounts of internal hemorrhage. **B,** AP pelvis radiograph after internal fixation with a plate and screws. Fracture reduction decreases pelvic volume, which both stabilizes and facilitates tamponade of bleeding fracture surfaces.

Compartment Syndrome

Muscles are surrounded by a relatively stiff fascial membrane composed of fibrous collagen. These fibrous envelopes separate various muscles into anatomically distinct compartments (Fig. 6-22). Bleeding and tissue swelling inside these membranes cause increased pressure within the fascial compartment. Under these circumstances, capillary blood flow to muscle and nerve is thus reduced, causing local acidosis, cell injury, and further edema. Compartment pressures can become so elevated that muscle and nerve necrosis result. Dead fibrotic muscle will cause joint contractures and the limb function will be severely impaired.

A compartment syndrome can be caused by fractures severe muscle contusions, crush injuries, and acute vascular occlusion. They may be aggravated by casts. Fractures that cause the most compartment syndromes are supracondylar distal humerus (Fig. 6-16), both bones (radius and ulna) of the forearm, and proximal third tibia fractures.

The classic signs of a compartment syndrome due to tissue ischemia are described by the four Ps: pain, paresthesia, paralysis, and pallor. Pain is the most useful clinical sign. It is intense and usually disproportionate to the injury. In addition, the pain is intensified on passive stretching of the muscles within the suspected compartment. If these symptoms and signs occur in the presence of one of the high-risk injuries, an urgent orthopaedic consultation should be obtained regarding possible fasciotomy. It is important to remember that a compartment syndrome can occur in the presence of normal pulses and sensation. Systolic arterial pulse pressures are usually much higher than the 30 mm Hg interstitial compartment pressure at which myonecrosis begins.

A high index of suspicion and pain out of proportion to the injury should lead to the removal of all circular bandages or casts. The clinician should not wait for paresthesia, paralysis, or pallor. Decompression by open fasciotomy is indicated if compartment pressure is greater than 30 to 40 mm Hg in an unconscious or paralyzed patient. (Compartment syndrome is also discussed in Chapters 10 and 23 in Lawrence's *Essentials of General Surgery*, 4th ed.)

Sports-Related Injuries

The recent emphasis on physical fitness has led to an increase in sports-related injuries. These injuries can be classified as those caused by acute trauma or repetitive stress. All musculoskeletal tissues are composed of living cells that are stimulated by physical stress to become stronger. When these tissues are not stressed, bones, ligaments, muscles, and tendons will atrophy. The goal of exercise is to produce beneficial increases in physical strength and endurance through the controlled application of stress. Tissues gain strength following stress-induced microscopic

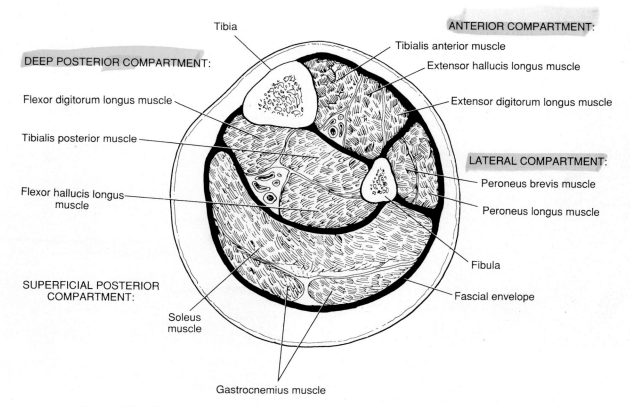

Figure 6-22 Four distinct leg compartments are separated by thick, unyielding fascial planes.

breakdown by a process of hypertrophic repair. When the stresses of exercise overwhelm the normal reparative process, tissues become chronically injured and inflamed and ultimately fail. There is much to be learned about the proper duration, frequency, and intensity of physical training. For example, the "no pain, no gain" attitude toward exercise often exacerbates many injuries. Although pain may be an annoyance, it is also appropriate biofeedback signifying injury and the need for rest.

It has been calculated that, while running, the foot strikes the ground between 800 and 2,000 times per mile at a force of 2 to 4 times body weight. An average 140-lb man generates between 110 and 560 tons of ground reaction force per mile. This tremendous amount of force is dissipated by the shoe, the small joints of the foot, and the bones and muscles of the leg. Any of these tissues can and do fail with injudicious exercise.

This section describes the more common injuries related to acute trauma and chronic, repetitive overuse. Many of these syndromes can occur as occupational injuries in which a given task is repeated with great frequency and without adequate periods of restorative rest.

Stress Fractures

Stress fractures are the classic overuse injury. They occur when individuals are subjected to increased activity levels or changes in habits and training methods. Historically, stress fractures were first identified in the metatarsals of military recruits who were expected to endure arduous marches (march fracture syndrome). Stress fractures have been identified in most bones of the body, including femur, tibia, calcaneus, and metatarsals in runners; humerus in throwers; ribs in oarsmen; and wrists and L5 vertebrae in gymnasts.

Stress fractures are postulated to occur as a consequence of muscle fatigue. Not only do muscles cause locomotion,

they also absorb shock. Eccentric muscle contraction, or controlled muscle lengthening, decelerates the body, absorbs shock, and diffuses stress away from bone. When muscles tire, this stress-shielding effect is negated and stress is transferred directly to bone. Repeated submaximal stress will cause bone as a material to fatigue. Microfractures result and may cause an achy discomfort. The traditional treatment of rest and stress protection permits these microscopic fractures to heal. Normal cellular bone healing mechanisms permit the bone to strengthen in response to increasing demands. If the bone's ability to heal itself is overwhelmed by repeated, unremitting stress, these microfractures will coalesce, resulting in a gross, macroscopic fracture. Because stress fractures are initiated on a microscopic level, radiographs lack diagnostic sensitivity and have high false-negative rates, missing as many as 70% of these injuries. Radioisotope-labeled technetium pyrophosphate bone scans, which detect cellular bone formation, can identify a stress fracture at an earlier stage of its pathogenesis (Fig. 6-23).

Lateral Epicondylitis (Tennis Elbow)

Lateral epicondylitis, or tennis elbow, is an overuse injury of the wrist extensor muscle origin. This condition affects players of racquet sports, as well as laborers who use their hand in repetitive forceful gripping. Wrist extension is necessary for power grip (try to grip with your wrist flexed!).

The wrist extensor muscles also dissipate force when a handheld object is used in striking. In tennis elbow, the common wrist extensors are damaged and inflamed at their lateral humeral epicondyle origin. The majority of these injuries respond to nonoperative methods that include rest, heat, anti-inflammatory agents, wrist extensor muscle stretching, and antagonist (wrist flexor) strengthening exercises. In the few cases that are managed operatively,

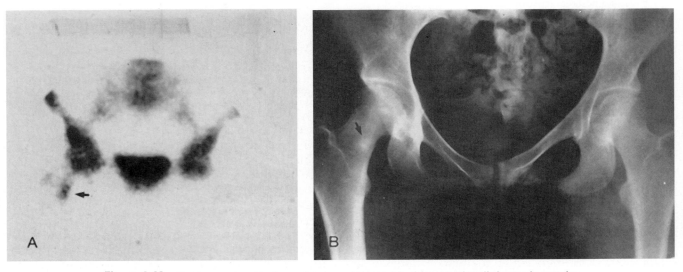

Figure 6-23   A, Femoral neck stress fracture detected by increased radioisotopic uptake on bone scan (*arrow*) 2 weeks before **B,** radiographic evidence of the fracture (*arrow*).

chronic granulation tissue is found in the origin of the extensor carpi radialis brevis and is resected.

Rotator Cuff Tendonitis (Shoulder Bursitis)

The glenohumeral joint of the shoulder is the most mobile joint in the body. The four rotator cuff muscles — subscapularis, supraspinatus, infraspinatus, and teres minor — all take broad origin from the scapular body and insert just lateral to the articular surface of the humeral head. These muscles act to stabilize the joint by pulling the humeral head into the shallow scapular glenoid fossa. The combined cross-sectional area of the rotator cuff musculature is equal to that of the deltoid muscle. Because cross-sectional area is directly related to muscle strength, it is interesting that the amount of shoulder muscle strength expended on joint stability through the rotator cuff is equal to that of the deltoid, which is responsible for joint mobility.

Rotator cuff tendonitis, or subacromial bursitis, is common to people involved in sports (e.g., swimmers, throwers) or who have jobs in which the arm is used overhead (e.g., mechanics). As the shoulder abducts away from the body, the rotator cuff muscles (especially the supraspinatus) contract under the coracoacromial arch. As the arm is raised, this arch becomes narrower, impinging on and mechanically irritating the tendons of the rotator cuff muscles. The subacromial bursa, which is a fluid-filled synovial sac, may become inflamed under these conditions of friction and can contribute to the pain. However, pathologic changes can also affect the tendon and run the gamut from edematous inflammation to calcific degeneration to tendon thinning and tearing (Fig. 6-24). Painful inflammatory changes may also affect the subacromial bursa. It is difficult to distinguish which structure is painful, the bursa or the tendon proper. A rotator cuff tear may show weakness of shoulder external rotation strength. Pain can mask the reliability of strength testing. A shoulder arthrogram, ultrasound, or MRI scan can diagnose a rotator cuff tear with good dependability.

Factors that contribute to rotator cuff pain include overuse, weakness, muscle imbalance, improper throwing technique, strenuous training techniques, and an unstable glenohumeral joint. Treatment consists of rest, eccentric rotator cuff strengthening exercises, and anti-inflammatory medication. Surgical decompression of the coracoacromial arch is indicated if the condition becomes chronic or if it is necessary to repair a torn rotator cuff tendon.

Plantar Fasciitis (Calcaneal Bursitis)

Plantar fasciitis is a problem common to runners. The plantar fascia is a thick, fibrous structure attached to the calcaneus that fans distally along the sole of the foot to envelop the metatarsal heads. It increases and stiffens the longitudinal arch of the foot during the propulsive toe-off phase of gait. When the inflexible plantar fascia is repeatedly impacted and stretched by running, it is injured at its calcaneal origin, becoming inflamed and painful. The inflammatory reaction can produce a traction spike of new bone, which on radiograph is called a heel spur. It is not clear how much of the heel pain can be attributed to the spur. Many patients who have had foot x-rays for other reasons have evidence of heel spurs but no symptoms of heel pain.

Classically, plantar heel pain is worse when gait is initiated in the morning, after sitting, or at the start of jogging. Contributory factors include both flat (planus) and high-arched (cavus) feet, toe or sand running, obesity, and improper shoe wear (e.g., slippers). Nonoperative treatment includes rest, medication, weight loss if applicable, proper shoe wear, heel padding, or cushioned shoe orthoses. If the condition has been of long-standing duration, recovery may be slow. Surgical release of the plantar fascia from its calcaneal origin is reserved for the most recalcitrant cases.

Patellar Overload Syndrome

Anterior knee pain is common to sports participants. The patella is embedded in the quadriceps muscle and glides through the femoral groove. The patella functions much like a pulley to increase the mechanical efficiency of the quadriceps in extending the knee joint. When the patella is abnormally loaded or malaligned, abnormal patellar wear and irritation can produce chondromalacia, or cartilage (*chondro-*) softening (*malacia*).

Patellofemoral knee pain is located anteriorly and is aggravated by climbing or descending stairs and hills, squatting, kneeling, arising from a chair, or after prolonged sitting. These activities all stress the knee extensor (quadriceps) mechanism. As the quadriceps muscle is inhibited by the discomfort, it may atrophy. Nonoperative treatment is often effective. Avoidance of aggravating activities, anti-inflammatory medications, and patellar orthotics known as "knee sleeves" are effective treatment adjuncts. Straight-leg raising and quadriceps-strengthening exercises are important to successful rehabilitation. Quadriceps exercises over a full arc of motion are to be avoided because they place excessive load on the patella and exacerbate the condition. The diagnosis of chondromalacia should be reserved for injury to the articular cartilage observed either by MRI or arthroscopy.

Exercise Compartment Syndrome (Shin Splints)

Shin splints are leg pain that is intensified during exercise. In recreational runners, the pain is usually localized to the anterior leg compartment (Fig. 6-22) containing the tibialis anterior extensor digitorum and extensor hallucis longus muscles. In competitive runners, the pain often emanates from the distal medial leg in the deep posterior compartment musculature (posterior tibialis, flexor digitorum, and flexor hallucis longus). Intramuscular pressures increase during contraction, which decreases blood flow. Muscle perfusion therefore occurs primarily during muscle relaxation. Sustained increases in compartment pressure decrease muscle perfusion, producing pain and the cessation of exercise. This phenomenon is known as an exercise compartment syndrome. When measured,

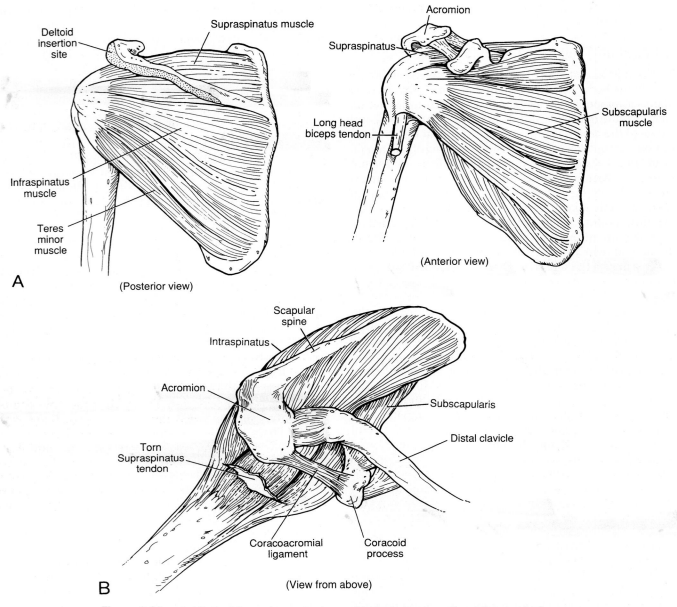

Figure 6-24   A, Viewed from the posterior and anterior perspectives, the cowl of rotator cuff muscles takes broad origin from the scapula and inserts close to the articular margin of the humeral head. The rotator cuff acts to pull the humeral head into the glenoid fossa as the arm is abducted away from the body. **B,** Viewed from its superior surface, the supraspinatus tendon is torn near its humeral insertion. The tear results from acromion and coracoacromial ligament attrition, when the shoulder is abducted and forward flexed. (**A,** Modified from American Academy of Orthopaedic Surgeons. *Athletic Training and Sports Medicine,* 2nd ed. Park Ridge, IL: American Academy of Orthopaedic Surgeons; 1991:235. **B,** Modified from Rowe CR. *The Shoulder.* New York: Churchill Livingstone; 1988:142.)

compartment pressures can increase to well over 100 mm Hg with exercise. In the asymptomatic individual, pressures return to normal levels very rapidly during periods of rest. In patients with exercise compartment syndromes, interstitial tissue pressures fall off slowly and have a delayed return to normal values. Tibia stress fractures, periostitis, nerve entrapment, and fascial muscle hernias have a similar clinical presentation. The diagnosis of exercise-related compartment syndrome is based on objective pressure measurements. When conservative treatments (e.g., rest, cushioned shoe orthotics, and changes in training patterns and running surfaces) fail, the condition can be successfully treated with a surgical fasciotomy of the involved leg compartment.

Sprains

A sprain is a ligament injury. Ligaments are collagenous structures that originate from and insert on bone. Ligaments stabilize joints, and they are injured under tensile or stretching loads. Sprains are classified according to the three grades of damage. Grade I sprains exhibit microscopic ligament damage, which produces ligament tenderness but no change in joint stability when the joint is subjected to stress. Grade II sprains show a greater degree of damage, with rupture of entire fascicles of ligament collagen. The ligament is in macroscopic continuity but is stretched or partially torn and therefore demonstrates joint laxity when stressed. There is a firm endpoint on clinical testing. When grossly disrupted with total loss of joint stability, the ligament injury is classified as a grade III sprain.

Ankle Sprains

The lateral ankle ligaments are the most commonly sprained ligaments in the body. The lateral ankle is supported by three discrete ligaments: the anterior talofibular, calcaneofibular, and posterior talofibular ligaments (Fig. 6-25). Because the longer fibular malleolus buttresses the ankle from abduction or eversion stress, the broad deltoid ligament that connects the medial tibial malleolus to the talus is not commonly injured.

When the ankle is subjected to an inversion stress, the anterior talofibular ligament is the first lateral ligament to be torn. With more severe injury, the calcaneal-fibular ligament will also be disrupted. These two ligaments resist anterior talar displacement on the tibia (anterior drawer test, Fig. 6-26) and abnormal inversion talar tilt, respectively.

The diagnosis of a lateral ankle ligament sprain and its severity are ascertained by the extent of ligament tenderness and by manual and radiographic stress tests. Treatment consists of ice, elevation, compressive wraps, and early weight bearing. Primary surgical ankle ligament repair is rarely indicated because most ankle sprains have no residual joint instability and the outcomes of early versus late ankle reconstruction are similar. Ligaments contain proprioceptive nerve endings that are also injured by a sprain. Recurrent ankle sprains may be the result of inadequate proprioceptive feedback. Balance board proprioceptor retraining is an effective component of ankle rehabilitation.

Knee Ligament Sprains

The knee is situated between the two largest bones, the femur and the tibia, and is spanned by the body's strongest muscles, the quadriceps and hamstrings. In general terms, the knee is stabilized by four ligaments: the two collateral ligaments that resist varus and valgus stress and the two cruciate ligaments that primarily resist AP motion (Fig. 6-27).

The collateral ligaments are usually damaged by trauma. The anterior cruciate ligament (ACL) can be injured in isolation in twisting with hyperflexion or hyperextension noncontact modes. The ACL is the only one of the four ligaments that is intrasynovial. In patients with bloody effusions (hemarthrosis) following knee injury, 70% have an ACL injury. In those with an acute ACL tear, 50% have a concomitant meniscus tear. The medial collateral and anterior cruciate ligaments are frequently injured in combination from a valgus stress (e.g., as occurs from a blow to the lateral thigh). When a collateral liga-

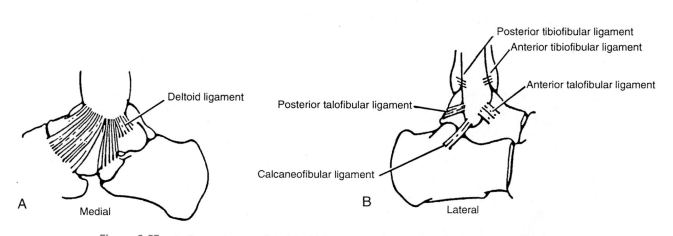

Figure 6-25 **A,** Extensive medial deltoid ligament of the ankle. **B,** The lateral ankle is supported by three discrete ankle ligaments. The most commonly sprained anterior talofibular ligament, the calcaneofibular, and the posterior talofibular ligaments. The anterior talofibular ligament resists anterior translation of the ankle (anterior drawer test); the calcaneofibular resists inversion stress (talar tilt). (Modified from Wilson FC, ed. *The Musculoskeletal System: Basic Processes and Disorders,* 2nd ed. Philadelphia: JB Lippincott; 1983.)

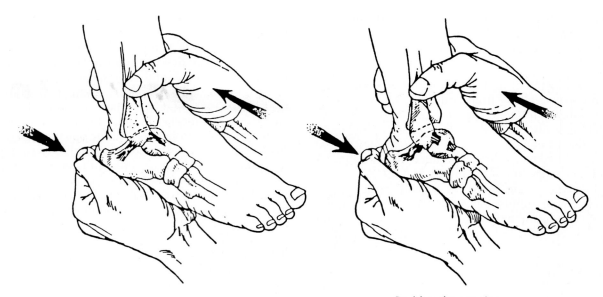

Positive drawer sign

Figure 6-26 Anterior drawer test. The anterior talofibular ligament resists anterior ankle stress. The anterior drawer test is positive when this ligament is disrupted and will detect excessive anterior translation of the foot on the leg. (Reprinted with permission from American Academy of Orthopaedic Surgeons. *Athletic Training and Sports Medicine,* 2nd ed. Park Ridge, IL: American Academy of Orthopaedic Surgeons; 1991:414.)

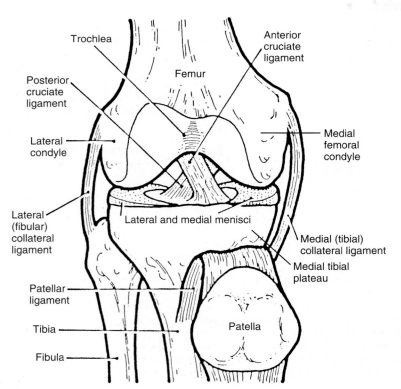

Figure 6-27 Knee joint stability depends on the two collateral and cruciate ligaments. The medial collateral ligament is broad and large and resists varus or abduction stress. The anterior cruciate ligament resists anterior tibial translation, while the posterior cruciate prevents posterior tibial shear.

ment is severely injured, the knee joint capsule and synovial lining are disrupted. The knee may not contain an effusion because hemorrhage leaks through the torn capsule.

Collateral ligament damage can be detected by local tenderness, pain, and laxity when the knee is manually stressed in a mediolateral (varus/valgus) plane. Laxity tests of an injured knee are always judged in comparison to the normal side. Valgus force on the knee will stress the medial collateral ligament, whereas varus force will test the integrity of the lateral collateral ligament. Full knee extension places the joint in a position of maximal geometric stability. Joint laxity in knee extension therefore implies a greater degree of collateral ligament damage. Subtle differences between the laxity on the normal versus the injured side can best be detected with the knee at 20 degrees of flexion.

The **anterior drawer test** is used to evaluate cruciate ligament integrity. With the knee flexed 45 degrees, the tibia is pulled forward like a drawer (Fig. 6-28). If there is abnormal anterior tibial translation, the anterior drawer test suggests that the anteromedial fibers of the ACL are torn. Conversely, abnormal posterior tibial translation to a posteriorly directed tibial force indicates a posterior cruciate ligament (PCL) injury. Anterior knee laxity may be better appreciated in the 20-degree knee-flexed position, which is called the Lachman test. This suggests injury to the posterolateral fibers of the ACL.

Isolated medial collateral ligament injuries heal well with immobilization in a hinged cast-brace, which protects the knee from valgus stress. An ACL injury is disabling to most athletes. With cutting and twisting movements, the knee will transiently sublux and give way. PCL-deficient knees are associated with patellar overload and arthritis, because the quadriceps muscle attempts to compensate for increased posterior tibial displacement. The less stout lateral collateral ligament (LCL) is often injured in conjunction with one of the two cruciate ligaments. Acute repairs of combination knee ligament injuries should be strong enough to tolerate early motion to prevent the common postoperative complication of joint stiffness.

The indications for surgical ligament repair and reconstruction are controversial. In general, younger patients whose activities cause symptoms of instability are candidates for surgery. The ACLs heal poorly and are generally reconstructed with soft tissue autografts from the patellar tendon, hamstrings tendon, or fascia lata.

Meniscal Injury

The knee joint is minimally constrained by virtue of its bony geometry. The medial and lateral meniscal fibrocartilages increase joint surface contact and aid in joint stability. In stance, the menisci transmit 40% to 60% of the weight-bearing load placed across the joint. The menisci also assist with joint lubrication and hyaline cartilage nutrition. The menisci move anterior to posterior as the knee is flexed. In flexion, the menisci are trapped between the

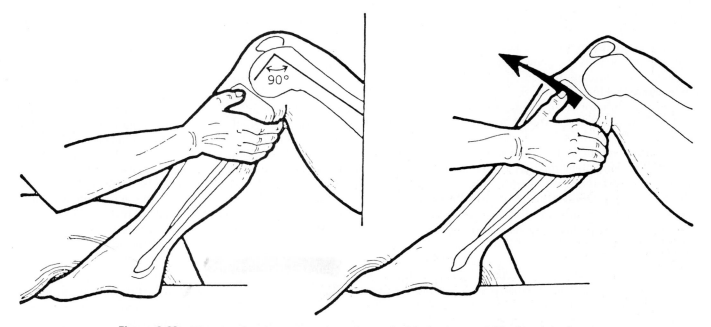

Figure 6-28 The anterior drawer test is performed with the foot stabilized and the knee flexed 90 degrees. With the examiner's thumb placed on the joint line, the tibia is pulled anteriorly. Excessive anterior tibial shift suggests that the anterior cruciate ligament is incompetent. The contralateral side can be used as a comparative reference. A similar test performed in 20 degrees of knee flexion is called the Lachman test and is more sensitive in the evaluation of acute injuries.

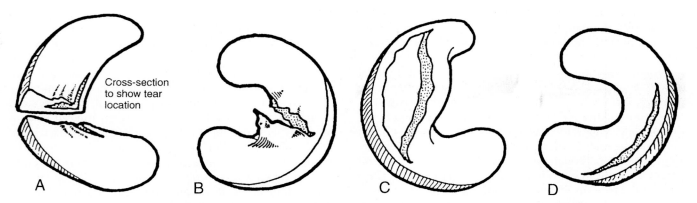

Figure 6-29   Meniscal tears. **A,** Degenerative horizontal tear. **B,** Radial tear. **C,** Displaced bucket handle tear. **D,** Longitudinal tear. (Reprinted with permission from American Academy of Orthopaedic Surgeons. *Athletic Training and Sports Medicine,* 2nd ed. Park Ridge, IL: American Academy of Orthopaedic Surgeons; 1991:365.)

femoral condyle and tibial plateau. If a twisting, rotatory motion occurs when the knee is flexed, the menisci may split longitudinally (Fig. 6-29C,D). Meniscal tissue loses hydration and becomes more brittle with age. Shearing, horizontal cleavage tears not seen on the meniscal surface are frequently found in older patients (Fig. 6-29A).

Patients with meniscal pathology may have pain and tenderness localized to the joint line (i.e., the palpable gap between femur and tibia). There may be recurrent effusion. A history of painful giving way suggests a tear located in the posterior portion of the meniscus. Symptoms of intermittent joint locking occur with displaceable and bucket handle tears (Fig. 6-29C), in which the torn component of the meniscus becomes trapped between the condyle and acts as a mechanical block to joint motion.

Clinical examination should check for loss of terminal extension (locking), localized joint line tenderness, and provocative test for displaceable meniscus (McMurray's test). McMurray's test involves flexion of the knee to 90 degrees, followed by internal rotatory movements of the tibia, and then followed by extension into valgus. The test is repeated with tibial rotation in the opposite direction followed by extension into varus. The test tries to trap a displaceable fragment of the meniscus between the articular surfaces of the tibia and femur. The test is positive if the patient experiences joint line pain and the examiner feels a snap or rub at the joint line.

Longitudinal tears (Fig. 6-29D) in the peripheral third of the meniscus will heal when repaired, because this zone is well vascularized. Total meniscectomy leads to the slow development of tibiofemoral arthritis. Irreparable and displaceable meniscal tears causing mechanical symptoms are best treated by arthroscopy and partial excision of the meniscus, leaving the stable, untorn meniscus in situ. Meniscal surgery is performed arthroscopically because it is less traumatic, is more precise, and can be performed on an outpatient basis.

Acromioclavicular (Shoulder) Separation

In addition to the glenohumeral articulation, the shoulder is composed of three other joints: the acromioclavicular, sternoclavicular, and scapulothoracic articulations. The acromioclavicular joint rotates approximately 20 degrees with flexion and extension of the shoulder. It is stabilized in this AP (horizontal) plane by the acromioclavicular ligaments (Fig. 6-1). In the craniocaudal direction (coronal plane), the joint is constrained by the stronger coracoclavicular ligaments.

The acromioclavicular joint is injured after a blow or fall onto the point (acromion) of the shoulder. The scapular acromion is driven caudally, whereas the clavicle remains fixed to the chest. If the acromioclavicular ligaments alone are torn and the coracoclavicular ligaments stretched, the injury is classified as grade II; the clavicle is partially displaced (subluxed) from the acromion (Fig. 6-1C). This may not be obvious but can be determined by stress radiographs taken with weights strapped to the patient's wrists. The distance between the clavicle and coracoid process will be widened on the affected side. When both acromioclavicular and coracoclavicular ligaments are disrupted (grade III), the joint will be dislocated. The distal clavicle will be elevated above the acromion, which is obvious to inspection (Fig. 6-1B). Treatment of a grade III shoulder separation is controversial. Both surgical and nonsurgical methods yield functional results.

Gamekeeper's Thumb

The ulnar collateral ligament of the thumb metacarpophalangeal (MCP) joint is a critical structure because it stabilizes the thumb during grip and index finger pinch. As the thumb is out of the plane of the hand, this ligament is vulnerable to abduction stress. It is injured in skiers who fall while still gripping their pole or in ball handling sports (Fig. 6-30). Loss of the stabilizing effect of the thumb MCP ulnar collateral ligament renders pinch weak and painful.

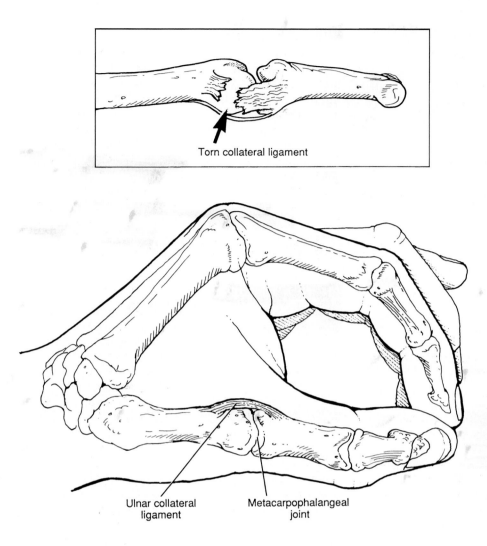

Torn collateral ligament

Ulnar collateral ligament

Metacarpophalangeal joint

Figure 6-30 **A,** Lateral depiction of a torn collateral ligament metacarpophalangeal joint. **B,** The ulnar collateral ligament of the thumb metacarpophalangeal joint is critical to opposable thumb function. Injury to this ligament (gamekeeper's thumb) renders the thumb unstable and weakens its contribution to pinch and grip strength.

To stress test the ligament, the thumb MCP joint is positioned in 35 degrees of flexion to relax the volar plate and the short thumb flexor. The adductor pollicis aponeurosis may be interposed between the ligament and the proximal phalanx, which can prevent ligament healing. Ligament exploration with repair or reattachment is performed. Good clinical results are also reported with use of a hand-based adduction splint for 6 weeks.

Mallet (Baseball) Finger

A sudden blow causing flexion to the tip of an extended finger can cause rupture of the digital extensor tendon. The finger distal interphalangeal (DIP) joint is in a flexed position and the patient cannot actively extend this joint (Fig. 6-31). This injury heals well if splinted in full DIP extension for 6 weeks.

Boxer's Fracture

The index and long finger metacarpals have limited mobility and act as rigid posts for the fine precision work of the

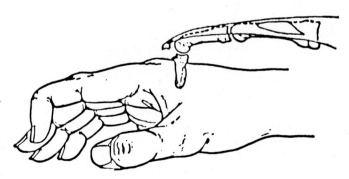

Figure 6-31 Mallet or baseball finger, which results from rupture of the extensor tendon. (Reprinted with permission from American Orthopaedic Association. *Manual of Orthopaedic Surgery,* 6th ed. Park Ridge, IL: American Orthopaedic Association; 1985:151.)

hand. In contrast, the ring and little finger metacarpals are more mobile and are important to power grip because motion is needed for these fingers to surround an object. For a fist to impart maximal kinetic energy, the more rigid radial side of the fist should strike the object. When the ulnar fist strikes an object the little finger metacarpal neck often fractures (**boxer's fracture**). With marked amounts of fracture angulation (>45 degrees), closed reduction and plaster immobilization is the preferred and usually successful treatment. Occasionally, percutaneous pins may be required to stabilize a very unstable fracture.

Achilles Tendon Rupture

Achilles tendon ruptures occur in the middle-aged athlete who stresses the tendon beyond its tolerance. Systemic and local steroid injections weaken tendinous tissue and predispose it to rupture. With an Achilles tendon rupture, the athlete feels a severe pain in the calf. There may be swelling, ecchymosis, and sometimes a palpable gap between tendon ends. Active plantar flexion of the ankle is weak but present because the tibialis posterior and long toe flexors are still functional.

The **Thompson test** (Fig. 6-32) verifies whether the gastrocnemius–soleus complex is intact. With the patient lying prone and the foot hanging free over this end of the stretcher, the examiner squeezes the calf muscle belly. Normally, the foot plantar flexes. Lack of plantar flexion indicates that the Achilles tendon is torn. The diagnosis can be easily confirmed by ultrasound.

Nonoperative treatment in a long leg cast with the foot in plantar flexion permits excellent tendon healing. This method is cumbersome. Surgical treatment may be more expeditious for athletes. Both types of treatment are effective.

Turf Toe

Turf toe is a hyperextension injury to the great toe metatarsophalangeal (MTP) joint (Fig. 6-33). The flexor hallucis brevis tendon is ruptured either at its proximal phalangeal insertion or by a fracture of its sesamoid bones. The plantar plate may also be torn. The injury occurs during football pile-ups, in which a player falls on the posterior aspect of a prone player's foot, hyperextending the great toe. The injured player experiences exquisite plantar great toe pain exacerbated by passive extension of the MTP joint. The toe-off, propulsive phase of gait is painful. Treatment consists of rest, taping of the toe in plantar flexion, and the use of a stiff forefoot, in-shoe orthosis. Untreated turf toe has been implicated as the cause of great toe MTP arthritis and loss of extension known as hallux rigidus.

Myositis Ossificans

Bone deposited in a muscle after a blunt injury is known as traumatic myositis ossificans (Fig. 6-34). When a deep muscle (often the quadriceps) is contused, the muscle closest to bone has the greatest amount of direct damage. Either a metaplasia of muscle cells or a release of osteogenic material from the underlying bone causes bone to form within the injured muscle. Early symptoms are deep muscle tenderness and loss of joint motion. The condition is self-limited and may be decreased by nonsteroidal anti-inflammatory agents. If the lesion is large or causes mechanical problems, surgical excision is indicated. When a lesion is resected early (i.e., before 18 months), there is a high rate of recurrence. A systemic form of myositis ossificans occurs in patients with traumatic paralysis or extensive burns.

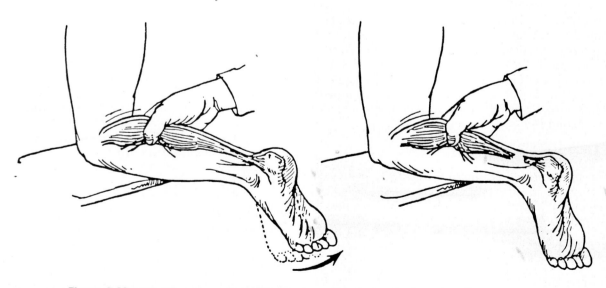

Figure 6-32   The Thompson test will provoke ankle plantar flexion when the gastrocnemius-soleus Achilles tendon complex is intact. Absence of this response indicates a tear of the Achilles tendon.

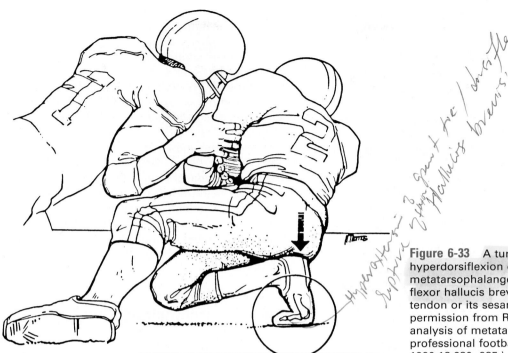

Figure 6-33   A turf toe injury occurs from hyperdorsiflexion of the great toe metatarsophalangeal joint and ruptures the flexor hallucis brevis mechanism through the tendon or its sesamoid bone. (Reprinted with permission from Rodeo SA et al. Turf toe: an analysis of metatarsophalangeal joint sprains in professional football players. *Am J Sports Med* 1990;18:280–285.)

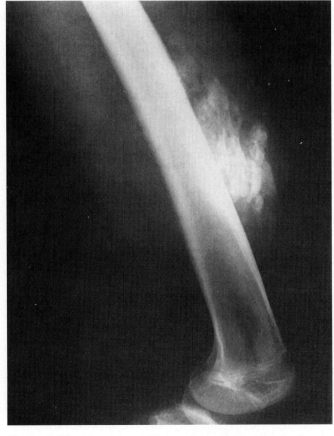

Figure 6-34   Myositis ossificans. Bone deposition in the quadriceps muscle after an anterior thigh contusion.

PEDIATRIC MUSCULOSKELETAL PROBLEMS

The term **orthopedic** is derived from the Greek word for straight, *orthos*, and the word for child, *pais*. The diagnosis and treatment of pediatric deformities thus represent the origin of the specialty of orthopedics. This section deals with common pediatric musculoskeletal disorders.

Lower Limb Torsion: In-Toeing and Out-Toeing

The most common childhood "deformities" are actually normal variations of musculoskeletal development. Flat feet, bowlegs, knock-knees, in-toeing, and out-toeing are commonly seen in young children but are unusual in adolescence. Because these conditions seem to resolve spontaneously, they must be considered part of the natural process of skeletal growth and development. The first 2 years of life are a remarkable period of physical growth. The average child attains almost half of its adult size and stature during these first 2 years. Body structure also changes radically as the skeletal frame is subjected to the demands of locomotion and bipedal gait.

The common rotational deformities of in-toeing and out-toeing can be ascribed to one of three lower limb sites: the femur (anteversion or retroversion), the tibia (internal or external torsion), or the forefoot (metatarsus adductus). Although rotational variations may run in families, the most common cause is the intrauterine positioning (Fig.

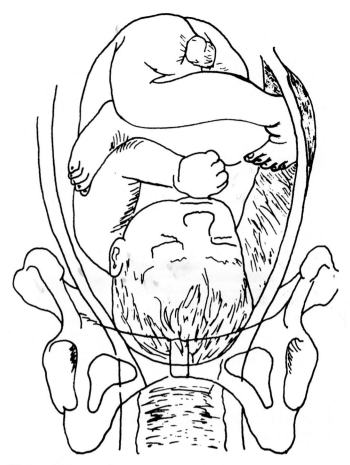

Figure 6-35 Cramped intrauterine confines often mold the child's plastic bone structure. Note that in utero fetal posture forces the tibias to be internally rotated and the forefeet adducted.

6-35). Certain sleeping or sitting postures may accentuate these conditions and delay their resolution. Femoral version describes the anatomic relationship of the femoral head and neck with the femoral shaft. The femoral neck is offset from the shaft in the coronal plane. This relation, called femoral anteversion, is seen if one looks down the shaft of the femur as one would a gun barrel: the femoral neck is canted an average of 10 to 15 degrees anterior (Fig. 6-36). At birth, femoral anteversion averages about 40 degrees. It decreases to 10 degrees by adulthood, with most of the change occurring in the first 3 years of life (Fig. 6-37).

All rotational deformities are best evaluated with the child placed prone. Femoral anteversion is present when medial or inward rotation of the femur is in excess of 30 degrees more than external femoral rotation (Fig. 6-38). When external (outward) femoral rotation is excessive, femoral retroversion is present.

When the prone child is viewed from above with his or her knee flexed, the angle that the sole of the foot makes with the thigh (i.e., the thigh–foot angle) allows

for assessment of internal versus external tibial torsion (Fig. 6-39A). The normal lateral border of the foot is straight. If it is curved inward or its lateral border is convex, metatarsus adductus is present (Fig. 6-39B). If the foot is flexible and can be passively corrected to neutral alignment, treatment is probably unnecessary. When the deformity is rigid, corrective serial casting is beneficial. Metatarsus adductus is often associated with internal tibial torsion. Both result from fetal positioning, the latter being the most common cause of rotational lower extremity problems (Fig. 6-35).

As the skeleton adapts to growth and bipedal posture, these torsional "deformities" resolve. A slight amount of in-toeing has been noted in the better athletes. In-toeing is advantageous during cutting maneuvers because a limb that is internally rotated will be aligned with the intended change of direction and is more effective in push-off acceleration.

Angular Limb Deformities: Bowlegs and Knock-Knees

Angular lower limb alignment, bowlegs and knock-knees (genu varum and valgum; Fig. 6-9), are another common cause for an orthopedic consultation. For most children, these conditions represent the spectrum of normal development. It is rare for limb malalignment to persist and cause functional or cosmetic impairment sufficient to require surgical intervention. Normal, nonambulatory infants have physiologic bowlegs with tibiofemoral angles of 20 degrees or more of varus (bow). At approximately 18 months of age, the angle corrects as the femur and tibia become collinear. After 3 years of age, the limbs assume the normal adult alignment of 7 degrees of skeletal valgus (Fig. 6-40).

Pathologic conditions can cause knee bowing, including growth arrest of the medial tibial metaphysis, chondrodysplastic dwarfism, and vitamin D–resistant (hypophosphatemic or renal) rickets. These systemic conditions also cause deformities of other bones and joints. If bowlegs persist beyond the 2 years of age, radiographic evaluation may be warranted.

Flat Feet

Flat feet are another common skeletal variation. The most common type is the flexible flat foot. The longitudinal arch of the foot is absent or flat in stance, but reconstitutes when the foot is non–weight bearing. Most flexible flat feet are asymptomatic and result from ligamentous laxity affecting the many small joints of the midfoot. A flat foot that is rigid and has little passive motion may be caused by a congenital coalition of the tarsal bones. A flat foot associated with a tight heel cord may be caused by muscular dystrophy or cerebral palsy. High arched feet (pes cavus) with clawed toes are the sequelae of peripheral neu-

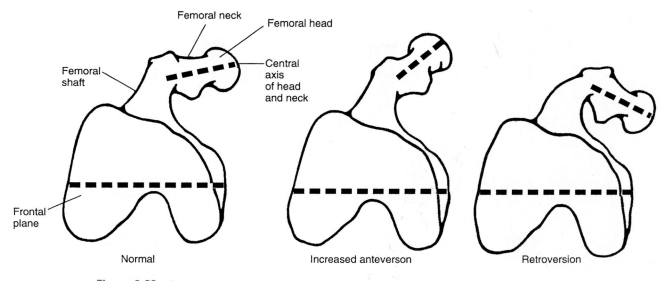

Figure 6-36 Femoral neck version or torsion as seen from the distal femoral condyles. (Reprinted with permission from Wilson FC, ed. *The Musculoskeletal System: Basic Processes and Disorders,* 2nd ed. Philadelphia: JB Lippincott; 1983.)

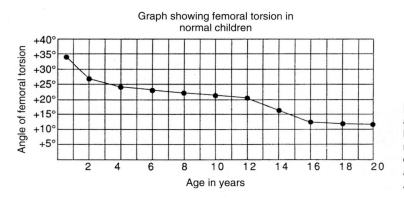

Figure 6-37 The average amount of femoral anteversion decreases from about 40 degrees at birth to the normal 10 degrees in adulthood. The most dramatic change occurs within the first 2 years of life. (Reprinted with permission from Dunlap K, et al. Congenital anomalies of hip and pelvis. *J Bone Joint Surg* 1953;35A:289.)

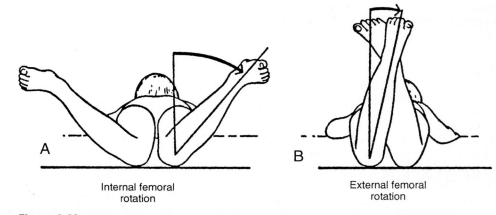

Figure 6-38 Clinical evaluation of a patient with intoeing caused by femoral anteversion. **A,** Internal femoral rotation is in greater excess than in part B. **B,** External femoral rotation. (Reprinted with permission from Staheli L. Rotational problems of the lower extremities. *Orthop Clin North Am* 1987;18:506.)

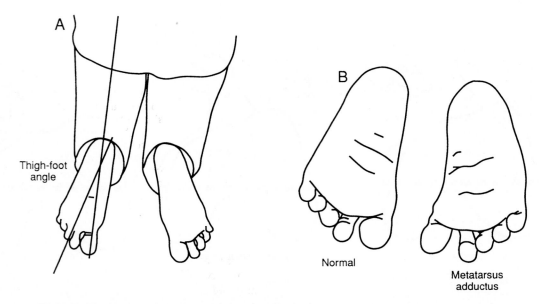

Figure 6-39 **A,** External tibial torsion is detected by a thigh–foot angle pointed away from the midline. **B,** Metatarsus adductus as a cause of in-toeing is noted by a convex lateral foot border. If the foot cannot be passively corrected to neutral, the deformity is rigid and may require serial casts for correction. (Reprinted with permission from Staheli L. Rotational problems of the lower extremities. *Orthop Clin North Am* 1987;18:506.)

ropathies, such as hereditary motor and sensory neuropathy (formerly known as Charcot-Marie-Tooth disease).

Developmental Dysplasia of the Hip

The incidence of developmental dysplasia of the hip, previously referred to as congenital dislocation of the hip, is 1.5 per 1,000 newborns. One third of cases are bilateral. The condition shows a familial predisposition and is associated with intrauterine breech presentations. Girls are affected much more often than boys, possibly because their ligaments are more sensitive to the relaxing effects of maternal estrogen released in preparation for birth.

The early diagnosis of developmental dysplasia of the hip allows early treatment. All newborns and infants must

be examined for hip instability. The diagnosis is never obvious, but must be sought by careful examination. Limited or asymmetrical thigh abduction suggests a hip abnormality (Fig. 6-41). The infant's thigh is gently grasped by the long finger and thumb. With the hip and knee flexed 90 degrees, the thigh is abducted while the greater trochanter is gently pressed forward in an anterior direction. A palpable jump or click during this maneuver—Ortolani's sign—signifies that the femoral head has been reduced into the acetabulum and that the hip was dislocated. An opposite, provocation maneuver, in which adduction and posterior pressure is applied by the thumbs over the femoral head, will lever the hip out of the acetabulum (Barlow's sign) if the hip is unstable. These two tests are useful in the first 2 weeks of life when the child's ligaments are

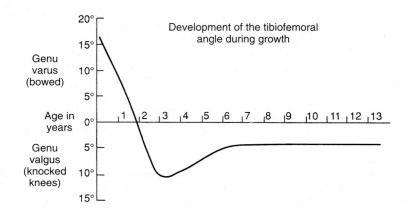

Figure 6-40 Changes in tibiofemoral alignment with growth shows that there is a natural progression from bowlegs at birth to physiologic knock-knees by the age of 3. (Modified from Kling T. Angular deformities of the lower limb in children. *Orthop Clin North Am* 1987;18:514.)

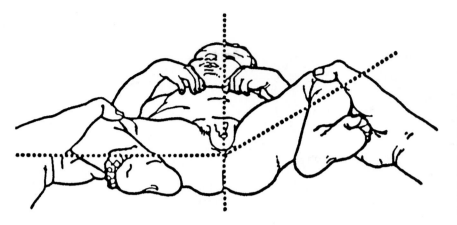

Figure 6-41   Limited hip abduction in congenital hip dislocation. The perineum should be perpendicular to the table. The limit of true hip joint motion is evidenced by concomitant movement of the perineum. (Reprinted with permission from American Orthopaedic Association. *Manual of Orthopaedic Surgery,* 6th ed. Park Ridge, IL: American Orthopaedic Association; 1985.)

under the relaxing influence of maternal hormones. Treatment is most successful early in life and is accomplished by manipulative reduction (Ortolani's maneuver) and immobilization with the hips in a stable position of flexion and abduction using a Pavlik harness. If the hip remains dislocated, the acetabular socket does not develop normally and remains shallow.

After 1 month of age, limited hip abduction is the most reliable sign of developmental dysplasia of the hip (Fig. 6-41). Asymmetry of thigh and buttock folds or telescoping of the flexed femur are other signs of late hip dislocation. When the condition is bilateral, all physical signs that depend on noting asymmetry will be absent, making diagnosis more difficult. When the child begins walking, a short leg limp is evident when the hip dislocation is unilateral. A waddling, hyperlordotic gait is apparent if the condition is bilateral. Treatment after walking age is more difficult. Contracted hip muscles are gradually stretched with traction or an adductor muscle release. Operative hip reduction is likely needed, and the reduced hip must be maintained in a cast.

The head of the femur is cartilaginous until almost 9 months of age and is not visible on radiograph. (Radiographs are therefore of limited early diagnostic value.) Ultrasonography shows cartilage well and is useful in the first 9 months. Hip joint ultrasound can dynamically evaluate the hip under positional stress. After the femoral head ossifies, radiograph shows a dislocated hip to be displaced lateral and superior to a shallow acetabulum.

The management of developmental dysplasia of the hip requires the prompt attention by an orthopedic specialist. When treatment is initiated early and followed closely, the prognosis for normal hip development and function is good.

Legg-Calvé-Perthes Disease

Legg-Calvé-Perthes disease is a condition of uncertain etiology that results in osteonecrosis of the femoral head in children 4 to 8 years of age. Boys are affected eight times more commonly than girls. Hip discomfort may be referred to the medial knee in the distribution of the obturator nerve. Therefore, pediatric patients complaining of knee pain should have their hip examined. The hip will display a subtle decrease in range of motion, especially in abduction and internal rotation. Hip abduction strength is also decreased and may cause a Trendelenburg limp, in which the child leans the torso over the affected hip.

Legg-Calvé-Perthes disease is self-limited and runs a 2- to 4-year course. Initial radiographs show minimal findings and may show disuse osteoporosis and hip joint-space widening. Later, when the dead bone is being resorbed and revascularized, new bone is laid down on dead bone, causing the femoral head to appear dense (sclerotic). During this revascularization stage, radiographic changes are most dramatic. Pathologic fractures of dead trabeculae may occur with weight-bearing loads, causing a flattening of the femoral head. The femoral head may appear fragmented and laterally displaced. The metaphysis may be rarefied and broadened. A child with Legg-Calvé-Perthes disease should be referred to an orthopedic surgeon. Treatment consists of traction to regain motion followed by bracing or surgical osteotomy to keep the articular portion of the femoral head within the weight-bearing portion of the acetabulum. This may involve femoral or pelvic osteotomies.

Slipped Capital Femoral Epiphysis

A cause of limping in adolescence is a fracture of the proximal femoral growth plate or slipped capital femoral epiphysis. A slipped capital femoral epiphysis is more common in boys than girls, is bilateral in approximately 33% of cases, and usually occurs during the prepubescent growth spurt (i.e., 10–14 years of age). Two distinctly different body types are susceptible to the condition. One group consists of obese children with delayed gonadal development; the other includes very tall children who have grown rapidly.

In addition to a limp, patients may have pain localized to the knee or, less frequently, to the groin. The affected leg is held externally rotated. Internal hip rotation is lim-

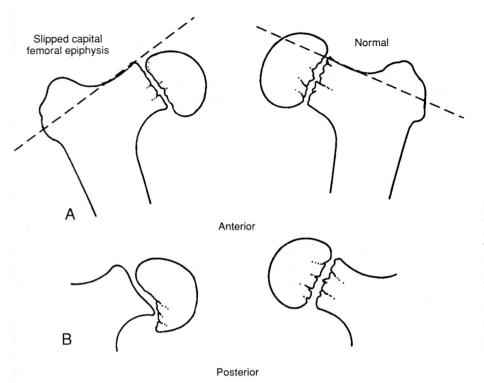

Figure 6-42   Slipped capital femoral epiphysis. The slipped capital femoral epiphysis on the left is compared to the normal hip on the right. **A,** On anterior-posterior radiograph, a line drawn tangential to the top of the femoral neck should pass through the normal femoral head (*right*). In a slipped femoral epiphysis the line does not intersect the head but passes above it (*left*). **B,** On a lateral radiograph, the head of the femur has slipped posterior to the femoral neck (*left*).

ited and painful. On AP radiographs, a line drawn tangential to the superior neck does not intersect the femoral head epiphysis as it does in a normal hip (Fig. 6-42A). Displacement is more apparent on the lateral radiograph, in which the femoral head appears posteriorly on the femoral neck (Fig. 6-42B). Untreated, this femoral head/neck slippage can continue until growth ceases. To prevent further displacement, the femoral head is fixed with multiple pins.

Osgood-Schlatter Disease

Osgood-Schlatter disease affects the insertion of the patellar tendon onto the tibial tubercle. It is believed to represent partial avulsion of the tibial tubercle in active children with avascular necrosis of the avulsed portion. The patient complains of pain over the tibial tubercle aggravated by kneeling, direct pressure, and running. The area is prominent and tender. Radiographs show irregular areas of bone deposition and resorption in the tibial tubercle. The condition is usually self-limiting and resolves as the growth plates close. Occasionally, a painful ununited nodule persists and is treated by excision.

Congenital Club Foot

The etiology of congenital club foot (**talipes equinovarus**) is unknown. It occurs in approximately 1:1,000 births and is twice as common in males as in females. Club feet are bilateral in 33% of cases. The condition is characterized

by three deformities: the ankle or talus is plantar flexed (equinus), the hindfoot or calcaneus is inverted into varus, and the navicular bone and forefoot is shifted medially and supinated (metatarsus adductus; Fig. 6-39B). Untreated, this deformity causes the patient to walk on the lateral border of the foot, not upon the sole. The posterior muscles of the leg are atrophic and contracted. Neuromuscular abnormalities must be excluded in children with a club foot. Corrective casts are applied immediately with the gradual application of force directed to correct each of the three deformities. When a club foot is refractory to serial cast correction, surgical release of the tight soft tissue structures of the posteromedial foot and ankle is indicated.

Scoliosis

Scoliosis is a curvature of the spine that is either flexible (correctable) or fixed (structural). A mobile form of scoliosis may be due to poor posture, the muscle spasm secondary to a prolapsed disc, or as compensation for a shortened leg. A fixed, structural scoliosis is accompanied by a rotational vertebral deformity that is not correctable by a change in posture. Scoliosis causes an asymmetry of the rib cage that is most noticeable when the patient bends forward. In stance, if the trunk is laterally shifted and not centered over the pelvis, the scoliotic curve is said to be decompensated. Decompensated scoliosis may be associated with a higher incidence of back pain.

Structural scoliosis can be caused by congenital vertebral deformities, neuromuscular diseases (e.g., myelomeningocele, cerebral palsy), or neurofibromatosis. Congenital scoliosis is due to abnormalities of vertebral formation. It is manifested at a young age and is rapidly progressive. These children frequently have associated neural tube, genitourinary, and cardiovascular malformations that occur at the same stage of embryologic development. A comprehensive assessment of these organ systems is mandated in the child in whom congenital scoliosis is identified. Neuromuscular scoliotic curves usually involve the full length of the spine. These curves result from paraspinal muscle imbalance produced by diseases such as polio, spinal muscle atrophy, cerebral palsy, and the muscular dystrophies. The scoliosis of neurofibromatosis is characterized by a short but severe curve.

The most common cause of scoliosis is idiopathic. It causes a painless progressive deformity of the thoracolumbar spine during adolescence. Girls are affected nine times more frequently than boys. The spinal deformity begins before puberty but increases most rapidly during the adolescent growth spurt. As the scoliotic curvature increases, the shape of the vertebrae and the attached ribs change. The vertebral bodies become wedge shaped, and the ribs prominent on the convex side of the curve. These changes of vertebral structure explain why the curves become inflexible over time. Aside from cosmetic concerns, severe thoracic spinal curves can compromise cardiopulmonary function. Some patients with large curves also develop degenerative spinal joint pain. Curve progression is more likely in young patients with larger curves. The goal of treatment is to prevent the scoliotic curve from increasing in magnitude. Spinal braces work well in smaller curves but must be worn until the cessation of growth. Larger curves or scoliosis that occurs with congenital or neuromuscular conditions that progress rapidly in severity despite bracing are managed with surgical correction and spinal fusion.

INFECTIOUS DISEASES OF THE MUSCULOSKELETAL SYSTEM

Musculoskeletal infection involves either bone (osteomyelitis) or joints (septic arthritis). Gram-positive organisms, primarily staphylococci, are usually the causative microbes. Gram-negative organisms have been increasing as a cause, especially in compromised hosts and in the nosocomial environment.

Osteomyelitis

Bacteria may infect bone by one of the following four mechanisms:

1 Hematogenous spread from a distant site
2 Contamination from an open fracture
3 After an operative procedure on bone
4 Extension from a contiguous infected foci

Acute Hematogenous Osteomyelitis

Acute osteomyelitis occurs most commonly in children and is due to hematogenous spread from a distant site of infection. In the 0- to 3-month age-group, the common causative organisms are coliforms from the maternal birth canal to which the infant is exposed during delivery. *H. influenzae* from otitis media and pharyngeal sources is common until age 3. *S. aureus*, which predominates in skin infections, is common in all age-groups.

Pathology

In children, metaphyseal capillaries turn back toward the diaphysis at the level of the growth plate, forming a turbulent area where organisms may be deposited. Due to this peculiarity of intraosseous vascular anatomy, the metaphyses of long bones are the most common foci of acute hematogenous osteomyelitis. Metaphyseal vessels cross the epiphyseal plate during a brief period of neonatal development, which permits epiphyseal infection to occur in infancy.

As trapped bacteria multiply and pus forms in metaphyseal tissue, the pressure within the unyielding bone causes intense pain, forcing the infection through the thin metaphyseal cortex to elevate and spread beneath the periosteum as a subperiosteal abscess (Fig. 6-43). Periosteal stripping stimulates new bone formation that is seen on radiographs. The infection may envelop the bone or burst through the periosteum into the soft tissues.

Clinical Presentation

The onset is acute, and progression can be rapid, even life-threatening. The child experiences severe pain near the end of a long bone and guards the limb, unwilling to move it. With septicemia, there may be fever, increased irritability, or malaise. Soft tissue swelling occurs late and indicates that the infection has spread beyond the bone. The white blood cell count and erythrocyte sedimentation rate are usually elevated. Radiographic changes occur late and may not provide evidence of infection for 1 week or more. A three-phase technetium pyrophosphate bone scan can distinguish among soft tissue cellulitis, rheumatic fever, and acute hematogenous osteomyelitis earlier in its clinical course.

Evaluation and Treatment

Blood cultures should be obtained along with a bone marrow aspirate for cultures and Gram stain. Parenteral antibiotic treatment should be initiated to cover organisms common to the child's age-group. Final antibiotic selection will depend on the results of bacteriologic cultures and sensitivities. If local and systemic manifestations of the infection have not improved within 24 hours, open surgical drainage of subperiosteal pus is indicated, as is bone drilling. Antibiotic therapy should be continued for at least 3 weeks to fully eradicate the organism. Serial sedimentation rates are useful in monitoring the therapeutic response: elevated rates should return to normal values as the infec-

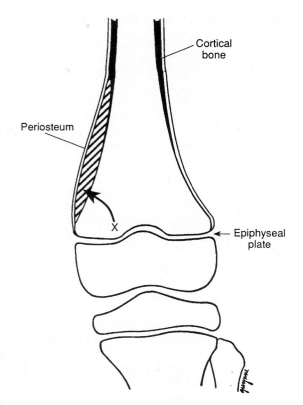

Figure 6-43   Osteomyelitis begins in the bony metaphysis, where hematogenous spread leaves bacteria entrapped in the end arteriolar system of interosseous blood vessels. With exponential bacterial reproduction, pressure within the unyielding bone causes pain and forces the infection through the thin metaphyseal cortex to form a subperiosteal abscess. The epiphyseal plate and periosteum provide a temporary barrier to the infection. *X,* infected foci; *arrow,* path of infection; *shaded area,* periosteum stripped from bone. (Modified from Salter RB. *Textbook of Disorders and Injuries of the Musculoskeletal System,* 3rd ed. Baltimore: Lippincott Williams & Wilkins; 1999.)

tion resolves. Late complications of hematogenous osteomyelitis include the development of persistent or recurrent chronic osteomyelitis, pathologic fractures, and growth disturbances from epiphyseal plate injury.

Adult osteomyelitis typically occurs after an open fracture or as a complication of surgery. Proper management of open fractures with aggressive and repeated debridement of devitalized tissue, wound irrigation, appropriate antibiotic coverage, fracture stabilization, and delayed wound closure serve to decrease the incidence of posttraumatic infection. A clean operative environment (e.g., room, air, personnel), nontraumatic tissue handling, adequate hemostasis, and prophylactic antibiotic administration — especially in implant surgery — are surgical methods that prevent postoperative infections. Effective treatment of an infected implant requires surgical removal of the implant, debridement, and parenteral antibiotics. *S. aureus* remains the leading cause of bone infection in adults. Some infections can result from less virulent organisms

such as *Staphylococcus epidermidis*. Diabetic foot infections tend to be due to mixed aerobic and anaerobic bacteria.

Chronic Osteomyelitis

The incomplete eradication of a previous bone infection results in chronic osteomyelitis. Bacteria that have been protected from leukocytes and antibiotics by a surrounding wall of avascular dead bone (sequestrum) remain dormant in the dead bone. Many years after the initial infection, the bacteria can suddenly multiply, form a sinus, and drain, or they can cause an acute recurrence of the osteomyelitis. Infected, sequestered bone needs to be surgically debrided (saucerized). Soft tissue coverage may be required to enhance local blood supply and antibiotic delivery. A bone graft or bone transport (distraction osteogenesis) may be necessary if radical amounts of infected bone have been resected.

Septic Arthritis

Pathology

When bacteria invade a synovial joint, the inflammatory process can cause rapid, severe destruction of the articular cartilage. In children, septic arthritis occurs as an extension of hematogenous osteomyelitis. The joints commonly involved are those in which the metaphysis resides within the joint capsule: the hip, elbow, and shoulder. Because the metaphysis is enclosed in the joint capsule, what begins as osteomyelitis can erupt through the cortex to involve the joint in the septic process (Fig. 6-44). Thus, in children, the causative organisms of septic arthritis are the same as those involved with osteomyelitis. *Staphylococcus* predominates in all age-groups. Gram-negative organisms affect children younger than 3 years. In adults, joint infections appear after penetrating wounds and rarely as a manifestation of disseminated gonorrhea.

Evaluation

If a newborn is profoundly ill and unresponsive, the diagnosis of septic arthritis may be difficult to establish. The major finding on physical examination is restricted, painful joint motion. The joint is also tender to palpation. Early radiographs and peripheral white blood cell counts are usually nonspecific. Because treatment delay has dire consequences, the clinical suspicion of a septic arthritis is enough to warrant emergency joint fluid aspiration for culture and Gram stain. To document that the joint has been entered, an arthrogram should be performed after aspiration. Joint aspiration through an area of cellulitis is contraindicated, because it may introduce organisms into the joint.

In the patient with active inflammatory arthritides on suppressive medications, acute septic arthritis can be mistaken for an acute flare of inflammatory arthritis. Joint aspiration for Gram stain and culture should be performed

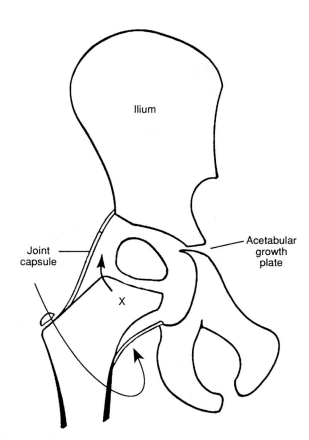

Figure 6-44 In children, septic arthritis occurs as a consequence of hematogenous osteomyelitis. The joints involved are those in which the bony metaphysis resides within a joint capsule such as the hip. When osteomyelitis erupts through the metaphyseal cortex, it will infect the joint space. *X*, infected foci; *arrow*, path of infection. (Modified from Salter RB. *Textbook of Disorders and Injuries of the Musculoskeletal System*, 3rd ed. Baltimore: Lippincott Williams & Wilkins; 1999.)

to rule out infection. The patient should be treated with antibiotics pending results of culture.

Treatment

To prevent the rapid degradation of articular cartilage by pyogenic toxins, treatment of a septic joint is an emergency. The most effective treatment is surgical incision of the joint capsule (arthrotomy), drainage, debridement of infected tissue, and joint irrigation. Intravenous antibiotic therapy is started and the wound is loosely closed over a drain. In the knee, arthroscopic drainage, irrigation, and synovectomy has proven equally effective in the treatment of joint sepsis. The potential complications from septic arthritis include arthritis, epiphyseal necrosis, pathologic joint dislocation, growth disturbances, leg length discrepancies, and limb deformity.

Infected Hand Flexor Tenosynovitis

Improperly treated hand infections can cause severe disability. A flexor tendon sheath infection is especially serious

because it can rapidly destroy the tendon's gliding mechanisms, create adhesions, and cause severe loss of joint motion. Tendon sheath infection can even cause tendon necrosis.

The prevailing infecting organism is *S. aureus*. Pyogenic flexor tenosynovitis is commonly caused by a penetrating palmar injury but can also occur by means of hematogenous seeding.

Kanavel described the four classic physical signs of infected flexor tendon sheaths, as follows:

1 The entire digit is enlarged and swollen (looks like a sausage).
2 The finger is held in a flexed posture.
3 There is tenderness over and limited to the course of the tendon sheath (tender with anterior-posterior pressure but not medial-lateral pressure).
4 There is exquisite pain with passive digital extension.

Pyogenic hand infections are limb threatening and require emergency care. If treated early with parenteral high-dose antibiotic therapy, the infectious process may be halted. Failure of symptoms and signs to improve over 24 to 48 hours warrants surgical drainage with irrigation. Early active range-of-motion exercise is needed to rehabilitate hand function.

INFLAMMATORY DISEASES OF THE MUSCULOSKELETAL SYSTEM

Arthritis means joint inflammation. The two common forms are **osteoarthrosis** and **rheumatoid arthritis**. The management of arthritis as it affects specific joints is well described in orthopedic and rheumatology texts. In this section, treatment will be discussed in general terms.

Osteoarthrosis

Osteoarthrosis is the most prevalent form of arthritis affecting adults. In the adult population older than age 65, there will be radiographic evidence of joint degeneration affecting one or more joints. Osteoarthrosis, also called degenerative joint disease, is characterized by the progressive narrowing of articular cartilage, sclerosis in the subchondral regions and a hypertrophic response of bone and cartilage (osteophyte formation). Its incidence increases with age and has no sex predilection. The etiology of osteoarthrosis is not clearly understood. Mechanical joint stresses are related to its development. Arthrosis results from joint surface incongruity, malalignment, and joint instability.

Pathology

Articular cartilage has physical properties that tolerate a limited amount of stress per unit surface area. When these forces are exceeded, the cartilage will show signs of wear. Pathologically, articular cartilage becomes softened, frayed, and eventually fibrillated. Focal cartilage erosions become widespread and expose the underlying subchondral bone. This bone becomes sclerotic and stiff as the trabeculae thicken and cysts form. At the periphery of the joint, spurlike bony outgrowths covered by hyaline cartilage (osteophytes) develop. Osteophytes are a biologic attempt to decrease joint stress by increasing joint surface area and decreasing motion.

The radiologic hallmarks of **osteoarthrosis** are as follows (Fig. 6-45):

Localized joint space narrowing
Subchondral bone sclerosis
Osteophytes
Subchondral cysts

Symptoms of degenerative joint disease begin gradually with joint pain brought on by activity and relieved by rest. The patient may report a history of joint swelling, stiffness and the slow, progressive loss of joint motion. Because the articular cartilage has no nerve supply, the pain of osteoarthritis is believed to originate in the periarticular structures. Pain and crepitus (a grinding sensation) occur with joint motion. Signs and symptoms often correlate with the degree and extent of radiographic abnormalities. It must be emphasized that osteoarthrosis is generally a local disease. Multiple joint involvement suggests a systemic process (inflammatory arthritis).

Degenerative joint disease in the hand commonly affects the thumb trapeziometacarpal joint. Pain occurs at the base of the thumb with pinching. Weight-bearing joints (e.g., hip and knee) are most frequently involved. Osteoarthritis can affect the great toe MTP joint.

Treatment

Nonsurgical Treatment

The goal of nonsurgical treatment of osteoarthrosis is to relieve pain and maintain strength and function. Reduction of joint load by means of activity modifications, weight loss, or walking aids (e.g., a cane) may provide some relief or symptoms. Physical therapy alleviates pain with the use of heat while attempting to maintain joint motion and muscle strength through exercise. Nonsteroidal anti-inflammatory drugs that interfere with the pain-producing products of inflammation (e.g., prostaglandins, lymphokines, kinins) can reduce pain and swelling. These drugs can have adverse effects including rashes, peptic ulceration, and tinnitus. Simple analgesics (e.g., acetaminophen) have been shown to be efficacious in the management of musculoskeletal pain. The chronic use of narcotics is to be avoided. Intra-articular steroid injections provide dramatic relief of acute arthritic symptoms. How-

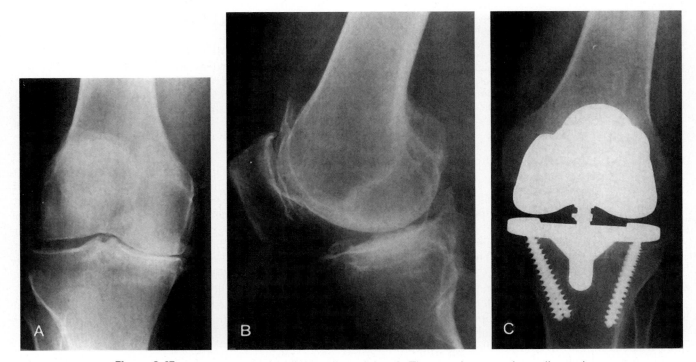

Figure 6-45   Osteoarthritis affecting the knee joint. **A,** The anterior-posterior radiograph shows joint space narrowing, subchondral sclerosis, and a hypertrophic osteophytic response of the bone at the joint margins. **B,** Osteophytes (seen better on this lateral radiograph) decrease joint motion and increase joint surface area, in a biologic attempt to decrease excessive joint surface stresses. **C,** The knee ultimately required total joint replacement.

ever, the repeated use of steroids may accelerate joint deterioration by deleterious effects on the metabolism of the cartilage. The role of intra-articular lubricating agents (hyaluronic acid) is not clear at this time. There are numerous dietary supplements (e.g., glucosamine and chondroitin sulfate) that claim benefits in the management of degenerative joint disease but have yet to be substantiated in scientific studies. One recently published study casts doubt on their efficacy.

Surgical Treatment

The selection of surgical procedures depends on the stage, site, and debility caused by the arthrosis. There are three categories of bony procedures: osteotomy for joint realignment, total joint replacement, and joint fusion (or arthrodesis). An osteotomy realigns the extremity, corrects deformity, and shifts weight-bearing forces from worn joint surfaces to healthier cartilage. This procedure should be considered in younger patients with degenerative arthrosis of the knee. An example would be a valgus-producing tibial osteotomy for a varus knee with symptomatic medial compartment arthrosis.

Total joint arthroplasty (Fig. 6-45C) involves the replacement of articulating surfaces with low-friction, metal, and high-molecular-weight polyethylene surfaces. Total joint arthroplasty is an extremely successful procedure that profoundly relieves pain in more than 90% of cases. Joint replacement is not without complications—prosthetic components wear out, loosen, become infected, and cause local osteoporosis and periprosthetic fractures. Therefore, joint replacement is reserved for patients with advanced **arthrosis** and a relatively sedentary lifestyle.

Joint arthrodesis is an effective procedure that converts painful arthritic joint motion into a painless, stable, stiff joint. Arthrodesis is a durable procedure that is indicated in young, very active patients with isolated joint involvement (e.g., great toe, spine, ankle). Large joint arthrodesis is contraindicated in patients with systemic multiple joint inflammatory arthritis.

Rheumatoid Arthritis

Rheumatoid arthritis is an inflammatory disorder of unknown etiology. It is a chronic symmetrical polyarthritis with a relapsing course that frequently leads to progressive joint destruction, deformity, and incapacitation.

Rheumatoid arthritis is a common illness with a female predominance of 3:1. The disease has a genetic basis. Individuals with the HLA-DR4 haplotype are at high risk for developing rheumatoid arthritis. Regardless of the inciting factor, the immune system is involved in the disease process. Of rheumatoid patients, 80% have autoantibodies to the Fc region of immunoglobulin G (IgG). The immunoglobulin M (IgM) autoantibody is termed the rheumatoid factor. Although the presence of the rheumatoid factor is not diagnostic of the disorder (1%–5% of normal subjects have it), high titers are associated with severe joint disease, multisystem involvement, and a poor prognosis.

Pathology

The pathology of rheumatoid arthritis results from synovial inflammation of joints and tendon sheaths. As the synovial membrane becomes infiltrated by macrophages and lymphocytes, it undergoes hypertrophy and causes joint swelling and effusions. The byproducts of the inflammatory process injure adjacent bone and cartilage. Hypertrophic synovial cells proliferate and damage the articular cartilage. This synovial overgrowth on to the joint surface is called pannus. Recurrent joint swelling stretches the capsule and supportive ligaments, which causes joint instability, deformity, and further mechanical injury. Adjacent inflammatory processes weaken tendons and cause muscle imbalance in the complex joint systems of the hand. Joint and tendon subluxation is common in rheumatoid hands that become weak and deformed (Fig. 6-46). The systemic nature of the disease is made evident by its extra-articular manifestations, which include vasculitis, neuropathy, iritis, lymphadenopathy, splenomegaly, and polyserositis.

Just as the pathophysiology of rheumatoid arthritis differs from that of osteoarthrosis, so do the radiologic pictures. Soft tissue swelling and periarticular osteoporosis are the early signs of rheumatoid arthritis. Diffuse cartilage destruction leads to generalized joint space narrowing and bone erosions at the site of synovial attachments (Fig. 6-46). Joint deformity, cystic bone destruction, and joint ankylosis mark end-stage disease. Hypertrophic osteophytes are rare in rheumatoid arthritis.

Treatment

The treatment of rheumatoid arthritis is directed toward pain relief, suppression of the inflammatory synovitis, prevention of joint deformities, and early joint reconstruction. In its early stages, the synovitis is inhibited by drug therapy or managed by surgical removal of the diseased synovium (synovectomy). Splinting the involved joints in functional positions during acute flare-ups rests the joint, prevents contractures, and minimizes deformity. Exercises to maintain range of motion and muscle strength—although painful and frustrating to the patient—are encouraged. With advanced joint destruction, tendon ruptures are repaired, and excisional or replacement arthroplasty helps to restore mobility and function.

To optimize the patient's function, it is often necessary to use mechanical aids and adaptive apparatus and to modify the physical layout of both the home and workplace. The proper management of rheumatoid arthritis requires the multidisciplinary teamwork of a rheumatologist, surgeon, physiotherapist, occupational therapist, and social worker.

More recently, anti–tumor necrosis factor (anti-TNF) preparations have been added to the treatment of patients with systemic inflammatory arthritis. There are reports of dramatic reduction in pain for some patients. The effects of long-term use of drugs of this class are not known.

Some arthritides are causes by infectious agents such as gonococcal arthritis and Lyme disease. Systemic gono-

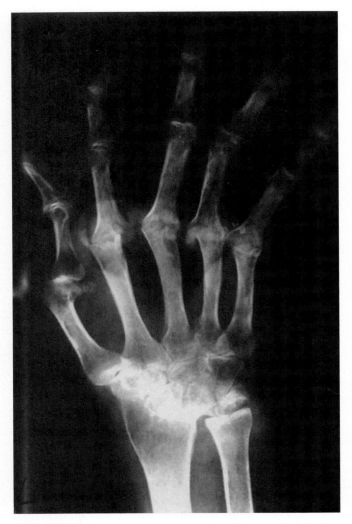

Figure 6-46   Radiographic evidence of rheumatoid arthritic joint involvement, with soft tissue swelling and multiple metacarpophalangeal joint palmar dislocations. Disuse osteoporosis is evident. Actual cartilage destruction causes joint space narrowing as exemplified at the proximal interphalangeal and wrist joints. Bone erosions occur at the site of synovial attachments. Osteophytic changes of bone hypertrophy typical of osteoarthrosis are unusual with rheumatic diseases.

coccal infection may be associated with petechial and pustular rashes on the palms and soles of the feet. Joint aspiration and culture should reveal typical Gram-negative diplococci. Infection usually involves small joints, especially of the hands and feet. Treatment usually leads to full recovery, because the organism does not produce collagenase. Antibiotic treatment includes cefuroxime 1 g intravenously daily for 7 days or penicillin 10 to 20 million units daily for 7 days, if sensitive.

Lyme disease is caused by the spirochete *Borrelia burgdorferi*. The infective agent is carried by ticks that live on deer. The clinical course tends to be a migratory polyarthralgia with or without a rash. The symptoms usually subside after antibiotic treatment with doxycycline 100 mg PO bid or amoxicillin 500 mg PO q6h for 10 days.

Other Arthritides

Although osteoarthrosis and rheumatoid arthritis are the most common arthritic conditions, there are a myriad of other arthritic diseases, including chronic juvenile arthritis, the spondyloarthropathies of ankylosing spondylitis, Reiter's disease, and psoriatic arthritis. In the arthropathies of gout and pseudogout, insoluble crystals are deposited in joints. With gouty arthritis, microscopic analysis of joint fluid under polarized light reveals splinterlike, monoclinic, negatively birefringent uric acid crystals, whereas in pseudogout, positively birefringent, rhomboid-shaped, calcium pyrophosphate dihydrate crystals are apparent. Radiographs of the latter may show typical articular cartilage or meniscal calcification. Acute flares of crystal-induced arthritis are treated with high doses of nonsteroidal anti-inflammatory drugs. Colchicine may be added to the acute treatment of gout. Long-term preventive treatment of gout involves use of allopurinol to decrease systemic uric acid levels. Neuropathies, hemophilia, and many other diseases have arthritic manifestations.

BONE NECROSIS

Interruption of the blood supply to bone results in bone cell death (osteonecrosis or avascular necrosis). Traumatic causes of osteonecrosis have been discussed and involve vascular injury or interruption of the blood supply to bones. The femoral head, talus, carpal lunate, and scaphoid are prone to avascular necrosis. These bones all are extensively covered by articular cartilage and have limited soft tissue attachments. Legg-Calvé-Perthes disease of the femoral head represents a form of avascular necrosis in developing skeleton. Nontraumatic causes of osteonecrosis involve intraosseous microvascular disturbances that result from either arterial emboli or impairment of venous outflow. Either of these mechanisms can compromise bone perfusion.

Patients on glucocorticoid therapy (especially those with systemic lupus erythematosus and or those who have had a renal transplant) are at higher risk of developing osteonecrosis. The thrombi of hemoglobinopathies (e.g., sickle cell disease), the nitrogen bubbles of decompression sickness (dysbarism), the glucocerebroside deposits of Gaucher's disease, hyperuricemic crystals, fat emboli of alcoholism, and pancreatitis may cause an occlusive form of bone infarction. Affected bones have a paucity of arterial anastomoses. The femoral head of the hip is the most frequently affected by avascular necrosis.

Pathology

Bone is a living tissue that is in a dynamic state of homeostasis involving bone resorption, replacement, and remodeling. Unlike other tissues, normal bone turnover occurs slowly. Following a loss of blood supply, bone cell and marrow necrosis occur within 24 hours. Although these changes can be detected microscopically by the absence of osteocytes from their lacunae, there is often a delay of as much as 5 years between the onset of symptoms and the appearance of radiologic abnormalities. MRI is the most sensitive method of detecting early osteonecrosis.

The revascularization process is slow. The living bone surrounding the infarction becomes hypervascular. The hyperemia of the surrounding bone causes local bone mineral resorption appearing as osteopenia on x-ray. Dead tissue retains its density and appears white (sclerotic) on x-ray. As vessels invade and try to repair the necrotic zone, new bone is laid down on the old trabeculae and dead bone is removed by osteoclasts. This reparative process weakens the femoral head at the margins of the infarct. With persistent weight-bearing stress, the necrotic subchondral bone may fracture, leading to severe pain and rapid joint degeneration (Fig. 6-47). Initially, the articular cartilage remains intact because it is nourished by synovial fluid. When a subchondral fracture occurs, the bone support is lost. The articular cartilage becomes separated from the subchondral bone and a process similar to osteoarthrosis causes joint destruction.

Evaluation and Treatment

The symptoms of osteonecrosis may not become manifest until a subchondral fracture occurs. Symptoms begin with painful limited active motion. Two thirds of patients complain of pain at rest. In the elderly, spontaneous osteonecrosis of the femoral condyle occurs with the sudden onset of severe knee pain not associated with trauma. Many cases show increased bone scan activity over the femoral condyle adjacent to the necrotic zone.

The prevention of joint loading until natural healing processes are completed is the basis of conservative treatment. Core decompression, in which dead cancellous bone is trephined from the ischemic segment, is best employed early in the disease process. Intraosseous pressure is decreased as the biopsy tract creates an avenue for revascularization.

Although the inciting agent is vascular, the joint deterioration results from loss of mechanical support for the articular surface. The management principles for advanced disease are similar to those employed in the treatment of osteoarthrosis. If the volume of dead bone is large, total joint replacement is a reasonable treatment option. Unfortunately, avascular necrosis occurs in younger patients, whose high activity levels place stresses that can exceed the design tolerance of implants.

DEGENERATIVE DISEASES OF THE SPINE

Lumbar Spine

Low back pain is the most common musculoskeletal complaint for the 30- to 65-year age-group. Eighty percent (80%) of adults experience an episode of low back pain severe enough to interfere with normal daily activities. In the United States, the annual cost of back-related medical payments is estimated at $16 billion. An additional $50 billion is attributed each year to lost worker productivity.

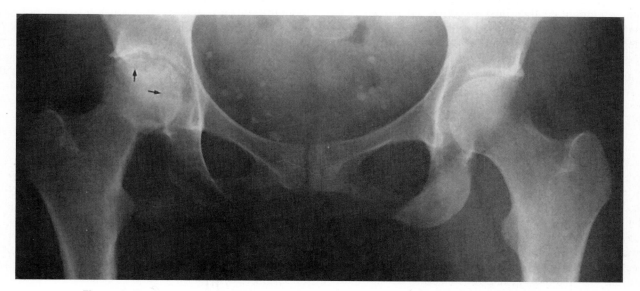

Figure 6-47   Advanced avascular necrosis of the femoral head in a patient with sarcoidosis who had been treated with systemic steroids. The femoral head is dense (sclerotic). There is evidence of a subchondral lucency (*arrows*) with joint surface flattening, collapse, and marginal osteophyte formation.

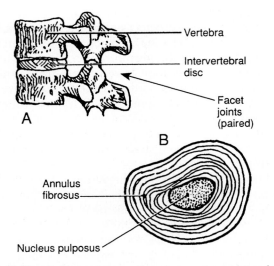

Vertebra

Intervertebral disc

Facet joints (paired)

A

B

Annulus fibrosus

Nucleus pulposus

Figure 6-48 **A,** The spinal motion segment consists of two vertebral bodies and the intervening disc. Motion occurs through two paired facet joints and the disc. The vertebrae rock or pivot over the disc in flexion and lateral bending. **B,** The disc comprises a central gelatinous nucleus pulposus and its peripheral fibrous encasement, the annulus fibrosus. (Reprinted with permission from American Academy of Orthopaedic Surgeons. *Athletic Training and Sports Medicine,* 2nd ed. Park Ridge, IL: American Academy of Orthopaedic Surgeons; 1991:515.)

Anatomy and Physiology

Degenerative joint disease is far more common to the joints of the spine than to the joints of the limbs. The spine is an articulated column of vertebrae that protects the spinal cord and nerve roots. The neural elements also can be affected by degenerative spinal pathology. The motion segment of the spine is composed of two bony vertebrae covered with cartilage end plates and the intervertebral disc. Vertebral motion takes place through a three-joint complex: the intervertebral **disc** and two posterior synovial facet joints (Fig. 6-48A). The disc is composed

of a central gelatinous nucleus pulposus and an elastic **annulus fibrosus** (Fig. 6-48B). In flexion–extension and lateral bending, the vertebrae moving through the spatial orientation of the paired facet joints directs spinal motion. The lumbar vertebral facets are in the sagittal plane and permit flexion and extension. The thoracic facets are oriented in more of a horizontal plane, allowing lateral bending and rotatory motion. Degenerative spine disease anatomically affects the two sites of spinal motion—the disc or the facet joints. The ligaments that tether the vertebrae together include the anterior and posterior longitudinal ligaments attached to the vertebral bodies. The ligamentum flavum connects the laminae with the interspinous and supraspinous ligaments between the spinous processes (Fig. 6-49). The paraspinal muscles are complex and span two to five vertebral segments. These muscles power spinal motion and help absorb the stresses of erect bipedal posture.

Etiology of Low Back Pain

Contrary to popular opinion, the vast majority of low back pain is not due to a "slipped disc." In 80% to 90% of patients with low back pain, the pain is of unknown etiology and the pathology remains obscure. Fewer than 10% of patients experience pain in the sciatic nerve (L5-S3) distribution ("sciatica"). Only 1% to 2% of patients require surgical treatment for a disc herniation. With symptomatic care, 50% improve in 2 weeks and 90% in 3 months.

Pathophysiology

Lumbar Strain (Mechanical Back Pain)
Most cases of back pain result from minor events, not from significant trauma. Many injuries involve myofascial strains, minor ligament injury, or overuse. Lack of exercise, poor muscle tone, and obesity contribute to minor postural injuries of the spine. This type of mechanical back pain is common in women during or after pregnancy. The pain of mechanical strain rarely radiates beyond the knee and remains localized to the spine and buttocks. More than

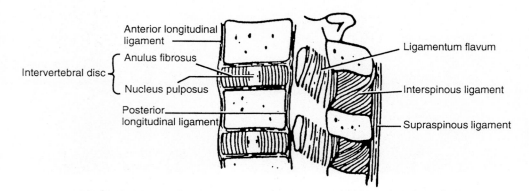

Anterior longitudinal ligament

Anulus fibrosus

Intervertebral disc

Nucleus pulposus

Posterior longitudinal ligament

Ligamentum flavum

Interspinous ligament

Supraspinous ligament

Figure 6-49   The ligaments of the spinal column. (Reprinted with permission from Wilson FC, ed. *The Musculoskeletal System: Basic Processes and Disorders,* 2nd ed. Philadelphia: JB Lippincott; 1983.)

80% of these back problems resolve within 6 weeks of onset.

Spondylolysis and Spondylolisthesis

The facet joints of the lumbar spine are oriented in the sagittal plane, which permits flexion and extension while resisting rotational and lateral bending motion. When the spine is hyperextended, the facet joints are engaged. If a rotational twisting force is added, the lamina may fracture, either after an acute injury or from the stress of repetitive microtrauma. The fracture occurs immediately caudal to the superior facet in a region called the pars interarticularis (Fig. 6-50A). This injury, **spondylolysis,** occurs 10 times more often in gymnasts than in age-matched controls and may result from back extension during dismount landings.

If the fracture is bilateral, the superior vertebral body, lacking facet support, may slide forward on the inferior vertebra. This anterior shift of one vertebrae on another is called spondylolisthesis (Fig. 6-50B). In young patients, the condition may be painful and the slippage can progress. Spinal fusion is the standard treatment for a progressive, painful spondylolisthesis.

Disc Herniation

Disc herniation is the result of extrusion of the nucleus pulposes through the annulus fibrosus. It occurs in adults 30 to 50 years of age (i.e., during the prime working years). The most frequently involved discs are at L4-L5 and L5-S1, the most mobile lumbar spinal segments. A ruptured L4-L5 disc will affect the L5 nerve root and a ruptured L5-S1 disc affects the S1 root. In adults, the nucleus pulposus loses proteoglycans and water content, making it less resilient. In the aging process, the annulus fibrosus loses its elasticity, especially posteriorly, where it is thinnest. The combination of age-related changes and repeated minor trauma can cause tears in the annulus. If an annular tear is large, it will permit the extrusion of the nucleus pulposus. In some cases, the herniated disc material causes minimal symptoms. In others, the herniated disc material exerts direct pressure on the nerve root (Fig. 6-51).

Clinically, patients complain of severe pain, often after bending to lift or while twisting with a heavy object. The pain emanates from the back or buttock and radiates into the leg and foot in a radicular (nerve root), dermatomal distribution. The pain is accentuated by bending, sitting,

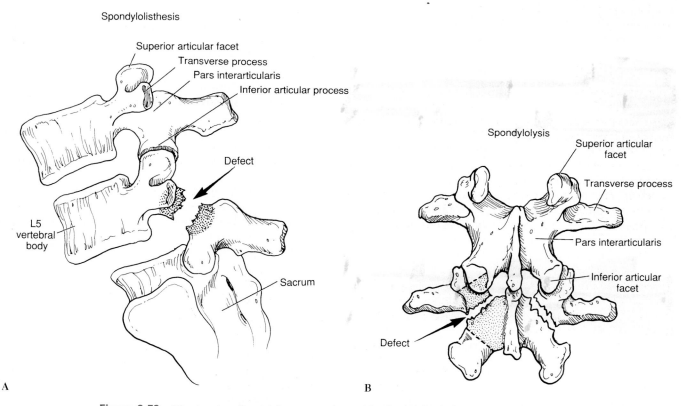

Figure 6-50   The lumbar facet joints are oriented in the sagittal plane and allow flexion and extension. With lumbar extension, the facet joints engage; when a significant rotatory force is added, the lamina just inferior to the facet may fracture. **A,** If spondylolytic fractures occur bilaterally, the unsupported superior vertebrae may translate anteriorly, producing spondylolisthesis. **B,** This fracture is called spondylolysis, which literally means spine lysis. (Modified from McNab I, McCullough J. *Backache,* 2nd ed. Baltimore: Williams & Wilkins; 1990.)

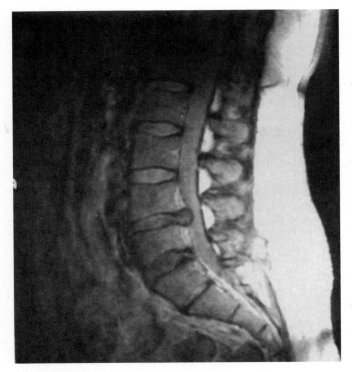

Figure 6-51   Magnetic resonance scan of a large L4-L5 herniated disc. The epidural fat plane is obliterated as the disc exerts extradural pressure on the thecal space.

Table 6-4	**Lumbar Lesions and Associated Radicular Abnormalities**
Location	**Abnormality**
L4 nerve root	
Pain/numbness	Medial leg and ankle
Sensory	Hypesthesia, medial leg and ankle
Motor	Weak ankle dorsiflexion or weak quadriceps (knee extension)
Reflex	Decreased knee jerk
L5 nerve root	
Pain/numbness	Lateral calf and dorsal foot
Sensory	Hypesthesia, dorsal foot
Motor	Weak extensor hallux longus
Reflex	Usually none; decreased posterior tibial tendon reflex possible (but that reflex present in only 20% of normal patients)
S1 nerve root	
Pain/numbness	Posterior calf, lateral and plantar foot
Sensory	Hypesthesia, lateral foot
Motor	Weak extensor hallux longus
Reflex	Weak toe and ankle flexors, foot evertor Decreased ankle jerk

and coughing. The supine straight-leg raising test places traction on the S1 nerve root and to a lesser degree, the L5 root. This test reproduces the pain, which should radiate below the knee to be considered positive. Ankle dorsiflexion accentuates the pain (Lasègue maneuver), whereas ankle plantar flexion should not affect it. The latter test is helpful to exclude malingerers. Radicular motor weakness, numbness, and reflex diminution provide objective evidence of nerve root compression (Table 6-4). When a large amount of disc is extruded into the spinal canal, it may compress more than one nerve root. When multiple nerve roots are involved, the clinical picture may be confusing because of overlapping patterns of pain and functional losses. Loss of bowel and bladder continence is a result of a central disc herniation compressing multiple S1-S4 roots. Called the **cauda equina syndrome,** this condition is a surgical emergency demanding decompression to prevent permanent incontinence.

MRI of the lumbosacral spine is the diagnostic test of choice to define the anatomic location of disc material for patients considered for surgery with unremitting leg pain or progressive neurologic deficit. CT is less sensitive and specific but may localize pathology. Myelography, the injection of water-soluble dye into the epidural space, is rarely used unless MRI is not available.

Spinal Stenosis

The spinal facets are synovial joints and are subject to degenerative arthritic changes. As the discs narrow, there are increased forces on the facet joints. The facet joints narrow and they develop marginal osteophytes. The development of hypertrophic facet joint osteophytes narrow the space available for existing nerve roots and may irritate or compress them. The narrowing of the disc may allow the ligamentum flavum to buckle into the spinal canal. This combination of folds of ligamentum flavum posteriorly and hypertrophic osteophytes anteriorly can cause encroachment of spinal canal or foraminal contents causing symptoms of **spinal stenosis.**

Spinal stenosis is a pattern of back and leg pain attributed to narrowing of the spinal canal. The pain tends to begin after being upright or walking for a period of time. It does not tend to diminish unless the patient sits down or lies down. This feature usually distinguishes it from vascular claudication. This pattern of pain is referred to as neurogenic claudication. It tends to affect people with extensive degenerative disc disease who are usually over 65 years of age.

Surgery for spinal stenosis involves decompression of the spinal cord and roots. Careful preoperative evaluation is necessary to properly identify the location and extent of pathology. CT and MRI scans of several spinal levels are needed to define the pathology and extent of neural canal and foraminal compromise. Each disc space is evaluated for herniation and each facet joint for stenosis of the lateral recess of the spinal canal.

Other Conditions

There are many other causes of back pain. The medical history is extremely helpful in identifying the etiology of low back disorders. The differential diagnosis includes the following:

1 Disc herniation with nerve root irritation or neurologic deficit
2 Spinal stenosis
3 Vertebral infection
4 Primary or metastatic neoplasms; especially thyroid, lung, breast, renal, and prostate.
5 Trauma (see Chapter 10 in Lawrence's *Essentials of General Surgery*, 4th edition)
6 Rheumatologic conditions (e.g., ankylosing spondylitis, rheumatoid arthritis, Reiter's disease)
7 Vascular disorders (e.g., aortic aneurysm, aortic dissection)
8 Psychogenic or malingering pain (vague history and bizarre gait with inconsistent physical findings suggest psychogenic causes)

Treatment

Nonsurgical Treatment

Most cases of back pain are mechanical. Nonsurgical measures that include analgesics, anti-inflammatories, and stretching and strengthening exercises are often effective. Patient education about the causes and nature of back pain is important. Instruction in proper postural mechanics and lifting techniques will prevent reinjury. Patients should be encouraged to take an active interest in and responsibility for their own back care.

Patients with back and referred leg pain may benefit from a short period of rest, analgesic and anti-inflammatory medications, and heat, followed by an active back exercise program. A brace may provide symptomatic relief. The brace acts as a proprioceptive device, reminding the patient to lift and bend properly. The excessive use of bed rest and back braces is to be avoided as both can cause paraspinal muscle atrophy.

Nonsteroidal anti-inflammatory medications are useful for their analgesic and anti-inflammatory effects. Narcotic analgesics and antispasmodic agents are used with caution, especially with chronic back pain. Both of these classes of drugs mask symptoms and may cause chemical dependency.

The two absolute indications for surgical decompression are as follows:

1 When disc herniation causes a progressive neurologic deficit
2 When cauda equina syndrome is suspected with loss of bowel or bladder continence

The majority (>80%) of patients with a symptomatic lumbar disc herniation will improve with conservative treatment and not require surgery.

Surgical Treatment

Approximately 10% of patients with leg pain do not respond to conservative treatment. If leg pain persists for more than 2 months of conservative care, surgery may be considered. The results are better if surgery is performed within 6 months of the onset of symptoms. After 6 months, the patient becomes physically deconditioned and psychologically dependent. The candidate for surgery should have consistent physical and radiographic findings. Spinal surgery treats symptoms and does not reverse the degenerative processes of spinal aging and arthritis. Operations for disc herniations should be precisely defined. In patients with spinal stenosis, decompression is more extensive. All structures causing nerve root pressure: herniated discs, osteophytic spurs, and calcified ligaments are surgically removed from each involved spinal level. The indications for spinal fusion in this setting are controversial. In patients with spinal instability from progressive spondylolisthesis or after anatomically extensive decompression, spinal fusion can be an effective stabilizing and palliative procedure.

Cervical Spine

Degenerative disc disease and disc protrusion also occur in the cervical spine. The erosive synovitis of rheumatoid arthritis has an affinity for the mobile cervical spine.

Cervical Disc Protrusion

The combined effects of age-related disc degeneration and abnormal stresses can cause cervical disc herniations. When disc material presses on the posterior longitudinal ligament, symptoms of stiffness and neck pain may be referred to the scapular region. When the herniated disc material protrudes posterior and lateral to the posterior longitudinal ligament, it may impinge on a cervical nerve root. Consequently, it may cause radicular pain, numbness, focal motor weakness, and diminution or loss of upper extremity deep tendon reflexes (Table 6-5). The

Table 6-5	Cervical Lesions and Associated Radicular Abnormalities
Location	**Abnormality**
C5 nerve root	
Sensory	Hypesthesia of the lateral arm
Motor	Weak deltoid, biceps
Reflex	Decreased biceps reflex
C6 nerve root	
Sensory	Hypesthesia of the lateral forearm and palmar thumb
Motor	Weak wrist extension
Reflex	Decreased brachioradialis reflex
C7 nerve root	
Sensory	Hypesthesia of the long finger
Motor	Weak finger extension, triceps
Reflex	Decreased triceps reflex
C8 nerve root	
Sensory	Hypesthesia of the medial forearm and little finger
Motor	Weak finger flexion
Reflex	None
Myelopathy	Diffuse hypesthesias
Sensory	Diffuse weakness, increased muscle tone, rigidity
Motor	Hyper-reflexia with clonus
Reflex	Positive Hoffmann or Babinski sign

most commonly ruptured discs are at the C5-C6 and C6-C7 interspaces, where cervical flexion–extension motion is the greatest. Likewise, the respective C6 and C7 nerve roots are most often affected by cervical disc pathology.

Nonoperative treatment involves rest, immobilization with a soft cervical collar, heat, and anti-inflammatory medication. Traction may help to alleviate nerve root pressure. Indications for surgical intervention are similar to those in the lumbar spine. Emergency decompressive surgery is indicated if there is spinal cord involvement (myelopathy) with hyper-reflexia, ipsilateral weakness, contralateral numbness, or the presence of pathologic long tract reflexes (e.g., **Babinski** or **Hoffmann sign**).

Cervical Spondylosis

Degenerative disc changes cause disc space narrowing and increases the forces on the facet joints and joints of Luschka. Osteophytes form at the posterior disc margin, creating a "hard disc." These bone spurs, called **Luschka's joints,** can encroach on the spinal cord or peripherally on an individual nerve root (Fig. 6-52). The clinical picture is similar to the herniation of the nucleus pulposus (soft disc), except that the onset of symptoms is more gradual. Treatment for degenerative cervical spondyloarthrosis is similar to that for cervical disc protrusion. When refractory to conservative treatment modalities, both conditions respond to anterior cervical discectomy with a fusion.

Rheumatoid Arthritis of the Cervical Spine

Rheumatoid arthritis often involves the synovial joints of the cervical spine. Progressive inflammatory destruction of bone, ligaments, and articular cartilage may cause cervical spine instability or neural compression.

Rheumatic cervical spine involvement usually takes one of the three following patterns:

1 Rheumatoid inflammation and swelling of the small synovial joint between the atlas and the odontoid process can stretch the stabilizing transverse ligament and cause the atlantoaxial joint (C1-C2) to subluxate with flexion. The two vertebrae no longer move in synchrony, which causes spinal canal narrowing and potential cord compromise by the posteriorly displaced dens.
2 Erosive synovitis between the atlas (C1 vertebra) and the occipital condyles causes cranial settling that may cause the odontoid process of the axis (C2) to protrude into the foramen magnum. This phenomenon is termed *occipitoatlantoaxial impaction* and can compress the spinal cord causing long tract signs.
3 Finally, facet joint synovitis affecting any cervical vertebrae below the axis can cause segmental instability known as subaxial subluxation. This instability is demonstrated on lateral radiographs by abnormal vertebral body tilt or displacement in the AP direction.

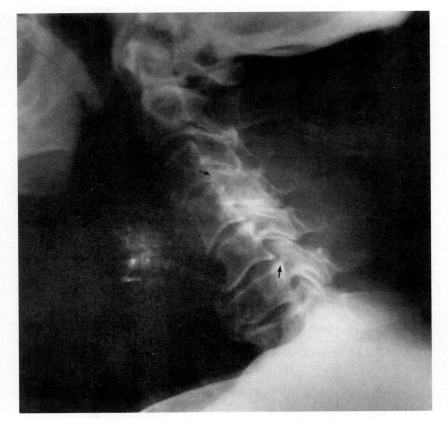

Figure 6-52 Osteoarthrotic cervical spondylosis with anterior vertebral body osteophyte formation and disc space narrowing. Posterior vertebral body osteophytes also called Luschka (or uncovertebral) joints (*arrows*) can cause encroachment on the spinal cord. This is known as a hard disc.

The prevalence of cervical instability in patients with polyarticular rheumatoid arthritis is such that flexion–extension lateral cervical spine radiographs must be obtained for any rheumatoid patient undergoing intubation for a general anesthetic. Neurologic involvement does not necessarily correlate with the degree of cervical vertebral subluxation. However, when neurologic impairment is caused by cervical instability, the treatment of choice is stabilization through surgical spine fusion. Most cases of rheumatoid neck pain, however, are successfully managed by nonoperative treatment modalities.

METABOLIC ENDOCRINE DISORDERS

Bone is a biphasic material consisting of an inert mineral and an organic matrix. The mineral is composed of calcium and phosphorous in a hydroxyapatite crystal $Ca_{10}(PO_4)_6(OH)_2$. The organic matrix (osteoid) is primarily composed of type I collagen, which has high tensile strength. The mineral phase of bone resists compressive forces, whereas the organic collagen fiber phase provides reinforcement and resistance to bending and twisting stress (like the meshed wire in cement). Normal bone is 70% mineral and 30% organic matrix.

Osteoporosis

Bone strength depends on the amount of bone mineral per unit volume. In osteoporosis, the chemical composition of the bone is normal but total bone mineral is more than 2 standard deviations below an age-matched control. The ratio of bone mineral to organic matrix is normal, but the absolute value of each is decreased. The bone is therefore weak, less dense, and predisposed to fractures with minimal trauma. The most common type of osteoporosis is the involutional senile type and is seen in postmenopausal, white females. The cause is unknown. Other conditions also result in osteoporosis (Table 6-6).

Table 6-6	Causes of Osteoporosis
Involutional	Postmenopausal age
Nutritional deficiencies	Scurvy
Endocrine disorders	Hypogonadism
	Hyperparathyroidism
	Cushing's disease
	Hyperthyroidism
Drug use	Corticosteroids
	Methotrexate
Disuse	Prolonged bed rest
	Weightlessness
Inflammatory arthritis	Rheumatoid arthritis
	Ankylosing spondylitis
	Chronic infection (tuberculosis)
Malignant disease	Multiple myeloma
	Leukemia
Idiopathic	

Osteoporosis is second to arthritis in causes of musculoskeletal morbidity in the elderly. The symptoms occur when bone mass is so compromised that the skeleton fractures as a result of the mechanical stresses of everyday life. Compression fractures of vertebral bodies or fractures of the proximal femur (hip; Fig. 6-18), humerus, and distal radius (Colles; Fig. 6-15) are often the first manifestations of osteoporosis. These patients should be screened for the medically treatable causes of osteoporosis. Exercise, dietary calcium, and vitamin D supplements (and estrogen in early postmenopausal women) can be effective prophylaxis against the bone loss of osteoporosis. Diphosphonates and calcitonin can be used to treat this condition and have been shown to increase bone mineral density and decrease fracture rates. Adequate calcium intake during the growing years as well as a healthy level of physical activity are the current long-term prevention strategies.

Osteomalacia

Osteomalacia is the result of a deficiency in the mineral content of bone. In contrast to osteoporosis, the amount of bone matrix per unit volume is normal. However, the matrix that is present is incompletely calcified. Clinically and radiographically, osteoporosis and osteomalacia are similar. Often the distinction is made by bone biopsy and histomorphometry, an analytic technique that requires ultrathin, nondecalcified, tetracycline-labeled bone biopsy specimens. In osteomalacia, wide osteoid seams of unmineralized bone are detected. The ratio of bone mineral to organic bone matrix is decreased because there is a mineral deficiency. In osteoporosis, the ratio of bone mineral to matrix is normal because the quantity of both is deficient.

Inadequate bone mineralization can result from inadequate dietary vitamin D or calcium intake, gastrointestinal malabsorption of calcium, problems with the enzymatic conversion of vitamin D, or defective renal calcium and phosphorous handling (Table 6-7). Correctable defects in the calcium pathway can be screened by obtaining levels of serum calcium and phosphorous, blood urea nitrogen, and creatinine, which may detect gastrointestinal, endocrine, or renal causes. In addition to the generalized de-

Table 6-7	Causes of Osteomalacia
Dietary	Vitamin D deficiency (rickets)
Hereditary	Hypophosphatemic rickets
Gastrointestinal	Biliary disease
	Pancreatitis
	Celiac sprue
	Milk alkali syndrome
	Cirrhosis
Drug use	Phenytoin
	Barbiturates
Chronic renal disease	

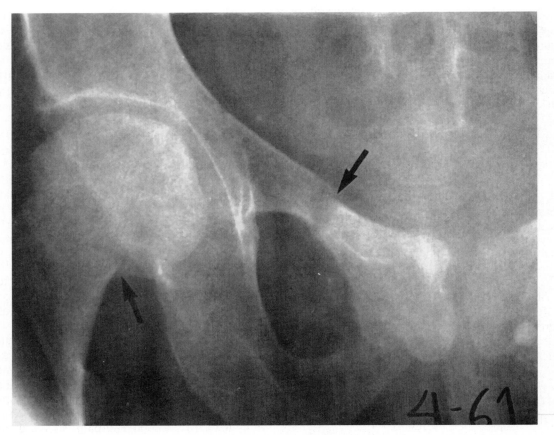

Figure 6-53   Looser line seen with osteomalacia. The band of rarefaction in the superior pubic ramus and in the femoral neck (*arrows*) represents a stress fracture and is due to inadequate bone mineralization.

crease in bone density seen radiologically, a band of bone rarefaction called a Looser zone is typical of osteomalacia (Fig. 6-53). The Looser zone represents a healing stress fracture and is most often noted in the femoral neck or pubic rami.

The pediatric form of osteomalacia is called rickets and is caused by dietary vitamin D deficiency and lack of exposure to sunlight. This disease was common during the industrial revolution before the advent of child labor laws. Today rickets is seen primarily in a genetic disease called vitamin D–resistant (hypophosphatemic) rickets, which is transmitted in an autosomal dominant pattern. In growing children, radiographs of osteomalacia (rickets) demonstrate widened growth plates and cupped metaphyses (Fig. 6-54). Soft, undermineralized long bones may be abnormally bowed.

Hyperparathyroidism

Hyperparathyroidism causes diffuse bony osteopenia. Parathyroid hormone is involved with the homeostasis of ionized calcium levels in the blood. In response to low serum calcium or high serum phosphorous concentrations, parathyroid hormone increases calcium release from bone, calcium absorption by the intestines, and calcium reabsorption by the kidney (while decreasing renal absorption of phosphate). These changes cause a net increase in plasma calcium and a decrease in plasma phosphate levels. Primary hyperparathyroidism is due to an adenoma or hyperplasia of the parathyroid gland. Secondary hyperparathyroidism is due to chronic renal insufficiency with decreased phosphate excretion. Radiographs of hyperparathyroidism show diffuse bony rarefaction but also include disseminated focal osteolytic lesions of cortical bone called osteitis fibrosis cystica (Fig. 6-55).

Paget's Disease

Paget's disease (osteitis deformans) is a disorder of unknown etiology characterized by excessive bone resorption and unregulated abundant bone formation. The involved areas of bone are highly vascular and can cause massive arteriovenous shunting with high-output cardiac failure. In the early (osteolytic) phase of the disease, bone resorption exceeds deposition. The bone is weak and may fracture and bend. Later, bone formation predominates (osteosclerotic phase) but is poorly organized. The bones become enlarged and thickened.

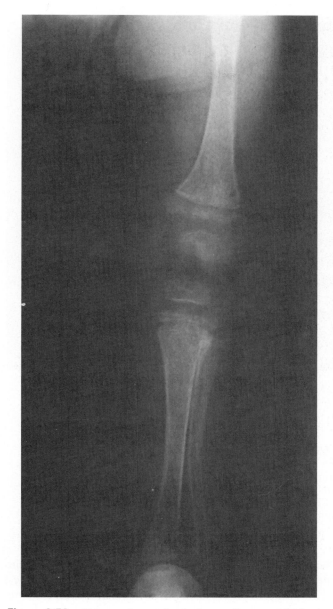

Figure 6-54   Rickets, the pediatric form of osteomalacia, is noted by diffuse osteopenia and abnormally wide growth plates. The soft bones may be bowed.

Patients with Paget's disease complain of bone pain, progressive lower limb bowing, or skull enlargement. Fractures through pagetic bone are prone to nonunion. Serum alkaline phosphatase levels secreted by bone-forming osteoblasts can be markedly elevated with Paget's disease. Microscopically, the bone is irregular, with a mosaic pattern of mature and immature bone. Radiographs show dense and irregular sclerotic bony trabeculae (Fig. 6-56). Long bone fractures are characteristically transverse and begin as a crack on the convex or tension side of the deformed bone. In less than 1% of all cases of Paget's disease, these bone-forming cells undergo malignant degeneration into osteosarcomas. The majority of cases are asymptom-

atic and are discovered incidentally on pelvic radiographs, the pelvis being a frequent site of Paget's disease. The medical treatment of Paget's disease with calcitonin or diphosphonates is reserved for intractable bone pain, malignant hypercalcemia, cardiac failure, or neural involvement from bony foraminal hypertrophy in the spine.

NEOPLASMS OF BONE

Tumors arising from musculoskeletal tissues are rare. However, bone involvement with metastatic tumor is common in patients older than the age of 50 years. Primary tumors of breast, prostate, lung, kidney, and thyroid often metastasize to bone. The sites of tumor metastasis are typically those bones involved with hematopoiesis and those with a rich blood supply, such as the spine, ribs, skull, pelvis, and long bone metaphyses. Metastases from breast and prostate may be either osteoblastic (inducing bone formation) or osteolytic (inducing bone resorption). Metastases from lung, kidney, thyroid, or gastrointestinal tract are usually osteolytic.

The most frequent primary bone tumors and their tissue of origin are listed in Table 6-8. Table 6-9 describes their salient features. The evaluation of primary or secondary bone tumors should be systematic and multidisciplinary. Before treatment is initiated, the physician must define the tumor according to its histology, its anatomic relationships to neuromuscular compartments and perivascular spaces, and the likelihood and mode of its metastatic spread.

The most common primary tumor of bone is multiple myeloma. It occurs in late adulthood. Patients may present with fatigue, bone pain, or, rarely, with a pathologic fracture. Clinical assessment involves general physical examination, routine blood work (including ESR), and urine for Bence-Jones proteins. Protein electrophoresis should also be carried out. A medical oncologist should be consulted as soon as the diagnosis of multiple myeloma is suspected.

Evaluation

The history is of great importance. It should include the patient's age, medical conditions associated with bone tumors (e.g., Paget's disease, dermatomyositis, prior radiation exposure), systemic symptoms (e.g., weight loss, bleeding diathesis, fever), and occupation (which may explain an unusual environmental exposure). Lifestyle and personal expectations are also important in selecting therapy. The physical examination should note the color and temperature of overlying tissues, and the size, degree of tenderness, and mobility of the tumor if it is palpable. A tumor that is confined to bone may have no abnormal physical findings.

A complete blood count and differential help to exclude infection and hematologic malignancies. Usually, laboratory studies can detect other organ system involvement and determine the patient's overall medical condition. Liver

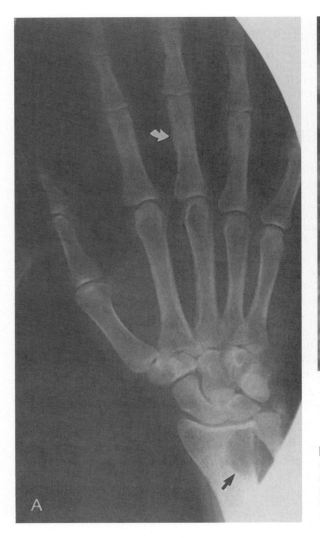

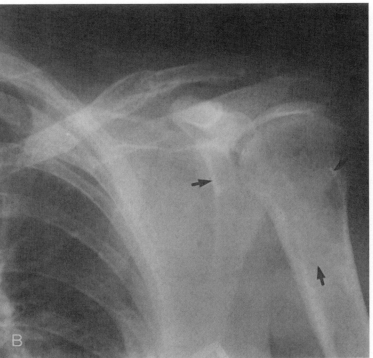

Figure 6-55 Primary hyperparathyroidism causes increased bone resorption to increase serum calcium levels. Radiographs of primary hyperparathyroidism show diffuse bone rarefaction. Note the phalangeal cortices (*curved arrow*) and multiple focal osteolytic lesions of cortical bone (*straight arrows*). This explains why the radiographic picture is described as osteitis fibrosis cystica.

function studies and measurements of uric acid (DNA turnover), alkaline phosphatase, calcium, and phosphorus are helpful in the evaluation of processes that form or destroy bone. With carcinoma of the prostate, a prostate-specific antigen (PSA) level is measured before a rectal examination is undertaken. If myeloma is suspected, serum protein electrophoresis is obtained.

The plain-film radiograph provides many clues about the behavior of the tumor. It may show a well-demarcated lesion with a reactive zone of bone formation or undemarcated lesion with bone destruction and little surrounding bone formation (Fig. 6-57). Defining the specific bone and region of involvement (epiphysis, metaphysis, or diaphysis) aids in diagnosis (Table 6-9) and staging. Subsequent radiographic investigation with bone scan, CT, MRI, or other specialized techniques is directed by suspicions generated from the plain-film radiograph. A bone scan is often an excellent screening test for metastatic disease. Radioactive, isotopically labeled technetium-99m pyrophosphate is incorporated into regions of active bone formation or increased vascularity. In multiple myeloma, however, the

bone scan is characteristically negative and shows no increased uptake. Computed tomography provides the best definition of cortical bone. It can detect cortical penetration and intraosseous detail. The CT scan is the preferred method of evaluating the lung for small pulmonary lesions. With contrast enhancement, a CT scan can define the relation between a tumor and the surrounding neurovascular structures. MRI is used to evaluate the intramedullary (marrow) extent of a tumor. The MRI also yields the best definition of soft tissue and neurovascular tumor relationships. Angiography is used to identify vascular lesions, which can then be embolized to shrink tumor mass and decrease blood loss before a surgical resection. These special imaging techniques are obtained before biopsy.

A surgical biopsy is performed to obtain tissue for histologic diagnosis. A biopsy may be obtained with open or closed (needle) techniques and should be performed by the surgical team responsible for definitive tumor treatment. The biopsy incision is placed so that it can be resected in total and not compromise the definitive procedure. An open biopsy incision is generally directed in the

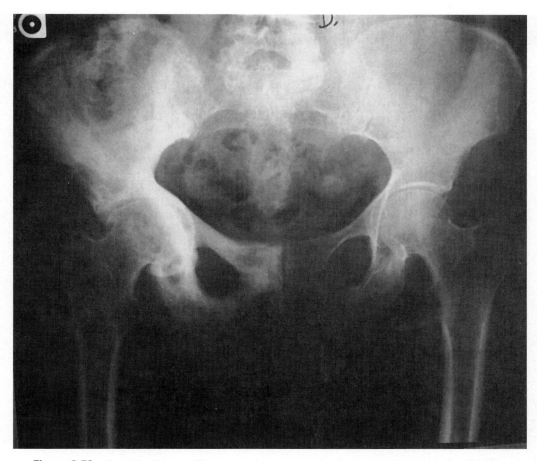

Figure 6-56 Paget's disease. The dense irregular sclerotic bony trabeculae signify the excessive, unregulated formation of bone. The bone is brittle and may fracture pathologically.

longitudinal bone axis over the tumor. To prevent contamination and tumor spread, extensive muscular dissection and neurovascular structures are avoided while meticulous hemostasis is maintained. When possible, an intraoperative frozen section is obtained to ensure that an adequate tissue specimen has been sampled. In closed biopsies, either a fine-needle aspiration is used to remove cells for

cytology or a tissue core is obtained for routine histologic preparation.

Treatment

The treatment of bone tumors depends on the tissue diagnosis, the degree of cell anaplasia, the extent of spread, the patient's medical condition, and the sensitivity of the tumor to treatment modalities. These modalities include surgery, chemotherapy, and radiotherapy.

Benign tumors are cured by local excision. If tumor resection will compromise the structural integrity of the bone (i.e., femoral neck), bone grafting or implant reinforcement will be necessary. Metastatic lesions may be palliated with local radiation. When a lesion occupies greater than 50% of a bone's cortical diameter, a pathologic fracture is imminent. Prophylactic fixation is preferable with impending pathologic fractures because patient morbidity and mortality is higher after fracture.

Generally, malignant bone tumors are resected with wide or radical surgical margins. Adjuvant chemotherapy and radiation therapy are used to eradicate tumor micrometastases that are assumed to be present. In some centers,

Table 6-8	Primary Bone Tumors and Their Tissue or Origin	
	Bone Tumor	
Tissue of Origin	**Benign**	**Malignant**
Bone	Osteoid osteoma	Osteosarcoma
Cartilage	Osteochondroma	Chondrosarcoma
	Enchondroma	
Fibrous tissue	Fibroma	Fibrosarcoma
Marrow elements	Eosinophilic granuloma	Myeloma
		Ewing's sarcoma
Uncertain	Giant cell tumor	Aggressive giant cell tumor

Table 6-9	Salient Features of Common Bone Tumors				
Tumor	**Main Symptoms**	**Age**	**Common Sites**	**Radiographic Appearance**	**Other**
Benign					
Osteoid osteoma	Pain, often relieved by aspirin	<30 yr	Femur and tibia	Small, radiolucent area <1 cm surrounded by zone of dense sclerosis	—
Osteochondroma	Palpable lump; may interfere with tendon function	Adolescence	Long bone metaphysis	Sessile or pedunculated bone excrescence; cartilage not seen unless calcified	Pain or increase in size suggests malignant change
Enchondroma (chondroma)	Swelling or pain with a pathologic fracture	Any age	Metaphysis of tubular bones of hands and feet; may be single or multiple (Ollier's disease)	Well-demarcated area of radiolucency that may contain specks of calcification	Malignant transformation is more common with multiple cartilage lesions (osteochondromas or enchondromas)
Nonossifying fibroma (fibrous cortical defect)	Asymptomatic unless pathologic fracture occurs through it	<30 yr	Cortical metaphysis of the distal femur or tibia	Well-demarcated, radiolucent, multilocular area adjacent ot cortex	Ossifies with skeletal maturation
Giant cell tumor (osteoclastoma)	Pain and swelling near joint	20–40 yr	Epiphyseal, especially distal femoral, radius, or proximal tibial epiphysis; after growth plate has closed	Epiphyseal, eccentric expanding; expands to involve metaphysis	Often aggressive; should be treated as a malignant lesion
Malignant					
Osteosarcoma	Tender mass; pain worse at night	Bimodal; before 30 yr and after 50 yr because of malignant change in Paget's disease	Metaphyseal; half affect distal femur and proximal tibia	Irregular, destructive lesion with radiodense osteoblastic or radiolucent osteolytic areas; periosteal new bone formation juxtaposed to a cortex that is permeated and destroyed; neoplastic bone spicules perpendicular to bone radiating in a sunburst pattern	Slightly more common in men than women
Chondrosarcoma	Increasing mass; dull, aching pain	40–60 yr	Central sites; pelvic and shoulder girdle	Permeative radiolucent lesion with calcific densities	Malignant transformation of preexisting enchondroma or osteochondroma, especially if multiple
Fibrosarcoma	Painful, destructive lesion	Adolescence and young adulthood	Metaphyseal regions of long bones	Poorly defined, destructive, radiolucent lesion	—
Myeloma	—	45–65 yr	Red marrow areas of the skeleton	Osteopenia, spinal compression fractures with minimal trauma	Most common primary malignant bone tumor of plasma cell origin; Bence Jones proteinuria, serum and urine protein electrophoresis
Ewing's sarcoma	Enlarging, painful, soft tissue mass	10–15 yr	Diaphysis of femur; ilium, tibia, humerus, fibula, ribs	Destructive bony lesion; onion skin layers of periosteal new bone formation	May be mistaken for osteomyelitis clinically and histologically

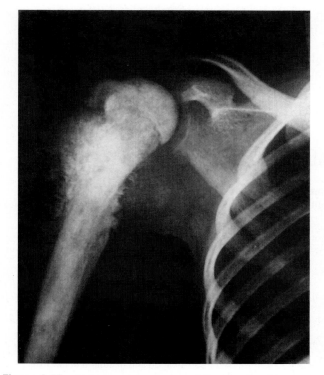

Figure 6-57   Osteogenic sarcoma of the proximal humerus metaphysis showing an aggressive, expanding, poorly demarcated, bone-forming lesion.

reconstructive techniques using bone and joint allografts alone or in combination with customized prosthetic joint replacement are used to salvage limbs (limb sparing) and maximize patient function. Limb salvage techniques should never compromise the eradication of the neoplasm.

GAIT

Normal ambulation is efficient and conserves energy. Abnormal ambulation is inefficient, requires increased energy expenditure, and usually is a manifestation of neuromuscular pathology. Gait observation and analysis is thus an essential part of the musculoskeletal examination. (A detailed analysis of normal and abnormal gait patterns is reviewed on videotape Program 9 in the series *Physical Examination of the Musculoskeletal System*; see Suggested Readings.)

A normal gait cycle (Fig. 6-58) extends from the heel strike of one foot to the next heel strike of the same foot. The normal cycle is divided into the stance phase (60% of the cycle), when the foot is in contact with the ground, and the swing phase (40% of the cycle), when the foot is off the ground. The stance phase begins at heel strike, is followed by foot flat, and ends with toe off. The swing phase is marked by advancement of the limb to the next heel strike. The stride length is the distance covered during one gait cycle (heel strike to ipsilateral heel strike). The step length is the distance between the heel strike of one

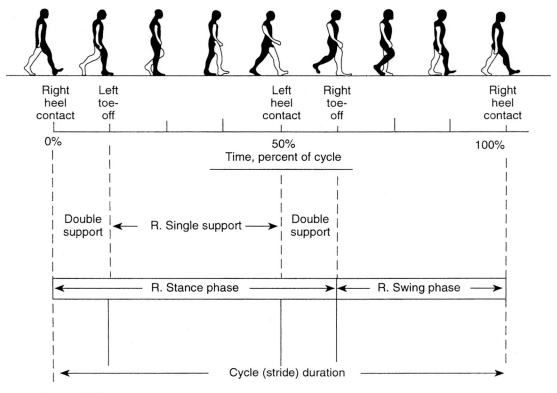

Figure 6-58   The gait cycle. (Modified from Phillips WA. The child with a limp. *Orthop Clin North Am* 1987;18:490.)

foot and the heel strike of the contralateral foot. Because the pelvis and trunk as well as the muscles and joints of the lower limb are involved in gait, abnormalities in these regions may indicate gait abnormalities.

An abnormal gait often is called a limp. Most gait abnormalities are detectable during the stance phase, when body weight is supported by one lower extremity. During stance, pain, muscle weakness, and joint abnormalities produce their maximal effect. The typical reaction to pain is to quickly unload the affected leg. Thus, an antalgic (pain-relieving) gait is manifest by a decreased stance phase of the affected limb. The swing phase of the limb opposite is also decreased, which results in a shortened step length.

Muscle weakness has significant effects on gait. Quadriceps weakness interferes with the ability to lock the knee in full extension before heel strike. To compensate, the patient will push the thigh backward with the hand. Weakness of the foot and ankle dorsiflexors will not allow the controlled placement of the foot after heel strike to the foot flat position. This results in a foot slap gait as the foot slaps to the ground after heel strike. Likewise, paralysis of the foot and ankle dorsiflexors due to peroneal nerve palsy will cause the patient to bring the knee up higher than normal during the swing phase so the toes clear the ground. This motion may result in a steppage gate. Other compensatory mechanisms for clearing a dropped foot include elevating the ipsilateral pelvis (hip-hike gait) or swinging the leg out to the side (circumduction gait). A weak gluteus maximus, which serves as a hip extensor, causes the trunk to collapse forward during midstance. The patient will compensate by thrusting the trunk posteriorly in what is called an extensor lurch or gluteus maximus gait. Weakness of the hip abductor muscles (gluteus medius and minimus) allows the contralateral pelvis to sink downward during stance. To compensate, the patient's torso lurches laterally over the weak hip in what is known as Trendelenburg or gluteus medius gait. Weakness of the calf muscles (gastrocnemius and soleus) prevents the normal propulsive toe-off push and is manifest as a flat-footed or calcaneal gait.

Joint abnormalities that interfere with the normal range of toe, metatarsophalangeal, ankle, knee, or hip joint motion also adversely affect gait. For example, an equinus (plantar flexion) ankle contracture causes knee hyperextension during the stance phase of ambulation.

Armed with a knowledge of gait mechanics and a critical eye, the clinician can distinguish many of these gait patterns when observing a group of people. An abnormal gait pattern may provide the first clue in the diagnosis of a neuromuscular disease process.

SUGGESTED READINGS

Books and Journals

American Academy of Orthopaedic Surgeons. *Athletic Training and Sports Medicine*, 2nd ed. Park Ridge, IL: American Academy of Orthopaedic Surgeons; 1991.

American Academy of Orthopaedic Surgeons. *Orthopaedic Knowledge: Update 5*. Park Ridge, IL: American Academy of Orthopaedic Surgeons; 1996.

Buckwalter JA, Martin J. Degenerative joint disease. *Clin Symp* 1995; 47:2.

Kaplan FS. Prevention and management of osteoporosis. *Clin Symp* 1995;47:1.

Kleinert HE, Kleinert JM, McCabe SJ, Berger AC. Replantation. *Clin Symp* 1991;43:2.

Lawrence PF. *Essentials of General Surgery*, 4th ed. Philadelphia: Lippincott Williams & Wilkins; 2006.

Mooney V, Saal JA, Saal JS. Evaluation and treatment of low back pain. *Clin Symp* 1996;48:4.

Netter FH. Musculoskeletal system: Part I. Anatomy, physiology and metabolic disorders. *The CIBA Collection of Medical Illustrations*. Vol. 8. Summit, NJ: CIBA Pharmaceuticals; 1987.

Netter FH. Musculoskeletal system: Part II. Developmental disorders and joint replacement. *The CIBA Collection of Medical Illustrations*. Vol. 8. Summit, NJ: CIBA Pharmaceuticals; 1990.

Netter FH. Musculoskeletal system: Part III. Trauma, evaluation and management. *The CIBA Collection of Medical Illustrations*. Vol. 8. Summit, NJ: CIBA Pharmaceuticals; 1993.

Salter RB. *Textbook of Disorders and Injuries of the Musculoskeletal System*, 3rd ed. Baltimore: Williams & Wilkins; 1999.

Schenck RC Jr, Heckman JD. Injuries of the knee. *Clin Symp* 1993; 45:1.

Schumaker HR, ed. *Primer on the Rheumatic Diseases*, 10th ed. Atlanta: Arthritis Foundation; 1993.

Videotapes

American Academy of Orthopaedic Surgeons, Association of Orthopaedic Chairmen, and McGill University. *Physical examination of the musculoskeletal system: A series of nine video programs*. Park Ridge, IL: American Academy of Orthopaedic Surgeons; 1987.

Carette S. *Intraarticular and soft tissue injection sites*. Montreal, Quebec, Canada: Roussel Canada; 1990.

JOEL GELMAN ■ BARRY P. DUEL ■ ISAAC YI KIM

Urology: Diseases of the Genitourinary System

4 Describe the pathophysiology, diagnosis, and treatment of bacterial cystitis and interstitial cystitis.

5 Describe the symptoms, evaluation, and treatment of bladder fistulae.

6 Discuss the physiology of normal bladder function and disorders of micturition (e.g., incontinence, neurogenic bladder).

7 Discuss the etiology, presentation, and treatment of bladder cancer.

Penis

1 Describe the etiology, clinical presentation, evaluation, and management of penile trauma.

2 Describe the etiology, clinical presentation, evaluation, and treatment of penile cancer.

3 Describe the clinical presentation and management of four acquired penile disorders.

4 Describe the clinical presentation and management of three congenital penile anomalies.

5 Discuss six sexually transmitted diseases. Demonstrate knowledge of their causative pathogens, clinical presentation, evaluation, and treatment.

6 Discuss the indications for and complications of circumcision.

Urethra

1 Describe the etiology, clinical presentation, evaluation, and management of urethral trauma.

2 Describe the natural history, evaluation, and treatment of male and female urethral cancer.

3 Discuss the etiology, presentation, evaluation, and management of urethral stricture disease.

4 Describe the clinical presentation, evaluation, and management of posterior urethral valves and hypospadias.

5 Name the common pathogens responsible for urethritis.

Testes, Male Infertility, and Impotency

1 Discuss three congenital anomalies involving the testes.

2 Discuss the evaluation and differential diagnosis of the patient with acute testicular pain.

3 Describe three scrotal infections.

4 Describe the evaluation of a patient with a scrotal mass.

5 Discuss germ cell tumors of the testicle, their staging, and their treatment.

6 Provide a concise evaluation plan for the infertile male.

7 List the four major categories of erectile impotency.

Urology is a surgical specialty that deals with disorders of the male and female urinary tracts, the male genital tract, and the adrenal glands. Diseases treated by urologists account for a substantial percentage of patient visits. For example, prostate cancer accounts for 29% of all diagnosed cancers in men, and urinary tract infections (UTIs) will affect approximately 10% to 20% of women during their lifetime.

PROSTATE

Anatomy and Physiology

The normal prostate gland is located just distal to the bladder neck and surrounds the urethra for a distance of 2 to 3 cm. The membranous urethra, which is surrounded by the external urinary sphincter, is located just distal to the prostatic urethra. The ejaculatory ducts empty into the prostatic urethra at the level of the verumontanum (pronounced *vee-roo-mon-tán-um*), a small midline portion of the prostate that protrudes into the prostatic urethra (Fig. 7-1). The prostate gland is anatomically divided into zones that can be distinguished both histologically and grossly. The transition zone enlarges substantially in men with be-

nign prostatic hyperplasia (BPH). The peripheral zone is the origin of nearly 90% of prostatic cancers.

The blood supply to the prostate originates primarily from branches of the hypogastric artery that enter the prostate posterolaterally (Fig. 7-2). A large dorsal vein complex is located on the anterior surface of the prostate. The puboprostatic ligaments anchor the prostate gland anteriorly to the pubic bone. Microscopically, the prostate gland is composed of glandular epithelium contained within a fibromuscular stroma.

Secretions from the prostate gland account for a major portion of the volume of a normal ejaculate. The prostatic fluid provides nutrients that are necessary for normal sperm motility and function. The prostate remains relatively dormant from birth until puberty and then begins to function as an exocrine gland. Enlargement begins in the fourth decade of life and may lead to BPH.

Inflammatory Diseases: Prostatitis

Prostatitis is an inflammatory condition of the prostate that may be bacterial in origin but often has no defined etiologic agent. Prostatodynia is a symptom complex that consists of an aching perineal discomfort, urinary frequency, urgency, and dysuria, in the absence of any known infec-

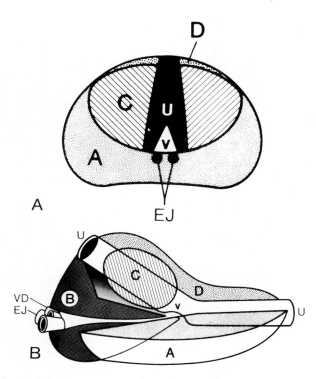

Figure 7-1 **A,** Schematic transverse image of the mid-portion of the prostate. *A,* peripheral zone; *C,* central zone; *V,*verumontanum; *U,* urethra; *EJ,* ejaculatory ducts; *D,* anterior fibromuscular stroma. **B,** Schematic longitudinal representation of the prostate. *A,* peripheral zone; *B,* central zone; *C,* transition zone; *D,* anterior fibromuscular stroma; *U,* urethra; *V,* verumontanum; *EJ,* ejaculatory ducts; *VD,* vas deferens.

tious etiology. More classic obstructive symptoms (e.g., urinary hesitancy, dribbling, difficulty emptying the bladder) may occur. A distinction between bacterial and nonbacterial prostatitis cannot reliably be made based on symptoms alone.

Acute Prostatitis

Acute prostatitis is a relatively unusual bacterial infection of the prostate that may have protean manifestations. The disease typically occurs after the second decade of life and is characterized by fever, back pain, chills, and dysuria. The symptoms are usually of relatively rapid onset. On physical examination, the prostate gland is swollen and often described as boggy, sometimes warm to the touch because of inflammation, and often exquisitely tender. The urine sediment shows white blood cells and the serum white blood cell count may be increased. Patients may present in acute urinary retention because of prostatic edema.

The infectious agent is usually a Gram-negative bacterium, most often *Escherichia coli*. Treatment consists of broad-spectrum antibiotics. When acute prostatitis is associated with urinary retention, catheterization of the bladder is required. Because placing a catheter transurethrally could lead to an exacerbation of the condition, it is usually recommended to place the catheter suprapubically. In some cases, infection of the prostate can progress, leading to the formation of an abscess. A prostate abscess can be diagnosed by fluctuance on digital rectal examination, or on imaging studies such as a computed tomography (CT) scan. The treatment of an abscess, in addition to that described previously, is transurethral unroofing of the abscess

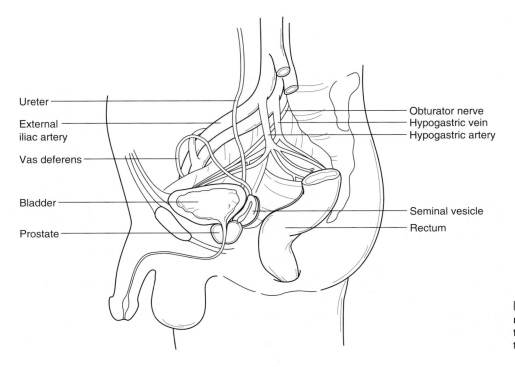

Ureter

External
iliac artery

Vas deferens

Bladder

Prostate

Obturator nerve
Hypogastric vein
Hypogastric artery

Seminal vesicle

Rectum

Figure 7-2 Sagittal view of male pelvic anatomy showing the relation of the prostate gland to adjacent pelvic structures.

with a resectoscope (most common treatment) or needle aspiration by transrectal ultrasonography (TRUS).

Chronic Prostatitis

Chronic prostatitis has a more indolent clinical course than acute prostatitis. It is uncertain whether chronic bacterial prostatitis is a consequence of recurring independent infections or of failure to adequately eliminate an initial infection. Most often, there is no antecedent history of acute prostatitis. Patients typically present with discomfort in the perineum, back, or pelvis that is associated with urinary frequency, hesitancy, and dysuria. A voided urinalysis may show white blood cells. Prostatic fluid obtained by "milking" the urethra after digital prostatic massage characteristically has more than 10 white blood cells per high-power field. Cultures of prostatic fluid should be positive for bacteria before a diagnosis of chronic bacterial prostatitis can be made. Treatment consists of oral broad-spectrum antibiotics (e.g., trimethoprim-sulfamethoxazole, quinolone), often for a 6-week course. Voiding symptoms usually improve on antibiotics, but may recur after antibiotics are discontinued.

Nonbacterial Prostatitis

Nonbacterial prostatitis is a common and often frustrating problem for patients and physicians. The subjective manifestations may be indistinguishable from those associated with chronic prostatitis. However, no bacterial or other etiologic agent is consistently identified, although *Chlamydia trachomatis* is isolated in some patients. Frequently, there are no objective findings and the prostatic fluid is normal on microscopic examination. Treatment options may include antibiotics (despite the absence of a documented bacterial etiology), prostatic massage, and symptomatic treatment consisting of sitz baths and nonsteroidal anti-inflammatory drugs.

Degenerative Diseases: Benign Prostatic Hyperplasia

Epidemiology

BPH is a process of hyperplasia (proliferation in the number of cells) and hypertrophy (enlargement of the prostate) associated with voiding symptoms. The pathologic process primarily occurs in the transition zone and can be demonstrated histologically as early as the third decade of life. Symptomatic manifestations of BPH are uncommon before 50 years of age. There is no apparent causal association between BPH and other pathologic conditions of the prostate (e.g., prostatitis, cancer). The natural history of BPH is poorly understood and variable. Significant spontaneous symptomatic improvement is relatively uncommon, but not all patients have progressive symptoms if left untreated. Histologic evidence of BPH is almost universal in aging men, but there is no direct correlation between prostate size and symptoms.

Clinical Presentation and Evaluation

Because of its anatomic position surrounding the urethra, enlargement of the prostate typically results in a relative bladder outflow obstruction. Classic obstructive symptoms are hesitancy in initiating voiding, a decrease in the force of the urinary stream, terminal dribbling, intermittence, or a feeling of incomplete bladder emptying. Because of bladder changes that may result from obstruction, typical irritating voiding symptoms (e.g., frequency, urgency, nocturia) are also common. The symptoms are usually of gradual onset and may progress to the point of acute urinary retention.

Digital rectal examination of the prostate often shows palpable enlargement. There may be some asymmetry of the prostate, but BPH characteristically has a smooth contour and a soft consistency. It is important to remember that marked enlargement of the prostate can occur without associated symptoms, and urologic consultation and evaluation is not indicated simply because of prostate enlargement on physical examination alone. Moreover, symptoms may occur without marked enlargement. In the absence of infection, a voided urinalysis is normal. A urine flow rate test shows diminished force of the urinary stream (usually less than 15 mL/sec in symptomatic patients). An abnormal amount of urine in the bladder after voiding, termed **postvoid residual** (PVR), may be demonstrable by direct catheterization or ultrasonography. Intravenous pyelography (IVP), when obtained for other symptoms or signs, may suggest thickening of the bladder detrusor muscle (trabeculation); it may also show J-hooking of the distal ureters, which is caused by cephalad displacement by the enlarged prostate. However, IVP is not routinely obtained or indicated in the evaluation of uncomplicated BPH. A decompensated bladder with poor emptying is a relatively unusual manifestation of long-standing BPH; it could result in **hydronephrosis** and renal failure because of the chronically increased intravesical pressure.

Treatment

Occasionally, patients may have objective indications for treatment (e.g., renal failure, poor bladder emptying resulting in recurrent infection or bladder stones). However, symptomatic relief is the best reason to pursue treatment of BPH. Patients should be counseled that symptomatic improvement can be achieved with treatment in most patients, but that a lack of treatment does not necessarily imply progressive symptoms or detrimental consequences. Symptoms may be quantified by administering the American Urological Association symptom score test. Improvement in symptom score is often used as an objective measure of treatment response. Because some patients tolerate marked symptoms with little bother, the degree of patient annoyance or bother with symptoms is most often the initiating factor for treatment.

Medical Therapy

Medical treatment for BPH can provide symptomatic benefit in many patients. With the advent of modern medical therapy for BPH, surgical treatment is much less frequently performed; surgery is usually reserved for patients who do not tolerate or are unresponsive to medical management. α_1-Adrenergic blocking agents are most commonly used in medical management of BPH. The exact mechanism of action is uncertain, although α-adrenergic receptors are present in the bladder neck and prostatic urethra. Three α blockers currently are used to treat lower urinary tract voiding symptoms: terazosin (Hytrin), doxazosin (Cardura), and tamsulosin (Flomax). Each agent is administered as a single daily dose. A favorable response can occur rapidly, sometimes within 24 hours of dose administration. Each of the available drugs is usually well tolerated, although drug-related weakness may occur and postural hypotension is occasionally observed.

Finasteride (Proscar) is a 5α-reductase inhibitor used for the treatment of symptomatic BPH. The usual dose is 5 mg/day. 5α-Reductase converts testosterone to the active intracellular metabolite dihydrotestosterone. Consequently, finasteride acts by blocking androgenic activity on the prostate cells. A modest decrease in prostatic size (20%–30%) occurs, and some patients have mild symptomatic improvement or a small increase in urinary flow rates. The drug is well tolerated, with very few side effects, although a small percent of patients notice sexual dysfunction (e.g., decreased libido, impotence). Finasteride usually lowers serum **prostate-specific antigen** (PSA), a marker for prostate cancer. When a patient is taking finasteride, serum PSA should be doubled to calculate a useful relative value. In comparative studies, finasteride was less effective than α-adrenergic blocking drugs in relieving lower urinary tract symptoms when the overall prostate size is less than 50 g. For men with large prostates, the drugs show equal efficacy, but response may not be observed with finasteride until after several months of usage.

Surgical Therapy

The surgical removal of obstructing prostatic tissue may be performed through an open or a transurethral route. An open surgical approach is usually chosen for patients with a very large (>60 g) prostate size. The prostate is approached through a lower midline abdominal incision or, rarely, a perineal incision. The enlarged prostatic adenomatous tissue is enucleated by sharp dissection with scissors and blunt finger dissection through either the bladder (suprapubic prostatectomy) or the prostatic capsule (simple retropubic prostatectomy). During open surgery for BPH, the capsule of the prostate is not removed and there is no disruption of urethral continuity.

More often, the transurethral route is chosen for the performance of **transurethral prostatectomy** (TURP). An electrocautery loop is used to successively remove prostatic tissue under direct visualization. The resection is usually carried to the level of the prostatic capsule, and all obstructing tissue is removed. Alternatively, a transurethral incision of the prostate may be performed in patients with smaller glands. With either technique, hemostasis is obtained with electrocautery.

Usually, the patient is hospitalized for one or two evenings after TURP; patients should be voiding well at the time of hospital discharge. The risk of incontinence is low (1%–2%) and treatment-related impotence occurs in less than 5% of patients. The risk of future prostate cancer is not affected by surgery for benign enlargement because the tissue removed is transitional tissue (the origin of most prostate cancers is the peripheral zone). In properly selected patients, treatment results are excellent and are usually marked by a substantial increase in urinary flow rate.

Minimally Invasive Techniques

Procedures for the treatment of lower urinary tract symptoms have proliferated. These procedures have fewer side effects than those of surgery, can be conducted on an outpatient basis, and are less expensive.

Transurethral microwave thermotherapy is performed on an outpatient basis and does not require anesthesia. This procedure involves delivery of microwave energy to the prostate. Long-term improvement in symptoms occurs in most patients, but objective measurements show less improvement than with surgery. Transurethral needle ablation uses radiofrequency energy transmitted through a specially designed needle inserted transurethrally into the prostate. Outpatient and even office-based treatment is feasible. Improvement in symptom score is observed in most patients.

Various methods are used for laser treatment of the prostate. Most commonly, neodymium:yttrium-aluminum-garnet (Nd:YAG) laser or Holmium:YAG energy is used to vaporize prostate tissue. Bleeding complications are reduced with laser treatment compared with electrocautery resection.

Malignant Diseases

Epidemiology

Carcinoma of the prostate is among the most common cancers in men in the United States. More than 95% of prostatic cancers are adenocarcinoma arising from the prostatic acinar structures. The incidence of prostate cancer increases with age. A familial pattern has been identified, and the disease is more common in African Americans than in Caucasians. A high-fat diet has been implicated as a contributing etiology in some studies. A pattern of autosomal dominant inheritance has been identified in some patients, especially those with an early age of onset.

Histologically, adenocarcinoma can be identified at autopsy in over 30% and 70% of men over the age of 50 and 80, respectively. Thus, there is a large discrepancy between histologic and clinically significant disease.

Clinical Presentation and Evaluation

Most men with early-stage prostate cancer have no disease-related symptoms. Prostate cancer and BPH may occur simultaneously, but there is no apparent causal relation. Obstructive voiding symptoms may be from BPH or, as the cancer enlarges, from malignant tissue. Patients with advanced disease may have weight loss, pelvic pain, ureteral obstruction, gross hematuria, or bone pain from distant metastasis.

Early Detection

Given the recent efforts to promote early detection by digital rectal examination and PSA testing, the current trend is for patients to present with an abnormality on screening. Although issues involving screening remain controversial, many feel that screening should begin at age 50 years. For those at high risk, African Americans, and those with a family history of prostate cancer, screening should begin at 40 years of age. In elderly patients and those with a life expectancy of less than 10 years, there may not be a significant benefit to prostate cancer screening.

Digital Rectal Examination. Digital rectal examination is an important method for early detection of prostate cancer. A normal prostate is smooth, symmetrical, and has a consistency similar to that of the muscles of the thenar eminence of the hand. Eighty percent of prostate cancers arise in the peripheral zone and, once they attain sufficient size, are palpable as an area of induration or nodularity within the substance of the prostate (Fig. 7-3).

For digital rectal examinations, patients are directed to lie in the knee–chest position or to stand while bending forward at the waist. A gloved and lubricated index finger is inserted into the rectum. The prostate gland is palpable beneath the anterior rectal wall (normal seminal vesicles are usually not palpable). The margins of the prostate should be distinct, and any areas of induration, nodularity, or asymmetry should be noted.

Prostate-Specific Antigen Testing. PSA is a serine protease enzyme whose function is to cleave the proteins in the postejaculatory semen. Serum PSA is specific for the pros-

tate but not prostate cancer because PSA is expressed by both benign and malignant prostatic epithelial cells. In normal conditions, PSA is secreted into the prostatic lumen. But with any conditions that destroy the normal prostatic architecture, the cellular polarity is lost and PSA is secreted both into the prostatic lumen and the blood vessels. Thus, the PSA level may be elevated in men with prostatitis, BPH, or prostate cancer.

PSA values differ somewhat, depending on the assay used. In general, a level less than 4.0 ng/mL is considered normal. However, prostate cancer is present in 20% to 25% of patients with "normal" PSA levels. A number of factors can be used to adjust PSA levels to increase specificity. The PSA level increases gradually with age, probably because of overall prostate enlargement. By age-adjusted PSA standards, a PSA level of 3.9 ng/mL is considered high for a man in the sixth decade of life, whereas a level greater than 4.0 ng/mL is within the normal range for older men.

PSA density (i.e., the amount of PSA per volume of prostate tissue) may also be measured. Men with a large prostate may have a higher PSA because of the benign component of the enlargement, even in the absence of cancer. PSA density may account for the age-adjusted variations that have been observed. A year-to-year comparison of PSA levels provides some useful information. A change of less than 0.75 ng/mL/yr is often considered acceptable, although this is both age dependent and related to the overall PSA level.

Serum PSA occurs in two forms, one conjugated to α_1-antichymotrypsin and the other unconjugated, or free. The relative proportion of the two forms can be used to improve the specificity of PSA testing. A greater proportion of free PSA is seen in men with a modest increase in PSA from BPH compared to those with prostate cancer. In general, a percent-free fraction of less than 20% to 25% is more commonly associated with prostate cancer than higher levels.

Evaluation

Transrectal Ultrasonography. The best imaging test for the prostate is TRUS, which can distinguish the zonal anatomy of the prostate and accurately measure the prostate size. Prostatic cancers typically are located in the peripheral zone and have a hypoechoic pattern (Fig. 7-4). Because of its lack of sensitivity and specificity, TRUS is not used as a screening test. It is used to direct prostate biopsy in men with a palpable abnormality of the prostate or an abnormal PSA reading.

Prostate Biopsy. Obtaining a biopsy for detection of prostate cancer is almost always performed via the transrectal route, although it can be accomplished through the perineum. Accurate needle placement is facilitated by TRUS but can also be performed with finger guidance. A spring-loaded automatic gun is used to obtain cores of tissue in a systematic fashion. Usually 10 to 12 cores are obtained.

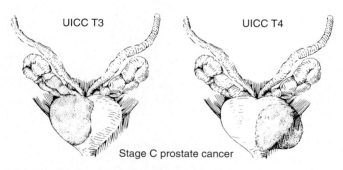

UICC T3   UICC T4

Stage C prostate cancer

Figure 7-3 Schematic representation of a palpable prostate cancer with extension into the seminal vesicle (*left*) and the levator ani muscle (*right*). Most prostate cancers arise in the peripheral zone, and once they attain sufficient size, are palpable by digital rectal examination as an area of induration or nodularity.

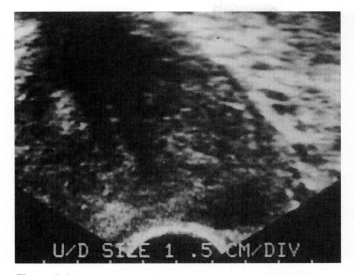

Figure 7-4 Transverse ultrasound image of the prostate showing a hypoechoic area in the peripheral zone and the left base, which is characteristic of prostate cancer. Ultrasound can help direct biopsies to specific areas of the prostate that may be suspicious for cancer.

Patients are usually given a Fleet enema on the morning of the examination. In addition, premedication with a broad-spectrum antibiotic for 1 to 2 days after the biopsy is required.

Tumor Grade. The degree of differentiation of the tumor provides important prognostic information. Most often, the Gleason grading system is used. This system assigns a number (1–5) to the dominant grade and a secondary number to arrive at a Gleason sum or score. Gleason scores of 2 to 4 are usually considered well differentiated, 5 to 7 moderately differentiated, and 8 to 10 poorly differentiated. Prognosis is strongly linked to grade. Most cancers found through early detection or screening programs are of an intermediate grade (i.e., Gleason 4 to 6).

Staging of Prostate Cancer

Staging of prostate cancer defines the local, regional, and distant extent of disease. The tumor-node-metastasis (TNM) system is currently the standard and allows categorization of nonpalpable tumors detected because of PSA or ultrasound abnormalities (Table 7-1).

The primary staging modality for local disease is digital rectal palpation. TRUS is used primarily to direct biopsy and is of limited value for staging. Serum PSA levels correlate only roughly with disease extent. However, bone metastasis is quite uncommon in patients with a PSA less than 20 ng/mL. Radionuclide bone scanning is the most sensitive method for detection of bone metastases (Fig. 7-5). Bone scan is not recommended if the PSA value is less than 10 ng/mL and the grade of the tumor is less than a Gleason sum of 7. Pelvic CT scanning is not routinely used because grossly positive nodes are detected rarely with

Table 7-1	Staging for Prostate Carcinoma

Primary Tumor, Clinical (T)

TX	Primary tumor cannot be assessed
T0	No evidence of primary tumor
T1	Clinically unapparent tumor not palpable nor visible by imaging
T1a	Tumor incidental histologic finding in 5% or less of tissue resected
T1b	Tumor incidental histologic finding in more than 5% of tissue resected
T1c	Tumor identified by needle biopsy (e.g., because of elevated PSA)
T2	Tumor confined within prostate[a]
T2a	Tumor involves one lobe
T2b	Tumor involves both lobes
T3	Tumor extends through the prostate capsule[b]
T3a	Extracapsular extension (unilateral or bilateral)
T3b	Tumor invades seminal vesicle(s)
T4	Tumor is fixed or invades adjacent structures other than seminal vesicles: bladder neck, external sphincter, rectum, levator muscles, and/or pelvic wall

[a]Tumor found in one or both lobes by needle biopsy, but not palpable or reliably visible by imaging, is classified as T1c.

[b]Invasion into the prostatic apex or into (but not beyond) the prostatic capsule is not classified as T3, but as T2.

PSA, prostate-specific antigen.

Used with the permission of the American Joint Committee on Cancer (AJCC), Chicago, Illinois. The original source for this material is the *AJCC Cancer Staging Manual,* 5th ed. Philadelphia: Lippincott-Raven; 1997.

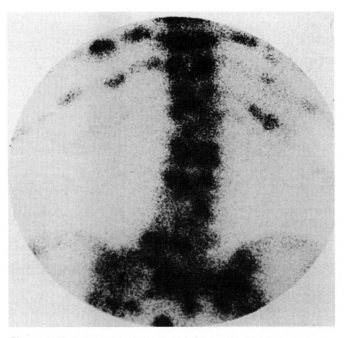

Figure 7-5 Radionuclide bone scan showing multiple areas of abnormal uptake in the pelvis and spine, typical of metastatic prostate cancer.

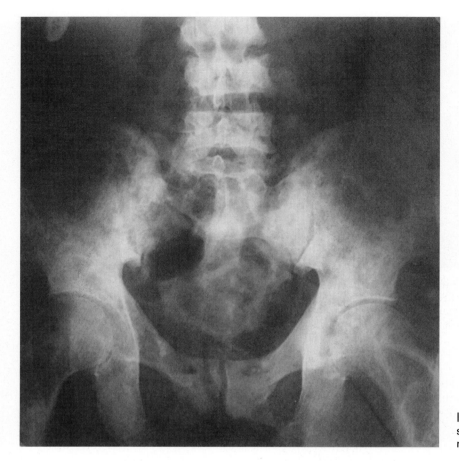

Figure 7-6 Radiograph of the pelvis showing characteristic osteoblastic metastases from prostate cancer.

a clinically localized tumor. Prostate cancer, when metastatic, typically affects the axial skeleton and forms osteoblastic metastases on plain radiograph (Fig. 7-6). Soft tissue metastasis may also occur but is unusual without concomitant bone metastasis.

Lymph node staging is of critical importance in selecting patients for therapy. CT scanning may show enlarged lymph nodes in patients with high-volume or high-grade primary tumors. Laparoscopic pelvic lymphadenectomy is technically feasible and, when indicated, can provide adequate sampling of the pelvic lymph nodes. Most often, though, lymph node dissection is performed through an open incision immediately before radical prostatectomy. The anatomic limits of a staging lymph node dissection for prostate cancer are the bifurcation of the common iliac artery proximally, the circumflex iliac vein distally, the midportion of the external iliac artery laterally, and the bladder wall medially. The dissection is carried posteriorly to the obturator nerve (Fig. 7-7).

In the past, patients who had a new diagnosis of prostate cancer usually underwent a metastatic workup that included a bone scan and lymph node dissection. However, studies have shown that when both the PSA level and Gleason grade are low the disease is almost always localized. Therefore, patients with both a PSA less than 10 and a

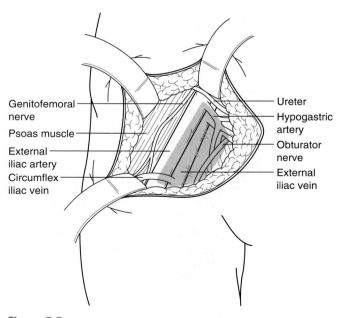

Genitofemoral nerve
Psoas muscle
External iliac artery
Circumflex iliac vein
Ureter
Hypogastric artery
Obturator nerve
External iliac vein

Figure 7-7 Anatomic boundaries of a staging pelvic lymph node dissection for prostate cancer.

Gleason score of 7 or less usually do not require a bone scan or lymph node dissection.

Treatment

Localized Disease

The optimal therapy for localized prostate cancer is uncertain and a point of continual controversy. For men with a life expectancy of less than 10 years, observation alone (i.e., "watchful waiting") may be appropriate. Surgical removal of the prostate (i.e., radical prostatectomy) and radiation therapy are the most commonly used treatments. Ten-year survival rates are similar after external beam radiation or surgery, but valid comparisons are difficult and follow-up beyond 10 years is important. Brachytherapy using interstitial implantation of either iodine-125 or palladium-103 is also used, but there is insufficient long-term follow-up to assess results adequately. Cryotherapy (i.e., freezing of the prostate) is being investigated in some centers, but results published to date indicate that this method is inferior to established treatments for intracapsular tumors.

Radical prostatectomy can be performed via a perineal approach (Fig. 7-8). An inverted U-incision is made anterior to the rectum. The dissection continues in the plane between the prostate and the rectum. The posterior layer of Denonvilliers' fascia is opened and the prostate gland, the capsule, and the seminal vesicles are dissected free entirely. The perineal route, associated with minimal postoperative pain, does not allow simultaneous lymph node dissection.

More often, radical prostatectomy is accomplished by a retropubic route. An incision is made from the umbilicus to the pubis. Usually, pelvic lymphadenectomy is performed. During radical retropubic prostatectomy, the entire prostate—including the prostatic capsule, the seminal vesicles, and the ampullary portion of the vas deferens—is removed. After the prostate is removed, a direct anastomosis is performed between the reconstructed bladder neck and the urethra (Fig. 7-9). In patients who are sexually active before therapy, potency can be retained in nearly two thirds by preservation of the neurovascular bundle that lies immediately posterolateral to the prostate and urethra. In patients with negative surgical margins, a 15-year, disease-free survival rate of nearly 50% can be anticipated. In patients who have positive surgical margins or histologically positive lymph nodes, adjuvant radiation treatment or hormonal therapy may be used.

A recent surgical advancement for prostate cancer is laparoscopy and robotic prostatectomy. These techniques remove the prostate using multiple small incisions. Currently, approximately 20% of prostatectomies are performed in this manner. It is anticipated that the percentage will markedly increase as more urologists and patients become familiar with the approach. Available data suggest that robotic and laparoscopic radical prostatectomies have the following advantages over the open surgery: (a) better cosmesis, (b) decreased risk of transfusion, (c) shorter time to recovery, and (d) earlier return to continence. Short-term results indicate that this technique is equivalent to open approach in controlling the cancer.

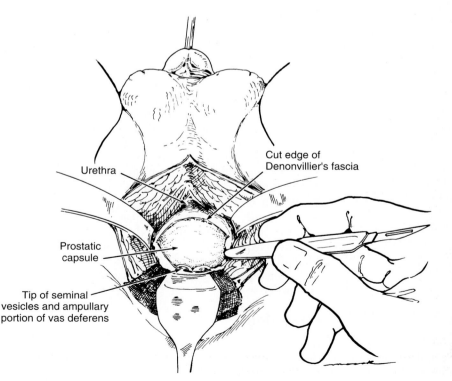

Urethra

Cut edge of Denonvillier's fascia

Prostatic capsule

Tip of seminal vesicles and ampullary portion of vas deferens

Figure 7-8 Radical perineal prostatectomy. The rectum is retracted posteriorly, and the posterior layer of Denonvilliers' fascia has been incised to expose the prostatic capsule.

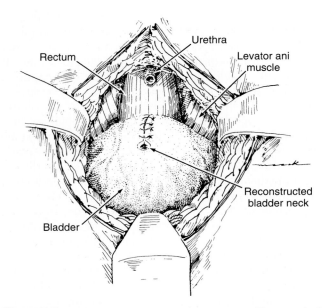

Figure 7-9 Radical retropubic prostatectomy. The surgical specimen has been removed and the bladder neck reconstructed. A direct anastomosis is performed with the stump of the urethra.

Serum PSA levels should decrease to an undetectable range after radical prostatectomy because all PSA-producing cells, both benign and malignant, ideally are removed. After radiation therapy, superior results are achieved in patients in whom the PSA level decreases to less than 1.0 ng/mL or, perhaps, 0.5 ng/mL. An increasing serum PSA is evidence of tumor recurrence, although other studies may not identify metastatic disease initially. There is controversy and uncertainty about when to initiate hormonal therapy in men with an increasing PSA level after treatment.

Metastatic Disease

Prostate cancer is a partially androgen-dependent disease. Therefore, the primary treatment for metastatic carcinoma of the prostate is deprivation of androgens from the cancer cell. Suppression of serum testosterone can be achieved by bilateral surgical orchiectomy or medical castration. Oral administration of estrogens effectively lowers serum testosterone, but is associated with cardiovascular side effects in up to 20% of patients. Estrogen therapy, common in the past, has been replaced by luteinizing hormone–releasing hormone (LHRH) analogs, which effectively suppress testosterone to the castrate range within 1 month of administration. LHRH analogs are associated with few serious side effects; however, they cause vasomotor hot flashes in approximately two thirds of patients. Loss of libido and impotence are consequences of orchiectomy or LHRH administration.

Less than 10% of circulating androgens in men are of adrenal origin. The contribution of these androgens to the growth of prostate cancer is uncertain. Some studies have shown that antiandrogen can prolong the duration of response when used in conjunction with LHRH analogs or orchiectomy. However, other studies have shown conflicting results. The drug is administered orally and can cause some degree of gynecomastia and gastrointestinal side effects (usually diarrhea). Hepatotoxicity is seen occasionally.

The duration of response to hormonal therapy in patients with metastatic prostate cancer is usually 18 to 24 months. After that time, disease progression occurs. Taxol-based chemotherapy has been shown to be moderately effective in hormone-refractory cancer. Radiation can be effective for isolated sites of bone metastasis. In the PSA era, the median survival of patients with hormone-refractory prostate cancer is 53 months.

THE KIDNEYS

Anatomy

The kidneys are paired retroperitoneal organs that lie on either side of the vertebral column, opposite the 12th thoracic and the first through third lumbar vertebrae. They are bordered by the diaphragm posteriorly and superiorly, and by the psoas and quadratus lumborum muscles posteriorly. The right kidney is bordered by the right lobe of the liver anteriorly and superiorly and by the right colon inferiorly (Fig. 7-10). The duodenum lies over the anteromedial portion of the right kidney. The left kidney lies adjacent to the spleen, with the left colon over its anterior lateral surface. The stomach borders the anterior surface of the upper pole, the jejunum overlies the anterior lower pole, and the tail of the pancreas overlies the hilum. Normally, the left kidney lies more cranially than the right one. The dimensions of the average kidney are approximately 11 cm in length, 6 cm in breadth, and 3 cm in anteroposterior thickness. The kidney typically weighs 150 g in the male and approximately 135 g in the female.

The kidney is covered by a renal capsule composed of fibrous tissue that is closely applied to the renal cortical surface. At the hilum, this layer becomes continuous with the fibrous sheaths of the renal and great vessels. The capsule is easily stripped from the parenchyma. The layer of adipose connective tissue surrounding the kidney and its vessels, the perirenal fat, is thickest at the borders of the kidney. Surrounding the perirenal fat is a layer of fibroareolar connective tissue, the renal fascia (Gerota's). Superiorly, the fascial layers envelop the adrenal glands. Inferiorly, the layers remain separate and surround the ureters. Medially, the layers fuse and adhere to the renal vessels and kidney pelves, limiting extravasation of urine, blood, or purulence.

Physiology

A clear understanding of renal and acid–base physiology is the basis for the management of many urologic disorders. Examples include hyponatremia as a complication of fluid

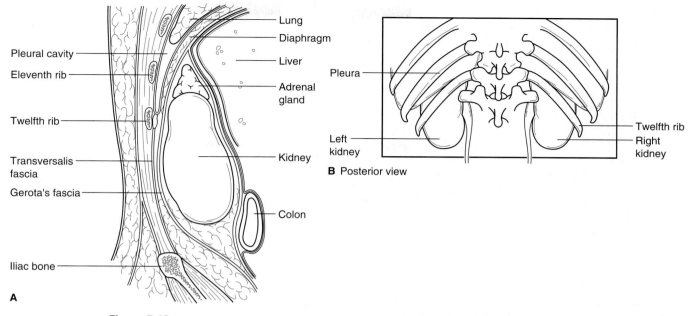

Figure 7-10 Anatomic relation of the pleural cavity and some intra-abdominal structures to the kidneys.

absorption during TURP (TURP syndrome), renal tubular acidosis, hyperchloremic metabolic acidosis after urinary diversion using intestinal segments, acute tubular necrosis after renal ischemia, and renal artery stenosis. A complete discussion of renal physiology should be reviewed in a physiology text.

Blood Supply

Twenty percent of cardiac output is directed to the kidneys. The renal vascular pedicle is anterior to the renal pelvis, entering at the hilum (Fig. 7-11). Usually, a single renal artery supplies each kidney. Later, this artery divides into branches that supply the various kidney segments. Variation in number and configuration of the renal arteries is extremely common. In one study, 65% of kidneys examined had at least one aberrant vessel. Interruption of these end arteries may result in ischemia and infarction of that portion of the kidney. The potential long-term sequela of this type of injury is hypertension. Additionally, aberrant lower pole arteries may be associated with congenital ureteropelvic junction obstruction.

Trauma

Blunt trauma accounts for 70% to 80% of all renal injuries. It usually results from motor vehicle accidents or, less commonly, from accidental falls or contact sports. The mechanism of injury is forces of rapid deceleration or actual impact on the upper abdomen, flank, or back. Hematuria occurs in many patients. Associated injuries can include rib fractures, vertebral body and transverse process fractures, and flank contusions and abrasions. Retroperitoneal

hematoma secondary to renal injury must be considered in patients who present in shock.

Evaluation

In the past, imaging was routinely performed when a renal injury was suspected based on mechanism of injury, microhematuria, or gross hematuria. It has subsequently been shown that adults with microhematuria after blunt renal trauma but no history of a major deceleration injury or hypotension do not necessarily need renal imaging. Children and patients with gross hematuria, hypotension, or a major deceleration injury require evaluation. A concern in children with rapid deceleration injury is an avulsion of the ureteropelvic junction; urinalysis can be negative in this situation.

A trauma patient with a suspected renal injury can be hemodynamically stable or unstable. The evaluation of a stable patient with a suspected renal parenchymal injury includes a CT scan. Any renal injury noted is classified as shown in Fig. 7-12. Minor contusions are the most common, and lacerations may be minor or major. In minor lacerations, the injury extends no further than the renal cortex, there is no urinary extravasation or large hematoma, and the capsule may remain intact. In major lacerations, there is a transcapsular rupture through the corticomedullary junction of the kidney and, often, associated urinary extravasation or a large perirenal hematoma.

An unstable patient should be taken to the operating room for an emergency laparotomy regardless of whether a renal injury is suspected. In this situation, renal imaging may be accomplished with a "one-shot" IVP. One protocol for this test involves administering an intravenous bolus of 2 mL/kg contrast, with a film taken 10 minutes later.

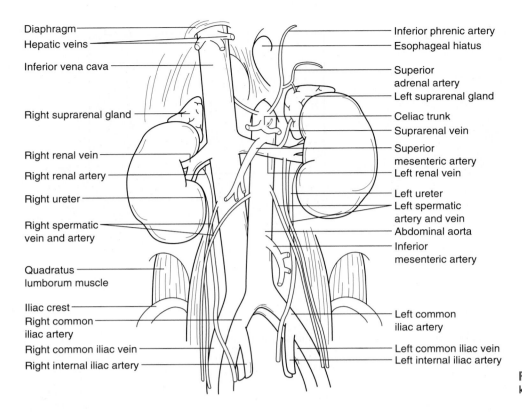

Diaphragm
Hepatic veins
Inferior vena cava

Right suprarenal gland

Right renal vein
Right renal artery

Right ureter

Right spermatic
vein and artery

Quadratus
lumborum muscle

Iliac crest
Right common
iliac artery

Right common iliac vein
Right internal iliac artery

Inferior phrenic artery
Esophageal hiatus

Superior
adrenal artery
Left suprarenal gland

Celiac trunk
Suprarenal vein

Superior
mesenteric artery
Left renal vein

Left ureter
Left spermatic
artery and vein
Abdominal aorta
Inferior
mesenteric artery

Left common
iliac artery

Left common iliac vein
Left internal iliac artery

Figure 7-11   Blood supply to the kidneys.

Treatment

In the stable patient who sustains blunt trauma, renal exploration is required only if the CT scan shows a major renal injury. There is no general agreement as to exactly what CT findings justify exploration. The trend is toward observation. In the unstable patient who undergoes surgery, indications for renal exploration include an expanding or pulsatile retroperitoneal hematoma or an abnormality on the IVP. The technical approach during renal exploration includes incision of the posterior peritoneum medial to the inferior mesenteric vein, anterior to the aorta, with isolation of the renal vessels before reflection of the colon and exploration of the kidney. This avoids exsanguinating hemorrhage.

The patient with penetrating trauma is managed similarly to the patient with blunt trauma. However, patients who have penetrating injuries more often require exploration, and the threshold to explore the kidney tends to be lower.

Congenital Disorders

Scores of congenital anomalies are found in the urinary tract. Some are symptomatic and discovered in children, others are asymptomatic and discovered serendipitously, and yet others do not become symptomatic until adulthood. Two common disorders that require intervention are horseshoe kidney and congenital obstruction of the urinary tract.

Horseshoe kidney occurs in 1:400 to 1:1,800 live births. It is the most common type of renal fusion anomaly and usually occurs at the lower pole. Symptoms are usually associated with obstruction or infection and include hematuria and vague abdominal discomfort. Diagnosis is usually made by IVP, although ultrasonography and CT are useful as well. When intervention is necessary, the renal isthmus connecting the kidneys is divided surgically (symphysiotomy). Revision of the ureteropelvic junction may need to accompany the symphysiotomy.

Congenital obstruction of the urinary tract occurs most often at the junction between the ureter and the renal pelvis, the ureteropelvic junction. The etiologic factors in this obstruction are myriad and complex and result in varying degrees of hydronephrosis. Bilateral involvement occurs in 10% to 40% of cases. An intrinsic obstruction caused by maldevelopment of the ureteropelvic junction is the likely cause of obstruction in children. In cases presenting in adulthood or late childhood, an aberrant vessel that crosses the ureteropelvic junction may also cause obstruction. The resulting stenosis or functional obstruction leads to hydronephrosis. Presenting signs and symptoms include palpable abdominal mass, pain, hematuria, urinary infection, fever, hypertension, and renal stones. Today, many cases of ureteropelvic junction obstruction are diagnosed by antenatal ultrasonography. Diagnosis is made by IVP or ultrasonogram. Nuclear scan (Lasix renography) is preferable to IVP in children because this type of scan is superior in quantifying renal function and obstruction. Surgical repair of

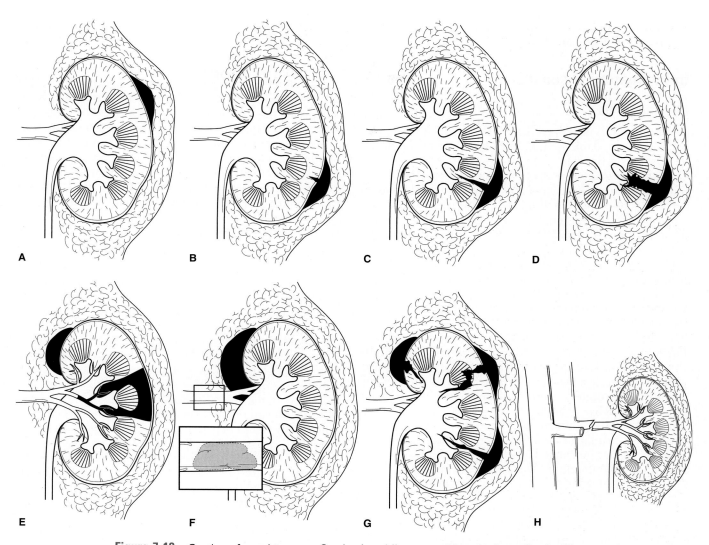

Figure 7-12   Grades of renal trauma. Grades I and II are considered minor. Grades III, IV, and V are considered major. **A,** Grade I trauma showing microscopic or gross hematuria. A contusion or a contained subcapsular hematoma is present. There is no parenchymal laceration. **B,** Grade II trauma showing a nonexpanding, confined perirenal hematoma or cortical laceration that is less than 1 cm deep. No urinary extravasation is present. **C,** Grade III trauma showing laceration of the parenchyma that extends less than 1 cm into the cortex. No urinary extravasation is present. **D,** Grade IV trauma showing laceration of the parenchyma that extends through the corticomedullary junction and into the collecting system. Laceration of a segmental vessel may also occur. **E,** Grade IV trauma showing thrombosis of a segmental renal artery. There is no laceration of the parenchyma, but there is ischemia of the corresponding parenchyma. **F,** Grade V trauma showing thrombosis of the main artery of the kidney. An intimal tear and a distal thrombosis are seen in the inset. **G,** Grade V trauma showing a kidney that is shattered because of multiple lacerations. **H,** Grade V trauma showing avulsion of the main artery or vein of the kidney. (Modified from Tanagho EA, McAninch JW, eds. *Smith's General Urology,* 13th ed. Norwalk, Conn: Appleton & Lange; 1992.)

the obstruction is performed to prevent loss of renal function and recurrent UTIs.

Inflammatory Diseases

Pyelonephritis

Pyelonephritis is usually a clinical diagnosis. Patients present with fever, flank pain, UTI, and costovertebral angle tenderness on the side of the involved kidney. In 80% of cases, *E. coli* is the causative organism. Chronic pyelonephritis often leads to renal failure and is a common reason for renal transplantation. Findings on IVP, usually nonspecific, include diffuse renal enlargement with calyceal distortion. If the infection is uncomplicated, treatment is outpatient oral antibiotic therapy. When the patient has evidence of sepsis or significant compromise requiring hospitalization, intravenous antibiotics are administered. It is not uncommon for fever and flank pain to persist for several days. If symptoms persist for a longer period, it is reasonable to image the kidneys with a CT or ultrasound to exclude an abscess. If ureteral obstruction is suspected, renal imaging must be immediately obtained and any obstruction must be emergently relieved (e.g., obstructive pyelonephritis associated with an obstructing ureteral stone) with a ureteral stent or a percutaneous nephrostomy. Obstructive pyelonephritis represents a urologic emergency because the infected urine proximal to the obstruction is similar to an abscess, but worse because the abscess is under pressure. These patients can become septic, and antibiotics alone do not represent adequate therapy. Treatment with removal of the stone is contraindicated as initial treatment because stone manipulation can lead to worsening of the sepsis. When emergently treating obstructive pyelonephritic, the goal is to relieve the obstruction. Treatment of a renal abscess is usually by percutaneous drainage in addition to antibiotics.

Emphysematous Pyelonephritis

Emphysematous pyelonephritis is a life-threatening infection in which bacteria, often *E. coli*, form gas in the renal parenchyma. The condition is associated with poorly controlled diabetes. Patients are usually septic and can deteriorate rapidly. A CT scan is diagnostic. Patients are managed with intravenous antibiotics, supportive measures, and an emergency nephrectomy. Percutaneous drainage of the affected area was recently reported as an alternative to nephrectomy. However, nephrectomy remains the standard treatment option.

Xanthogranulomatous Pyelonephritis

Xanthogranulomatous pyelonephritis (XGP) is another inflammatory disease of the kidney. Females are affected more often (75% of cases). Patients with XGP, a disease generally involving patients in the fifth to seventh decades of life, often have a history of failure to thrive and chronic UTI. The diagnosis can be difficult because the symptoms

are usually nonspecific. There is often a delay in the diagnosis of XGP, and it is important for primary care physicians to consider this disease with the described presentation. When urine culture shows UTI, *E. coli* and *Proteus* species are the most common causes. Currently, the CT scan is the imaging test of choice used to diagnose XGP. The lesions in the kidney, which may be quite large, are characterized by diffuse enlargement, central nephrolithiasis, and spherical areas surrounding the kidney in a hydronephrotic pattern. The affected kidney is usually nonfunctional. The treatment is usually a nephrectomy. The kidney can be adherent to adjacent structures, and the nephrectomy is frequently technically challenging.

Genitourinary Tuberculosis

Painless frequency, especially at night, is a common complaint in patients with genitourinary tuberculosis (TB). In a patient with sterile pyuria, TB should be suspected. A PPD skin test can help establish the diagnosis. A positive test does not necessarily indicate active disease. A definitive diagnosis is made by urine culture with isolation of *Mycobacterium tuberculosis*. Further testing includes chest films and spine imaging. When genitourinary TB is diagnosed, an IVP is mandatory. Findings may include calcifications at any point along the genitourinary tract, and extensive renal calcifications can be seen. Ureteral obstruction can occur secondary to stricture of the ureter. The management of genitourinary TB begins with antituberculosis drugs. Subsequent nephrectomy may be indicated in some cases when extensive renal destruction and nonfunction are present. Ureteral stricture management options may include temporary internal stenting, corticosteroids, or ureteral reimplantation in distal ureteral strictures. Treatment depends on the location and length of the stricture and the response to medical management.

Neoplasms

Renal masses are classified as benign or malignant; malignant tumors are primary or metastatic. The most commonly encountered renal mass lesion is a simple cyst (70% of cases). Renal cell carcinoma is the most common primary neoplasm of the kidney and accounts for more than 85% of all primary renal cancers in adults. This chapter discusses only the most frequently encountered tumors.

Clinical Presentation and Evaluation

Patients with renal cancer often have painless hematuria, but the cancer is being discovered with increasing frequency on CT scans and ultrasound as an incidental finding. Many texts refer to the classic triad (a complex of flank pain, abdominal mass, and hematuria) as characteristic of renal cancer. However, patients seldom have all three findings.

CT scanning plays a prominent role in the workup of solid renal masses and may be valuable in characterizing some atypical cystic masses. Cystic lesions are often identified by IVP and confirmed by ultrasound. Arteriography, once a standard preoperative study, is recommended only in selected cases where the diagnosis is in doubt or aberrant vasculature is expected. If tumor invasion of the inferior vena cava is suspected, a magnetic resonance image (MRI) or inferior venacavogram is indicated to define the extent of involvement.

Benign Neoplasms

Most simple cystic lesions are asymptomatic and benign and require no intervention. However, some are complex (e.g., septations, wall thickening, or calcifications) and require further investigation to rule out malignancy. Benign simple renal cysts are usually asymptomatic. Simple cysts are found in as many as 33% of adults. A simple cyst noted on imaging (e.g., CT, ultrasound) is managed by observation. A complex cyst is usually considered cancerous until proven otherwise, and partial or radical nephrectomy may be indicated. A needle biopsy or cyst aspiration is usually of little value in most cases because a negative result may be a false negative and does not rule out malignancy. Benign solid tumors of the kidney are encountered occasionally. An angiomyolipoma is usually diagnosed by the characteristic appearance of fat within the lesion on CT scan. Fat is black on CT, and when fat is seen within a renal mass, angiomyolipoma is almost always the diagnosis.

Malignant Neoplasms

Renal Cell Carcinoma

Renal cell carcinoma, a tumor that usually arises from the proximal convoluted tubules, is by far the most common primary solid tumor affecting the kidney. Although etiologic factors are not well documented in human beings, nitrosamines are implicated in animal studies. Carcinogens found in cigarette smoke have also been implicated, but no specific carcinogen has been identified. Renal cell carcinoma has a 2:1 male-to-female preponderance. Typically unilateral, this lesion is spherical with a pseudocapsule of parenchyma and fibrosis. Five percent of renal carcinoma may be bilateral.

Hematuria is the single most common sign, occurring in 29% to 60% of reported cases. Flank pain and palpable flank mass occur next most often, but the classic triad of hematuria, flank pain, and a palpable abdominal mass are reported in only 4% to 17% of cases. Other common signs and symptoms are fever, anemia, and elevated sedimentation rate. Although serum lactate dehydrogenase and alkaline phosphatase may be elevated, there are no reliable tumor markers for renal cell carcinoma. Renal cell cancers can cause only nonspecific symptoms such as weight loss, fever, or weakness.

In later stages, this tumor invades the renal vein and vena cava and may even extend into the right atrium. A staging system such as the TNM system (Table 7-2) is used to determine the extent of the primary lesion, the involvement of contiguous structures, the extent of vascular involvement, and whether the tumor has metastasized. Renal cell carci-

Table 7-2	TNM Classification of Renal Carcinoma

Primary Tumor (T)

TX	Primary tumor cannot be assessed
T0	No evidence of primary tumor
T1	Tumor 7 cm or less in greatest dimension limited to the kidney
T2	Tumor more than 7 cm in greatest dimension limited to the kidney
T3	Tumor extends into major veins or invades the adrenal gland or perinephric tissues, but not beyond Gerota's fascia
T3a	Tumor invades the adrenal gland or perinephric tissues but not beyond Gerota's fascia
T3b	Tumor grossly extends into the renal vein(s) or vena cava below the diaphragm
T3c	Tumor grossly extends into the renal vein(s) or vena cava above the diaphragm
T4	Tumor invades beyond Gerota's fascia

Regional Lymph Nodes (N)[a]

NX	Regional lymph nodes cannot be assessed
N0	No regional lymph node metastases
N1	Metastases in a single regional lymph node
N2	Metastasis in more than one regional lymph node

Distant Metastasis (M)

MX	Distant metastasis cannot be assessed
M0	No distant metastasis
M1	Distant metastasis

[a]Laterality does not affect the N classification.

Used with the permission of the American Joint Committee on Cancer (AJCC), Chicago, Illinois. The original source for this material is the *AJCC Cancer Staging Manual,* 5th ed. Philadelphia: Lippincott-Raven; 1997.

noma metastasizes most often to lungs, bone, and brain, in that order. Metastatic lesions may appear in both the ipsilateral and contralateral kidney, and late metastasis may occur to the liver. Five-year survival rates for stages I and II are 80% to 90%, and for stages III and IV are 40% to 60%.

Treatment for renal cell carcinoma is radical nephrectomy (Fig. 7-13). However, partial nephrectomy is now considered a reasonable alternative for small tumors, even in the presence of a normal contralateral kidney. As with radical prostatectomy, laparoscopy has significantly reduced the perioperative and postoperative morbidity associated with the traditional open approach. Preoperative evaluation should include a chest radiograph and liver function tests. A bone scan is required in the presence of bone pain or elevated alkaline phosphatase. The kidney, perinephric fat, Gerota's fascia, ipsilateral adrenal gland, and ipsilateral regional lymph nodes are removed during a radical nephrectomy. The renal vessels should be controlled before manipulation and dissection. In cases of vena cava involvement, the incision may need to be extended or a median sternotomy performed for adequate exposure. The vena cava, which is controlled superiorly and inferiorly, may need to

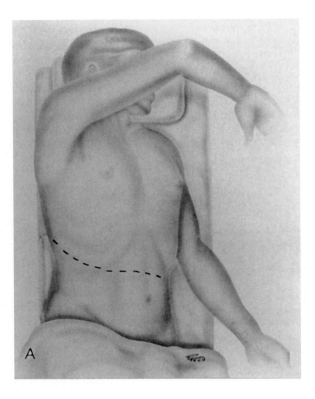

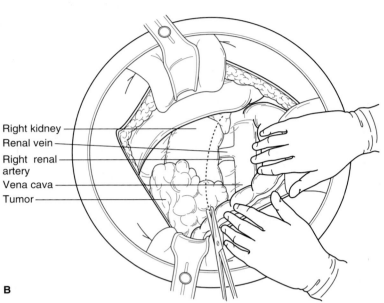

Right kidney
Renal vein
Right renal artery
Vena cava
Tumor

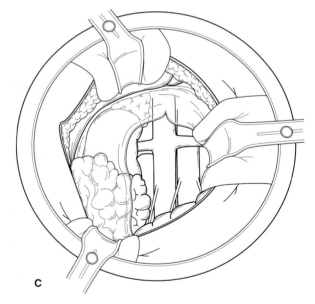

Figure 7-13   **A,** Eleventh rib surgical approach for radical nephrectomy. **B,** Right kidney, renal artery, and tumor identified. **C,** Line of incision in retroperitoneum to expose right kidney.

be incised to remove a tumor thrombus. The lumbar and contralateral renal veins must be controlled as well. Postoperative complications include bleeding, retroperitoneal abscess, ileus, and wound infection, as well as recognized complications of abdominal surgery (e.g., pulmonary embolism).

Transitional Cell Carcinoma

Transitional cell carcinoma of the renal pelvis may present as a renal mass or a filling defect on IVP. Urine cytology may be negative, but usually shows abnormal cells. Small lesions are hard to see by CT. Ureteroscopy can be used to visualize or biopsy suspicious lesions. Many upper urinary tract lesions seed the lower urinary tract, making upper tract evaluation paramount when transitional cell carcinoma is found in the lower tract. Treatment is nephroureterectomy, with removal of a cuff of bladder at the ureteral orifice because of the high incidence of ipsilateral ureteral orifice and bladder involvement.

Urinary Stone Disease

Urinary tract calculi represent a significant cause for morbidity in the United States: more than 500,000 people are affected yearly. Men are affected more often than women, and the 30- to 50-year age-group has the highest incidence. The majority of stones are composed of calcium oxalate.

Risk factors are associated with specific types of stone formation. Factors that lead to the formation of calcium stones include underlying metabolic disorders (e.g., renal tubular acidosis, hyperparathyroidism). Other risk factors include poor hydration, immobilization, and a family history of renal stones. Risk factors for uric acid stones include high dietary intake of purines, history of gout, poor hydration, and hyperuricosuria. Cystine stones are usually seen in families with a history of cystinuria, an inherited disorder affecting the renal reabsorption of four amino acids including cysteine. Cysteine, ornithine, lysine, and arginine are the four involved amino acids. Cystine stones represent a true inherited disorder, in which the renal tubules do not transport four amino acids. These patients develop stones early in life. Struvite (magnesium ammonium phosphate) stones (infection stones) develop in patients with chronic UTIs. Patients with chronically indwelling catheters are at particular risk for the development of these stones. When these stones grow to occupy the entire collecting system, they are termed Staghorn stones.

A number of theories have been proposed to describe the mechanism of calcium stone formation. A widely accepted theory proposes that urine becomes supersaturated with calcium oxalate. Normal urine contains substances that inhibit crystallization. If an individual has an inadequate amount of one or more inhibitors, or an inhibitor does not function properly, spontaneous crystallization follows. Moreover, if there is a high calcium concentration in the urine through increased calcium absorption from the intestine, or increased excretion (renal leak), crystallization is promoted. These crystals either are passed harmlessly through the kidney into the ureter or become lodged in the collecting system. Once they lodge, the crystals develop rapidly, forming a stone. If the stone obstructs the ureteropelvic junction or ureter, hydronephrosis can result.

Clinical Presentation and Evaluation

Urinary tract stones are usually diagnosed in the emergency room. Renal colic is the presenting symptom in most patients with symptomatic stones. It is described as a constant pain in the flank often radiating to the groin, accompanied by nausea and vomiting. The pain can be acute and so severe that even large doses of narcotics cannot completely control it. The cause of the pain is usually not the stone itself, but the obstruction caused as the stone passes from the collecting system into the ureter. Actual passage of the stone through the urethra is relatively uneventful.

Emergency room evaluation always includes urinalysis.

Microhematuria is commonly associated with stone disease. The diagnosis of stone disease requires an imaging study. The traditional study used to image the upper urinary tracts is an IVP. A scout film is obtained, contrast is injected intravenously, and multiple radiographs are obtained over time. This test provides excellent anatomic and functional information. For example, a delayed nephrogram and delayed excretion confirms a functional obstruction. Uric acid stones are seen on IVP as a filling defect. A uric acid stone is lucent on a plain film, but is bright white on a noncontrast CT. A renal ultrasound is noninvasive but lacks the anatomic detail of an IVP, especially along the ureters, and does not provide functional information.

The elective metabolic workup for renal stones is usually obtained in children with stones and patients with recurrent stones, but may be obtained in any patient with stones. This evaluation is obtained after passage of the stone, when the patient is on a regular diet. There is no standard metabolic evaluation. Some urologists obtain a more comprehensive evaluation initially, whereas others obtain screening laboratory data and obtain further testing if the initial studies are abnormal. Laboratory testing includes determining values for serum calcium, parathyroid hormone, electrolytes, urine pH, and 24-hour urine collections to measure calcium and other electrolyte concentrations.

Treatment

Treatment of urinary calculi depends on the size, location, and composition of the stones. Obstructive pyelonephritis is one situation that deserves particular attention. This condition occurs when a patient has an obstructing stone associated with infection of the affected upper urinary tract, causing "pus under pressure"; it is a true urologic emergency. Patients come to the emergency room with flank pain, fever, and infected urine. This is similar to the presentation of a patient with pyelonephritis not associated with stone disease. In this setting, it is important to rule out obstructive pyelonephritis by imaging the kidney. When a patient has obstructing pyelonephritis, antibiotics alone do not effectively treat the problem. The treatment must include relief of the obstruction, with emergency placement of an internal stent (placed cytoscopically) or a percutaneous nephrostomy. No attempt is made to manipulate or remove the stone because manipulation can lead to septic complications. The goal of emergency intervention is to promote drainage.

Ureteral stones smaller than 5 mm usually pass spontaneously. Larger ureteral stones, especially stones larger than 8 mm, often do not pass without urologic intervention. When intervention is indicated for ureteral stones, which are often obstructing, treatment may involve stent placement alone because a stent in the ureter can lead to passive dilation of the ureter and subsequent stone passage. Another option is flexible or rigid ureteroscopy with stone fragmentation and extraction. When ureteral stones are approached endoscopically and require fragmentation before removal, devices used to fragment the stone include electrohydraulic lithotripsy and a new modality, the Holmium laser.

Selected ureteral stones can be managed with **extracorporeal shock wave lithotripsy** to fragment the stones into pieces small enough to pass spontaneously. The technology involves transmission of a focused shock wave from outside the body to the calculus. A high-voltage underwater spark gap initiates the shock wave. The gap or discharge, occurring in approximately 1 microsecond, results in vaporization of the fluid surrounding the arc, developing a plasma-like state. This explosive vaporization of fluid propagates a high-energy shock wave, which is focused by surrounding the spark gap with a semi-ellipsoid, allowing concentration of the energy at a second focal point, F2 (Fig. 7-14). By placing the calculus at this second focal point, the destructive energy is transmitted to the stone, causing it to fragment.

Management of stones in the collecting system usually is accomplished with extracorporeal shock wave lithotripsy. Alternatively, percutaneous removal is an option, especially when there is a large stone burden. Unlike calcium stones, uric acid stones can be treated medically be-

cause they dissolve when the pH is increased. The treatment of uric acid stones therefore consists of urinary alkalization and increased fluid intake. Open surgery, commonly performed in the past, is rarely indicated today.

THE URETERS

Anatomy

The ureters are the conduits for urine between the kidneys and the bladder. Each ureter enters the bladder posterolaterally on its inferior portion and courses obliquely for 1.5 cm through the bladder wall. For half that distance, the ureter traverses the muscularis; for the other half, it is submucosal. The lower portion of the ureter is anchored and supported by special fibromuscular tissue called Waldeyer's sheath. The normal anatomy of the ureter allows free efflux of urine into the bladder but prevents reflux. This one-way flow depends on the complex relation between the ureteral muscle, the bladder base, and the ureteral route through the bladder wall. In its upper portions, the ureteral muscle has an irregular helical pattern. Near the bladder and in its intramural portion, the muscle fibers run parallel to the lumen. Peristalsis of the ureteral wall propels urine toward the bladder. As the contraction approaches the bladder, the longitudinal fiber arrangement causes the intramural ureteral lumen to open and shorten, allowing urine to enter. When a ureteral contraction is not present, increasing bladder pressure compresses the submucosal ureteral lumen against the underlying bladder muscle and prevents reflux (Fig. 7-15).

Ureteral Obstruction

Ureteral obstruction can be caused primarily by diseases directly involving the ureters, including stone disease, extrinsic masses (e.g., tumors of the colon), gynecologic malignancy, vascular aneurysm, inflammatory disease of the colon, and retroperitoneal fibrosis. The IVP is an excellent test to diagnose ureteral obstruction because it provides both anatomic and functional information. Treatment depends on the underlying etiology. In patients with nonurologic malignancy causing ureteral obstruction, treatment is influenced by the overall prognosis. Initial management usually includes stenting of the ureter.

Ureteral obstruction also can be secondary to other diseases. When there is bladder outlet obstruction secondary to BPH, prostate cancer, urethral stricture, or other lower tract pathology, the effects are transmitted to the upper tracts. Ultrasound findings often include bilateral hydronephrosis with bilateral hydroureter along the entire length of both ureters. The patient is usually initially managed with bladder catheterization.

Iatrogenic Injuries to the Ureters

Iatrogenic injury to the ureters can occur during general, vascular, and gynecologic surgery. Diverticulitis, aortic

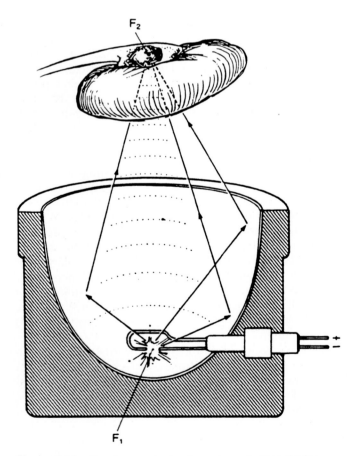

Figure 7-14   Spark gap electrode and semi-ellipsoid for focusing shock waves. Electrode is placed at first focus inside ellipsoid with stone placed at second focus.

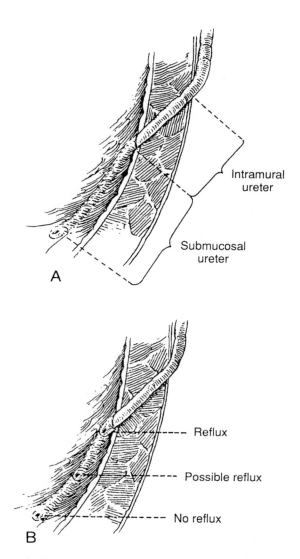

A

Intramural
ureter

Submucosal
ureter

Reflux

Possible reflux

No reflux

B

Figure 7-15 **A,** Normal ureterovesical junction. **B,** Refluxing ureterovesical junction and ureterovesical junction showing inadequate submucosal tunnels.

or iliac artery aneurysms, and ovarian or uterine tumors often exist in close proximity to the distal third of the ureter. The ureters are occasionally injured inadvertently during surgery for a large pelvic mass. Ureteral stents may be temporarily placed through the bladder before surgery to help with intraoperative identification of the ureters when the risk of injury is considered high. A ureteral injury can be repaired with an end-to-end anastomosis and then stented. When the injury occurs to the distal ureter, a ureteral reimplantation is usually performed. If a ureter is injured in a contaminated surgical field, however, proximal urinary diversion with percutaneous nephrostomy or open nephrostomy becomes necessary. If the ureter is injured during repair of an intra-abdominal aortic aneurysm, the ureter is often repaired primarily and then wrapped with omentum.

THE BLADDER

Anatomy

The bladder is a hollow muscular organ that functions to store urine and then evacuate it. When empty, the bladder lies just behind the pubic symphysis. As it fills, its superior portion protrudes into the peritoneal cavity and can often be palpated suprapubically. It is lined with transitional epithelium that lies on a loose, elastic connective tissue bed, the lamina propria. The muscle of the body of the bladder, the detrusor, is composed of interlacing smooth muscle bundles with no distinct layers. An exception is the trigone, a triangular area that lies between the ureteral orifices and the urethral opening. In this area, the muscle wall has two layers, a superficial one fusing with the ureteral musculature and a deeper one indistinguishable from the detrusor. Although only the superiormost portion of the bladder is covered with peritoneum, the entire bladder is covered with the loose fascia of the pelvic cavity. The bladder is firmly attached to the posterior aspect of the pubic bone by condensations of this fascia, called the puboprostatic ligaments in males and the pubovesical ligaments in females. The median umbilical ligament, the fibrotic remnant of the urachus, attaches the bladder to the anterior abdominal wall. Condensation of the pelvic fascia in the dorsolateral aspect of the bladder also serves as an anchor and neurovascular conduit. Blood is supplied by the superior, middle, and inferior vesical arteries, branches of the hypogastric artery. In females, blood is also supplied by the vaginal and uterine arteries. The bladder is surrounded by a rich plexus of veins that drains into the hypogastric veins. Bladder lymphatics drain to the external iliac, hypogastric, common iliac, and sacral lymph nodes.

Evaluation

Endoscopic Evaluation: Cystourethroscopy

The bladder and urethra are evaluated endoscopically by flexible and rigid cystoscopes. These contain an optical fiber–lens system for visualization, fibers to carry illumination and ports for instruments, catheters, and irrigation fluid. The rigid cystoscope consists of a telescope, a bridge, and a sheath available in various sizes, with input and output ports for irrigation. The bridge, forming a watertight connection between the sheath and telescope, may have one or two ports for the introduction of tools, catheters, or electrodes. The telescopes vary in viewing angles from 0 degrees (straight ahead) to 120 degrees (retroview). Flexible cystoscopes have a maneuverable tip for examining the bladder.

An examination regimen is used during **cystoscopy** to avoid oversights. The entire bladder mucosa is examined systematically for mucosal irregularities, tumors, lesions, or unusual vascularity. Trabeculation (i.e., the formation of bands of muscle tissue) of the bladder wall, cellule formation (i.e., the formation of small diverticula that have not yet protruded beyond the bladder wall), and diverticula are noted. Ureteral orifices are checked for position and configuration. Ureteral urine, as it effluxes into the bladder, can be observed for color to rule out blood coming from either ureteral orifice. In addition, the bladder neck is evaluated for contracture, the prostatic fossa is checked for mucosal lesions and anatomic occlusion from prostatic tissue, and the urethra is examined for stricture formation, mucosal lesions, and tumors. Retrograde pyelography can be performed through the cystoscope by inserting a catheter into the ureteral orifice and injecting radiographic contrast to evaluate ureteral and renal pelvic anatomy. Although cystoscopy provides information concerning the anatomy of the lower urinary tract, its ability to assess lower urinary tract function is extremely limited.

Urodynamic Evaluation

Urodynamics is a collection of studies used to evaluate the reservoir and micturition function of the lower urinary tract. Urodynamic tests include PVR urine volume, cystometrogram (CMG), urinary flow rate (**uroflow test**), urethral pressure profile, sphincter electromyography (EMG), and fluoroscopic cystography. The PVR is the volume of urine that remains in the bladder after voiding. One way to measure the PVR is to catheterize the bladder immediately after voiding and record the output. Ultrasound is a less invasive but less precise test that also can be used to measure the amount of residual urine. Normal individuals void to completion; significant residual urine occurs with bladder outlet obstruction, cystocele, and neurogenic bladders. The CMG evaluates intravesical pressures during filling and voiding. The CMG measures bladder sensation, capacity, compliance, and voiding pressures; it can also detect premature detrusor contractions. The normal bladder should fill to a capacity of 350 to 500 mL without a significant increase in pressure or detrusor contraction. The first sensation of needing to void occurs around 150 to 250 mL of filling, and definite fullness is sensed at 350 to 450 mL.

Urinary flow rate measures the rate of urine flow from the urethra. Normally, flow rates occur around a tight, bell-shaped curve. Men have a peak flow rate of 20 to 25 mL/sec and women 20 to 30 mL/sec. Low flow rates indicate either bladder outlet obstruction or poor detrusor function. Urethral pressure recordings, a test not commonly performed, measures intraluminal pressures of the urethra. EMG is used to evaluate sphincter activity. Normally, sphincter EMG activity increases with filling and decreases just before voiding. Fluoroscopic cystoscopy can visualize the bladder neck and sphincter and can also detect cystocele, descensus (bladder prolapse), and reflux.

Congenital Anomalies

Vesicoureteral Reflux

Primary vesicoureteral reflux (VUR) is the result of an abnormally short intramural ureteral tunnel. Develop-

mentally, this is thought to be due to a laterally placed origin of the ureteral bud from the fetal bladder. This anomaly allows potentially infected urine to reflux up the ureter, resulting in kidney damage. The ensuing inflammatory reaction causes permanent tubular damage and loss of renal function.

The degree of reflux can be graded to correlate with the possibility of spontaneous resolution or renal damage (Fig. 7-16). Lower grades of reflux (grades I and II) usually resolve as a child grows and the ureterovesical junction matures. Because higher grades of reflux are less likely to resolve spontaneously and present an increased risk of renal damage, surgical correction is recommended. Secondary reflux can occur after resection of the ureteral orifice during removal of an overlying tumor, after ureteral meatotomy to aid in stone removal, after kidney transplantation, or after dilation of the intramural ureter for ureteroscopy. Occasionally, secondary reflux may require operative intervention. During episodes of cystitis, marginally competent ureteral orifices may reflux, but this transient reflux usually subsides after resolution of the bladder inflammation.

Clinical Evaluation

VUR is most often discovered during the investigation for UTI. In children, the prevalence of VUR is inversely proportional to age; it is associated with 29% to 50% of children evaluated for UTI. The voiding cystourethrogram (VCUG) is the primary diagnostic test for reflux. The bladder is filled with contrast and visualized fluoroscopically to detect reflux as the bladder fills and voids. The VCUG may be performed as soon as the urine has been sterilized after an acute infection. This study also can be performed with a radioisotope (radionuclide cystogram), which allows a smaller total dose of radiation and can detect smaller degrees of reflux. However, the anatomic detail is inferior to that obtained with a fluoroscopic VCUG. Renal ultrasound and IVP detect upper tract dilatation but cannot alone diagnose reflux. Cystoscopy is not indicated routinely in children with reflux. However, it may be useful if there is suspicion of an associated anatomic abnormality (e.g., an ectopic ureter).

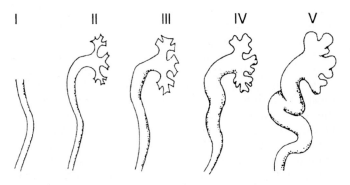

Figure 7-16 Grading of reflux based on findings on voiding cystourethrogram.

Treatment

The therapeutic goal in VUR is prevention of UTIs and renal damage. In children with reflux but without dilated ureters (i.e., grade I or II reflux), reflux disappears in 20% to 30% of cases every 2 years, with 80% resolving eventually. Continual low-dose antibacterial agents can be used prophylactically to prevent UTI and protect the kidneys until reflux stops. It is essential that the antibacterial prophylaxis is not interrupted and that careful follow-up is conducted. The child should have a culture obtained every 3 months, with each febrile illness, and with urinary symptoms. A VCUG or radionuclide cystogram should be performed yearly, as well as a renal ultrasound to detect hydronephrosis or upper tract scarring. If there is suspected new renal scarring, a radionucleotide **renal scan** is more sensitive than ultrasound. Serum creatinine, blood urea nitrogen, height, weight, and blood pressure should also be checked yearly.

Surgical repair is undertaken in patients who have severe reflux or in those who fail medical management, either by poor compliance, repeated UTIs despite prophylaxis, or loss of renal function. The goals of ureteral reimplantation include lengthening the intramural portion of the ureter four to five times its diameter, immobilizing the ureteral meatus by anchoring it to the underlying detrusor, and supporting the intramural ureter with the firm underlying bladder wall. In cases with severe reflux and marked ureteral dilation, the ureter may require plication or tapering before reimplantation.

A new mode of therapy for reflux is the transurethral injection of dextranomer/hyaluronic acid copolymer (Deflux) into the bladder wall just within the ureteral orifice. This is an outpatient procedure done under general anesthesia and generally takes less than 30 minutes. Early results for grade 2 to 4 reflux show that between 70% and 91% of patients are cured after a single injection. Although this therapy may be emerging as a "middle ground" between antibiotic prophylaxis and open surgery, long-term data are lacking. A new mode of therapy for reflux is the transurethral injection of collagen or Teflon into the bladder wall just below the ureteral orifice. Although this method is effective in milder forms of reflux or after failed reimplantations, it is too new to have yielded long-term results or to have received FDA approval for general use. Concern also exists regarding migration of Teflon particles to distant sites, such as the brain, lungs, and lymph nodes.

Several techniques are used to perform a ureteroneocystostomy, allowing the operation to be tailored to fit the patient's needs and anatomy. Ureteral advancement procedures (e.g., Glenn-Anderson technique) can be applied when the ureteral meatus is high and lateral enough to allow creation of a tunnel of adequate length without placing the new meatus too close to the bladder neck. The ureteral meatus is approached transvesically and the surrounding mucosa circumscribed. A stent is placed up the ureter and sutured to the mucosa next to the meatus (Fig. 7-17). The Cohen procedure, the most commonly performed repair, is a cross-trigonal tunneling of the ureter

that can be used when there is insufficient space between the ureteral hiatus and the bladder neck (Fig. 7-18). The Politano-Leadbetter technique is often used when reoperation is required. Although originally a transvesical procedure, it is now most often approached as a combined transvesical and extravesical procedure, in which the ureter is completely mobilized from the bladder. The submucosal tunnel is lengthened by creating a new hiatus superolaterally. The old hiatus is closed, and the new orifice is created nearer the bladder neck. The ureter is then brought through the new hiatus and passed submucosally to the new orifice and secured there (Fig. 7-19). Ureteral reimplantations also can be done laparoscopically, with results similar to those with open surgery.

Other Anomalies

Exstrophy of the bladder is the result of improper development of the anterior abdominal wall, pelvic girdle, and anterior wall of the bladder. It results in exposure of the posterior wall of the bladder through the abdominal wall and a separation of the symphysis pubis. It is an uncommon anomaly, occurring in 1:30,000 births, and has a 3:1 male predominance. Besides disfigurement and total incontinence, bacterial colonization and UTIs are common. Often, total urinary tract reconstruction including bladder augmentation and bladder neck reconstruction is necessary to preserve renal function and provide urinary continence. There is an increased risk of adenocarcinoma of the bladder in patients with exstrophy, and they need lifelong follow-up by a urologist.

Urachal persistence can occur as umbilical sinus, abdominal wall cyst, diverticulum at the bladder dome, or fistula from bladder to umbilicus. These are best treated with simple excision. Persistent urachal remnants are also associated with adenocarcinomatous changes. Congenital diverticula are difficult to differentiate from acquired ones. Previously, presence of muscle in the wall of the diverticulum was considered to indicate a congenital origin, but this is no longer believed to be true. Excision of the symptomatic diverticulum is the treatment of choice in most situations.

Trauma

Bladder injury can occur as a result of penetrating or blunt trauma. Common causes of penetrating bladder injuries are gunshot wounds, stab wounds, and instrumentation. Pelvic fractures can cause puncture of the bladder wall either by sharp fracture edges or fragments. Blunt trauma, as occurs in motor vehicle accidents, causes a sudden increase in intravesical pressure, resulting in a bladder wall contusion or rupture. Bladder contusions often result in hematuria, whereas bladder tears may result in intraperitoneal or extraperitoneal extravasation. Traumatic bladder ruptures are often associated with damage to other pelvic and intra-abdominal organs.

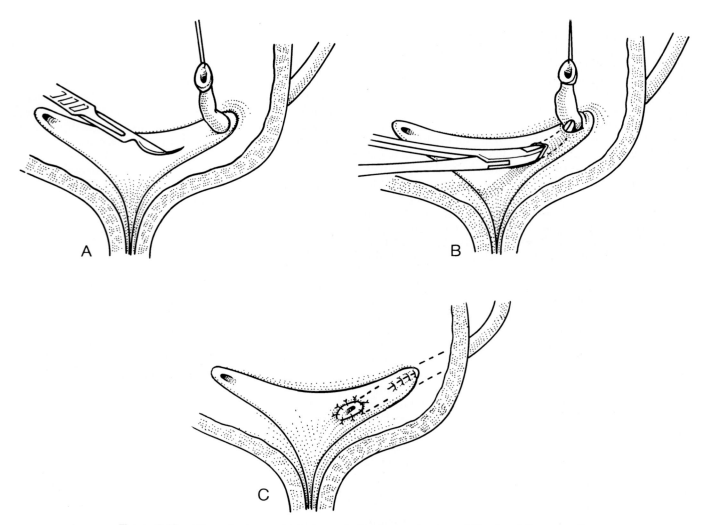

Figure 7-17 Glenn-Anderson technique. **A,** Ureter has been mobilized and the new site for the meatus is incised. **B,** Ureter is brought through a new, longer submucosal tunnel to the new meatus site. **C,** Completed procedure showing the longer submucosal tunnel.

Evaluation

Conscious patients with a bladder rupture often complain of severe suprapubic or pelvic pain with an inability to void. In unconscious patients, however, a high degree of suspicion is essential to make the diagnosis. Bladder ruptures almost invariably cause hematuria, and, if associated with pelvic fractures, a urethral disruption must be suspected. The most dependable diagnostic study for a bladder rupture is a cystogram. However, if accompanying urethral damage is suspected (e.g., because of blood at the meatus), a **retrograde urethrogram** must be performed to exclude a urethral tear before catheterization (Fig. 7-20). To perform a cystogram, a scout film is taken: approximately 350 mL sterile contrast is instilled into the bladder (adults), the catheter is clamped, and films are taken (Fig. 7-21). Views may include oblique and lateral films in addition to a posterior-anterior image. A postdrainage film must

be obtained because approximately 15% of bladder ruptures are diagnosed on the postdrainage film.

Treatment

Small, extraperitoneal ruptures can be managed with 1 to 2 weeks of Foley catheter drainage, with complete healing anticipated. Intraperitoneal bladder ruptures and large or complicated extraperitoneal bladder ruptures require surgical repair.

Repair consists of exploration through a midline intraperitoneal incision, with care taken to avoid the pelvic hematoma, careful inspection of the bladder, closure of the bladder with absorbable suture, and placement of a catheter to provide adequate urinary drainage. Because bladder ruptures are often associated with damage to other intra-abdominal organs, repair is often part of an exploratory laparotomy.

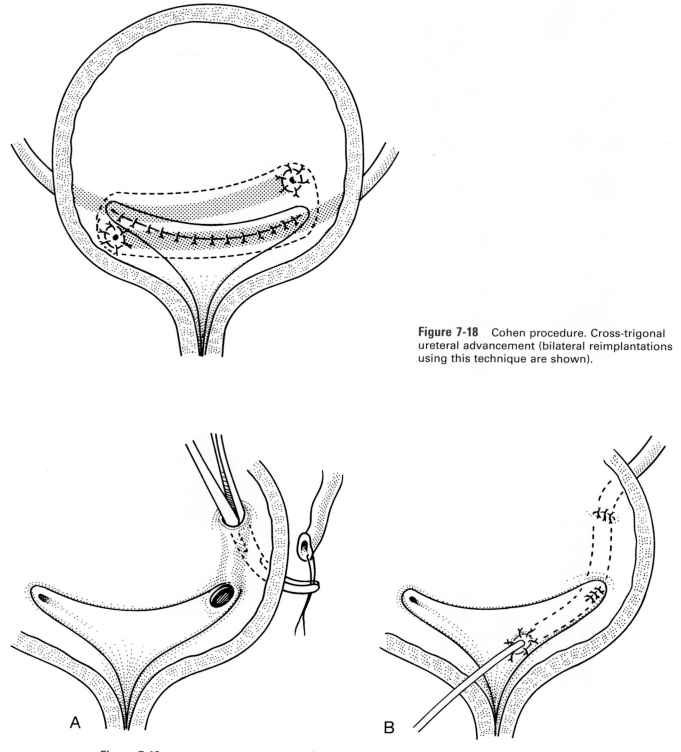

Figure 7-18   Cohen procedure. Cross-trigonal ureteral advancement (bilateral reimplantations using this technique are shown).

A

B

Figure 7-19   Politano-Leadbetter procedure. **A,** The ureter has been dissected completely and a new hiatus made superolaterally. **B,** The finished procedure with stent in place.

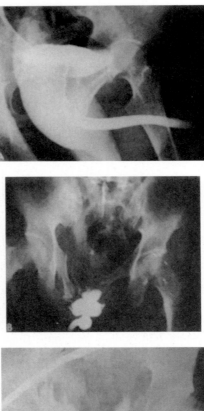

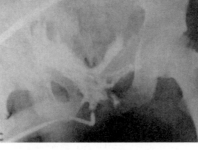

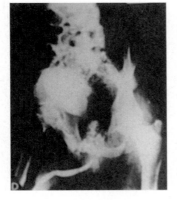

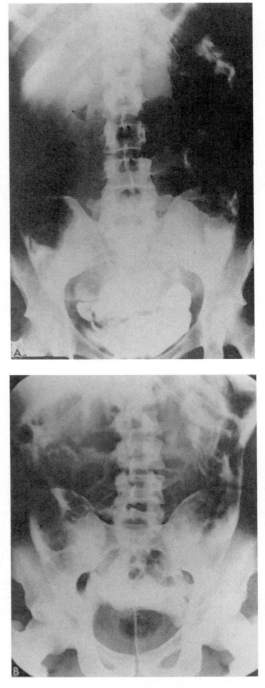

Figure 7-20 **A,** Normal retrograde urethrogram. The contrast material has been injected during the exposure to ensure delineation of deep bulbar, membranous, and prostatic urethra. **B–D,** Disruption of the posterior urethra in the male.

Figure 7-21 Intraperitoneal urinary bladder rupture. **A,** Pooling of contrast media in the right upper quadrant of the peritoneum. **B,** The contrast material outlines the peritoneal surface that the bowel interfaces.

Inflammatory Diseases

Bacterial Cystitis

Patients who have bacterial cystitis have irritative voiding symptoms, including dysuria, frequency, urgency, nocturia, and, if the inflammation is severe enough, gross hematuria. Fever is not common with uncomplicated cystitis, and if present may indicate an upper tract infection. Bacterial cystitis is much more common in women, with bacteria ascending to the bladder by way of their shorter urethra. Studies indicate that the vaginal introitus becomes colonized with fecal organisms before cystitis. Women who are prone to recurrent UTIs may be predisposed to infections because of increased vaginal and bladder mucosal bacterial adherence. In men, bacterial cystitis is usually the result of incomplete emptying of the bladder. The most common bacteria involved are the Gram-negative rods of the family Enterobacteriaceae. *E. coli* causes more than 80% of all urinary tract infections.

Evaluation includes a urinalysis to determine the presence of bacteria, leukocytes, and red blood cells. A properly collected urine specimen (i.e., a "clean catch") for culture and sensitivity is necessary for accurate diagnosis. The initial antibiotic is chosen empirically, usually a drug effective against a broad range of Gram-negative organisms. Antibiotic therapy is then adjusted depending on the culture and sensitivity results. With appropriate therapy, symptoms should resolve in 3 to 5 days.

Further evaluation of the urinary tract, including cystoscopy and radiologic studies, is indicated in children, in men, and in women who do not respond to antibiotic therapy or have multiple recurrent infections. The purpose of evaluation is to detect correctable causes of recurrent infections (Table 7-3). Carcinoma should be considered in patients whose irritative voiding symptoms persist even after sterilization of the urine. To prevent bacteremia, manipulation of the urinary tract should be delayed until after the acute infection has resolved. Evaluation in adults includes IVP or renal ultrasound, urinary cytology, cystoscopy, and possibly a voiding cystourethrogram when reflux is suspected. Children are usually evaluated with a renal ultrasound and a voiding cystourethrogram. Although cystoscopy aids little in diagnosing bacterial cystitis, it can detect the presence of a neoplasm or stone and may suggest anatomic bladder outlet obstruction.

Interstitial Cystitis

Interstitial cystitis is a syndrome of unknown etiology that is characterized by lower abdominal pain and irritative voiding symptoms. It predominantly affects women and is a difficult problem to manage. Urinalysis occasionally shows microhematuria. Typically, urine cultures for bacteria, fungi, and viruses are negative. Cytoscopically, submucosal petechiae (glomerulations) may be seen. Rarely, a mucosal ulceration (Hunner's ulcer) is seen. Interstitial cystitis is a diagnosis of exclusion. Symptoms wax and wane. In some patients, the pain and urinary frequency become debilitating. Histologically, the bladder is chronically inflamed, and in severe cases the bladder becomes fibrotic and contracted. Carcinoma in situ, which can also cause irritative symptoms in patients with sterile urine, is excluded by urinary cytology and bladder biopsy. Cystoscopy may show a Hunner's ulcer or glomerulations after hydrodistention of the bladder. Biopsies often show evidence of chronic inflammation, mast cell infiltration, and fibrosis. Therapeutic options may include bladder dilatations under general anesthesia and instillation of various substances (including dimethyl sulfoxide, heparin, and amitriptyline). This therapy often brings temporary relief of symptoms. A subtotal cystectomy and augmentation with bowel or a cystectomy with diversion may be necessary in patients with a severely contracted bladder whose symptoms are incapacitating.

Degenerative Diseases

Bladder Fistulae

A fistula between the bowel and the bladder most commonly is caused by sigmoid diverticulitis, neoplasm, Crohn's disease, or penetrating abdominal injury. Patients often present with symptoms of UTI, hematuria, pneumaturia, or fecaluria. Tests that can detect a fistula include water-based contrast enemas, cystogram, cystoscopy, and CT scan without bladder catheterization (air in the bladder confirms the diagnosis). Treatment usually involves resection of the involved portion of the bowel, with either reanastomosis or colostomy, depending on the etiology. The edges of the bladder fistula are debrided and closed. Vesicovaginal fistula can occur from pressure necrosis during prolonged labor or from surgical injury. Incontinence, the usual presenting symptom, is typically continuous. Diagnosis is made by a cystogram and cystoscopy. IVP or

Table 7-3	Correctable Urologic Causes for Recurrent Urinary Tract

Infections

Prostatic hypertrophy
Urethral stricture
Calculus
Chronic bacterial prostatitis
Ureteral reflux
Foreign body
Infected dysplastic or atrophic kidney
Urethral diverticulum
Papillary necrosis
Vesicovaginal or vesicointestinal fistula
Urachal cyst
Ureteral duplication or ectopy
Perivesical abscess

Adapted from Dairiki L, Stamey T. Infections of the urinary tract. In: Walsh PC, et al, eds. *Campbell's Urology,* 7th ed. Philadelphia: WB Saunders; 1998.

bilateral retrograde pyelography is sometimes necessary to evaluate the upper tracts for obstruction or a ureterovaginal fistula. Small fistulae may be particularly difficult to delineate and may require additional maneuvers, including instillation of methylene blue into the bladder followed by insertion of a vaginal tampon to detect leakage. Repair of a simple vesicovaginal fistula can often be performed by a vaginal approach.

Urinary Incontinence

Urinary incontinence is the involuntary loss of urine. It is classified as stress, urge, overflow, or total incontinence, according to the symptoms associated with the leakage of urine.

Stress incontinence occurs when a rise in intra-abdominal pressure from coughing, sneezing, laughing, or straining causes urine leakage. The etiology is low resistance between the bladder neck and the urethra. Urge incontinence is an irritative symptom in which leakage is preceded by an urge to urinate, but the patient cannot "make it to the restroom in time." Bladder instability with involuntary contraction is the cause. Overflow incontinence occurs when the bladder overfills, usually from urinary retention, and uncontrollably empties. Urinary retention can be caused by obstruction to outflow or inability of the bladder to contract. Total incontinence occurs when there is continuous leakage of urine. This type of incontinence is characteristic of a fistula (e.g., a vesicovaginal fistula).

Evaluation

Taking an accurate history is essential in the evaluation of incontinence. The amount of leakage, associated activities, and voiding symptoms should be characterized. A voiding and incontinence diary that records the frequency, timing, and severity of episodes is helpful. In particular, when a patient wears pads, it is helpful to document the number of pads used daily and the degree of saturation that occurs. The medical history should be reviewed for medications, trauma, pelvic or urinary tract surgery, difficult deliveries, malignancy, neuromuscular disorders, diabetes, UTIs, and abnormal bowel habits. In men, a review of erectile and ejaculatory function may show neurologic dysfunction.

The physical examination should include special attention to the abdomen, back, pelvis, and rectum. Perianal sensation, anal sphincter tone, as well as lower extremity motor and sensory function and reflexes should be evaluated. Women with suspected stress incontinence should be examined in the lithotomy position. Laboratory evaluation should include urinalysis, urine culture, and cytology (when indicated). Other studies that can be performed include a PVR measurement, cystoscopy, and urodynamic evaluation. Upper tract evaluation should be done when indicated but is not a routine part of an incontinence workup.

Treatment

The cause of incontinence dictates the mode of therapy. Detrusor instability without associated obstruction, blad-

der malignancy, infection, or neurogenic pathology adversely affecting bladder contractility may be treated effectively with anticholinergic medications such as oxybutynin (Ditropan), which causes detrusor relaxation.

Stress urinary incontinence is treated by restoring the bladder neck and urethra to proper anatomic position using one of a number of procedures. The Marshall-Marchetti-Krantz procedure uses an anterior abdominal approach. The bladder and urethra are dissected off the posterior aspect of the pubic symphysis. Heavy, absorbable sutures are placed into the vaginal fascia on either side of the bladder neck and the urethra. These sutures are then placed in the posterior aspect of the symphysis to reposition and anchor the bladder and urethra superiorly and anteriorly (Fig. 7-22).

Elevation of the bladder neck into the proper position also can be accomplished with a suspension procedure using a combined vaginal and suprapubic approach. The Stamey, Raz, and other similar procedures place nonabsorbable sutures through a vaginal incision into the tissue on each side of the bladder neck. In the Stamey procedure, a small piece of Dacron vascular graft placed on the suture near the bladder neck serves as a bolster to prevent the suture from tearing out. In the Raz procedure, the suture is passed several times helically through tissue lateral to the bladder neck, including the urethropelvic ligament. In both of these procedures, suprapubic incisions are used and a needle ligature carrier is passed from the suprapubic incision immediately behind the pubic symphysis through the vaginal incision. Both ends of the bladder neck sutures are passed by this needle into the suprapubic incision. The suspension sutures are then tied over the anterior rectus fascia with enough tension to correct the anatomy but not kink or obstruct the urethra. A suprapubic tube, placed at the time of surgery by some surgeons, serves postoperatively as the primary bladder drainage. Later, as the patient begins to void, it serves to empty any PVRs until normal voiding returns (Fig. 7-23).

Stress urinary incontinence in women, which can be associated with urethral sphincter incompetence and poor coaptation of the urethra leading to poor urethral resistance, is usually treated with a transvaginal "sling" procedure. This procedure can be thought of as a modification of a bladder neck suspension procedure in which fascia or anterior vaginal wall is fashioned as a sling around the urethra. The upward traction of sutures attached to the sling bilaterally reestablishes coaptation and increases urethral resistance. There is a trend toward an increase in the use of sling procedures for the treatment of female stress urinary incontinence, Commercially available "off-the-shelf" materials are now favored as slings in the treatment of female incontinence. In men, poor urethral resistance can be managed with an artificial urinary sphincter, which is a prosthetic device that includes a cuff that encircles the bulbar urethra, a reservoir that contains fluid, and a pump in the scrotum. The cuff provides adequate urethral resistance. When the patient wishes to void, he uses the pump to transfer fluid from the cuff to the reservoir.

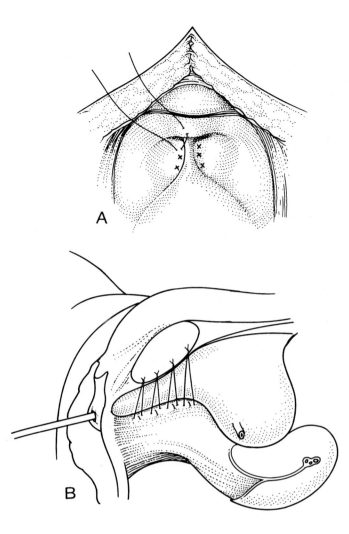

Figure 7-22   Marshall-Marchetti-Krantz procedure. **A,** Placement of absorbable sutures lateral to urethra and bladder neck as seen intraoperatively. **B,** Lateral view of completed repair with bladder neck and urethra in proper position.

Neurogenic Bladder Dysfunction

Micturition is a complex event requiring coordination between different levels of the central nervous system, the somatic and autonomic systems, and the detrusor and sphincter muscles of the bladder. During the filling phase, the bladder "relaxes" to accommodate an increasing urine volume. This ability to store larger amounts of urine without a significant increase in pressure is called compliance. Also, during bladder filling, sphincter muscle tone is increased. Normal micturition, a voluntary event involving complex coordination of the detrusor and sphincter muscles, begins with relaxation of the external sphincter followed by relaxation and opening of the bladder neck and contraction of the detrusor. The normal detrusor contraction lasts long enough to empty the bladder. In the central nervous system, there are highly integrated interrelations between the cerebral motor cortex, basal ganglia, cerebellum, pontine nuclei, and sacral cord nuclei that control voiding. Peripheral detrusor innervation is parasympathetic, mostly from S3 and some from S4. The trigone and bladder neck receive sympathetic output from T11 to L2. The external sphincter (somatic) receives most of its input

from S2 via the pudendal nerve. Disruption of any one of these pathways can result in a neurogenic bladder (Table 7-4).

Classification

Attempts to categorize the various neurologic bladder disorders have resulted in multiple systems of classification. The system devised by Lapides is one of the most useful for urologists because it characterizes bladder dysfunction according to urodynamic evaluation.

The uninhibited neurogenic bladder is one that has uncontrolled detrusor contractions with filling. This "overactive" detrusor is often accompanied by decreased capacity but normal sensation and appropriate sphincter coordination. Patients complain of frequency, urgency, and urge incontinence. Neurologic lesions associated with this type of bladder interfere with the cerebral inhibition of bladder reflexes and include cerebral vascular accidents, tumors, cerebral palsy, dementia, and multiple sclerosis.

The reflex uninhibited bladder occurs as the result of suprasacral spinal cord lesions from trauma, transverse myelitis, cord tumors, or multiple sclerosis with cord involve-

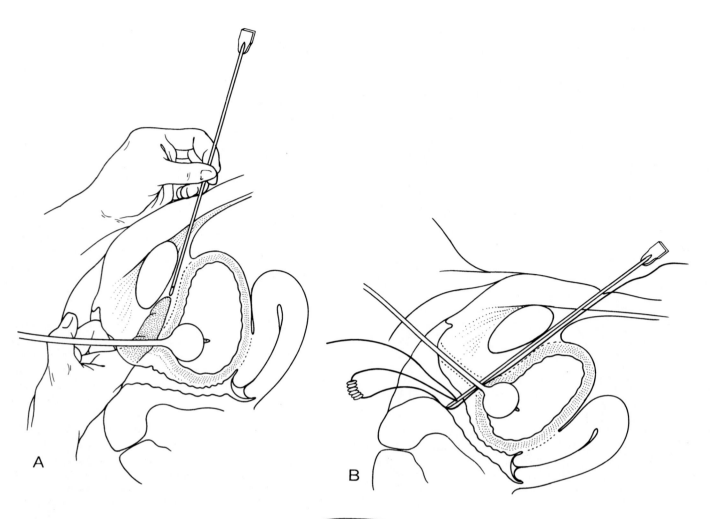

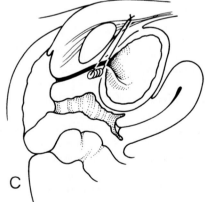

Figure 7-23   Stamey cystourethropexy. **A,** Lateral view showing passage of ligature carrier from the suprapubic incision, behind the pubic symphysis, and down to the vaginal incision (surgeon's finger is in the vaginal incision). **B,** Lateral view of ligature carrier with ready-to-pass second end of a suspension suture (note Dacron bolster). **C,** Lateral view of completed Stamey procedure with corrected position of bladder neck.

Table 7-4	Effects of Neurologic Lesions on Bladder Function
Neurologic Lesion	**Urodynamic Findings**
Lesions above the brain stem	Involuntary bladder contractions
Complete lesions of the spinal cord above S2 dyssynergia	Involuntary bladder contractions with smooth sphincter synergia and striated sphincter
Brain tumors	Detrusor hyperreflexia, urinary incontinence
Parkinson's disease	Detrusor hyperreflexia, urgency, frequency, urge incontinence
Shy-Drager syndrome	Detrusor hyperreflexia
Lesions above T6	Autonomic dysreflexia
Multiple sclerosis	Detrusor hyperreflexia, urgency, frequency
Diabetes mellitus	Impaired bladder sensation, decreased bladder contractility, impaired urinary flow, residual urine
Tabes dorsalis	Loss of bladder sensation, decreased bladder contractility
Herpes zoster	Urgency, frequency, urinary retention
Disc disease	Detrusor areflexia
Radical pelvic surgery	Urinary retention
Myelodysplasia	Urinary retention, bladder dysfunction

ment. In these patients, phasic uninhibited detrusor contractions occur and may be triggered by intrinsic or extrinsic stimulation. In certain situations, such as a high thoracic or cervical spinal cord injury, the sphincter is often dyssynergic. This is called detrusor sphincter dyssynergia. Detrusor contractions can be unsustained, resulting in inefficient emptying. These patients can have no sensation of bladder filling but may have autonomic reflex reactions to bladder distention, such as sweating, headache, severe hypertension, or lower extremity spasticity. Bladder compliance may be normal or decreased.

The autonomic neurogenic bladder shows no efficient voluntary or involuntary detrusor contractions on CMG. Voiding may be aided by increasing intra-abdominal pressure, but usually residual urine volume is large. Sensation is decreased or absent and compliance is variable. This type of neurogenic bladder results from damage to the sacral cord, conus medullaris, cauda equina, or sacral plexus from trauma, myelomeningocele, or pelvic surgery.

The sensory neurogenic bladder is one with diminished or absent sensation, no detrusor hyperreflexia, and a large capacity. It results from interruption to sensory pathways from the bladder either in the sacral reflex arc or in the long afferent spinal tracts. It is associated with tabes dorsalis, diabetes, syringomyelia, and pernicious anemia.

A motor paralytic bladder occurs only rarely. Patients with this condition have no detrusor function but have normal sensation and either normal or increased capacity. This type of neurogenic bladder can be caused by poliomyelitis, trauma, meningomyelocele, or other congenital abnormalities.

Evaluation

Urodynamic evaluation of the neurogenic bladder takes several forms. Detrusor function is determined by CMG to evaluate the strength and timing of detrusor contraction and bladder compliance. The CMG also shows uninhibited or hyperreflexic detrusor contractions. Sphincter function is evaluated with urethral pressure studies and EMG. Efficiency of voiding is assessed by PVR measurements. Fluoroscopic voiding studies show the anatomic position of the bladder and urethra, assess bladder neck function and coordination, and detect the presence of VUR. Sensory function is appraised by questioning the patient about the sensation of filling and urgency during a CMG. In addition to urodynamics, renal ultrasound should be performed to check for hydronephrosis or stone disease, particularly in spinal cord injured patients who are at risk for stones. Serum creatinine should be obtained to evaluate renal function.

Treatment

The therapeutic goals in the management of neurogenic bladder dysfunction are to preserve renal function by preventing renal damage and to normalize urinary tract function as much as possible, especially with respect to continence, bladder emptying, and infection prevention. Anticholinergics (e.g., tolterodine tartrate and oxybutynin chloride) can be useful in suppressing uninhibited detrusor contractions and improving compliance. Clean intermittent catheterization has proven to be an efficient, relatively easy, and safe method of ensuring bladder emptying with a wide range of applications. Because it has a significantly lower rate of infection, it is preferred over chronic urethral or suprapubic catheter drainage. Many patients require a combination of medicines and manipulations. Some patients have bladders that empty poorly and have high intravesical pressures. If these pressures are elevated over the long term, reflux and infection can lead to renal damage and even renal failure.

It is important to identify patients who have poorly compliant bladders that fill and store at a high pressure, causing ureteral reflux. Intervention is mandatory to prevent the patient from developing irreversible renal damage. Treatment options include anticholinergic medication and intermittent catheterization; if these options fail, augmentation of the bladder with bowel is used. Alternatively, high-pressure filling and storage can be treated in certain cases with a sphincterotomy, an endoscopic procedure that cuts the sphincter. This usually promotes incontinence, which is managed with a condom catheter external drainage device; this device connects through tubing to a drainage bag. In the past, sphincterotomy or chronic indwelling catheterization were common treatments for neurogenic bladder dysfunction from spinal cord injury; they remain treatment options. The current trend is toward bladder augmentation and intermittent catheterization.

Regardless of the regimen used, patient compliance and close follow-up are essential. These patients need an annual evaluation of renal function and upper tract anatomy and possibly cystoscopy. Urodynamic evaluations are repeated as necessary to detect deleterious changes in bladder function that require a change in management.

Malignant Diseases

Bladder carcinoma, the fifth most common malignancy in the American population, is 2.5 times more common in men. It is about five times more prevalent among cigarette smokers and is associated with known carcinogens in rubber and oil refinery workers. Transitional cell carcinoma represents approximately 85% to 90% of tumors. Adenocarcinomas also occur, often in association with a patent urachus and tumors of the bladder dome. Chronic bladder inflammation, which occurs with chronic indwelling Foley catheters or with bladder infections caused by *Schistosomiasis*, is associated with squamous cell carcinoma.

Evaluation

Gross, painless hematuria is a common presenting sign. However, approximately 20% of patients may present with only microscopic hematuria. Irritative voiding symptoms may also suggest a bladder tumor. The evaluation of gross hematuria usually includes imaging of the upper tracts (e.g., IVP or a CT urogram, which is a study that combines CT scanning with a postcontrast abdominal film to outline the ureters), cystoscopy, and urine cytology. Bladder cancer is staged primarily according to depth of tumor invasion, as follows:

Tis = Carcinoma in situ
Ta = Noninvasive papillary tumor
T1 = Extension to lamina propria
T2 = Invasion of detrusor muscle
T3 = Perivesical fat invasion
T4 = Adjacent organ involvement

Treatment

Management of bladder carcinoma depends on tumor stage. For Ta and T1 bladder carcinoma, transurethral resection of the tumor is often the only treatment required. However, if the tumor is recurrent, intravesical chemotherapy with agents such as thiotepa, bacillus Calmette-Guérin (BCG), and mitomycin-C may be useful. BCG has also been very effective in treating Tis. Use of these agents may reduce the recurrence rate by 50%. Patients with transitional cell carcinoma of the bladder have an increased incidence of tumors occurring at other sites in the bladder, ureter, or renal pelvis. Surveillance is mandatory because the recurrence rate in the bladder may be as high as 50% at 5 years. Surveillance protocols include cystoscopy and urinary cytology every 3 to 4 months for the first 1 to 2 years, followed with declining frequency.

Bacillus Calmette-Guérin is the most commonly used intravesical therapy to prevent recurrence. Usually, a 6-week induction course is given followed by a maintenance regimen for 2 to 3 years. Systemic infection occurs in a small percentage of patients, but fever, dysuria, and hematuria are common during treatment. The risk of progression to muscle invasive disease is relatively low (<10%) for Ta tumors, but increases as tumor stage advances (T1) or with high-grade lesions.

For tumors that invade the bladder muscle, radical cystectomy is recommended. In men, this entails removing the bladder, prostate, perivesical fat, and pelvic lymph nodes; in women it involves removing the bladder, anterior vaginal wall, uterus, and lymph nodes. Five-year survival rates are approximately 60% after cystectomy for T3 bladder cancer.

Urinary reconstruction may be accomplished with ileal conduit diversion to the skin, which subsequently requires the patient to wear a collection appliance. A continent cutaneous diversion may be created, most often using the right colon, with a tapered and catheterizable efferent limb of ileum. An orthotopic neobladder allows creation of a reservoir using detubularized bowel with direct anastomosis to the urethra. This procedure avoids any cutaneous diversion or need for catheterization.

THE PENIS

Anatomy

The penis is composed of two corpora cavernosa and the corpus spongiosum, which are bound by fibrous tissue and covered by skin (Fig. 7-24). Each corpus cavernosum has a thick fibrous capsule, the tunica albuginea, which forms around the cavernous sinuses. Distal to the symphysis pubis, the corpora cavernosa run side by side, divided by a septum. More proximally, the corpora cavernosa separate and fuse to the ischial rami. The corpus spongiosum is positioned ventrally, with its distal portion expanding to form the glans penis. The urethra is enclosed by the corpus spongiosum, traverses the glans penis, and opens as the external urethral meatus. The corpora cavernosa and corpus spongiosum are enveloped by Buck's fascia and covered with skin that is virtually hairless and devoid of fat. The penile skin extends over the glans to form the prepuce or foreskin.

The major blood supply of the penis is from branches of the internal pudendal artery, which in turn is a branch of the internal iliac artery. Venous drainage from the penis is into the iliac veins by way of the deep and superficial dorsal veins. The lymphatics of the glans penis, corpus spongiosum, and distal corpus cavernosum drain into the external iliac, superficial, and deep inguinal lymph nodes. The proximal corpus cavernosum and posterior urethra drain into the internal iliac lymph nodes.

Trauma

Penile injury may result from blunt or penetrating trauma, avulsion, strangulation, burns, fracture, and, occasionally, biting. When the mechanism of injury indicates that there is a possibility of urethral injury, assessment of urethral integrity with a retrograde urethrogram is mandatory. A

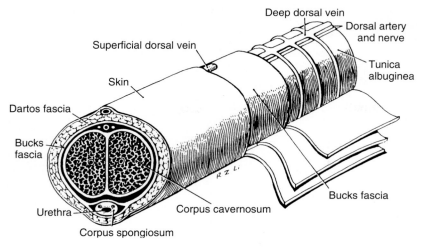

Figure 7-24   Anatomy of the penis.

careful physical examination is of prime importance. Retrograde urethrography is indicated in all cases of suspected urethral injury, and testicular ultrasound is helpful when testicular injury is suspected.

The management of penetrating penile injuries is variable depending on the presence, extent, and location of urethral or corporal injury. Knife injuries resulting in superficial lacerations may be closed if the wound is clean. Urethral injuries along the anterior urethra can occasionally be immediately repaired or can be managed with suprapubic catheter placement and delayed urethral repair. Repair of complete penile amputations using microsurgical techniques can be attempted if the penis has been properly preserved in cold saline. If repair of the amputated penis is not feasible, then partial penectomy is performed. Injuries that involve the testis require surgical exploration.

Avulsion injury to the skin of the penis may be caused by the patient's clothing and penis becoming entrapped in industrial machinery. Usually, the skin and loose areolar tissue superficial to Buck's fascia are avulsed and deeper tissues are left intact. When sufficient skin remains, the injury can be treated with primary closure. With circumferential penile avulsions, complete interruption of the lymphatic drainage results in chronic lymphedema of skin distal to the injury. Superior cosmetic results are obtained if the skin distal to the injury is removed up to the coronal sulcus and replaced with a split-thickness skin graft.

Penile burns may be caused by thermal, chemical, or electric injury and are managed similarly to burns in other areas of the body. Because penile preservation is the prime objective, extensive debridement should be approached cautiously. One consideration is to avoid prolonged urethral catheterization because this can result in urethral sloughing. When bladder drainage is indicated, especially for longer than 72 hours, a suprapubic tube should be placed.

Fracture of the penis involves rupture of the tunica albuginea of the corpus cavernosum. Penile fracture usually occurs during intercourse. The patient typically reports experiencing a cracking sensation or noise in association

with a misguided thrust followed by pain, detumescence, and rapid penile shaft swelling. The immediate management of penile fracture consists of surgical exploration with evacuation of the hematoma and repair of the tunica albuginea.

Malignant Diseases

Premalignant Lesions

Four penile lesions have been identified as premalignant: leukoplakia, Bowen's disease, erythroplasia of Queyrat, and giant condyloma acuminatum (Table 7-5). Leukoplakia appears grossly as a white plaque and is characterized microscopically by acanthosis, hyperkeratosis, and parakeratosis. The treatment is local excision. Bowen's disease typically appears as a solitary, erythematous plaque on the penile shaft. Approximately 25% of patients with Bowen's disease will have a concomitant visceral malignancy. Erythroplasia of Queyrat consists of raised, red, velvety, well-marginated areas of the glans penis or coronal sulcus. Both Bowen's disease and erythroplasia of Queyrat histologically appear as carcinoma in situ and may be treated by Nd:YAG laser fulguration, local excision, or topical application of 5-fluorouracil. Giant condyloma acuminatum (Buschke-Löwenstein tumor, verrucous carcinoma) is a large, exophytic lesion often grossly indistinguishable from squamous cell carcinoma. Histologically, these lesions are similar to condyloma acuminatum except that the tumor extends into the underlying tissue. Local excision is required, often necessitating partial or total penectomy. Balanitis xerotica obliterans (BXO), also referred to as lichen sclerosus et atrophicus, has been classified as a "premalignant" condition, but is generally benign. BXO presents as white, atrophic, edematous lesions involving the glans penis or prepuce. Histologically, the dermis is composed of abundant amorphous collagen and a lymphocytic infiltrate in the underlying reticular dermis. BXO is often associated with urethra stricture disease that can become progressive to involve the entire anterior urethra. Treatment of BXO consists of topical steroids, and, if there is associated

Table 7-5	Premalignant Penile Lesions		
Penile Lesion	**Gross Characteristics**	**Microscopic Characteristics**	**Treatment**
Leukoplakia	White plaque	Acanthosis, hyperkeratosis, and parakeratosis	Excision
Balanitis xerotica obliterans	White, atrophic red lesion of glans or prepuce	Abundant, amorphous collagen and lymphocyte infiltrate of reticular dermis	Excision, topical steroids
Bowen's disease	Solitary, red plaque on penile shaft	Carcinoma in situ	Laser fulguration, excision, topical 5-fluorouracil
Erythroplasia of Queyrat	Raised, red velvety lesion of glans or coronal sulcus	Carcinoma in situ	Laser fulguration, excision, topical 5-fluorouracil
Giant condyloma acuminatum	Large, exophytic lesion	Similar to condyloma acuminatum with invasion into underlying tissue	Excision

urethral stricture disease, extended meatotomy or open staged urethral reconstruction is the current standard of care.

Squamous Cell Carcinoma

Although rare in the United States, penile cancer is common in men living in hot, humid regions. Poor personal hygiene and retained phimotic foreskin have been implicated in the etiology of penile carcinoma. Penile cancer is extremely rare in men circumcised at birth, with fewer than 10 cases reported. Squamous cell carcinoma of the penis occurs most commonly in the sixth decade. The symptoms are related to ulceration, necrosis, suppuration, and hemorrhage of the penile lesion. The clinical evaluation of patients with penile cancer includes physical examination with palpation of the inguinal region, liver function tests, chest radiograph, CT of the abdomen and pelvis, and bone scan. The most widely used staging system is the TNM staging system (Table 7-6).

Small penile cancers limited to the prepuce can be treated by circumcision alone. Partial penectomy with at least a 2-cm margin of normal tissue is used to treat smaller (2–5 cm) distal penile tumors (Fig. 7-25). The remaining penis should be long enough to permit voiding in the standing position. The 5-year cure rate for patients treated with partial penectomy is 70% to 80%. Larger distal penile lesions or proximal tumors require total penectomy and perineal urethrostomy. If the scrotum, pubis, or abdominal wall is involved, radical en bloc excision may be necessary.

Many patients have inguinal lymphadenopathy at presentation. However, inguinal lymph node enlargement before excision of the primary tumor may be the result of infection and not metastatic disease. Thus, clinical assessment of the inguinal region should be delayed 4 to 6 weeks, during which time the patient is treated with antibiotics. If inguinal lymphadenopathy persists or subsequently develops, there is a high likelihood of metastatic lymph nodal disease and ilioinguinal lymphadenectomy should be performed. However, if inguinal lymphadenop-

athy resolves, prophylactic lymph node dissection may not be necessary.

Radiation of the primary tumor and regional lymph nodes is an alternative to surgery in patients with small (<2 cm), low-stage tumor. The advantage of radiotherapy over surgery is preservation of the penis. However, control rates are slightly lower than those of surgical excision. Similarly, radiation therapy can cure some patients with ingui-

Table 7-6	TNM Classification of Penile Carcinoma
Primary tumor (T)	
TX	Primary tumor cannot be assessed
T0	No evidence of primary tumor
Tis	Carcinoma in situ
Ta	Noninvasive verrucous carcinoma
T1	Tumor invades subepithelial connective tissue
T2	Tumor invades corpus spongiosum or cavernosum
T3	Tumor invades urethra or prostate
T4	Tumor invades other adjacent structures
Regional lymph nodes (N)	
NX	Regional lymph nodes cannot be assessed
N0	No regional lymph node metastasis
N1	Metastasis in a single superficial, inguinal lymph node
N2	Metastasis in multiple or bilateral superficial inguinal lymph nodes
N3	Metastasis in deep inguinal or pelvic lymph node(s) unilateral or bilateral
Distant metastasis (M)	
MX	Distant metastasis cannot be assessed
M0	No distant metastasis
M1	Distant metastasis

Used with the permission of the American Joint Committee on Cancer (AJCC), Chicago, Illinois. The original source for this material is the *AJCC Cancer Staging Manual,* 5th ed. Philadelphia: Lippincott-Raven; 1997.

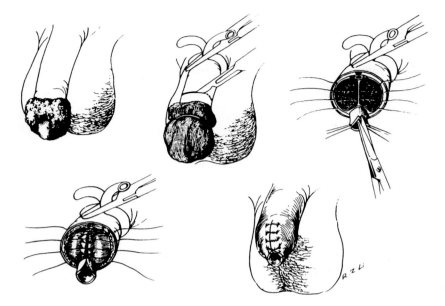

Figure 7-25   Technique of partial penectomy.

nal nodal metastases, but at a lower rate than with ilioinguinal lymphadenectomy.

Acquired Disorders

Priapism

Priapism is the pathologic prolongation of penile erection. Unlike normal tumescence, in priapism only the corpora cavernosa are turgid, whereas the corpus spongiosum (including the glans penis) remains flaccid. Priapism is characterized as either low-flow or high-flow. In low-flow priapism, the penile venous outflow is obstructed, which produces sludging and thrombosis of cavernosal blood. Left untreated, the corpora cavernosa become fibrotic and the patient becomes impotent. Etiologies include sickle cell anemia, leukemia, metastatic disease, and intracorporeal injection of vasoactive substances for the treatment of impotency. In high-flow priapism, there is increased blood flow to the penis. It can be caused by injury to the pelvic vasculature, as in pelvic trauma, with increased blood flow to the penis secondary to a vascular fistula.

The treatment of patients with sickle cell anemia should be directed at the underlying cause. Sickle cell patients should be treated with hydration, alkalinization, analgesics, and exchange transfusions.

Patients with priapism caused by intracorporeal injection of vasoactive substances may respond to intracorporeal injection of phenylephrine, especially when the duration of priapism is less than 6 hours. Otherwise, treatment requires aspiration of the corporal blood with a large needle and corporal irrigation with saline. If this treatment fails, another option is a Winter procedure, as illustrated in Figure 7-26. This procedure involves placing a biopsy needle into the corpora through the glans bilaterally and removing a core of tissue. In this way, a communication between the corpora cavernosa and the corpus spongiosum is created, allowing the blood trapped in the corpora to drain through the unobstructed outflow of the corpus spongiosum. In the rare patient for whom the above maneuvers fail, open surgery is an option: a formal communication is made between the corpora cavernosa and the corpus spongiosum.

When high-flow priapism is suspected, a corporal blood gas determination should be obtained. In low-flow ischemic priapism, the P_{O_2} is low. In high-flow priapism, the P_{O_2} is high and management is pudendal arteriography with selective embolization of the fistula.

Phimosis

Phimosis is the fibrotic contracture of the foreskin, prohibiting retraction of the prepuce over the glans penis. The etiology is poor hygiene or infection beneath redundant foreskin, resulting in chronic irritation. Diabetes mellitus is a predisposing factor. Phimosis is often effectively managed with improved hygiene. Elective circumcision is often indicated.

Paraphimosis

When mild preputial contracture is present, the retracted foreskin forms a constricting band proximal to the coronal sulcus that over a prolonged period of time results in edema. The inability to place the foreskin back over the glans is termed paraphimosis. Initially, venous occlusion results in edema, which leads to arterial occlusion and eventually glandular ischemia. Paraphimosis is a urologic emergency. Manual compression of the glans usually decreases the edema, allowing the foreskin to be reduced (Fig. 7-27). If manual compression fails, the constricting preputial band of tissue requires incision. Circumcision should follow resolution of edema and inflammation.

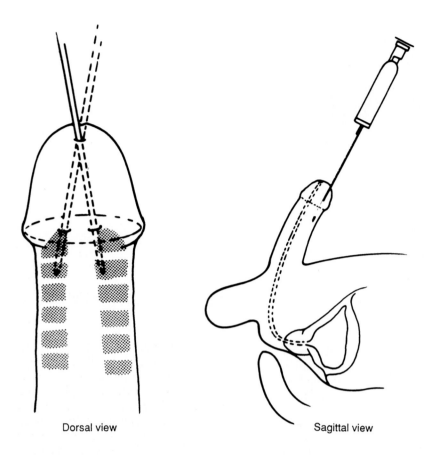

Dorsal view   Sagittal view

Figure 7-26   Winter shunt for the treatment of priapism. A Travenol biopsy needle is used to create fistulae between the glans penis (corpus spongiosum) and the corpora cavernosa. **A,** Dorsal view. **B,** Sagittal view.

Peyronie's Disease

Peyronie's disease is a process involving scarring of the tunica albuginea of the corpora cavernosa, resulting in plaques. Peyronie's plaques are typically located on the dorsal penile surface. The disease is associated with variable degrees of penile curvature that may be sexually incapacitating. The disease is initially termed "immature." This period, which is variable but often lasts longer than 6 months, is characterized by painful erections, progressive curvature, and induration of the plaque on physical examination. During this immature phase, surgery is absolutely contraindicated. The management is conservative. No one medical treatment of Peyronie's disease is very successful. Conservative approaches include vitamin E, and perhaps potassium *p*-aminobenzoate (Potaba) or colchicine. Peyronie's disease can often resolve spontaneously. If conservative management fails and a patient has mature disease (generally defined as unchanged curvature for a 6-month duration with resolution of pain) and curvature that prevents satisfactory intercourse, the erectile function is assessed. If the patient has good erectile function, surgical options to correct the curvature include plication opposite the plaque or incision/excision of the plaque with grafting (e.g., dermis or saphenous vein, or other biomaterials). Erectile dysfunction is often associated with Peyronie's; when this occurs, therapy is directed at treating the erectile dysfunction. As a last resort in a patient with erectile dysfunction, a penile prosthesis is sometimes placed to correct impotency and ensure penile straightening.

Circumcision and Dorsal Slit

Circumcision is the most common operation performed on males in the United States (Fig. 7-28). Indications include parental decision, phimosis, cosmetic effect, and malignancy. Contraindications to circumcision include myelodysplasia and hypospadias (because the foreskin may

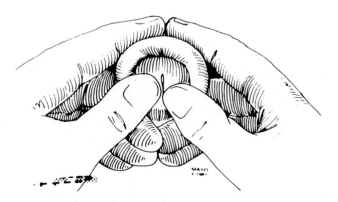

Figure 7-27   Manual reduction of paraphimosis.

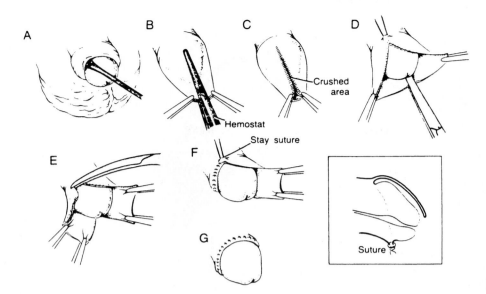

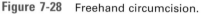

Figure 7-28   Freehand circumcision.

be needed for use during hypospadias repair). In the newborn, a Gomco clamp or Plastibell is usually used without anesthesia. Adults often obtain excellent anesthesia from a local penile block; circumcision may be performed as an outpatient procedure.

After appropriate preparation and draping, a straight hemostat is placed on the middle of the dorsal surface of the prepuce. The hemostat is removed, and a dorsal slit is performed by cutting the crushed foreskin proximally to within 1 cm of the coronal sulcus. The prepuce should now easily retract to expose the glans penis. If only a dorsal slit is to be performed, the cut edges are hemostatically approximated by absorbable interrupted sutures. If a circumcision is to be done, the cut edges of the dorsal slit are not sutured. A similar incision is made in the ventral surface of the prepuce to the frenulum. Occasionally, bleeding from a frenula artery will require ligature. With the foreskin divided in two, redundant prepuce is excised. Hemostasis is secured with electrocautery or absorbable sutures. It should be stressed that cautery should not be used in conjunction with Gomco or similar metal clamps because severe cautery injuries to the glans penis could result. The mucosal and cutaneous surfaces of the foreskin are then approximated using interrupted absorbable sutures.

THE URETHRA

Anatomy

The male urethra is divided into posterior and anterior portions (Fig. 7-29). The posterior portion includes the prostatic urethra and the membranous urethra (which is the location of the external striated sphincter). The anterior portion consists of the urethral meatus, the fossa navicularis, the penile urethra, and the bulbar. The prostatic urethra is lined by transitional epithelium; the membranous, bulbous, and penile sections of the urethra are lined by pseudostratified or stratified columnar epithelium; the external urethral meatus is lined by squamous epithelium. Paired bulbourethral (Cowper's) glands, located in the membranous urethra, produce a clear viscous fluid (sometimes called the pre-ejaculatory fluid) and secrete into the bulbous urethra. Multiple glands of Littre, which also produce a pre-ejaculatory fluid, line the penile urethra. The lymphatic drainage of the posterior urethra is directly into the obturator and iliac nodes, whereas that of the anterior urethra is through the deep inguinal nodes into the iliac nodes.

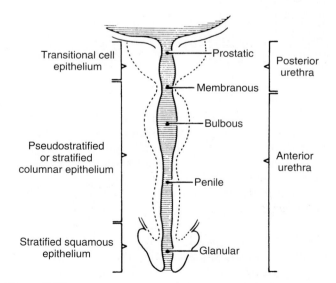

Figure 7-29   Anatomy and cell types lining the male urethra.

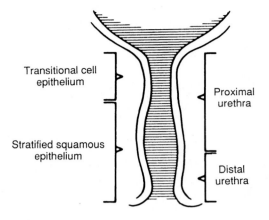

Figure 7-30   Anatomy and cell types lining the female urethra.

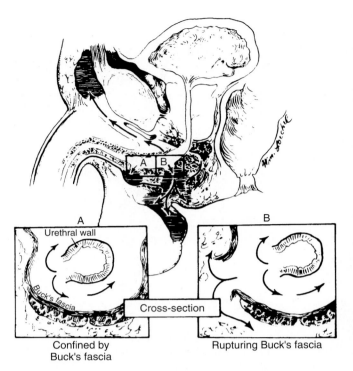

Figure 7-31   Straddle injury to the bulbous urethra demonstrating pathways of blood and urine extravasation.

The female urethra, about 4 cm long (Fig. 7-30), lies immediately anterior to the vagina; its external urethral meatus opens 2 cm posterior to the clitoris. Transitional epithelium lines the proximal third of the female urethra and stratified squamous epithelium lines the distal two thirds. The periurethral glands of Skene are homologs of the male urethral glands and empty into the distal urethra. The proximal female urethra drains into the iliac lymph nodes and the distal portion into the inguinal lymph nodes.

Trauma

Anterior urethral injuries usually result from blunt trauma, such as straddle injuries, in which the bulbous urethra is injured. Prostatomembranous urethral injuries occur in approximately 10% of patients who sustain pelvic fractures in motor vehicle accidents or occupational injuries. Urethral injury should be suspected in patients with blood at the urethral meatus, inability to void, or penile or perineal edema and ecchymosis. If Buck's fascia remains intact, extravasation of blood and urine are confined to the penile shaft (Fig. 7-31).

Evaluation

When urethral injury is suspected, radiographic evaluation must precede urethral catheterization. On retrograde urethrography, a partial urethral rupture is suggested when there is both urethral extravasation and passage of contrast into the bladder. Extravasation without passage of contrast into the bladder suggests a complete urethral rupture (Fig. 7-32).

Treatment

Small, incomplete anterior urethral ruptures with extravasation limited by Buck's fascia are initially treated by draining with a urethral catheter or by performing a suprapubic cystostomy. Patients who sustain a posterior urethral injury

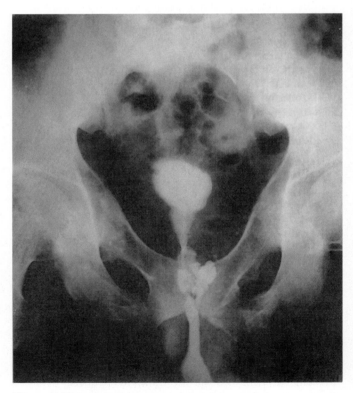

Figure 7-32   Retrograde urethrogram showing retroperitoneal extravasation of contrast due to a traumatic posterior urethral rupture.

associated with a pelvic fracture require a suprapubic tube. In addition, an aligning urethral catheter can be placed, if possible, but this procedure is controversial. In general, posterior urethral disruptions are managed by a minimum of 3 months of suprapubic diversion, and delayed urethral reconstruction via a perineal approach with excision of the stricture and a primary anastomosis. Infrapubectomy may be needed to achieve exposure of a patent urethra proximal to the obliteration.

Malignant Diseases

Male Urethral Carcinoma

Urethral carcinoma is rare and usually occurs after 60 years of age. Approximately 80% are squamous cell cancers. In the absence of metastatic disease, partial or total penectomy is the treatment of choice when the distal urethra is involved. Proximal urethral cancers are managed with urethrectomy and cystoprostatectomy.

Female Urethral Carcinoma

Urethral cancer is the only genitourinary malignancy that occurs in women more often than in men. The usual presenting symptom is a papillary or fungating urethral mass or urethral or vaginal bleeding. Local tumor extension into the vagina and bladder neck is common. Lymphatic spread of distal urethral lesions is by way of the inguinal nodes, whereas that of proximal urethral tumors is by way of the iliac nodes. When present, inguinal lymphadenopathy usually indicates metastatic disease. Noninvasive distal urethral lesions are often squamous cell cancers and can be managed with distal urethrectomy. Proximal and panurethral cancers are managed by chemotherapy or radiation therapy followed by radical excision. The above represent general guidelines for the management of localized disease. The treatment of an individual patient may vary depending on a number of factors, including general health status, nodal status, and extent of involvement of the primary tumor.

Urethral Strictures

Urethral strictures were once considered to be most often caused by gonococcal urethritis. The most common causes of anterior urethral strictures today are straddle injury (e.g., a bicycle accident long ago) and instrumentation of the urethra. Obstructive voiding symptoms (e.g., those encountered with prostatism) are common complaints. Occasionally, UTI or inability to pass a urethral catheter may lead to the initial diagnosis.

Evaluation

When a urethral stricture is suspected, cystoscopy will diagnose a stricture. However, the urethra is usually only seen up to the point of narrowing and the scope cannot be passed proximally. A retrograde urethrogram along with a voiding cystourethrogram will outline the exact location, caliber, and length of a urethral stricture.

Treatment

In the past, most strictures, regardless of the length, were initially managed with one or more dilations or endoscopic incisions (direct visual internal urethrotomy) of the strictures. These treatments were often performed without preoperative imaging studies. The modern management of urethral stricture disease requires complete diagnostic evaluation with retrograde and antegrade imaging and urethroscopy before a discussion of treatment options. The treatment that is best for a patient depends on the length and location of the stricture. If the stricture is truly discrete (<1 cm) and mucosal in character, dilation or urethrotomy may be curative. Longer strictures and recurrent strictures can also be managed with the above modalities. However, the recurrence rate is high, approaching 100% when multiple prior endoscopic treatments have failed. The advantages of dilation and urethrotomy are that they are less invasive than open surgery. These procedures are an excellent option when the patient wants to "manage" the stricture.

When the goal is to permanently cure the disease, open urethral reconstruction offers the highest success when properly performed using dedicated equipment and instruments. For example, a short bulbar urethral stricture (Fig. 7-33) can be treated with open excision and primary anastomotic repair, with a permanent cure rate of more than 98%. When strictures are long or more distally located, open repair requires tissue transfer. Tissues that can be used to enlarge the narrowed urethra include preputial skin as a flap or graft, or a graft of buccal mucosa.

Congenital Disorders

Posterior Urethral Valves

The most common type of posterior urethral valve anomaly (type I) consists of paired folds of mucous membranes that extend from the distal portion of the prostatic verumontanum and meet anteriorly in the membranous urethra (Fig. 7-34). Posterior urethral valves cause a variable degree of urethral obstruction, with resultant bladder distention, VUR, hydroureteronephrosis, and renal damage. Today, it is commonly diagnosed on antenatal ultrasound, with bladder distention, echogenic hydronephrotic kidneys, and oligohydramnios. In severe cases, placement of a vesicoamniotic shunt may reverse the oligohydramnios, allowing the lungs to develop and the pregnancy to be carried to term. The diagnosis is suggested in newborns with poor urinary streams or inability to void, and suprapubic or flank masses. VCUG may show the valves, but a more consistent finding is a dilated posterior urethra, with secondary findings of bladder and upper urinary tract obstruction.

Initial treatment consists of placing either an 8-French

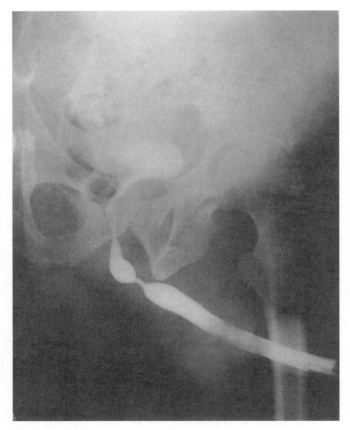

Figure 7-33 Retrograde urethrogram showing bulbar urethral stricture.

infant feeding tube as a urethral catheter or a percutaneous suprapubic tube. Fluid, electrolyte, and acid–base status must be optimized. After the patient is stable, endoscopic valve ablation may be performed; alternatively, the bladder dome may be opened onto the lower abdomen (cutaneous vesicostomy) and endoscopic valve ablation performed another time.

Hypospadias

Hypospadias is one of the most common congenital anomalies, occurring in 1:300 live male births. In hypospadias, the urethral meatus is located on the ventral penile surface proximal to its normal position at the tip of the glans penis (Fig. 7-35). Classification is based on the location of the meatus, which may be perineal, penoscrotal, shaft, coronal, or glanular. Usually the prepuce is incompletely developed and is present as a dorsal hood. Additionally, remnants of the corpus spongiosum distal to the urethral meatus form fibrous bands termed chordee, producing ventral penile curvature. When the chordee is released during hypospadias repair, the meatus often retracts more proximally, resulting in a greater distance between the hypospadiac and normal meatal positions. In boys with perineal hypospadias, the scrotum is bifid (resembling labia majora), the testes are often undescended, and the penis

is small (resembling a hypertrophied clitoris); gender assignment may be difficult.

The goals of hypospadias repair are twofold. First is the correction of penile curvature, which is usually accomplished by releasing the chordee, either by simply degloving the phallus or placing dorsal plication sutures in the dorsal corpora cavernosa. Second is the creation of a new urethra to bridge the gap between the hypospadiac meatus and the tip of the penis. Numerous techniques of hypospadias repair exist, including dorsal urethral incision with ventral urethral tubularization (Snodgrass repair), penile skin flap repairs, and in complex and revision cases, reconstruction with the use of buccal or split thickness skin grafts. To minimize the psychological effects of genital surgery, it is best that hypospadias repair be performed before the child is 1 year old.

Infectious Diseases

Gonococcal Urethritis

Gonorrhea is caused by the pathogen *Neisseria gonorrhoeae*, an anaerobic Gram-negative diplococcus, which is transmitted during sexual intercourse. After an incubation period of 2 to 14 days, most men present with a yellowish urethral discharge caused by anterior urethritis. Other symptoms may include dysuria, urethral itching, and urinary frequency. About 25% of infected males remain asymptomatic and serve as a reservoir. Diagnosis is made by obtaining a urethral specimen (swab) for culture using Thayer-Martin medium. If rectal or oral intercourse is suggested by the history, rectal and pharyngeal cultures are recommended. If a presumptive diagnosis of gonococcal urethritis is made, patients and their sexual contacts are treated without waiting for the culture reports. Ceftriaxone 250 mg given once intramuscularly is considered the treatment of choice.

Nongonococcal Urethritis

Nongonococcal urethritis is characterized by dysuria, urinary frequency, periurethral itching, and a clear or white mucoid discharge. *Chlamydia trachomatis* is the most common causative agent. The incubation period is 1 to 3 weeks. The diagnosis of nongonococcal urethritis is made by cultures of the urethral swab, not the exudate. *C. trachomatis* and *U. urealyticum* are sensitive to doxycycline; 100 mg is given orally twice daily for 7 days. It has recently been shown that a single dose of azithromycin (1 g orally) is equivalent in efficacy to a 7-day course of doxycycline and is currently the treatment of choice. In clinical practice, patients suspected of having a sexually transmitted disease from gonorrhea or chlamydia are usually managed for both agents with swabs for both pathogens and then treated with both ceftriaxone and azithromycin.

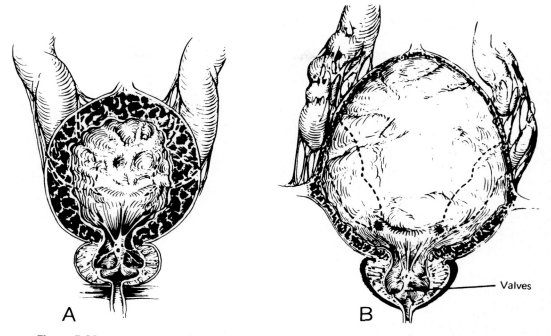

Figure 7-34 Posterior urethral valves. **A,** Dilation of the prostatic urethra, hypertrophy of vesical wall, and trigone in stage of compensation; bilateral hydroureters due to trigonal hypertrophy. **B,** Attenuation of bladder musculature in stage of decompensation; advanced ureteral dilation and tortuosity, usually secondary to vesicoureteral reflux.

THE TESTES, MALE INFERTILITY, AND IMPOTENCY

The Testes

Embryology and Anatomy

The testes develop embryologically from a long band of mesoderm on the posterior abdominal wall (retroperito-

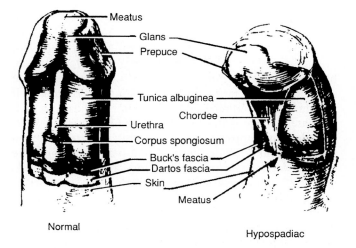

Figure 7-35 Comparison of normal and hypospadiac penis showing chordee.

neum), the genital ridge. Due to differential growth, by the seventh month of gestation the testicle lies just inside the internal inguinal ring. The gubernaculum (rudder) is a thick, inelastic structure connecting the lower pole of the testicle to the genital eminence, which leads the testicle through the inguinal canal into the scrotum during the eighth month of gestation. During its descent, the testicle becomes invested with a number of coverings (Fig. 7-36). The peritoneum surrounds the anterior four fifths of the testicle and becomes the tunica vaginalis. The superior portion remains as the tubular processus vaginalis, which shortly collapses and obliterates. The internal oblique fascia becomes the cremasteric (suspender) fibers, which act as a thermoregulator, elevating the testicle during periods of cold.

The main arterial supply to the testicle, the internal spermatic artery, arises from the aorta below the renal artery. Additional arterial inflow arises from the deferential artery, a branch of the inferior vesical artery, and from the external spermatic (cremasteric) artery, a branch of the inferior epigastric artery. The venous drainage parallels the arterial supply. A deferential vein drains into the hypogastric vein, an external spermatic vein drains into the epigastric vein, and an internal spermatic vein drains into the vena cava on the right and the renal vein on the left. Because of the juxtaposition of the mesonephric and genital ridges, the lymphatic drainage of the testicles is to the preaortic and precaval region, not, as commonly thought, to the inguinal or pelvic nodes. This knowledge is essential in considering the spread of testicular malignancy.

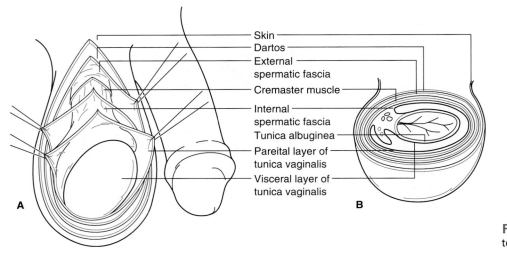

Skin
Dartos
External
spermatic fascia
Cremaster muscle
Internal
spermatic fascia
Tunica albuginea
Pareital layer of
tunica vaginalis
Visceral layer of
tunica vaginalis

A

B

Figure 7-36   Coverings of the testicle.

Congenital Disorders

Testicular Abnormalities

One of the more common abnormalities seen in newborn boys is cryptorchidism, which is a nonpalpable testicle. The incidence of this abnormality decreases with age, from 3.4% seen in term infants to 0.7% seen in infants at 9 months of age. The incidence is high with prematurity. If an empty scrotum is found, anorchia, nondescent, or retractile testis is possible. (See Chapter 12 in Lawrence's *Essentials of General Surgery*, 4th ed.)

Anorchia occurs in 3% to 5% of all cases explored for nonpalpable testes. Most are caused by prenatal torsion or vascular accidents, rarely by agenesis. At exploration, a vas deferens is found adjacent to the spermatic vessel, with a bud of scar representing the infarcted testicle (blind ending vas). Unilateral anorchia is of minimal concern; the contralateral testicle is usually larger, and spermatogenesis and hormonal function do not appear to be affected. Bilateral anorchia leads to sterility and the need for hormone replacement at puberty.

Retractile testes are caused by overactivity of the cremasteric musculature. They are easily pulled into the scrotum, but retract promptly into the groin. Most descend properly at puberty. This phenomenon underlines the need to examine the infant in a warm environment with gentle manipulation of the inguinal region.

Undescended testicles usually lie along the usual course of descent, from the retroperitoneum to the external inguinal ring. Rarely, the testicular descent is aberrant and the testicle may be found in the perineum in front of the anus. Most commonly, if the undescended testicle is not palpable within the inguinal canal, it is found just inside the internal inguinal ring. If neither testicle is palpable, but present, a stimulatory test with human chorionic gonadotropin (hCG) will cause an increase in serum testosterone. If no surge is noted, the diagnosis of intersexuality should be entertained. If a surge is noted with bilateral and sometimes unilateral cryptorchidism, treatment with exogenous

hCG may occasionally lead to descent. In general, studies such as CT and ultrasound are not useful for locating nonpalpable testicles. Laparoscopy is often useful to locate intra-abdominal testes or to confirm the diagnosis of an absent testis. An intra-abdominal testicle must be brought down because the undescended testicle has 48 times greater incidence of testis malignancy. The contralateral descended testicle also has an increased risk of malignant degeneration. Unfortunately, surgical orchidopexy (movement of the testicle into its normal position) does *not* decrease these risks, but does allow earlier diagnosis of future malignancies. Men with a history of testicular maldescent also have an increased risk of subfertility. A number of epididymal abnormalities are also seen with testicular nondescent, including an elongated epididymis, detachment from the testicle, and partial disruption.

Patent Processus Vaginalis

The processus vaginalis, the tube of peritoneum extending from the abdominal cavity to the tunica vaginalis, usually closes and involutes before birth. When it does not, the child presents with an inguinal hernia. A patent processus vaginalis is found in 4.4% of full-term and up to 13% of premature infants. If the processus is completely open, herniation of abdominal viscera may occur with possible strangulation, dictating emergency surgical correction. If the processus partially closes, a hydrocele forms, which increases in size if the infant is upright or cries. If a hydrocele is not apparent, gentle examination may show a fuller cord on one side. During examination, rubbing the cord between the thumb and forefinger may give the sensation of silk rubbing on silk (i.e., the "silk glove" sign) when the peritoneal sac is palpated. Spontaneous obliteration of the processus vaginalis may occur after birth. If the hydrocele persists after 1 year of age, varies in size (communicating hydrocele), or is symptomatic, repair is necessary. Repair consists of simple high ligation of the patent processus vaginalis at the internal inguinal ring.

Testicular Cord Torsion

Neonates who present with an acutely hard, enlarged scrotal mass that does not transilluminate may have incarcerated inguinal hernia, torsion of a testicular appendage, trauma-induced scrotal hematoma, or testicular torsion. In the newborn, torsion is extravaginal; that is, the epididymis, testicle, and tunica vaginalis all twist within the internal spermatic fascia with resultant organ infarction. Examination of the scrotum in the early phase of torsion will sometimes demonstrate a testicle lying in the transverse plane rather than in the normal longitudinal position. Occasionally, the epididymis may be palpable in the abnormal anterior position rather than in the normal posterior medial position. Loss of cremasteric reflex can be seen in 95% of patients with testicular torsion. An incarcerated hernia is sometimes diagnosed with ultrasound or stethoscope. Auscultation of bowel sounds in the scrotum indicates trapped bowel contents.

Intravaginal torsion occurs more commonly in the adolescent period. In this entity, the tunica vaginalis surrounds the testicle instead of being fixed posterolaterally. The testicle is then free to twist inside the tunica, similar to the clapper within a bell. The patient presents with an acutely swollen, tender testicle that may preclude examination. The testicle may be retracted high in the scrotum, or the epididymis may be in an abnormal position. A thorough history may elicit previous episodes of transient testicular pain. Torsion may follow vigorous activity, but it is rarely caused by it. Differential diagnosis includes trauma, epididymo-orchitis, torsion of a testicular appendage, scrotal insect bites, viral orchitis (chickenpox, mumps, coxsackievirus, infectious mononucleosis), or testicular cord torsion. Torsion of a testicular appendage may have a blue dot sign, in which the infarcted appendage is seen through the scrotal skin as a blue infarcted area. Epididymo-orchitis is extremely rare in the adolescent age-group and in the absence of pyuria should not be considered.

If the diagnosis is in doubt, color Doppler ultrasonography should be performed to evaluate testicular blood flow and intrascrotal anatomy. If testicular cord torsion is a possible diagnosis, the patient should undergo surgical exploration. Temporizing maneuvers of icing the scrotum, blocking the cord with an anesthetic, or attempting manual detorsion may be used while awaiting operating room availability. Because prolonged torsion (>6 hours) may lead to irreversible testicular damage with resultant subfertility, correction should proceed quickly. If a bell clapper deformity is noted at surgery, it should be assumed to be present bilaterally and simultaneous contralateral testicular fixation can prevent subsequent contralateral torsion.

Trauma

Although the testicles hang freely within the scrotum and are relatively resistant to trauma, a direct blow to the organ may lead to injury. It is important to determine if the tunica albuginea of the testicle is intact because this influences the management. If a patient has a scrotal hematoma and an intact testicle, conservative management is the standard of care. If a tunica albuginea is torn, the patient is managed with scrotal exploration, with removal of defunctionalized seminiferous elements and closure of the tear. An ultrasound examination is often helpful in assessing the integrity of the tunica albuginea.

Scrotal Infections

Infections involving the scrotal skin include cellulitis due to Gram-positive bacteria, treated with antibiotics such as cefazolin or cephalexin, and candidal fungal infection, treated with a topical antifungal medication.

A rare but dreaded infection involving the scrotum is necrotizing fasciitis (Fournier's gangrene), a process associated with a mixed infection involving the subcutaneous tissue. Associated conditions may include diabetes, obesity, urethral stricture, and perirectal disease. The scrotum becomes erythematous, tense, and moist. The gangrene spreads rapidly and can progress along the anterior abdominal wall with associated crepitus. Wide debridement and drainage of the affected area, as well as administration of broad-spectrum antibiotics, are essential. Without immediate aggressive surgical management, the disorder can lead to the patient's death.

Malignant Diseases

Testicular cancer is the most common solid malignancy in men between the ages of 18 and 35. Finding a scrotal mass is a frightening experience for a young man, and fear of malignancy may lead to denial.

Evaluation

The patient presenting with a scrotal mass should be questioned as to how long the mass has been present and whether it is increasing in size or painful or has been preceded by infection, trauma, or surgery. After the scrotum is examined manually, a bright light is placed behind the mass in an attempt to transilluminate it. Transillumination implies fluid with probable hydrocele or spermatocele as the etiology. If the testes are seen to float in the middle of the cystic mass, the mass is a hydrocele, caused by decreased absorption of fluids by the parietal layer of the tunica vaginalis, leading to a fluid collection between the two leaves of the tunica. If, however, the mass sits above or below the testes, it is probably a spermatocele. Both entities are benign, but the distinction is important if surgical correction is entertained. If the mass is adjacent to the spermatic cord and is tubular with a bag of worms sensation, it is probably a varicocele: a dilated segment of internal spermatic vein. Varicoceles are seen in approximately 15% to 20% of all men and need correction only if there is ipsilateral pain, testicular atrophy, or subfertility. The etiology of this abnormality is unknown, but because of its predilection for left-sided occurrence, a valve abnormality is a common explanation. If the mass does not transilluminate but appears to be localized to the head or tail of the epididymis, it most likely is a sperm granuloma, an epididymal cyst, a benign epididymal adenomatoid tumor, or rarely, a mesothelioma of the epididymis, which has malignant potential.

A mass that involves the testicle has a high probability of malignancy. Real-time ultrasonography of the mass can be performed to help differentiate the various causes of scrotal masses, but surgical exploration is usually necessary for both diagnosis and treatment. Because of the lymphatic drainage of the testicle, a scrotal incision is contraindicated. If a malignancy is present, lymphatic drainage patterns are altered and future treatment compromised. Therefore, a groin incision should be made in the region of the midinguinal canal. The spermatic cord is atraumatically occluded and the testicle brought into the surgical field and exposed. If a tumor is present, the cord structures are ligated with a silk suture and the testicle is removed.

Treatment

Testicular malignancies can be divided into germ cell (which arise from the germinal elements) and non–germ cell tumors (which arise from the mesodermal elements of the testicle). Germ cell tumors, the most common, are discussed the following section.

Germ cell tumors of the testicle are divided into seminomas and nonseminomas. Seminomas do not undergo further neoplastic transformation, whereas nonseminomas differentiate along extraembryonic lines (e.g., in choriocarcinoma or yolk-sac tumors) or intraembryonic lines (e.g., in a teratoma). Before radical orchiectomy, certain tumor markers are obtained. α-Fetoprotein (AFP) has a half-life of 5 to 7 days and, when elevated, is diagnostic of nonseminomatous tumor components. β-hCG has a shorter half-life and may be elevated in either seminoma or nonseminomatous tumor. Because AFP is produced by endodermal cells lining the yolk sac, it will not be elevated in a pure seminoma. β-hCG, however, is produced by the syncytiotrophoblastic cell and may be found in 30% to 40% of seminomas.

Tumor markers are important in the management of testicular cancer. For example, if the AFP (made by a nonseminomatous tumor only) is elevated after orchiectomy and the testicle has pure seminoma, either the pathologist missed nonseminomatous cells in the specimen or there are nonseminomatous cells elsewhere. If the AFP or β-hCG is elevated before orchiectomy, extragonadal cancer is indicated.

After radical orchiectomy (removal through an inguinal incision), tumor staging is performed with retroperitoneal CT scanning (supplanting lymphangiography), chest radiographs (with or without CT scan), and postoperative tumor markers. Clinical and pathologic staging is complicated, but usually follows the outline in Table 7-7.

Seminomas usually cause diffuse enlargement of the testis. The cut tissue is glistening white. Microscopically, there is a monotonous overgrowth of large round cells with clear cytoplasm. Lymphocytic infiltration is found in 20% of cases. After the histologic diagnosis is made, staging is completed (according to Table 7-7).

Table 7-7	Staging of Germ Cell Tumors
Stage I	Metastatic workup negative; preoperative markers, if positive, normalize; tumor isolated to the testicle
Stage IIA	Microscopic retroperitoneal disease
Stage IIB	Minimal retroperitoneal disease on radiographic studies (<5 cm)
Stage IIC	Bulky retroperitoneal disease (>5 cm)
Stage III	Disease beyond retroperitoneal lymph drainage, or positive markers after retroperitoneal lymph node dissection

Seminoma is an exquisitely radiosensitive tumor. Stages I and IIa seminoma are usually treated with moderate doses of retroperitoneal radiation therapy. For bulky retroperitoneal or distant metastatic disease, platinum-based chemotherapy is the first-line treatment.

For stage I nonseminomatous disease, retroperitoneal lymph node dissection is usually indicated. In this procedure, lymph node packets adjacent to the aorta and vena cava medial to the ureters are removed. (Additional details regarding this technique, including templates of the dissection, can be found in the urologic atlas and textbooks listed at the end of this chapter.) Preservation of sympathetic nerve fibers within the dissection preserves ejaculatory function in most men. Careful surveillance without node dissection is an option for some men, but is usually not recommended.

For more advanced or metastatic tumors, platinum-based chemotherapy is used. A 5-year survival rate exceeding 70% is achieved, even in the presence of metastatic disease. Resection of any abdominal mass is required after chemotherapy to identify any residual cancer or to remove mature teratoma, which may gradually enlarge.

Male Infertility

Of all newly married couples, 15% experience difficulty conceiving a child. Statistics show that 60% of fertile couples will conceive within 3 months of unprotected intercourse, and 90% within 1 year. Therefore, each partner merits evaluation if no pregnancy occurs within 1 year of unprotected intercourse. This section will limit itself to male infertility. A male factor is causative in 40% of cases, and partially responsible in an additional 20%.

Evaluation

A complete history should include obtaining information about the following:

Childhood illnesses (e.g., mumps) and previous groin, scrotal, or bladder surgical procedures
Problems with delayed or premature puberty
Previous viral illnesses (because spermatogenesis takes approximately 90 days)
Medications that may cause fertility abnormalities (e.g., cimetidine, Macrodantin, Azulfidine)

Toxin exposure and marijuana or cigarette smoking
Knowledge of fertility timing (the couple may be having intercourse too often, not often enough, or timing it incorrectly)
Use of lubricants (some are spermicidal)

Physical Examination

The physical examination includes the following: examining the genitalia; the body habitus for Klinefelter's syndrome; the visual fields and olfactory sense to ascertain possible pituitary or hypothalamic lesions; the chest for gynecomastia; the penis for lesions; the urethral meatus for position and size; the vas deferens and epididymis (palpated for abnormalities); the testicles (palpated and sized with an orchidometer, noting consistency and abnormalities). The presence of a varicocele should be documented.

Semen Analysis

The mainstay of male evaluation is semen analysis. Because the findings of this analysis may vary, three fresh ejaculates, obtained after 24 hours of sexual abstinence, are examined within 1 hour of collection. The complete ejaculate is collected in a wide-mouthed glass jar (plastic may be spermicidal). Semen analysis results should be discussed in terms of adequacy as determined by the World Health Organization (Table 7-8), rather than in terms of average or normal. Parameters measured include sperm density, motility and morphology, and ejaculate volume. Problems with fertility can occur when there is a low volume. Causes of a low volume include a decreased serum testosterone, retrograde ejaculation into the bladder, and ejaculatory duct obstruction.

Treatment

Patients with retrograde ejaculation can be diagnosed by an evaluation of a postejaculatory urine specimen for the presence of sperm. The treatment of retrograde ejaculation is sympathomimetic medication, such as pseudoephedrine. If this fails, sperm can be harvested from the bladder, washed, and used for intrauterine insemination. Tests for ejaculatory duct obstruction include fructose ejaculatory analysis, because fructose is normally produced by the seminal vesicles. Its absence in the ejaculate indicates a lack of seminal vesicle fluid in the ejaculate. TRUS is now used more often to evaluate patients for ejaculatory duct

obstruction, which can often be successfully treated with transurethral resection of an ejaculatory duct stenosis.

Patients with azoospermia without the above etiologies may have vasal agenesis, a condition that warrants an evaluation to rule out cystic fibrosis. These patients may be candidates for microsurgical epididymal sperm aspiration. Patients with azoospermia, atrophic testicles, and a high follicle-stimulating hormone level usually have intrinsic testicular failure. Testicular biopsy may show sperm that can be extracted. Unfortunately, these patients are usually infertile and adoption may be the best option. Normal testicular biopsy findings and azoospermia with a normal ejaculate volume suggest obstruction at the level of the vas deferens or epididymis. These patients may be candidates for scrotal exploration, vasography, and vasovasostomy or vasoepididymostomy.

If a varicocele is present in a patient with a low sperm count or abnormal functional parameters (oligoasthenospermia), varicocele repair is an option.

Impotency

In the past, most men with erectile dysfunction were thought to have an underlying psychological abnormality. However, recent advances in knowledge of the mechanisms of erections have led to findings of organic impairment in over 85% of these men.

Erections involve neurological, endocrine, and vascular events. The ability to obtain and maintain an erection requires adequate arterial inflow, smooth muscle relaxation in the erectile corporal tissues, and storage of blood within the corpora cavernosa at high pressures. Sexual stimulation and arousal, associated with libido that is in part mediated by testosterone, lead to neurologic events with nitric oxide release from nonadrenergic, noncholinergic neurons. This leads to increased cyclic guanosine monophosphate (cGMP) production, leading to corporal smooth muscle relaxation. Dilation of arteries and arterioles and blood flow to the penis increase, and venous outflow decreases, trapping the blood in the corporal tissue. A disturbance of one or more of the above processes causes erectile dysfunction. Erectile impotence is classified according to four main categories: vasculogenic, endocrinologic, psychogenic, and neurogenic. However, several of these components are often present in a given patient.

Vasculogenic

Vasculogenic disorders probably are the most common cause of erectile dysfunction. Arterial insufficiency is worsened by hypertension, hyperlipidemia, diabetes mellitus, and cigarette smoking. Pelvic trauma can lead to a focal arterial injury. An inability to store venous blood in the corporal tissue may occur secondary to a venous leak, where inflow is adequate, but the blood does not become trapped.

Endocrinologic

Endocrinologic syndromes associated with a low serum testosterone, decreased libido, and erectile dysfunction in-

Table 7-8	Standards for Adequate Semen Analysis[a]
Ejaculate volume	1.5–5.0 mL
Sperm density	>20 million/mL
Motility	>60%
Grade of motility	>2 (scale 1–4)
Morphology	>60% normal

[a]As determined by the World Health Organization.

clude hypogonadotropic hypogonadism and pituitary adenoma. The first hormonal test in the evaluation of impotence is a serum testosterone level, keeping in mind the circadian nature of testosterone release. If the testosterone level is low, gonadotrophins and prolactin levels are drawn. Hyperprolactinemia (associated with a low testosterone) may be caused by a pituitary lesion; when this condition is found, an MRI of the sella turcica is indicated. Although rare, a pituitary adenoma can present as erectile dysfunction.

Psychogenic

Psychogenic factors may be a component contributing to erectile dysfunction or may be entirely responsible. Testing to determine if impotence is psychogenic is performed selectively. One test, nocturnal penile tumescence, uses REM sleep erections, which occur in otherwise healthy men. The absence of erectile function during normal sleep suggests organic impairment, whereas normal erectile function at night indicates psychogenic impairment.

Neurogenic

The most common neuropathic lesions are caused by spinal cord injury, multiple sclerosis, alcoholism, and diabetes. Surgery (e.g., radical prostatectomy) may lead to injury to the neurovascular bundles as they course posterolaterally between the prostate and the rectum.

Evaluation

A number of tests can be performed to evaluate erectile dysfunction. Nocturnal tumescence testing, duplex ultrasound of the penis before and after a pharmacologically induced erection, cavernosometry/cavernosography, and pudendal arteriography are used for evaluation. These tests are not routinely performed in most patients, because the results may not affect treatment decisions. Exceptions include young patients with pelvic trauma who may benefit from revascularization if a discrete arterial injury is the etiology of impotence.

Treatment

Treatment options in patients without specific problems, such as pelvic trauma or an endocrine disorder as described previously, include observation and a vacuum erection device (pump placed over the penis that can cause an erection as a vacuum is created), with or without use of a constriction band at the base of the penis to maintain the erection induced by the vacuum pump. Another option is the administration of a urethral suppository of alprostadil or the intracavernous injection of vasoactive medications. These treatments involve the administrations of medications that cause smooth muscle relaxation in the penis. An option that should be considered as a last resort is a penile prosthesis.

Recently, sildenafil citrate (Viagra) was approved as an oral medication to treat erectile dysfunction. Sildenafil works by inhibiting phosphodiesterase, a compound that breaks down cGMP, which is necessary for smooth muscle relaxation in the penis. The result is that cGMP is increased, promoting smooth muscle relaxation and erectile function. This medication is highly effective in most patients and has made a remarkable impact. The demand for sildenafil is high, and its introduction has revolutionized the management of erectile dysfunction. Many patients are now initially treated with sildenafil, with alternatives considered only if it fails. Sildenafil is contraindicated in patients taking nitrates. There are now two additional oral mediations available for the treatment of erectile dysfunction—vardenafil (Levitra) and tadalafil (Cialis).

SKILLS

Bladder Catheterization (Male)

1 Have all materials to be used opened and ready to use before beginning any aspect of the procedure. Once the procedure is initiated, one hand is always holding the penis or spreading the labia; therefore, it is essential that everything be ready for use and available within reach of the other hand. Items needed are the catheter (usually 16 French) and a drainage bag, lubrication (to coat the tip of the catheter or inject into the urethra), a cleansing agent (e.g., povidone-iodine [Betadine]) and an applicator, a 10-mL syringe filled with water, drapes, and sterile gloves.

2 Drape the field with the patient in the supine position. With one hand, grasp the penis with upward traction, retracting the foreskin completely if the patient is uncircumcised. With the other hand, clean the meatus and glans with antiseptic solution. The hand that is not holding the penis is used to perform the remainder of the procedure.

3 Coat the catheter tip with a water-soluble lubricant. Excellent lubrication of the urethra facilitates catheter passage. Injecting 10 mL of lubricant into the urethra, as well, is recommended. Prefilled tapered-tip syringes that contain a lubricant and lidocaine are commercially available (Uro-jet). Alternatively, a 10-mL syringe can be filled with lubricant during the setup.

4 Slowly pass the catheter until only the portion of the catheter in the area of the balloon port remains visible (2–3 inches) (Fig. 7-37).

5 Look for urine return, then inflate the balloon with 7 to 10 mL water.

6 Connect the catheter to the drainage bag, and tape the catheter to the thigh.

Bladder Catheterization (Female)

1 Place the patient in the frog-leg position. When practical, the lithotomy position is preferred.

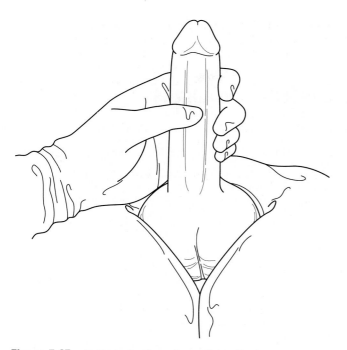

Figure 7-37   Catheterization of a male patient.

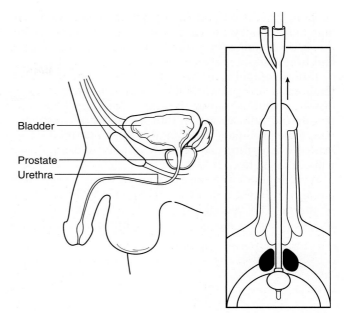

Figure 7-39   Difficulty in passage of the catheter because of the prostate.

2 Perform the procedure as above, except for the following: use one hand to spread the labia (Fig. 7-38). Alternatively, have an assistant perform this maneuver. When the catheter is placed, it needs to be advanced for only half its length before the balloon is inflated.

Bladder catheterization is also described and depicted in Lawrence's *Essentials of General Surgery*, 4th ed., pp. 559–560.

Difficulties

The main problem encountered is resistance to passage of the catheter in the male. This commonly occurs at the level of the prostate where the urethra courses upward toward the bladder (Fig. 7-39). If the catheter cannot negotiate this curve, it will poke into the median lobe of the prostate. Moreover, enlargement of the lateral lobes of the prostate inhibits efforts to pass the catheter. When resistance is encountered, do not use force because doing so will only cause urethral trauma. Instead, attempt to overcome the resistance by injecting additional lubricant into the urethra and placing a larger (18–20 French) **coudé catheter** (Fig. 7-40), which has an upwardly curved tip. As the catheter is advanced, orientation is maintained by

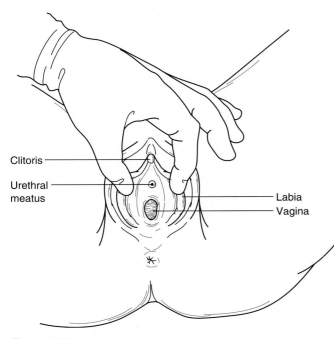

Clitoris

Urethral meatus

Labia

Vagina

Figure 7-38   Catheterization of the female patient.

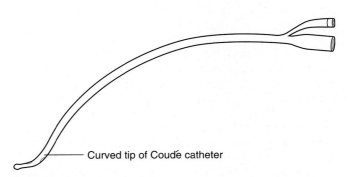

Curved tip of Coudé catheter

Figure 7-40   Coudé catheter.

keeping the balloon port facing upward. The most important points are never force the catheter in and never inflate the balloon unless the catheter advances all the way in and urine output is seen.

If urine output is not seen, the catheter lumen may be temporarily blocked with lubricant. The lubricant usually dissolves within a minute. If urine output is still not seen, irrigate the catheter with 60 mL saline using a catheter-tip syringe (Toomey). Appropriate catheter position is confirmed when saline can be easily instilled and withdrawn without resistance.

A urethral stricture can also cause resistance to catheter passage. At times, a smaller catheter (12–14 French) can be placed. However, the urethral lumen in the area of a stricture is often too narrow to permit the passage of a catheter. In such a case, urologic consultation is mandatory.

SUGGESTED READINGS

Hinman F. *Atlas of Urologic Surgery*, 2nd ed. Philadelphia: WB Saunders; 1998.

Lawrence PF. *Essentials of General Surgery*, 4th ed. Philadelphia: Lippincott Williams & Wilkins; 2006.

Macfarlane MT. *House Officer Series: Urology*, 2nd ed. Baltimore: Williams & Wilkins; 1985.

Tanagho EA, McAninch JW, eds. *Smith's General Urology*, 14th ed. Norwalk, Conn: Appleton & Lange; 1995.

Walsh PC, Retik AB, Vaughan ED Jr, Wein AJ, eds. *Campbell's Urology*, 7th ed. Philadelphia: WB Saunders; 1998.

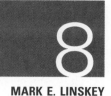

MARK E. LINSKEY

Neurosurgery: Diseases of the Nervous System

OBJECTIVES

Cranial and Cerebrovascular Disease

1 Describe the basic anatomic organization of the central nervous system in terms of hierarchical control and functional segregation.

2 Develop a common vocabulary to describe accurately the clinical findings and sites of localization to consultants and colleagues.

3 Describe the basic anatomic organization of the blood supply to the brain and the cerebrospinal fluid circulation.

4 Apply the Glasgow Coma Scale to assessment of level of consciousness.

5 Describe the clinical findings that lead one to suspect each of the herniation syndromes.

6 List the steps in the determination of brain death, and explain their significance.

7 List and explain the indications for and contraindications to lumbar puncture.

8 Discuss the treatment alternatives and sequential steps in medically stabilizing elevated intracranial pressure, the risks associated with hyperventilation, as well as the indications for, and different types of, intracranial pressure monitors.

9 Describe the initial evaluation of a comatose patient with a head injury.

10 List the different types of intracranial lesions seen on early neuroimaging for closed head injury; discuss their significance for patient outcome and their potential for surgical reversal.

11 List the features of a basilar skull fracture that would raise one's suspicion for a traumatic vascular injury to the carotid artery.

12 Describe the typical setting and clinical and neuroimaging findings associated with pediatric shaken-whiplash syndrome and understand the physician's responsibility in reporting this syndrome for child abuse investigation.

13 Describe the management of scalp lacerations and penetrating injuries.

14 Define transient ischemic attack, list the most common sources, and describe its relationship to cerebral infarction.

15 List the clinical and radiologic features that differentiate ischemic stroke from hemorrhagic stroke. List the disorders that can produce each type.

16 Describe the role and timing of carotid endarterectomy and endovascular thrombolysis in patients with cerebrovascular disease.

17 Describe the danger associated with aneurysmal subarachnoid hemorrhage, define and discuss the frequency of sentinel bleeds, and describe the relative roles of CT scanning and lumbar puncture in diagnosing subarachnoid hemorrhage.

18 List the common brain tumors that affect adults and children, the prognosis for each, and the symptoms that herald a brain tumor.

19 Based on the history and physical examination, choose and interpret the diagnostic tests needed to establish the site and nature of the tumor.

20 List examples of tumors and clinical circumstances that might benefit from stereotactic biopsy, open surgical excision, stereotactic radiosurgery, fractionated radiotherapy, and chemotherapy for brain tumors.

21 Describe the symptoms, evaluation, and treatment of a patient with a brain abscess.

22 Describe the role and alternative techniques of diagnostic brain biopsy for patients with nonbacterial central nervous system infections.

23 Describe the symptoms and evaluation of a patient with suspected hydrocephalus.

24 Describe the complications of ventricular shunting.

25 Describe the shape of the head with premature closure of the cranial sutures: the sagittal suture, one coronal suture, both coronal sutures, and the lambdoid suture.

26 Describe the signs and symptoms of Chiari I and Chiari II malformation and the goals of surgical intervention for these conditions.

27 Describe the significance of a new-onset seizure in an adult and distinguish this circumstance from epilepsy.

28 Define intractability for patients with epilepsy, list at least two invasive epilepsy monitoring techniques, describe the most common surgical epilepsy procedures, and list the resulting benefits of the procedures from the standpoint of seizure control, cognitive function, employability, and quality of life.

29 Describe the role of surgery in patients with Parkinson's disease, and list the lesional and stimulator surgical options available for these patients.

30 Describe the symptoms of normal pressure hydrocephalus, as well as the diagnostic procedures that correlate with improvement after ventricular shunting.

Spine and Spinal Cord Disease

1 Describe the clinical findings that lead one to suspect each of the spinal cord syndromes, and compare and contrast cauda equine and conus medullaris syndrome.

2 List the most common causes of each of the spinal cord syndromes.

3 Describe the three-column theory of for inferring spinal column stability based on anatomic disruption.

4 List the important steps in the evaluation and management of acute spinal cord injury. Consider bodily injury, spinal instability, and spinal cord damage.

5 Describe the diagnostic name, anatomy of the break, and findings on neuroimaging of three stable C1–2 fractures.

6 Describe the diagnosis and significance of Spinal Cord Injury Without Radiographic Abnormality (SCIWORA) in the pediatric population.

7 Describe the initial imaging findings, initial stabilization methods, early reduction steps, and indications for surgery for subaxial C3–C7 fractures.

8 Describe the difference between a compression and burst fracture, and list the indications for surgical stabilization.

9 Define dermatome and myotome, describe the symptoms and findings of radiculopathy, and list the most common causes of radiculopathy.

10 Describe the signs and symptoms of neurogenic claudication and describe its relationship to lumbar stenosis.

11 Describe the clinical manifestations, diagnostic workup, conservative management, and surgical indications for a patient with cervical disc herniation and lumbar disc herniation.

12 Describe the clinical manifestations, diagnostic workup, conservative management, surgical indication, and different surgical approaches for a patient with degenerative cervical stenosis and lumbar stenosis.

13 List the pathologic features, clinical symptoms and signs, and surgical corrective measures for spondylolisthesis.

14 Describe the vascular supply to the anterior and posterior spinal cord, as well as the differential supply to the cervical and upper thoracic versus lower thoracic and lumbar-sacral spinal cord.

15 Describe the differential clinical signs and symptoms that distinguish anterior spinal artery spinal cord infarction from compression by epidural hematoma.

16 Describe the common route of spread for metastatic carcinoma and the corresponding findings on neuroimaging, and compare this with the common route of spread to the spine and imaging findings for lymphoma.

17 Describe the relative and appropriate roles for steroid treatment, emergent fractionated radiotherapy, surgical decompression, and surgical fusion for metatstatic cord compression.

18 Describe the single most important prognostic factor for determining whether a patient will have functionally independent ambulatory function after surgical decompression for metastatic spinal cord compression.

19 List the common intradural intramedullary and extramedulalry spinal cord tumors, and compare their typical modes of presentation.

20 List the social and medical risk factors for spontaneous discitis, and describe the typical radiographic findings for this condition.

21 Describe the differences seen on neuroimaging between bacterial discitis and osteomyelitis and tuberculous spine disease.

22 Describe the medical and surgical treatments for common spine infections.

23 Differentiate between meningocele and myelomeningocele according to deficits and appearance. Describe and compare them with respect to associated neural and other problems.

24 List at least two other central nervous system conditions associated with spina bifida, and describe the significance of folate for changing the incidence of this developmental anomaly.

25 Describe the relative growth features of musculoskeletal somites and central nervous system spinal cord segmental innervation during development as it relates to the formation of the cauda equine and its significance for tethered cord syndrome.

Peripheral Nerve Disease

1 Describe the cross-sectional anatomy of a peripheral nerve.

2 Describe the role of the brachial and lumbar-sacral plexus in mixing dermatomes and myotomes into peripheral nerve distributions.

3 Define neuropraxia, incomplete nerve transection, and complete nerve transection. Describe the means to differentiate them.

4 Compare the healing of a crushed nerve, a transected nerve, and a surgically joined nerve.

5 List the factors that affect the timing of peripheral nerve repair.

6 Describe the role of electromyography in distinguishing between radiculopathy and peripheral neuropathy, defining the level of traumatic peripheral nerve or plexus injury, as well as the course of recovery after injury or surgical repair.

7 Describe the features that distinguish carpal tunnel syndrome, tardy ulnar palsy, and cervical disc disease.

8 List the treatable medical risk factors for potentially medically reversible nerve entrapment neuropathies.

9 Describe the role of electromyography and nerve conduction studies in confirming and localizing pathologic nerve entrapment.

10 Describe the relationship of neurofibromatosis to schwannomas and neurofibromas and the worrisome signs and symptoms for malignant degeneration in patients with neurofibromas.

Pain

1 Describe the characteristic signs and symptoms, typical natural history, as well as early medical treatment of trigeminal neuralgia and glossopharyngeal neuralgia.

2 Describe the potentially curative as well as palliative surgical options available for treating patients with trigeminal neuralgia, as well as the general efficacy and recurrence rates for each.

3 Describe the surgical options available for treating patients with glossopharyngeal neuralgia.

4 Describe the gating control theory of pain.

5 Describe the potential downside of peripheral deafferentation procedures for pain syndromes.

6 Describe the surgical options for treating painful neuromas.

7 Describe at least two chronic pain syndromes that may respond to sympathectomy.

8 List and describe surgically implantable pharmacologic and stimulatory spinal cord strategies for treating chronic neuropathic and terminal cancer pain syndromes.

9 List and describe stereotactic lesioning and stimulatory deep brain strategies for treating chronic neuropathic and terminal cancer pain syndromes.

10 List at least three chronic pain syndromes that have shown therapeutic response to motor cortex stimulation.

Neurological surgery is a relatively young specialty field that evolved as a separate discipline from general surgery during the early 1900s. While often referred to as "brain surgery," modern practice management surveys reveal that general community neurosurgical practice comprises approximately 75% to 80% spinal surgery, 20% cranial and cerebrovascular surgery, and 5% to 10% peripheral nerve surgery. Academic and university practices average roughly 50% to 60% spinal surgery, 35% to 45% cranial and cerebrovascular surgery, and 5% peripheral nerve surgery. This chapter will present an overview of neurosurgical diseases and interventions that includes cranial and cerebrovascular, spinal, peripheral nerve, pain, adult and pediatric, and congenital and acquired conditions.

CRANIAL AND CEREBROVASCULAR DISEASE

Anatomy and Physiology

Unlike other organs such as liver, lungs, kidneys, and muscles, in which cells are organized into repetitive identical units (e.g., lobules, alveoli, glomeruli), the central nervous system (CNS) is heterogeneous and is hierarchically organized at many different levels. Involuntary motive force for activities such as consciousness, breathing, blood pressure, and heartbeat have intrinsic pacemakers within the brain stem, which is divided into the midbrain, pons, and medulla (see Figs. 8-1 and 8-2; shown in Fig. 8-12). Voluntary activities including thinking, communicating, motor movements, and behavior have their origin in the lobes of the cerebral hemispheres (frontal, parietal, temporal, and occipital), which send motor efferent and receive sensory afferent signals down through the brain stem and the spinal cord to reach the rest of the body via the cranial and peripheral nerves, as well as the autonomic nervous system. These afferent and efferent connections are modulated and modified by superimposed secondary circuitry from the cerebellum, striatum, subthalamus, and red nucleus. The thalamus serves as a relay station and connection module for afferent primary and all secondary circuitry. Through its control of the pituitary gland, the hypothalamus serves as the source of autonomic tone and impulses, the modulator of body homeostasis (temperature, serum osmolarity), and the master regulator of hor-

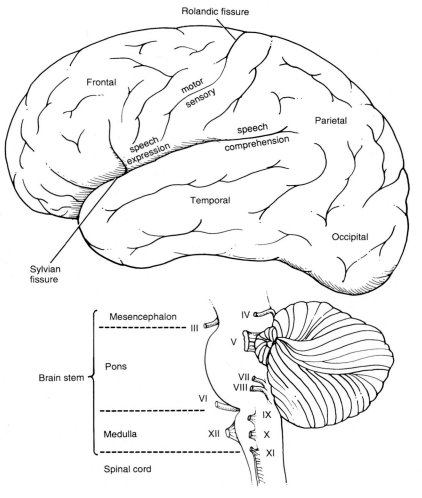

Figure 8-1 Medial aspect of the left side of the brain. The brain stem is displaced caudally for purposes of illustration.

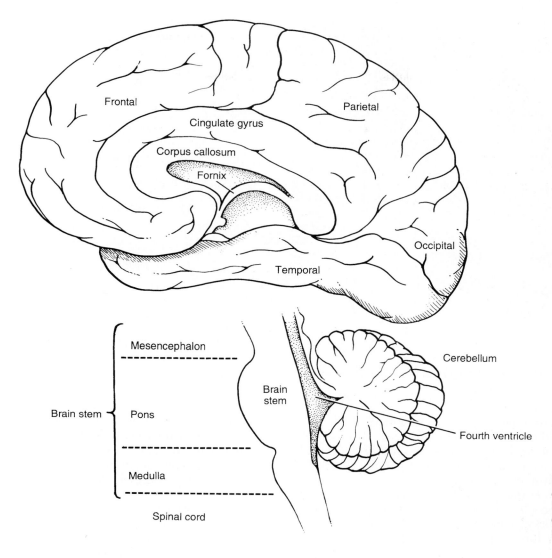

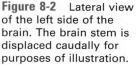

Figure 8-2 Lateral view of the left side of the brain. The brain stem is displaced caudally for purposes of illustration.

monal levels and temporal rhythms. Knowledge of CNS functional organization and regional specialization, along with a thorough neurologic examination, are the keys to determining the level and location of a CNS lesion.

The intracranial cavity is divided into two chambers by a fibrous curtain called the tentorium. The tentorium has an opening (tentorial incisura) through which the brain stem travels to connect with the cerebral hemispheres. Both cerebral hemispheres occupy the **supratentorial** space. The supratentorial space is divided into two lateral compartments by an incomplete curtain of dura called the falx cerebri, which extends the length of the interhemispheric fissure. The hemispheres are composed of an outer cortical layer (gray matter — containing neurons), a middle layer of white matter (containing axons), and an inner mass of gray matter (diencephalon, thalamus, and hypothalamus — containing neurons) (Figs. 8-1 to 8-3). The outer cortex is folded into ridges (gyri) separated by fissures (sulci). The frontal lobe, which occupies the anterior cranial fossa, is separated from the parietal lobe by the Ro-

landic fissure (i.e., central sulcus — see Fig. 8-1) and from the temporal lobe, which sits in the temporal bone and the tentorium, by the sylvian fissure (Fig. 8-1). The occipital lobe occupies the posterior pole of each hemisphere.

The frontal lobe is the primary source of motor function. Lesions in the posterior portion cause contralateral weakness and hyperreflexia. The primary motor strip lies just in front, and the primary sensory strip just behind, the central sulcus. Lesions of the anterior parietal lobe cause contralateral sensory dysfunction. The visual pathways course from the optic nerves through optic chiasm and tracts to the lateral geniculate body of the thalamus. From there, the white matter connections course through the posterior temporal lobe (Meyer's loop) and through the parietal lobe to finally end on the primary calcarine cortex in the interhemispheric surface of the occipital lobe. Lesions of the temporal lobe visual pathways lead to a contralateral superior visual field defect (superior quadrantanopsia), lesions of the parietal visual connections cause an inferior visual defect (inferior quadrantanopsia),

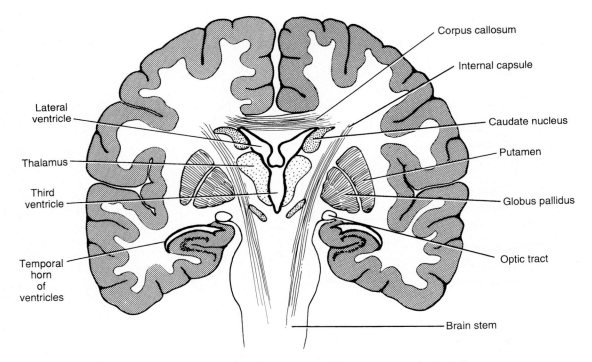

Figure 8-3   Coronal section of the brain showing the gray matter (*stippled*).

and lesions of the primary visual cortex cause a contralateral complete visual field defect (hemianopsia).

Although primary motor and sensory functions are symmetrically organized bilaterally, some higher cortical functions are represented only in one hemisphere or the other. Speech dominance is an example. Ninety-five percent of naturally right-handed people have speech located in the left hemisphere, while 50% of naturally left-handed people have speech located in the right hemisphere. For left brain–dominant people, lesions of the inferior-lateral left frontal lobe, just above the root of the sylvian fissure (Broca's area), cause an **expressive (nonfluent) aphasia.** Lesions in the posterior-superior temporal lobe, just below the end of the sylvian fissure (Wernicke's area) cause loss of speech comprehension and a fluent aphasia consisting of meaningless sounds or words. Lesions of the connection between the two areas lead to a conductive aphasia, in which speech is understood but the patient is unable to repeat the understood phrase. Other examples include calculations, which localize to the right parietal lobe, and pattern recognition and spatial orientation, which localize to the right parietal lobe in left brain–dominant people

Some functions do not respect lobar boundaries, but involve connections throughout all four. An example is the limbic system, which consists of concentrically paired looping circuits involving the medial temporal lobe (amygdala, hippocampus, and parahippocampal gyrus), the medial parietal lobe (posterior cingulated gyrus), the inferior medial occipital lobe (posterior occipital-temporal gyrus), the medial and inferior frontal lobe (anterior cingulated gyrus and the medial septal nuclei), the fornix, and the

hypothalamus. The limbic system is the entry portal for short-term memory and is intimately involved in learning, as well as regulating mood and affect. However, only bilateral lesions are usually symptomatic. Still other functions such as long-term memory are diffusely stored in ways we have yet to fully understand.

The cortical functions of the four lobes within one hemisphere connect with one another via subcortical white matter tracts oriented anteriorly-posteriorly, including the superior and inferior longitudinal fasciculi. They connect one hemisphere to the other by way of laterally oriented white matter tracts across the corpus callosum, as well as the anterior and posterior commissures. They connect with the brain stem and spinal cord by way of a condensation of white matter tracts called the internal capsule (Fig. 8-3; shown in Fig. 8-9E), which are oriented in a rostral-caudal direction. The internal capsule passes through the diencephalon between the basal ganglia. The caudate and putamen (striatum) lie laterally and the thalamus medially to the internal capsule (Fig. 8-3; shown in Figs. 8-9E and 8-10). Even very small vascular lesions in this tight condensation of white matter connections can lead to severe weakness (lacunar strokes). The nonspecific nuclei of the thalamus are extensions of the reticular formation of the brain stem and are involved with arousal and alertness. When they are damaged (e.g., thalamic hemorrhage), coma occurs. The thalamus acts as a relay point for sensation. Somatosensory input from the spinal cord and brain stem is processed in the ventral posterior thalamus and relayed to the parietal lobe. Special sensory afferent information is relayed to the cortex from the posterior thalamus (hearing from the medial geniculate nucleus to the temporal lobe and vision from the lateral geniculate nucleus to the occipital lobe). Input from the limbic system related to memory and emotion is also connected through the thalamus. The anterior nuclei receive limbic input from the mamillary bodies of the hypothalamus (to which the hippocampus projects) and project to the medial cortex of the frontal lobe (cingulate gyrus).

The infratentorial compartment of the cranium (the **posterior fossa**) contains the brain stem and the cerebellum. The brain stem connects inferiorly with the spinal cord byway of an opening in the skull called the foramen magnum. The cerebellum lies on the back of the brain stem like a papoose and connects with the brain stem by way of three axially oriented white matter tracts on each side (the superior, middle, and inferior cerebellar peduncles, respectively—Fig. 8-1; shown in Fig. 8-12). The cerebellum is involved with modulation and coordination of motor movements by means of inhibitory modulatory inputs. The paired lateral hemispheres control the limbs, and lesions here lead to dysmetria. The central vermis controls the axial musculature, and lesions here cause ataxia. The inferior tonsils as well as the inferior-lateral flocculus and nodulus control vestibular-ocular coordination, and lesions here cause nystagmus.

The brain stem is divided into a dorsal component (tectum) that contains the reticular formation, cranial nerve nuclei, and lemniscal sensory tracts. The ventral component (tegmentum) contains the motor white matter connections, the cerebellar modulatory connections, and the cranial nerve roots. The motor pyramidal tract is densely compacted and lies very close to the ventral surface of the brain stem at two locations. In each of the locations it is susceptible to dysfunction form external pressure. The first is in the midbrain cerebral peduncle, where contralateral hemiparesis occurs with compression by the medial hippocampus during transtentorial herniation. The second is the decussation of the pyramids in the ventral medulla, where ventral skull-base tumors can cause confusing motor weakness patterns (cruciate paralysis). Most of the long white matter tracts that pass between the spinal cord and the brain stem cross from side-to-side at the spinal medullary junction. The level of lesions in the brain stem can be determined from the level of cranial nerve involvement. Cranial nerves 3 and 4 arise from the midbrain. Cranial nerves 5, 6, 7, and 8 come from the pons. Cranial nerves 9, 10, 11, and 12 arise from the medulla (Fig. 8-2). All cranial nerves exit the brain stem ventral-laterally except for the fourth cranial nerve, which exits dorsally. The reticular formation of the brain stem controls respiration, heart rate, blood pressure, and consciousness.

Blood Supply

The brain receives 20% of the stroke volume of each heartbeat. Four major blood vessels course through the neck from the apical chest vessels to supply the brain. The two common carotid arteries divide at the carotid bifurcation into the internal carotid artery (ICA) and external carotid artery (ECA). The ECA supplies blood to the face, the scalp, and the meningeal covering of the brain by way of several terminal arteries, including the middle meningeal artery (MMA). The major ECA scalp terminal branches are the superficial temporal artery (STA) coursing just in front of the ear and the occipital artery coursing just behind the ear. The ICA courses through the petrous canal of the skull base to the cavernous sinus located on either side of the pituitary gland. It supplies the ophthalmic branch to the orbit and then penetrates the dura covering of the brain. The carotid system supplies 80% of the blood supply to the brain, with each ICA supplying approximately 40%. The two vertebral arteries (VA) together supply 20% of the brain's blood volume. Most people have a left-brain dominant VA, fewer have a balanced vertebral system, and a small number have a right-dominant VA. The VAs enter the transverse foramen of the cervical vertebra at C6 and segmentally course through each transverse foramen all the way up through C2. They penetrate the dura between the arch of C1 and the posterior-lateral rim of the foramen magnum. The VA is susceptible to injury (dissection or occlusion, with subsequent ischemia or embolization) with sudden spinal movements or with spine fractures involving the transverse foramen.

The posterior fossa is the only location in the human body where vessels (in this case the VAs), instead of branching as they extend further from the heart, join to form a single distal posterior circulation artery, the basilar artery (BA). Before joining to form the BA, each VA gives off a posterior inferior cerebellar artery (PICA), which supplies the lateral medulla and the inferior-lateral cerebellum. At the mid pons level, the BA gives off bilateral anterior-inferior cerebellar arteries (AICA), which supply the lateral pons and cerebellum. Near its terminus, the BA gives off bilateral superior cerebellar arteries (SCA), which supply the lateral brain stem and the superior and superior-lateral cerebellum. The BA ends in a bifurcation consisting of the initial segments of the posterior cerebral arteries (PCA), which supply the inferior temporal lobe, the occipital lobe, and the posterior-medial parietal lobe. The ICAs give off posteriorly coursing posterior communicating arteries (pCom A) on each side, which join with the PCAs at the level of the midbrain. They then continue, bifurcating into the middle cerebral artery (MCA) and the anterior cerebral arteries (ACA). The ACAs course medially under the frontal lobes and connect with each other by way of an anterior communicating artery (aCom A), before continuing up the interhemispheric fissure to supply the frontal pole and the medial frontal and medial anterior parietal lobes. The MCA courses up the sylvian fissure to supply the whole lateral portion of the frontal, temporal, and parietal lobes. Because it carries the largest volume of blood flow and supplies the largest volume of brain, the MCA distribution is the most common distribution to receive a vascular embolus (embolic stroke or metastatic brain tumor). Normal, average, mixed cortical cerebral blood flow (CBF) to the brain is 55 mL/100 g/min (SD $\pm$ 12); white matter values are approximately 22 mL/100 g/min.

The base of the brain in the arachnoid cisterns contains a unique collateral supply system called the circle of Willis. It consists of the ICA, the first segments of both ACAs, the aCom A, both pCom As, and the first segments of both PCAs. These segments connect in a geometric pentagon, with the short aCom A segment constituting the blunted apex. Through the circle of Willis any one ICA and one VA could theoretically supply blood to any area of the brain. In reality, the circle of Willis is quite variable in integrity and symmetry, and even angiographic demonstration of an intact ring does not guarantee adequate collateral potential. Only 75% to 80% of people will tolerate the sudden loss or occlusion of one ICA without stroke. Five percent will become symptomatic within 5 to 15 minutes of occlusion from flow-related ischemia, and 15% to 20% will initially be asymptomatic, but will have marginal reserves that carry a high risk of delayed stroke with any subsequent episode of dehydration or hypotension.

Venous drainage of the brain has both deep and superficial components. Deep in the brain, the two paired thalamostriate and intracerebral veins drain the diencephalon and join the two basal veins of Rosenthal, which drain the upper brain stem to form the single, short, and deep vein of Galen. The inferior sagittal sinus, which runs along the inferior edge of the falx cerebri dural reflection separating the hemispheres, joins the vein of Galen. Here, the falx joins the tentorium to form the straight sinus. The straight sinus runs along the falx-tentorium insertion to join the torcula. Superficially, the sylvian vein (the vein of Labbé), coursing in the sylvian fissure, drains the brain. This vein runs from the top of the sylvian fissure down along the posterior-lateral aspect of the temporal lobe to join the transverse sinus. The vein of Trolard runs upward from the top of the sylvian fissure along the central sulcus to join the sagittal sinus. Together, the sylvian vein, vein of Labbé, and vein of Trolard form a crude venous Mercedes-Benz symbol on each side of the brain. Multiple smaller lateral cortical veins run upward to join the sagittal sinus by bridging across the subarachnoid space to the dura. These "bridging veins" are particularly prone to tearing with lateral shear forces. They are a major source of both acute traumatic and spontaneous chronic subdural hematomas. Ultimately, the sagittal sinus flows back to join the two transverse sinuses, along with the straight sinus at a junction called the torcula. The two transverse sinuses then flow laterally to join the sigmoid sinuses behind each ear, which then flow down to finally become the internal jugular veins bilaterally. A minor anterior venous drainage collateral system courses through the cavernous sinus and the pterygopalatine plexus of the face.

Cerebrospinal Fluid Circulation

During life, the brain has the texture and consistency of uncooked tofu. Thus, it is susceptible to deformation and shearing forces with sudden accelerations and decelera-tions. Fortunately, it has an internal structural skeleton in the form of fluid-filled cerebral ventricles and an external fluid cushioning layer in the form of the subarachnoid space and the basal arachnoid cisterns. Cerebrospinal fluid (CSF) performs this structural and cushioning role; it also forms a second circulation for the brain, helping to maintain and regulate cerebral and systemic homeostasis. It is produced by choroid plexus in an energy-dependent, carbonic anhydrase–dependent, active process at the rate of 0.3 mL/min (totaling 432 mL/day). Because the total volume of CSF in the cranium and spinal canal is approximately 150 mL, this means that the total volume of CSF is completely replaced 3 times per day.

The cerebral hemispheres contain paired lateral ventricles that form the internal core of all four lobes. They form a large medial-leaning "C" with a posterior extension into the occipital lobe (occipital horn). The two lateral ventricles drain into a single midline third ventricle, which lies between the two diencephalons just above the midbrain by way of the paired foramen of Monroe (Fig. 8-4). Only the anterior horn of the lateral ventricle does not contain choroid plexus. The third ventricle drains through the midbrain by way of the single narrow aqueduct of Sylvius to join the fourth ventricle, which lies in the posterior fossa between the brainstem in front and the cerebellum behind. Fluid then exits the ventricular system either by way of the single medial foramen of Magendie (located between the paired tonsils of the cerebellum), draining into the cisterna magna, or laterally via two foramina of Luschka, draining into the cerebellopontine angle on either side. The CSF flows down the spinal canal, under the brain through the basal arachnoid cisterns, and over the convexity of the brain in the subarachnoid space. It is absorbed into the venous system at the dural venous sinuses by way of arachnoid villi. These villi serve as one-way communication valves, with absorption driven by the pressure gradient between the subarachnoid space and the venous pressure in the dural sinuses.

Intracranial Pressure, Cerebral Perfusion Pressure, Cerebral Autoregulation, and Brain Herniation

The skull is a closed, rigid chamber with both fixed and variable content volumes. Under normal conditions, the cranial cavity contains only brain, CSF, and blood. Normal intracranial pressure (ICP) in an adult is less than 10 to 15 cm of H_2O (14–20 mm Hg). In children, before skull growth-plate fusion, it is much lower. According to the Monroe-Kellie hypothesis, in a fixed, enclosed space adding additional masses to the fixed volume (e.g., blood clots, swollen contusions, tumors, large strokes, excess CSF) will lead to stable intracranial pressure only so long as the buffering capacity of increased CSF absorption can keep up. At some point, this buffering capacity is saturated, and at this point even small extra volume increases will lead to very large increases in ICP. Indeed, ICP will rise

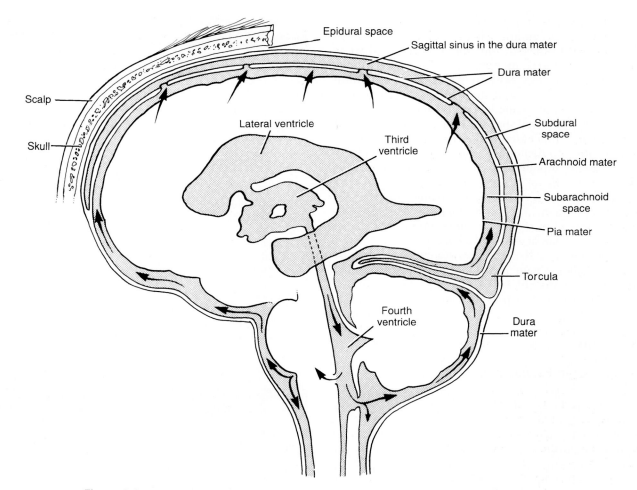

Figure 8-4   Circulation of the cerebrospinal fluid.

exponentially with additional volume increases from this point onward.

The brain volume is fixed in both the supratentorial and infratentorial compartments. It is also fixed in each lateral compartment of the supratentorial space (separated by the falx cerebri). The CSF volume is relatively fixed, with only small increases in CSF absorption possible by increasing the pressure gradient across the arachnoid villi–dural sinus interface. The blood volume is the most variable of the three because elevated ICP can prevent inflow of blood into the cranial cavity. It is therefore the most susceptible to pathologic derangement resulting from conditions that raise ICP, with the potential for secondary ischemic injury to the brain. Cerebral perfusion pressure (CPP) is the difference between mean systemic arterial pressure (MAP) and ICP (CPP = MAP − ICP). Normal CPP is >50 mm Hg (usually in the range of 55–65 mm Hg). In general, when CPP falls below 45 mm Hg, the brain is at risk for developing areas of reduced CBF, depending on local-regional conditions for the area of brain at risk.

Cerebral autoregulation is a vasoconstriction-dilatation compensation mechanism that normally keeps CBF constant over a wide range of blood pressures (MAP 40–140 mm Hg). In addition to the actual CBF, the arterial level of CO_2 is the second main arbiter of the degree of cerebral vascular tone (vasoconstriction with low levels of CO_2 and vasodilatation with high levels). Intracranial pressure can be lowered by hyperventilating the patient and lowering arterial CO_2, but only at the expense of lowering CBF to a brain that may be very susceptible to secondary injury with any further ischemia. With brain injury from trauma or ischemia, autoregulation can be disrupted in local regions of the brain, and with repeated or prolonged elevations of CPP, autoregulation can fail throughout the brain. When this occurs, CBF is dependent on CPP in a linear manner.

A hernia is the physical displacement of tissue from one compartment into another due to a pressure gradient across the opening between the chambers in question. This definition and concept is the same for the inguinal canal, the diaphragm, or the cranial cavity. Because the cranium has several compartments, several types of herniation are possible, including: (a) transtentorial herniation (tissue moving downward from the supratentorial space through the tentorial incisura into the infratentorial space); (b) tonsillar or downward herniation (tissue moving from the posterior fossa through the foramen magnum); (c) subfalcine herniation (tissue moving from one side of the supratentorial space to the other under the falx cerebri); (d) upward central herniation (tissue moving upward from the infratentorial space through the tentorial incisura into the supratentorial space); and (e) herniation of tissue outside the skull through a craniotomy or traumatic skull defect. With herniation syndromes, it is the physical mass effect from the herniating tissue pressing on the tissue in the recipient compartment that causes dysfunction and damage. High ICP alone will not lead to herniation so long as the pressures are equal across compartments. Patients with pseudotumor cerebri routinely exhibit ICPs in the 20 to 30 cm H_2O range without herniation because the pressures are equal across all compartments.

Evaluation

The Neurologic Examination

An organized and systematic approach to the neurologic examination is the best way to ensure thoroughness. The examination should include assessment of: (a) mental status, (b) cranial nerves, (c) cerebellar function, (d) motor and reflex function, and (e) sensory function. Initial elective evaluations require detail and depth in each portion. Subsequent follow-up examinations and emergency evaluations should be tailored to go into clinically relevant detail as necessary.

Mental status examination includes assessment of level of consciousness; orientation to person, place, and time; speech comprehension and expression (best tested with repetition of phrases); immediate and short-term memory; mental arithmetic; writing; and drawing. Descriptions should include the specifics of both stimulus attempted and the response obtained. For patients with head injury, the Glasgow Coma Scale (GCS) with scores extending from 3 to 15 is very useful and has been verified for reproducibility and interobserver variability (Table 8-1). A patient with a score of 8 or less is considered to be comatose. For nontrauma patients, a useful objective and quantifiable format is the Mini-Mental Status Examination (Table 8-2).

Olfaction is tested in conscious and cooperative patients in each nostril separately with a nonvolatile, nonirritating odor (e.g., coffee grounds, cinnamon, vanilla). Eyes are checked for pupil size, shape, and reactivity; fullness of visual fields; presence of atrophy, papilledema, or hemorrhages on funduscopic examination; ptosis of the eyelids; fullness and absence of diplopia on extraocular movements (EOMs); and the presence or absence of nystagmus. Trigeminal nerve examination includes testing facial sensation in all three trigeminal divisions, symmetry of the

Table 8-1	Glasgow Coma Scale
Activity	**Score**
Eye opening	
Spontaneous	E4
To speech	3
To pain	2
Nil	1
Best motor response	
Obeys	M6
Localizes	5
Withdraws	4
Abnormal flexion	3
Extensor response	2
Nil	1
Verbal response	
Oriented	V5
Confused conversation	4
Inappropriate words	3
Incomprehensible sounds	2
Nil	1
Glasgow Coma Scale score (E + M + V) = 3 to 15	

Table 8-2	Mini-Mental Status Exam	
Maximum Score	**Score**	**Mini-Mental State**
		Orientation
5	( )	What is the (year) (season) (date) (day) (month)?
5	( )	Where are we: (state) (county) (town) (hospital) (floor)?
		Registration
3	( )	Name 3 objects: allow 1 second to say each. Then ask the patient all 3 after you have said them. Give 1 point for each correct answer. Then repeat them until the patient has learned all 3. Count trials and record.
		Attention and calculation
5	( )	Count by serial 7s. Give 1 point for each correct answer. Stop after 5 answers. Alternatively, spell "world" backwards.
		Recall
3	( )	Ask for the 3 objects named above. Give 1 point for each correct answer.
		Language
9	( )	Name a pencil and a watch (2 points). Repeat the following: "No ifs, ands, or buts" (1 point). Follow a 3-stage command: "Take a paper in your right hand, fold it in half, and put it on the floor" (1 point). Read and obey the following: "Close your eyes" (1 point). Write a sentence (1 point). Copy a design (1 point).
30	___	Total score
Assess level of consciousness along a continuum		

muscles of mastication, and presence and symmetry of corneal reflex. Facial nerve testing includes distinguishing between peripheral cranial nerve weakness (all branches) and central CNS upper motor neuron weakness (weakness limited to the mid and lower face). Hearing can be tested with a 712-Hz tuning fork for both bone conduction symmetry (midline—Weber test) and an air–bone conduction gap on either side (mastoid tip versus ear canal—Rinne's test). In an unconscious patient, vestibular function can be assessed with the oculocephalic reflex ("doll's eyes") or caloric testing. In a normal state, rotating the head suddenly from side-to-side leads to the eyes maintaining a straight-ahead gaze. If they move with the rotation of the head, then they have an abnormal oculocephalic reflex. With caloric testing, cold water irrigated through a small tube in one ear canal, with the patient's head elevated 30 degrees, depresses vestibular function of that ear, permitting unopposed function of the opposite ear and conjugate deviation of the eyes toward the irrigated ear. Absence of response is pathologic. Glossopharyngeal function is tested by both symmetry of the uvula with palate elevation and gag reflex on either side. In patients who are intubated, vagal nerve function can be tested by presence of cough reflex to deep tracheal suctioning. Shoulder shrug symmetry and tongue protrusion symmetry assess cranial nerve XI and XII function, respectively.

Cerebellar function testing includes stance and gait assessment, stability of stance with eyes closed and arms extended (Romberg's sign), as well as appendicular assessments for dysmetria (finger-to-nose with eyes closed) and dysdiadochokinesia (finger-nose-finger with eyes open and changing target positions). The cerebellum does not function in isolation. Thus, abnormal gait can also be seen with motor hemiparesis, and nystagmus or poor balance can also indicate vestibular dysfunction.

Motor assessment in conscious patients includes analysis of symmetry of muscle bulk and tone as well as muscle strength on a scale of 0 to 5. Zero means no palpable muscle contraction, while 5 is normal strength. Three means strength enough to resist gravity but no additional resistance. Two and 4 are any assessment between 0 and 3 or between 3 and 5. In patients with altered consciousness, motor response is assessed in response to stimuli (localization, purposeful coordination, symmetry of response). A pathologic flexor response (**decorticate**) must be distinguished from a pathologic extensor response (**decerebrate**). Reflexes are rated on a scale of 0 to 4. Zero is absent reflexes, 1 is a weak reflex, and 2 is a normal reflex. Three is an overly active reflex with up to 1 to 3 beats of clonus. Four is a reflex associated with more sustained clonus. Pathologic reflexes associated with upper motor neuron lesions include extensor plantar responses (**Babinski reflex**), finger flexion response with sudden flexion of the distal interphalangeal joint (**Hoffmann response**), and ankle clonus.

Sensory examination includes both the spinothalamic pathway (pain—pin response) and the lemniscal pathway (joint position sense and symmetry of vibration sensation).

Testing for pronator drift (Barrés sign—arms extended, palms up with fingers spread, with eyes closed) is a rapid way to test for both asymmetry of motor strength and integrity of joint position sense. A pathologic response includes both unilateral pronation and asymmetrically dropping one arm.

For supratentorial cerebral lesions, bilateral symmetry of examination takes on paramount importance and "lateralizing signs" (either motor, reflex, or sensory) are key findings assisting in hemispheric localization. For brain stem lesions, the level of cranial nerve involvement and the presence of decorticate or decerebrate posturing in comatose patients are critical for localizing the level of the lesion. For cerebellar lesions, lateral asymmetry of findings for hemispheric lesions and defining truncal versus appendicular findings is critical for distinguishing midline vermis versus lateral hemispheric lesions. Coma (GCS score ≤8) occurs only with diencephalic or brain stem reticular activating system dysfunction, or with global, bilateral, and diffuse cortical dysfunction.

Herniation Syndromes

Four of the five CNS herniations described above are associated with distinct clinical syndromes. Since each represents a neurologic emergency, it is very important that they be quickly recognized and addressed.

Transtentorial herniation (i.e., uncal herniation) is the most common CNS herniation syndrome. It involves the movement of the uncus and hippocampus of the medial temporal lobe medially and downward through the tentorial incisura to compress the third cranial nerve and the upper midbrain on the same side (Fig. 8-5A). The herniation results from a pressure differential between the supratentorial and infratentorial compartments and is usually associated with a lateral hemisphere mass lesion. Downward pressure on the third nerve affects the outer papillary fibers, leading to a dilated pupil on the side of the lesion (Fig. 8-5B). Pressure and torsion on the midbrain affect the reticular activating system and rapidly lead to unconsciousness. Pressure on the cerebral peduncle usually leads to contralateral hemiparesis and eventually to contralateral decorticate and then decerebrate posturing, as consciousness is lost. Rarely, pressure on the peduncle pushes the midbrain over to impact the contralateral peduncle on the edge of the tentorium without ipsilateral dysfunction (Kernohan's notch—see Fig. 8-5C). This phenomenon occurs in <10% of transtentorial herniation syndromes, but leads to motor findings on the same side as the pupillary change. Thus change in the size of the pupil is always the most reliable lateralizing sign.

Central upward herniation also arises from a pressure differential between the supratentorial and infratentorial compartments. However, in this case the superior medial cerebellum moves upward through the tentorial incisura to symmetrically impact upon the upper brain stem. The result is sudden loss of consciousness from reticular activating system dysfunction and symmetrical bilateral brain stem pathologic motor findings.

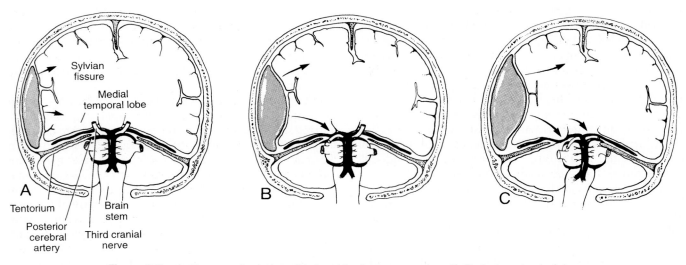

Figure 8-5 **A,** Extracerebral clot with local brain compression. **B,** Early transtentorial herniation. **C,** Late stage of herniation.

Central downward herniation (i.e., tonsillar herniation) arises from a pressure differential between the infratentorial compartment and the spinal canal. The cerebellar tonsils move downward and forward to put pressure on the lower medulla. In addition to sudden loss of consciousness from reticular activating system dysfunction and bilateral brain stem extensor posturing, medullary cardiorespiratory center dysfunction leads to bradycardia and hypertension (Cushing's reflex), as well as disrupted breathing patterns (e.g., Cheyne-Stokes respiration).

Each of the three herniation syndromes described above involves compression of the brain stem, with effects on level of consciousness through the reticular activating system. Because the brain stem is the primary involuntary respiratory and vasomotor control center for the body, all of these syndromes usually lead to death if not recognized and rapidly treated. Although the initial effects on level of consciousness can develop slowly and insidiously, each of these syndromes is characterized by rapidly accelerating clinical progression once consciousness is impaired. For this reason, consciousness and mental status remain the most important component of the neurologic examination in brain-injured patients, and medicines that affect level of consciousness (pain medications, sedatives, and other CNS depressants) must be carefully considered in these patients, unless an intracranial pressure monitor is in place.

With subfalcine herniation, the cingulated gyrus moves underneath the falx cerebri over the corpus callosum. Pressure on the ACA, which runs in this space, leads to distal ischemia in the distal distribution of that artery including the medial portion of the primary motor strip. Because this portion of the primary motor strip somatotopically maps to the leg, the patient is often symptomatic with a contralateral lower-extremity monoparesis.

Brain Death

Brain death is a legal definition of death that recognizes an irreversible physiologic state in which the brain has no function, but heartbeat and blood pressure are maintained. The determination is best made by a neurologist or neurosurgeon. At the time of examination, there should be no evidence of significant hypothermia or potential pharmacologic cause of CNS suppression. Brain stem reflexes (pupillary, corneal, oculovestibular, caloric, gag, and respiratory) should be absent. There should be no response to trigeminal painful stimuli and no more than local motor responses (spinal) to body or limb stimulation. Disconnection of the respirator to test for the absence of spontaneous respiration is essential. This determination is carried out after a period of ventilation that allows the P_{CO_2} to normalize. When the respirator is disconnected, adequate, steady flow of oxygen is delivered through a catheter that is introduced well down the endotracheal tube. The patient is observed for absence of spontaneous respirations. The determination is carried out until the arterial P_{CO_2} is greater than 59 mm Hg.

Laboratory tests (electroencephalographic silence; cerebral radionuclide brain scans, cerebral angiography, or, possibly, transcranial Doppler confirmation of absent CBF) are usually considered optional, unless hypotension occurs and forces discontinuation of apnea testing. Usually, two complete examinations, which are separated in time and show no evidence of brain activity by the previously described criteria, are performed by licensed physicians before the patient is pronounced dead.

Electrolyte Disturbances of Cental Nervous System Origin

The hypothalamus is the main arbiter of systemic serum osmolality and sodium concentration, which are sensed via osmoreceptors present in areas of the hypothalamus where the blood–brain barrier is not present. The two hormones involved in this control are antidiuretic hormone (ADH) and either brain natriuretic peptide (BNP) or an upstream hormone controlling the release of BNP. Both of these hormones possibly are released from the posterior lobe of the pituitary gland (a direct extension of the hypothalamus) into the systemic blood stream. Oversecretion of either hormone leads to hyponatremia. It can precipitate herniation in a patient with a CNS mass lesion, and it can lead to seizure activity as well as make any subsequent seizure activity refractory to pharmacologic control. Loss of basal tonic ADH secretion leads to a dangerous condition known as diabetes insipidus (DI). With DI, the kidneys cannot reclaim water in the distal collecting tubules and the serum sodium and osmolarity can rise extremely fast. Sudden shifts in serum sodium (usually either up or down ≥ 3 mEq/L/hr) can lead to a clinically devastating demyelination syndrome of brain stem at the tegmentum-tectum junction in the pons known as central pontine myelinolysis (CPM). For reasons that are not clear, patients are most susceptible to CPM if they have concomitant liver disease (e.g., hepatitis, liver failure, liver transplant). Rapid rises in serum sodium can also lead to seizure activity, as well as make any subsequent seizure activity refractory to pharmacologic control. Thus, evaluation of serum sodium and osmolality is a very important component of the evaluation of a patient with CNS pathology.

Nonspecific brain pathology is second only to nonspecific pulmonary pathology (pneumonia, lung cancer, congestive heart failure) as the most common cause of syndrome of inappropriate ADH secretion (SIADH). SIADH can be seen in CNS conditions as diverse as meningitis, abscess, brain tumor, stroke, and intracerebral hemorrhage. The mechanism leading to hypothalamic dysfunction is poorly understood. With SIADH, the distal tubules of the kidney maximally resorb free water despite a low serum osmolarity and sodium level. The hallmark of SIADH is a high urine sodium level (>20 mEq/L). The urine sodium level indicates the severity of the SIADH episode (mild 20–99, moderate 100–150, severe >150). It is also the most sensitive indicator of syndrome resolution because it will reduce and then normalize well in advance of the serum sodium. In the absence of loop diuretics or severe kidney disease, SIADH and cerebral salt wasting are the only two conditions that will lead to abnormally high urine sodium. With SIADH the patient is hyponatremic due to hemodilution with free water and is relatively volume-overloaded, despite the common presence of intense thirst (also hypothalamically controlled). Treatment is fluid restriction for mild cases (800–1200 mL/24 hr) and/or intravenous 3% NaCl, with or without diuresis in patients in critical CNS condition or in those who have severe forms of the syndrome.

Cerebral salt wasting (CSW) is a unique syndrome that, so far, has only been described for patients with subarachnoid hemorrhage (SAH). Atrial natriuretic peptide (ANP), a hormone first described as arising from the heart, is se-

creted in response to atrial distention due to volume overloading. It leads to natriuresis in the kidneys. Because sodium obligates a minimum volume of water as solvent, natriuresis leads to intravascular volume reduction through natural diuresis. Recently, ANP has been found to be exactly the same as a protein derived from brain called BNP. It is not yet clear whether the hypothalamus is actually secreting the BNP by way of an atrial distention autonomic feedback loop from the heart or whether the hypothalamus can control the heart's secretion of BNP by means of an upstream releasing factor. Either way, in patients with SAH, BNP levels can rise precipitously, leading to significant hyponatremia. The presumed mechanism of hypothalamic dysfunction is vasospasm of the perforating small arteries that supply the hypothalamus from the basal cisterns in reaction to the SAH. CSW also leads to elevated urine sodium; however, unlike patients with SIADH, patients with CSW are volume *contracted*. Fluid restriction in this setting is inappropriate and potentially dangerous. Treatment often requires intravenous 3% NaCl infusion. Because SIADH and CSW can occur in the same patient, often the conditions can be distinguished, and the correct measures instituted, only after inserting central venous catheters to asses patient intravascular volume status. Because CSW is seen only with SAH, many internists and medical and surgical critical care physicians are not familiar with it. It is important that neurosurgeons and neurologists carefully ensure that low serum sodium situations with high urine sodium are not all automatically treated as cases of SIADH.

The most common cause of DI is iatrogenic disruption of the hypothalamus or pituitary stalk function after surgery for hypothalamic or pituitary tumors. However, DI can also be seen in the setting of severe brain injury (trauma, intracerebral hemorrhage, major stroke, or other high ICP condition). Presumably caused by hypothalamic ischemia or infarction in these settings, it is a very dire sign that usually portends severe permanent brain damage, and often occurs as a preterminal event. Treatment of DI involves intravenous or intranasal desmopressin acetate (DDAVP), which is a short-acting ADH analog. Iatrogenic DI can be either temporary or permanent, so careful serum sodium monitoring is mandatory until the situation is more clearly defined. Patients with iatrogenic DI and relatively normal brain function can lead normal lives with administration of exogenous DDAVP, once the correct dosage and schedule is titrated.

Coagulation Disturbances of CNS Origin

The CNS has the highest concentration of tissue thromboplastin per gram of tissue homogenized of any other organ in the body. Indeed, rodent or rabbit brain was the original standard reagent utilized to trigger the prothrombin (PT) clotting test in laboratories before pure chemical reagents became available. Since tissue thromboplastin triggers the extrinsic clotting pathway, any condition in which brain tissue can become homogenized and exposed to the intravascular contents can lead to a consumptive systemic coagulopathy known as disseminated intravascular coagulation (DIC). With DIC, platelets, clotting factors, and fibrinogen are rapidly consumed, and fibrin degradation products rapidly rise. DIC is a life-threatening systemic coagulopathy that can be temporized by transfusions of platelets, clotting factors (fresh frozen plasma [FFP]), and fibrinogen (cryoprecipitate), but can only halt when the cause of the syndrome is removed, is cured, or exhausts itself naturally. DIC is most commonly seen in cases of severe traumatic brain injury. Rarely, it has been seen in cases of large stroke or intracerebral hemorrhage, as well as in cases of large-volume brain tumors removed through homogenation using an instrument known as a cavitronic ultrasonic aspirator. Because a large volume of tissue thromboplastin is needed to trigger systemic DIC, DIC is a marker for a major brain injury. DIC can lead to progression in a patient's brain injury through enlargement of preexisting hematomas, conversion of contusions into hematomas, and conversion of ischemic strokes into hemorrhagic strokes. Its presence underlines the severity of the situation and usually portends a poor prognosis. Indeed, cynical students of neurology and neurosurgery often suggest that DIC in these settings stands for "death is coming." All patients with major head injury, significant intracerebral hemorrhage, or stroke should be carefully assessed for coagulopathy.

Neuroendocrinology

The brain, through the hypothalamus, is the master controller of all hormones in the body, either through direct secretion into the systemic circulation (from posterior pituitary), or through sending releasing factors into the hypothalamic-pituitary portal circulation. Releasing factors stimulate the anterior pituitary to release its own stimulating hormones into the systemic circulation, which ultimately stimulate hormone secretion at the terminal gland (e.g., adrenal gland, thyroid, testes, ovary). It is the site that contains "thermostat" receptors, which constantly monitor the systemic levels of hormones as well as the site that integrates and coordinates hormone release with the body's natural circadian rhythms. The previous discussion of electrolyte section covered the role of the posterior lobe of the pituitary in secreting ADH, dysfunction of which can lead to DI.

With the exception of prolactin, which is tonically suppressed by dopamine (except in women immediately postpartum, when lactation occurs), the hypothalamus and anterior pituitary gland stimulate the ultimate end-organ secretion of cortisol thyroid hormone, growth hormone, somatomedin-C (i.e., insulin-like growth factor-1 [IGF-1]), and the sex hormones (testosterone, estrogen, and progesterone). Traumatic brain injury as well as pituitary and parasellar masses can lead to varying forms and severity of hypopituitarism, which can be assessed only by measuring the hormone levels concerned. Cortisol and thyroid hormone can be particularly problematic in the neurocritical

care and emergency care settings. Patients can go into Addisonian crisis because of inability to mount a stress steroid response and can have serious anesthetic consequences if they are severely hypothyroid. If there is any doubt, patients should be empirically treated intravenously with stress doses of steroids (100 mg of hydrocortisone or its equivalent every 8 hours) until their hormone status can be better defined. Pituitary tumors (adenomas) can lead to hormone hypersecretory syndromes (e.g., Cushing's disease, acromegaly, or prolactinemia), and, in these settings, hormone testing can be diagnostic.

Lumbar Puncture

The CSF is a separate homeostatically regulated physiologic fluid unique to the CNS. Laboratory evaluation of CSF is just as important as systemic blood work in evaluating patients with CNS pathology. It is usually accessed by means of a lumbar puncture (LP) at either L4-5 or L5-S1. At these levels there is no danger of spinal cord injury, because only the cauda equina lies in the thecal sac at these levels. An LP can give a diagnostic opening pressure, which will be elevated in cases of pseudotumor cerebri, CNS infection, or high ICP from mass lesion. Standard CSF examination includes measurement of glucose level (lowered in the setting of infection), protein level (elevated in many pathologic settings), Gram stain and culture (infection), and cell count (both white cell and red cell). In the emergency room, if community acquired and potentially infectious meningitis is suspected, the CSF can be screened for antigens to the common community-acquired infectious meningitis agents. The CSF cell count assessment is particularly important. Although white cells will be elevated (>5) in the setting of many infections, a neutrophil predominance suggests bacterial process, while a mononuclear predominance suggests a viral, fungal, or noninfectious inflammatory condition. An elevated CSF red blood cell (RBC) count may be the only indication that a patient has had an SAH. CT scans are only 90% sensitive for SAH in the acute setting, but a CT scan coupled with an LP increases sensitivity to approximately 98%. It is important in this setting to send both the first and fourth tubes of fluid sample for cell count, because a high RBC count in the first tube that clears by the fourth tube suggests a traumatic LP rather than an SAH. The CSF should also be assessed for xanthochromia (straw color), which indicates a prior SAH (minimum 2–3 days previously) with subsequent RBC lysis, a high protein content, or both.

Many very useful additional specialty tests can be run on CSF. Because they are expensive and often somewhat esoteric, they should only be ordered when clinical circumstances and differential diagnosis evaluation specifically dictate. Among others, these tests include CSF cytology tests for malignant cells; polymerase chain reaction (PCR) tests for tuberculosis (TB) and certain CNS viruses; India ink staining for cryptococcus; antigen titers for viruses and cryptococcus; special TB, fungal, and viral cultures; Venereal Disease Research Laboratories (VDRL) tests for syphilis; immunoglobulin and protein electrophoresis for detecting immune complexes and pathologic proteins; and myelin basic protein and multiple sclerosis testing battery to assess for multiple sclerosis and other demyelinating syndromes.

The LP can be used to introduce dye into the CSF to augment diagnostic studies such as a contrast CT cisternogram for the head or a myelogram or myelogram CT scan for the spine. Myelography was invented by neurosurgery and initially performed predominantly by neurosurgeons. It can also be used therapeutically to relieve ICP by withdrawing CSF on a one-time basis or as a first step in inserting a lumbar drain for chronic spinal CSF withdrawal over days. Care must be taken when contemplating an LP to ensure that the act of LP does not lead to a compartment pressure gradient differential that could lead to herniation and clinical deterioration from a herniation syndrome. The most common scenario is an LP performed in a patient with high ICP due to an intracranial mass lesion leading to either transtentorial or central downward foramen magnum herniation. In general, all patients should be assessed for papilledema with an ophthalmoscope before LP, if possible, and, if doubt persists, a CT or magnetic resonance imaging (MRI) scan should be performed. Rarely, an LP performed below a partial or complete spinal canal CSF block from mass lesion can lead to neurologic deterioration. To rule out spinal canal lesions in patients with a known diagnosis of systemic cancer, an MRI scan of the spine generally should precede diagnostic CSF cytologies performed by LP

Neuroimaging

Before 1976, the only modalities other than the neurologic examination and blood and CSF tests available to the neurosurgeon to diagnose CNS pathology were the cerebral angiogram (dye injected within the cerebral arteries to visualize them on x-ray films), the pneumoencephalogram (air injected into the ventricular system to visualize it on x-ray films), and radionuclide brain scans (injected radioactive tracers sometimes taken up by brain tumors). Both the cerebral angiogram and pneumoencephalogram were invented and were initially performed by neurosurgeons, while the brain scan came from radiology. In 1976, CT revolutionized the ability to see directly brain lesions and brain and skull anatomy. MRI followed in the late 1980s, offering even better resolution of CNS tissue. Few medical disciplines are as critically dependent on imaging for best clinical practice benchmarks as neurosurgery. Neurosurgeons are experienced at interpreting CT and MRI neuroimages and usually work closely with their affiliated neuroradiologist(s).

Currently, nuclear brain scans are rarely performed. The exceptions are to distinguish recurrent primary malignant brain tumor from radiation necrosis after a course of radiation therapy and to trace the flow of CSF after injection of a tracer by LP or CSF device injection. Complete

diagnostic pneumoencephalography is no longer performed. However, limited air ventriculography still has a role in acute trauma settings, when the patient is too unstable to go to the CT scanner or has to be taken directly on arrival to surgery for life-saving abdominal or thoracic surgery. In this setting a ventricular catheter can be placed through a burr hole in the skull to serve as an ICP monitor. The catheter can also serve a diagnostic function by using it to withdraw 1 to 2 mL of CSF and then replace it with 1 to 2 mL of air. A subsequent anterior-posterior (A-P) portable skull film will often (but not always) indicate whether midline is shifted to either side and suggest the appropriate side for emergent empiric cranial exploration if clinically indicated.

Cerebral Angiography, Embolization, Thrombolysis, and Embolectomy

Although MR angiography and CT angiography are less invasive and can usually be obtained more quickly, nothing compares with cerebral angiography for detailed resolution of CNS vascular anatomy and definition of CNS vascular lesions. Such lesions include cerebral aneurysm, arteriovenous malformation (AVM), arteriovenous fistula, and arterial embolus. Originally performed by direct needle stick of the cervical CCA and VA, it is now routinely performed by catheters introduced into the femoral artery in the groin and navigated cephalad. Diagnostic cerebral angiography is a very powerful tool; however, it is an invasive test and carries an approximately 1% risk of stroke for anterior circulation assessment, increasing to a 1% to 3% stroke risk for posterior circulation assessment. Diagnostic cerebral angiography can be used to visualize CNS lesions and to assess collateral circulation by assessing the status of the circle of Willis. It can also be used to perform a temporary balloon test occlusion of an artery while the patient is assessed clinically, electrophysiologically, or with CBF imaging.

Cerebral angiography can even be used therapeutically. Endovascular embolization of CNS vascular lesions (e.g., aneurysms and AVMs) was developed by neurosurgeons and is currently performed by both endovascular neurosurgeons as well as interventional radiologists. With endovascular access, selected cases of aneurysms can now be partially or completely occluded by either coil embolization or glue casting. Some AVMs and vascular tumors can now be temporarily (in preparation for microsurgical excision) or permanently embolized with resorbable particles, permanent coils, or casting glue. Endovascular applications of treatment for cerebrovascular disease have now expanded to include angioplasty and stenting for cervical and intracranial carotid, VA disease, and arterial dissections. Intraluminal chemical and mechanical cerebral angioplasty for post-SAH vasospasm, catheter-directed chemical thrombolysis, and endovascular embolus retrieval for stroke are also frequently performed.

CT Scanning

CT scans are the study of choice for neurosurgical emergencies, because they are readily available at most hospitals (even after hours), can be obtained very quickly, and provide a wealth of important information for emergent decision making. They can show bone more clearly than MRI and therefore are excellent when used in evaluating cases for skull fracture. They are very sensitive for detecting acute blood (which appears white), and are therefore useful in assessing patients for SAH, intraparenchymal hemorrhage, hemorrhagic stroke, spontaneous or posttraumatic extra-axial blood clot (**epidural** or **subdural hematoma**), or traumatic contusion. They show the ventricular system very well (hypodense) and thus aid in detecting communicating or obstructive hydrocephalus. They can show differentiation between ventricular system displacement and a space-occupying mass lesion. They are useful in detecting abnormal calcium deposits in a blood vessel or brain mass. They are moderately sensitive for detecting swelling or vasogenic edema surrounding a pathologic lesion. CT scan disadvantages include poorer resolution of parenchymal brain structures than MR scanning, less sensitivity for identifying brain tumors (even with intravenous contrast agents), and an inability to show an acute stroke (hypodensity can take 12–36 hours to develop on CT scans). Administration of iodine-based intravenous contrast dye improves the sensitivity of the CT scan for detecting brain tumors and areas of focal infection. Administration of dye into the CSF (CT cisternography) improves its ability to show lesions in the CSF compartments and detect CSF leaks. The development of CT angiography has been a major step forward in assessing suspected SAH for the presence of an aneurysm without the time delay and risks of more invasive cerebral angiography. CT angiography at many centers has now become so good that in some cases neurosurgeons are able to take patients directly to the operating room to clip an aneurysm microsurgically without ever performing a preoperative cerebral angiogram.

Magnetic Resonanc Imaging

MRI scans do not show bone well, and thus are inferior to CT scanning for assessing patients for fractures or osseus involvement of tumors or infection. Although MRI is very sensitive for detecting subacute or chronic bleeding, it is relatively insensitive compared with CT scanning for detecting acute bleeding and is therefore not the best study for ruling out acute hemorrhage or assessing acute head trauma.

MR scanning provides the best resolution of intracranial soft tissue. Gray matter, white matter distinctions, deep gray matter structures, major cerebral vessels, the meninges, the ventricular lining, and even cranial nerves are very well shown. Flow attenuated inversion-recover (FLAIR) sequences and long time-to-response (TR), or "T2-weighted," sequences provide excellent sensitivity to even small amounts of vasogenic cerebral edema or demyelination. Gradient response sequences with long TRs provide very good sensitivity to even small amounts of deposited extracellular blood products. Administration of contrast leads to significant improvements in sensitivity over contrast CT scanning for detecting meningeal, ventricular, or cranial nerve pathology, as well as brain tumors and areas of cerebritis and abscess. MRI diffusion studies can almost immediately detect the early cytotoxic edema associated with a stroke, well before the area becomes hypodense on CT scan. As a result, MRI scanning has become the diagnostic procedure of choice for both neuro-oncology and stroke neurology and for assessing patients for inflammatory lesions and multiple sclerosis. MR angiography also serves as an excellent noninvasive screening tool without iodine dye load for assessing patients for cerebral aneurysm, AVM, atherosclerotic cerebrovascular disease (both cervical and intracranial), and vascular dissection.

Further advances in MRI are rapidly progressing and have exciting potential for clinical neuroscience. High-field 3–tesla magnets have increased soft tissue resolution still further while allowing the high signal-to-noise ratios necessary to perform metabolic tissue sampling through single- and multivoxel MR spectroscopy (MRS). MRS is an excellent technique for distinguishing a mass lesion from tumor, radiation necrosis, infarction, or infection. It can also assess the likelihood of tumor invasion beyond imaging apparent tumor borders into surrounding normally appearing brain. Functional MR can localize sensory and motor speech areas as well as primary motor strip and determine their relationship and degree of direct involvement versus displacement in regard to adjacent mass lesions. Diffusion tensor imaging is a way of mapping the major CNS white matter association tracts (corpus callosum, side-to-side, superior and inferior longitudinal fasciculus, anterior-to-posterior, and the primary motor and sensory long tracts, rostral-to-caudal). It does this by detecting the integrity of selective movement of water within the parallel-oriented cleavage planes along these white matter tract connections. It has the potential for determining whether a mass lesion has invaded and disrupted these cleavage planes within the relevant tracts or merely compressed or displaced them (and if so, demonstrate where they are located relative to the lesion in question). All of this information is very important for clinical decision making and preoperative surgical planning.

Head Injury

Head injury is very common. In the United States, approximately 2 million people each year suffer a head injury and approximately 150,000 people per year become comatose from head injury. Annually, head injury accounts for approximately 1% to 2% of all deaths in the United States, 25% of all trauma-related deaths, and up to 60% of all motor vehicle-related deaths. Head injuries can be acute, subacute, or chronic. Acute head injuries include scalp lacerations, contusions, and abrasions, skull fractures (basal and cranial vault), CSF leakage, extraparenchymal hematomas (subdural and epidural hematomas), brain contusions and intraparenchymal hematomas, traumatic arterial dissection leading to SAH or stroke, and axonal connection shear injuries. Subacute and chronic problems include postconcussive syndrome, chronic subdural hematomas, persistent CSF leak, growing skull fracture, arteriovenous fistulae, infection from retained foreign body, hydrocephalus, posttraumatic epilepsy, and permanent cognitive and neurologic deficits. The initial postresuscitation GCS score is highly predictive of head injury. Patients with GCS scores of 3 to 4 on admission have a 50% to 100% mortality rate. Those with scores of 5 to 6 have a 25% to 65% mortality rate. Patients with scores of 7 to 8 have a 10% to 25% mortality rate. Older patients do worse than younger patients with the same GCS score. Patients who have acute subdural hematomas do worse than other patients with similar GCS scores without subdural hematomas.

Evaluation of Acute Injuries

Evaluation of an acutely head injured patient begins with a primary survey that focuses on the ABCs (airway, breathing, and circulation). Neurologic examination is not reliable or predictive until the patient has been stabilized from the standpoint of ventilation, hypoxemia, and circulatory shock. Careful note should be taken of the need to administer pharmacologic paralytic agents or sedatives during initial resuscitation, because these will significantly affect neurologic assessment. The neurologic assessment begins with a rapid initial survey that determines the patient's GCS score (Table 8-2), pupillary response, and the symmetry of motor and papillary findings on either side. The degree of impairment and the presence or absence of pending herniation syndrome determines the need to proceed immediately to CT scan for head examination versus the ability to proceed with a secondary neurologic survey before the CT scan. Often, portions outlined in this paragraph are assessed simultaneously or in parallel to save time and expedite the logistics of transport and imaging acquisition. If the patient has a GCS score of 12 or less, the operating room and anesthesiologist should probably be notified to be standing by for possible emergent craniotomy or ICP monitoring procedure.

During the secondary neurologic survey, a careful history from the emergency medical technicians is desirable. The mechanism of injury provides valuable information regarding associated injuries and severity of force transmission to the patient. Whether the patient had a safety belt on, whether the airbag deployed, the structural state of the car, the location the patient was found in the car, and whether the patient was ejected from the car (if the incident was a motor vehicle accident) is very useful information. Knowing whether the patient had a predisposing medical event (e.g., myocardial infarction, drug ingestion) and whether there was a period of hypotension, hypoxemia, or even cardiac arrest is very important. The timing of intubation, if required (in the field versus on arrival), may give valuable clues as to potential secondary hypoxemic injury. During this portion of the evaluation a more detailed systematic neurologic examination is obtained if the patient is conscious and cooperative. If the patient

is unconscious or sedated, cranial nerve reflexes (pupils, corneas, gag, and cough) are assessed. The scalp is assessed for signs of bleeding form laceration or abrasion, subgaleal hematoma, projectile wound, or palpable fractures. If an open wound is located, it is noted but is not probed or explored for fear of causing further bleeding and increasing the risk of infection. The patient's mastoid and periorbital areas are assessed for ecchymosis indicating basilar skull fracture (mastoid—Battle's sign; periorbital—raccoon eyes). The nose is assessed for signs of CSF rhinorrhea, and, if noted, the trauma surgeon or emergency room physician is instructed (a) to be careful with any subsequent bag-mask pressure ventilation for fear of introducing intracranial air and raising ICP due to ball-valve cranial air entry, and (b) not to insert a nasogastric tube if stomach decompression is required, but to decompress the stomach using an orogastric tube (danger of intracranial penetration by way of an anterior basal skull fracture). The ear canals are examined bilaterally for otorrhea, and the tympanic membranes are assessed for hemotympanum. If the patient is unconscious, has no signs of otorrhea, otorrhagia, or hemotympanum, and if sufficient time is available, caloric testing as an additional brain stem reflex test can be done. Given the risk of cervical spine injury in a patient with an acute head injury, oculocephalic reflex testing is usually deferred until ervical spine injury is excluded.

An unconscious patient should be assessed for history of loss of consciousness, as well as anterograde or retrograde amnesia, which correlate with degree and risk of concussion. Any patient with a history of head injury and a GCS score less than 13 should probably be assessed by CT scan if it is readily available. Patients with GCS score of 13 to 15 can be assessed with CT scan or observed for at least 23 hours (the time a patient can be held in the emergency department before that patient must be admitted to the hospital). Observation consists of repeated neurologic examinations every 2 hours, with a CT scan obtained rapidly if the patient worsens clinically. A patient with a history of a head injury, a GCS score of 15, and a normal neurologic examination has a normal CT scan of the head can probably be discharged home so long as the patient is returning to a stable social situation with an identified responsible adult who has been instructed in how to monitor and assess the patient for the next 23 hours. The patient should return to the hospital if there is hemiparesis, pupillary inequality, increase in headache, sleepiness, decrease in consciousness, or persistent vomiting.

Stabilization

If the patient is exhibiting clinical signs and symptoms of high ICP or herniation syndrome, acute temporizing medical measures to control ICP and maintain CPP should be instituted immediately. Acute or persistent elevations of ICP are treated as described in Table 8-3. Blood pressure and CPP need to be maintained with volume and systemic pressures. In severely injured patients, pharmacologic paralysis with muscle relaxants combined with con-

Table 8-3	Medical Treatment of Increased Intracranial Pressure
Method	**Treatment**
Osmotic diuretics	Mannitol 20%, 1 g/kg IV single dose or 0.25 g/kg every 8 hr as needed for repeated usage
Renal diuretics	Furosemide 1 mg/kg IV single dose or 0.25–0.5 mg/kg every 8 hr or more as needed
Maintain normovolemia[a]	IV infusion of crystalloid
Hyperventilation	P_{CO_2} 30–35 mm Hg
Elevation of the head	

[a]Some protocols favor normovolemia or even hypervolemia and hypertension rather than dehydration and normotension.

IV, intravenous

trolled respiration is necessary to prevent additional increases in ICP because of coughing and straining. Mannitol and furosemide given intravenously are effective in transiently lowering ICP and can be given if the patient's systemic blood pressure will allow. Hyperventilation does lower ICP, but at the expense of potential ischemia to already injured brain. It is therefore used only on a temporary basis in an acute herniation situation until the cause of the herniation can be identified and rectified or until the ICP can be lowered by pharmacologic or CSF drainage means. Even then, only temporary periods of moderate hyperventilation to CO_2 levels of 28 to 30 are recommended. Surgically correctable mass lesions identified on trauma CT scans require urgent neurosurgical intervention if the patient is neurologically compromised and the lesion is sufficiently large. Patients without major surgically reversible mass lesions on CT scan and who have GCS scores of 8 or less are candidates for invasive ICP monitoring as they continue to be treated with neurocritical care measures and assessed for changes in neurologic status by regular examination, ICP and CPP monitoring, and interval neuroimaging reassessment. Careful attention is paid to evaluating the patient's electrolyte status, serum osmolality, and coagulation status. Intravenous fluids are switched to normal saline from lactated Ringer's solution as soon as resuscitation of systemic shock is completed.

Once a patient is stabilized but does not improve over time despite normal ICP and CPP, consideration should be given to the possibility of concomitant global ischemic brain injury due to delay in transportation from the scene of injury, severe hypoxemia or hypotension before resuscitation initiation, or delay in some aspect of resuscitation (usually intubation). Another possibility is diffuse axonal shear injury with axonal connection breakage due to lateral shearing forces caused by rapid acceleration–deceleration of the head and intracranial contents. These shear injuries can sometimes be seen on cerebral MRI scans taken several days after the injury. On MRI, they appear to be multiple focal areas of high FLAIR or T2-weighted

signal or even multiple areas of petechial hemorrhage on T2-weighted gradient response sequences. They tend to localize to areas of maximal torquing forces (the upper brain stem and diencephalon) and to the point of maximal differential tissue shearing movement (the cortical gray matter–white matter interface). Both conditions leave the patient with a poor prognosis for functional recovery and eventual independence. Any recovery that does occur tends to take place over a long period of time (generally 6–18 months).

Intracranial Pressure Monitoring and Control

In general, monitoring of ICP is indicated for patients with a GCS score of 8 or less. ICP monitors usually take the form of either a ventriculostomy or an intraparenchymal fiberoptic pressure probe. A ventriculostomy consists of a percutaneous Silastic tube inserted through a burr hole in the skull that courses through the brain tissue to the lateral ventricle. The tube provides a continuous column of fluid from the ventricular CSF to an external drainage system and can be transduced like an arterial line. A ventriculostomy is the preferred means of ICP monitoring because it is therapeutic at the same time that it provides the necessary ICP data. Given the conditions of the Monroe-Kellie hypothesis, outlined previously, nothing reduces ICP faster or more effectively than actual CSF drainage. Unfortunately, some ventricular systems are too small to safely intubate, and ventricular chambers can collapse to the point where the ventriculostomy no longer effectively transduces pressure. There are also borderline situations in which the need for ICP monitoring is equivocal or uncertain. In these situations, an intraparenchymal fiberoptic ICP monitor is another option. It provides accurate readings of ICP. However, it cannot drain CSF and becomes increasingly less accurate over time due to zero baseline "drift," which can gradually lead to inaccuracies of approximately 5 mm Hg over the course of 5 to 10 days. With the ICP known and tracked, the actual CPP for the patient can be determined at any given time (CPP = MAP – ICP), and adjustments made to maintain it on a running basis.

Acute or persistent elevations of ICP are treated as described in Table 8-3. Once CT scanning has ruled out the presence of an acutely reversible surgical mass lesion, and other measures have had a chance to take effect, hyperventilation to even moderate degrees is avoided whenever possible, to prevent secondary ischemic CNS injury. The mainstay of ICP management in the acute head injury situation is CSF drainage through a ventriculostomy. In the presence of reduced brain compliance, even intermittent removal of volumes as small as 1 to 2 mL can have a dramatic and sustained ICP reduction effect. Mannitol is given in intermittent intravenous boluses of 0.125 to 0.25 g/kg (usually 12.5–25 g at a time) every 4 to 6 hours as needed, taking care to follow serum osmolality closely (not allowing it to rise above 315 mOsm/L). The ICP-reducing effects of mannitol can be accentuated by premedication with small intravenous doses of furosemide

(10–20 mg/bolus) given 5 to 10 minutes before the mannitol dose. Intravenous infusion sedation with an agent that is short-acting and that can be quickly stopped to allow for neurologic examination (e.g., fentanyl or propofol) will reduce the incidence of struggling against the ventilator, endotracheal tube, or other Valsalva maneuvers, and thus help keep ICP down. Both intravenous sedation and pharmacologic paralysis will reduce muscular tone, thereby increasing venous return from the head and reducing CO_2 production from muscle contractions, all of which will help with ICP control. Physiologic levels (up to 5 mm Hg) of positive end expiratory pressure (PEEP) are not likely to have major negative effects on cerebral venous return and ICP, but higher levels of PEEP should be avoided when possible. Serum sodium needs to be carefully monitored because SIADH and resulting hyponatremia can accentuate cerebral edema and ICP problems. Maintenance fluids should consist of normal saline solution with consideration given to judicious use of intravenous 3% NaCl solution if SIADH is confirmed by urine sodium measurement in the presence of low serum sodium (<135 mEq/L) and elevated ICP. When all else fails, induction of barbiturate coma by bolus injection, followed by continuous infusion, is sometimes necessary. When utilized, the minimum infusion necessary to maintain electrical activity burst-suppression should be confirmed by electroencephalogram (EEG). Induction of barbiturate coma must be considered carefully because it tends to lead to hypothermia, systemic hypotension due to cardiac suppression (which fights against CPP maintenance efforts), and impaired pulmonary ciliary function, which leaves patients susceptible to pneumonia. It also can take some time to wear off.

Cerebral Perfusion Pressure, Tissue Metabolism, Glucose, and Oxygenation

In general, under normal autoregulatory conditions, CBF is not impaired with normal ICP down to MAP as low as 40 mm Hg (CPP ~30–32 mm Hg). Even within the globally high ICP situation of pseudotumor cerebri (in which ICP is routinely 27–34 mm Hg), the brain functions normally with a CPP of approximately 36 to 43 mm Hg. However, in head injury, cerebral autoregulation has been shown to be dysfunctional and impaired both globally and in the microenvironment at the site of injury so that CBF can become directly dependent on CPP. Although normal CPP is 50 to 60 mm Hg, in the setting of head injury a desirable target is a minimum CPP of 60 to 70 mm Hg. CPP is maintained by ensuring adequate cardiac preload (CVP 8–10 mm Hg, or pulmonary artery wedge [PAW] pressure 12–15 mm Hg) without volume overload (which could accentuate cerebral edema). Early use of systemic vasopressors is implemented once preload is optimized if a CPP of 60 to 70 mm Hg is not spontaneously achievable. Dopamine has the added advantage of dilating cerebral surface collateral vessels; however, epinephrine or norepinephrine can also be used and may need to be used if dopamine is insufficient.

Another important consideration for maintaining tissue function in the presence of marginal CBF nutrient supply is neuronal metabolic demand. Theoretically, a high metabolic demand situation should lead to greater supply–demand mismatch and potential neuronal injury in the setting of marginal nutrient supply. Given this theoretical observation, efforts are made to control and treat fevers, because elevated temperature increases metabolic demand. Phenytoin is given to prevent seizures, which can markedly increase neuronal metabolic demand and increase ICP. Attempts to purposefully reduce metabolic demand through therapeutic moderate hypothermia have been tried, but have yet to demonstrate improved survival or outcome for major head injury. In addition to reducing ICP, pharmacologically induced barbiturate coma has the added benefit of potentially reducing neuronal metabolic demand and may provide some biochemical free-radical scavenging role at potential sites of continued injury.

In experimental models of CNS ischemia, elevated serum glucose levels before ischemic injury are positively correlated with larger subsequent strokes and worse neurologic outcome. Given the potential role of subsequent ischemia as a major mechanism for secondary CNS injury, glucose levels are carefully controlled and monitored in the patient with head injury. For the first 24 to 48 hours, normal saline solution maintenance fluids do not contain dextrose and the serum glucose level is tightly controlled, even if an insulin infusion is required. This level of tight glucose control continues even after nutrition has been started for the patient and 5% dextrose returned to the intravenous solutions.

Early data suggest that fiberoptic tissue oxygenation probes may prove useful in the management of patients with severe head injury. These fiberoptic probes continuously monitor the extracellular tissue oxygen tension and can be inserted through the same burr hole as a fiberoptic ICP monitor. Responding to low oxygen tension readings with increasing FiO_2 has been shown to improve cerebral tissue oxygen tension. Furthermore, it is possible that luxurious cerebral tissue oxygen tension measurements may help identify cases in which moderate hyperventilation (CO_2 28–32) may potentially be safely performed, if necessary, to reduce ICP without risking secondary ischemic injury. It should be remembered, however, that these O_2 tissue tension monitors only measure local microenvironment oxygenation, which may not reflect oxygenation status at the site of primary and potential secondary injury. Their use has yet to be correlated with improved survival or neurologic outcome from head injury. Other tissue parenchymal monitors such as microdialysis monitors that can measure and follow tissue lactate and amino acid levels are currently being utilized as part of clinical experimental protocols in studying head injury, but have yet to achieve a defined clinical role.

Closed Head Injury

Closed head injury (CHI) describes conditions in which the intradural contents of the cranium are not exposed to the outside environment and are not herniating out through a traumatic cranial defect. CSF leak from a basilar skull fracture is one exception that is still considered a CHI. In the civilian sector, and certainly in times of peace, CHI is the dominant form of head injury seen in the U.S. health care system.

Concussion

Concussion is a clinical syndrome of temporary global brain dysfunction that can be inferred from a history of brief loss of consciousness or a period of anterograde or retrograde amnesia surrounding a CHI. A patient with a history suggestive of a concussion and a history of head injury with a GCS score of 13 to 15 is classified as having a minor closed head injury. Very few of these patients, if imaged, will be found to have a pathologic lesion on CT scan, and the vast majority of these will be nonsurgical in consequence. A concussion does, however, imply significant force transmission to, and absorption by, the brain. Given the delicacy of the CNS, it is not surprising that many of these patients will continue to have annoying symptoms for weeks to months (occasionally for up to 6–12 months after injury) until they finally resolve. The condition is known as postconcussive syndrome. To prevent unwarranted anxiety in patients and assist them in coping with it, counseling should be offered regarding the likelihood of syndrome symptoms. These symptoms include persistent recurring headaches, difficulty concentrating, reduced attention span, short-term memory and learning dysfunction, disturbance in normal wake–sleep rhythms, social disinhibition, emotional lability, depression, and social withdrawal. These symptoms tend to be self-limited and usually resolve given sufficient time.

Closed Skull Fractures

Skull fractures can occur in the skull base or the cranial vault. Skull base fractures involving the anterior cranial fossa may manifest with unilateral or bilateral periorbital swelling and ecchymosis (raccoon eyes). If they involve the orbit roof, floor, and walls, vision acuity and extraocular movements should be carefully checked to rule out extraocular muscle entrapment by the bone fragments. Involvement of the posterior wall of the frontal sinus, cribriform plate, or planum sphenoidale, could indicate risk of early or delayed anterior CSF leak. Anterior cranial fossa skull-base fracture is a relative contraindication for positive pressure bag-mask ventilation and for nasogastric tube placement. The potential risks are intracranial air introduction, elevation in ICP if introduced air cannot subsequently escape (ball-valve mechanism), and intracranial passage of the gastric tube. Basal skull fractures involving the middle cranial fossa are at risk for damaging the ICA in its parasellar/cavernous sinus location. Fractures that extend through the petrous carotid canal exit into the cavernous sinus, or lateral sphenoid sinus wall fractures with sphenoid sinus air-fluid levels may warrant further investigation with CT angiography, MR angiography, or conventional cerebral angiogram. Fractures of the temporal bone can lead to

CSF leak through the tympanic membrane (otorrhea) or down the back of the throat via the middle ear and eustachian tube. Visualization of fluid within the mastoid air cells on CT scan should lead to careful search for a temporal bone fracture. Horizontal temporal bone fractures run parallel to the course of the internal auditory canal. Although they can cause CSF leak, they rarely cause cranial nerve dysfunction. Transverse temporal bone fractures run perpendicular to the course of the internal auditory canal. They imply a much larger transmission of force to the skull base and are much more likely than horizontal fractures to be associated with facial, vestibular, and cochlear nerve dysfunction. They are also occasionally associated with mechanical disruption of the middle ear ossicles. Every patient with a temporal bone fracture should be carefully evaluated for facial nerve function, nystagmus, and hearing loss, as well as CSF leak. Fractures that extend through the petrous carotid canal of the temporal bone may warrant further investigation to rule out ICA injury with CT angiography, MR angiography, or conventional cerebral angiogram (see Chapter 5).

Cranial vault fractures can be linear or comminuted (several fragments). They can be diastatic (gap between the fracture edges) or even depressed. Closed cranial vault fractures require surgical exploration only if they are depressed and the depression is greater than the cross-sectional width of the skull (unlikely to heal cosmetically through remodeling alone), if they occur in a cosmetically obvious area (e.g., forehead), if they are associated with an underlying mass lesion that needs to be excised, or are associated with an area of intracranial air suggesting dural penetration. Diastatic fractures in very young children can lead to a special situation called a growing skull fracture. In this situation, dura gets trapped between the edges of the skull fracture and begins to act as a new skull growth plate, preventing proper healing and promoting further diastasis. Growing skull fractures are detected with a 4- to 6-week follow-up skull x-ray and require surgical exploration.

Subdural Hematomas

Subdural hematomas can be acute, subacute, or chronic. Acute subdural hematomas can be spontaneous or traumatic. Subdural hematomas occur between the arachnoid of the brain and the dura of the meninges (Fig. 8-6). They are hyperdense on CT scans (white) due to the presence of fresh blood. On CT scan, they appear to follow the curve of the hemispheric surface like the rind of a watermelon. Spontaneous subdurals usually occur because of tearing of a parasagittal bridging vein due to shearing forces associated with even minor CHIs or cerebral acceleration–deceleration. They are more common in elderly patients who have an accentuated distance between their brain and dura due to cerebral atrophy. They are also more common in patients taking anticoagulant medications (e.g., warfarin, aspirin, dipyridamole, clopidogrel bisulfate). Post-traumatic subdural hematomas are usually associated with an underlying cortical brain injury (e.g., cortical laceration

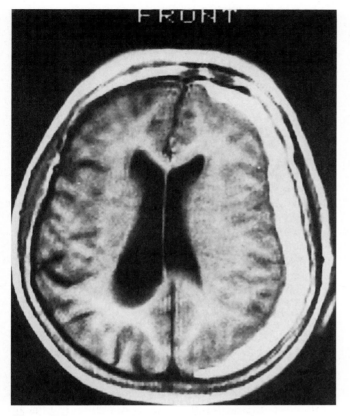

Figure 8-6 Magnetic resonance imaging scan of a subacute subdural hematoma.

or contusion). As a result, they can be either venous, arterial, or mixed in origin. They carry a significantly worse prognosis than their spontaneous counterparts. Not all subdural hematomas require surgical evacuation. If they are small enough (e.g., <30 mL volume) and the patient is doing well clinically, the patient can be treated conservatively with careful follow-up, neurologic examination, and serial CT scanning. The majority of subdural hematomas will naturally resorb.

Within 7 to 14 days the RBCs in the clot begin to lyse and the hematoma may appear as a mixed density mass or even isodense compared with brain. At this subacute stage, the hematoma can sometimes be difficult to see on CT scan, but its presence can usually be detected with careful image windowing, inferred from unilateral loss of gyral surface pattern, or inferred by mass effect on the ipsilateral lateral ventricular. If the hematoma has not been absorbed by approximately 4 to 6 weeks after formation, the body will have walled it off by forming an enclosing membrane of fragile neovascularity, which can easily rebleed with minor trauma. The clot itself is fully lysed, is liquid in consistency (either straw-colored fluid or crank-case-oil appearance grossly, depending on age), and can usually be effectively drained through one or two burr holes.

Epidural Hematomas

Epidural hematomas are acute in origin. They occur between the skull and the dura (Fig. 8-5). They are usually associated with adjacent skull fractures. On CT scan they tend to appear biconvex (lenticular) in shape because they can only extend to the next point of dura attachment to the cranial vault (usually a suture line, i.e., coronal or squamosal suture). In adults, fractures of the temporal squama are worrisome because they can be associated with epidural hematomas from damage to the MMA. Given the size of the artery involved and the direct lateral vector the associated clot places on the supratentorial temporal lobe, they are at great risk for rapid enlargement (even in a delayed fashion in a normal-appearing patient) and early herniation syndrome. Fractures in other locations and fractures in the vascular calvarium of children more commonly lead to venous epidural hematomas. Not all epidural hematomas require surgical evacuation. If they are small enough (e.g., <30 mL volume), the patient is doing well clinically. If the location and skull fracture do not suggest MMA involvement, they can be followed conservatively with careful neurologic examination and serial CT scanning. The majority will go on to naturally resorb. Given the fact that the dura remains intact as a protective layer and the fact that they are not routinely associated with underlying direct brain, epidural hematomas carry a much better prognosis than subdural hematomas of the same size and location.

Contusions and Intraparenchymal Hematomas

Cerebral contusions are literally tissue bruises of the brain. Following acceleration–deceleration forces, they tend to occur on the inferior surface of the brain (inferior frontal lobes and inferior temporal lobes) due to abrasion of the brain against the irregular anterior cranial fossa and middle cranial fossa bony floor. The rapid acceleration–deceleration forces lead to translational brain movements within the CSF-filled cranial cavity. The forces also tend to act on the anterior poles of the brain (frontal pole, temporal pole, and occipital pole), as these surfaces impact against the inner surface of the cranium during the same translational brain movements. With direct blows to the head, they can occur directly underneath the point of impact (coup injury) as a result of overlying skull fracture or transmission of percussive force. Coup injuries are often associated with contracoup injuries involving the brain on the opposite side of the head. Injury occurs when that opposite area is suddenly translated against the inner skull surface as a result of translational brain movement or a fall to that side, leading to a second cranial impact on the opposite side. If the contusion is associated with disruption of a moderately large tissue blood vessel, a frank intraparenchymal hematoma can develop. Contusions can also lead to brain tissue homogenation and are thus at risk for causing coagulopathy from tissue thromboplastin release, which can lead to conversion of a contusion into a hematoma or enlargement of the contusion. Most contusions can be managed conservatively without operation, and smaller traumatic hematomas can also be managed conservatively so long as the patient does not have a coagulopathy and is doing well clinically. Most contusions and intraparenchymal hematomas warrant a follow-up CT scan 12 to 24 hours later to rule out lesion evolution or enlargement.

Vascular Dissection, Stroke, and Carotid-Cavernous fistula

Arterial dissection can occur in the cervical segments of the ICA or VA or in the course of the ICA through the skull base to enter the dura. Cervical ICA traumatic dissections are associated with sudden neck acceleration–deceleration movements and are more common in children than adults. Skull-base ICA dissections are associated with basal skull fractures that traverse the petrous canal of the ICA, the lateral wall of the sphenoid sinus, or the anterior clinoid process. Cervical VA dissections are associated with sudden acceleration–deceleration neck movements (e.g., manual cervical manipulation), as well as cervical fractures that extend through the transverse processes of C2–C6. Extradural arterial dissection can extend up to the intradural penetration of the ICA (near the anterior clinoid process up to the ophthalmic artery take-off) or the intradural portion of the VA (up to the take-off of the PICA). In either case, if the false intramural lumen dissects outward through the adventitia instead of ending in a blind alley, a traumatic basal arterial cistern SAH can occur. This can sometimes be confused with an aneurysmal SAH if the initial neck injury history was not obvious. A more common end point for arterial dissection is either partial lumen obstruction with a raised intimal flap or complete vessel occlusion. From a CBF standpoint, depending on the status of the patient's collateral cerebral circulation potential, this occlusion can be immediately symptomatic, symptomatic in a delayed fashion with subsequent episodes of dehydration or hypotension, or remain completely asymptomatic. Both vessel occlusion and intimal flap elevation can also lead to symptoms from distal embolization. Typically, this occurs in a delayed fashion (usually 12 to 48 hours after initial injury). Occasionally, patients with cervical or petrous ICA dissections will manifest clinically with an ipsilateral Horner's syndrome (ipsilateral miosis, mild ptosis, and facial anhydrosis). A search for vascular dissection by CT angiography, MR angiography, or cerebral angiography should be considered in a trauma patient with Horner's syndrome, with neurologic deficits out of proportion to the damage seen on CT scan, with high-risk basal skull fractures as described above, or with cervical fractures through the transverse foramen. It should also be considered in a patient who experiences a sudden, severe neurologic deficit in a delayed fashion. Treatment of incomplete dissections includes endovascular stenting or endovascular permanent arterial occlusion, if tolerated. Preexisting occlusions with embolization are treated with anticoagulation, if other associated injuries permit. Preexisting occlusions with inadequate CBF are treated with vascular bypass grafting.

In addition to SAH or dissection leading to flow-related or embolic stroke, ICA injury in the cavernous sinus can lead to a carotid-cavernous fistula, where arterial blood empties directly into the cavernous sinus venous spaces. This can occur acutely or in a delayed fashion, days to weeks after injury. This condition leads to injection and chemosis of the conjunctiva, pulsating exophthalmos with a bruit, elevated intraocular pressure from venous congestion, and cranial nerve dysfunction (e.g., ptosis, diplopia, ophthalmoplegia, visual loss). Treatment is usually endovascular embolization by an arterial or venous route.

Pediatric Shaken-Whiplash Syndrome

Infants and very young children have very large heads relative to their body size, have poor cervical basal muscular tone to resist rapid flexion–extension or lateral flexion stress forces, and have soft brains due to incomplete myelination. Their brains are thus susceptible to injury when impacted against rigid dural reflections. Thus, infants and very small children are susceptible to major CHI as a result of degrees of physical shaking that would not affect older children or adults. Infants and very young children also have unfused skulls that allow for cranial expansion to temporarily accommodate rising ICP, allowing the syndrome to progress to full maturation before brain stem dysfunction. Infants and very small children with shaken-whiplash syndrome usually present with listlessness and respiratory suppression; signs of external injury may be minimal or absent. Funduscopic examination usually reveals retinal hemorrhages. The fontanelle is usually full and tense. CT scan often shows SAH, subdural hematomas, diffuse cerebral edema, and major vascular distribution hypodensities from infarctions. This pattern of injury is evidence of child abuse until proven otherwise. The proper authorities should be notified and a proper investigation initiated. Prognosis is extremely poor despite aggressive measures.

Penetrating Head Injury

Penetrating head injury includes open skull fractures and projectile injuries. They are much more common in military conflicts than in peacetime and more common in urban than suburban or rural civilian settings.

Open Skull Fractures

Open skull fractures require operative exploration if they are associated with brain herniation, significant underlying hematoma or other surgical mass lesion, CSF leak, localized intracranial air on CT scan, or fragments of bone driven into the brain or if they are significantly depressed. The goal in these explorations is to restore dural integrity, debride intraparenchymal foreign bodies, deal with any associated brain injury or intracranial hematoma, and repair depressed or comminuted skull fractures. Simpler open skull fractures can be treated with local irrigation, antibiotics, and scalp closure in layers in the emergency department.

Cerebral Gunshot Wounds and Other Projectile Injuries

Cerebral gunshot wounds (GSWs) can be very serious injuries. Indicators of a very poor outcome even with surgical intervention include a GCS score of 8 or less, as well as bihemispheric involvement, transventricular passage, multilobar dominant hemisphere involvement, and brain stem involvement. These injuries often involve tremendous energy transmission to the brain, often associated with extensive cavitation and homogenation of brain tissue. They are also associated with a high incidence of DIC and coagulopathy. The decision whether to explore surgically is based on the patient's age, neurologic status, and extent of anatomic damage. Goals of surgery include obtaining hemostasis, debriding obviously dead brain and hematomas, removing superficial and readily accessible bone fragments, and restoring dural integrity. Deeper explorations in an attempt to retrieve additional bone fragments or the bullet itself will not reduce the incidence of subsequent infection or posttraumatic seizures, may cause further brain damage, and are no longer generally recommended. The patient is treated with intravenous antibiotics and anticonvulsants.

A GSW is caused by high-velocity projectiles with tremendous force transmission ($E = MV^2$). Shrapnel fragments or other foreign body projectiles may or may not have a larger mass than a bullet, but they usually are not traveling at as great a velocity. As a result, the prognosis for patients injured with these projectiles is generally better than those with cerebral GSWs, and the surgical outcomes are usually better as well. The surgical principles and goals remain the same

Traumatic Cerebrospinal Fluid Leak

Traumatic CSF leaks associated with open cranial injuries usually require surgical exploration for debridement and dural closure. CSF leaks associated with basilar skull fractures are another matter. These patients are kept on bed rest with their head elevated to 30 to 45 degrees. Most of these CSF leaks will spontaneously cease and heal within 3 to 5 days. If they do not, a trial of lumbar drainage may allow the major subset of the remainder to go on to heal without surgery. Prophylactic antibiotics to prevent meningitis have not been shown to be effective and may select for resistant organisms. If the patient develops a fever, an LP is performed if safe according to associated injuries, and antibiotics started only after the CSF culture has been sent to the laboratory. Broad-spectrum antibiotics are tailored by organism identification and antibiotic sensitivities once they are known. Only those who fail conservative management acutely or because of delayed recurrent CSF leak require surgery to repair the defect. Goals of surgery include restoration of dural integrity with dural patch grafting and treatment of any predisposing hydrocephalus that may be present. Skull-base surgical techniques including vascularized, pedicled, pericranial grafts (for anterior cranial fossa leaks), endoscopic or microscopic trans-sphenoidal approaches (for sphenoid sinus leaks), or transmastoid temporal bone approaches (for temporal bone origin leaks) are often the most effective. Preoperative precise definition of the probable leak site by CT cisternography can be most helpful.

Scalp Lacerations

The scalp is very vascular, and scalp lacerations can lead to significant blood loss, particularly in children. All scalp blood vessels lie between the galea and the dermis. As a result, scalp bleeding can be easily controlled by placing the galea under tension by grasping it with a hemostat or a suture. Scalp lacerations require generous irrigation, occasional debridement, and careful closure. The scalp may be closed in a single layer. However, placing a few interrupted absorbable stitches to reapproximate the galea before closing the skin controls scalp bleeding, takes the tension off the epithelial closure, and leads to a more cosmetically acceptable scar.

Long-Term Residua

The potential residua of head injury include motor deficits (an early clue to ultimate functional independence), cognitive deficits, behavioral changes, and emotional problems. Traumatic brain injury rehabilitation, including cognitive rehabilitation and vocational retraining, offers some hope and promise. Pharmacologic therapy with amitriptyline, β-blockers, or bromocriptine may assist with behavioral and affect issues. Rehabilitation has been shown to progress faster if the patient can be weaned off anticonvulsants within 2 to 8 weeks of the initial injury. Family group counseling and couples marriage counseling and support may help during the process, as well as once the situation has become stable. However, even subtle cognitive and personality changes may be sufficient to interfere with employment, social activities, and relationships. The effect on productivity, disability, and societal financial support of major CHI is profound.

Brain Attack and Cerebrovascular Disease

"Stroke" is a term that reflects a sudden ictus (being struck down). Strokes are sudden cerebrovascular events that can be classified as ischemic infarction or intracerebral hemorrhage (ICH). ICH can be further divided into spontaneous intraparenchymal hemorrhage (IPH) and SAH. Ischemic infarction is the most severe and permanent form of symptomatic atherosclerotic cerebrovascular disease that also includes transient ischemic attacks (TIAs—reversible ischemic neurologic deficit lasting <24 hours) and reversible ischemic neurologic deficits (RINDs—transient focal neurologic deficits that last more than 1 day but less than 1 week). Risk factors for cerebral atherosclerotic disease include family history, hypertension, smoking, diabetes mellitus, and hyperlipidemia. Risk factors for IPH include hypertension, drug use (especially cocaine and methamphetamine), dementia, and coagulopathy. Risk factors for aneurysmal SAH include family history and prior history of a berry aneurysm.

Transient Ischemic Attacks

TIAs often precede the onset of permanent ischemic stroke, and they can serve as a warning sign to allow intervention to prevent a stroke. Seventy percent of TIAs last less than 10 minutes. Common symptoms include transient monocular visual obscuration (amaurosis fugax), unilateral motor weakness, unilateral sensory paresthesias or numbness, or speech deficit. Most TIAs result from either artery-to-artery emboli or cardiac origin emboli. The most common source of artery-to-artery emboli is an atherosclerotic plaque at the carotid bifurcation. The MCA distribution is the one most commonly affected by both TIAs and ischemic infarctions. Patients with TIAs should be assessed for carotid bruits (2% per year stroke risk with a symptomatic carotid bruit, 0.1% to 0.4% annual stroke risk for an asymptomatic carotid bruit). Their superficial temporal artery (STA) pulses should be assessed for asymmetry (increased STA pulse may indicate near occlusion of the ipsilateral ICA). Funduscopic examination should be done to assess for cholesterol plaques and central retinal artery occlusion. They should also be assessed for treatable cerebral atherosclerotic risk factors. In general, the risk of cerebral ischemic infarction after a TIA is approximately 5% per year. Rapid repetitive or clustering of TIAs (crescendo TIAs) is a particularly risky and ominous situation that should lead to aggressive search for a treatable source with consideration given to anticoagulation with heparin until the workup can be completed. Initial workup for cause should include cervical carotid imaging (carotid duplex ultrasonography, MR angiography, CT angiography, or cerebral angiography), 12-lead electrocardiogram (ECG), 24-hour Holter monitoring, and echocardiography (transesophageal is superior to transthoracic). A vascular coagulopathy panel, lipid screening panel, and basic screening studies to assess for arteritis should be considered.

Surgery should be considered in patients with ICA distribution or minor completed strokes, with 70% or greater stenosis of the internal carotid artery or a deeply ulcerated plaque carotid endarterectomy (CEA) (see Chapter 23 in Lawrence's *Essentials of General Surgery*, 4th ed). The patient should have no other major health problems, and the surgeon should have combined morbidity and mortality rates with angiography and surgery of less than 5%. If the patient was initially diagnosed by less invasive screening studies, the actual degree of stenosis should be confirmed by cerebral angiography. Prospective randomized studies have shown that patients with TIAs and 70% or greater ipsilateral internal carotid stenosis have much lower stroke and mortality rates after endarterectomy than those treated medically. The results are less impressive in asymptomatic patients. Occlusions are not usually correctable. More recently, encouraging results have been reported for endovascular angioplasty and stenting to treat patients with ICA distribution TIAs and critical ICA steno-

sis. Angioplasty and stenting have yet to show results equivalent to those of CEA, but can be considered in symptomatic patients with major medical problems or at high risk for stroke with CEA due to cerebral collateral circulation deficiencies. Endovascular angioplasty and stenting can also be considered for intracranial artery-to-artery embolic sources, although the procedure is riskier in these locations, particularly in the posterior circulation.

Ischemic Infarction

Ischemic infarction can occur from loss of CBF due to cervical ICA or VA occlusion or cerebral embolus. Embolic infarction is overwhelmingly more common and can occur from artery-to-artery emboli (carotid bifurcation is the most common source), a primary cardiac source (due to atrial fibrillation, postmyocardial infarction mural thrombus, or cardiac valvular disease), or transmission of a venous emboli resulting from deep venous thrombosis through a patent foramen ovale. Small, flow-related strokes can occur from progressive hypertension-related arteriolar sclerosis affecting the small perforating end arteries of the diencephalon (basal ganglia, thalamus, and internal capsule), brain stem, and deep cerebellar nuclei. These lacunar strokes can be either silent or surprisingly symptomatic given their small size relative to the eloquence and redundancy of function of the deep cerebral areas affected. Unlike ICH patients, who usually present with sudden-onset headache with or without alteration of consciousness, nausea, or vomiting, patients with ischemic infarction usually present with rapid onset of neurologic deficit, with little or no headache and only rarely effects on the level of consciousness. CT scan may appear normal and is primarily obtained to rule out ICH or hemorrhagic conversion of an ischemic infarction, but MRI will show a diffusion defect in the area of intracellular cytotoxic edema. Medical workup is similar to that described for TIAs.

If the patient has an appropriate neurologic assessment, does not show blood on the CT scan, and presents for initiation of therapy within 3 hours of ictus, intravenous tissue plasminogen activator (TPA) has been shown in prospective randomized clinical trials to improve patient neurologic outcome with a finite but acceptable risk of ICH. For selective endovascular delivery of thrombolytics, this 3-hour therapeutic window can be extended to 6 hours for ICA distribution emboli or thrombosis and to 12 to 24 hours for posterior circulation vertebrobasilar disease.

A completed ischemic infarction contains a central area of irreversibly dead brain surrounded by an ischemic penumbra region of brain with persisting marginal CBF. This ischemic penumbra region is susceptible to secondary ischemic injury with subsequent stroke enlargement if blood flow is not maintained to this region. Thus, overly strict blood pressure control is generally unwise in the setting of ischemic infarction, particularly for a patient whose brain is used to basal levels of hypertension. Generally, as long as coagulopathy is not present, and the spontaneous pressure levels are not malignant (roughly ≥200 mm Hg systolic), blood pressure should be allowed to seek its own desired level and hypotension should be avoided and treated.

The early mortality rate from completed and irreversible ischemic infarction is generally less than 20%, but can be as high as 33% for complete MCA distribution infarctions and as high as 50% for complete ICA distribution (ACA + MCA) infarctions. Death in these large strokes is usually from progressive edema, mass effect, elevated ICP, and herniation syndrome. Maximal edema and risk of death generally peaks 3 to 5 days after the initial event. Decompressive craniectomy can be a lifesaving measure in these situations. All the previously mentioned methods of dealing with elevated ICP are employed.

Intraparenchymal Hemorrhage

IPH can result from hypertensive arteriolar disease, amyloid angiopathy, drug abuse, coagulopathy, AVM rupture, hemorrhage into a brain tumor, cerebral infection, or vasculitis. Hypertension, amyloid angiopathy, and drug abuse (especially cocaine and methamphetamine) are currently the most common causes. IPH usually presents with symptoms of headache, with nausea or vomiting associated with a sudden new neurologic deficit. Level of consciousness is much more likely to be affected in these patients than in patients with ischemic infarctions. The mortality rate for IPH is much higher than that for ischemic infarction and currently exceeds 50%, despite aggressive efforts at intervention.

Hypertensive Hemorrhage

Hypertensive hemorrhage typically occurs in patients with a prior history of hypertension. Patients usually have systolic blood pressures of 190 mm Hg or higher (often ≥200 mm Hg systolic). Common locations for hypertensive hemorrhage parallel the locations for lacunar infarctions and include, in decreasing order of frequency, the basal ganglia (putamen most common), thalamus, brain stem, deep cerebellar nuclei, and deep hemispheric white matter. Multiple prospective randomized clinical trials, including the recent STICH trial, have shown that the neurologic damage is done by the tissue trauma caused by the initial hemorrhage, and that routine surgical primary clot evacuation does not improve neurologic outcome or survival. Generally, most neurosurgeons currently reserve primary clot surgical evacuation for three special circumstances: (a) when the clot is in the cerebellum and is large enough to cause direct brain stem compression, as well as obstructive hydrocephalus; (b) when the patient has a normal level of consciousness, deteriorates while an inpatient, and can be in the operating room with surgery initiated in less than an hour; and (c) younger, healthier patients with good neurologic function who present with clots 300 mL or greater in volume. Short of primary clot evacuation, surgical insertion of a ventriculostomy is often indicated to relieve or prevent obstructive hydrocephalus

in cases of smaller cerebellar clots and cases of IPH with intraventricular extension and to serve as an ICP monitor to guide best medical therapy. Unlike in ischemic infarctions, there is no significant at-risk ischemic penumbra area surrounding the IPH. The major risk is of clot enlargement through rebleeding. Thus, careful blood pressure control with titrated intravenous dinfusions and strict control of coagulopathy are critical steps. Encouraging preliminary results are also being reported for using concentrated recombinant factor VII as a means of preventing clot enlargement over the first 24 to 48 hours after presentation.

Amyloid Angiopathy

Amyloid angiopathy is a vasculopathy characterized by fragile cerebral arteries due to amyloid protein deposition in the vessel wall, which appears as apple-green birefringence with polarized light under the microscope. It predominantly occurs in the elderly and is positively associated with Alzheimer's disease. Indeed, at least 50% of patients with amyloid angiopathy IPH have a prior history of symptomatic dementia. Amyloid hemorrhages tend to be subcortical and lobar in location. The parietal lobe at the parietal-occipital junction is most common followed by the frontal lobe. The hemorrhages can be quite large, but are often remarkably well tolerated because of preexisting cerebral atrophy. Surgical intervention is generally reserved for clots 30 mL or greater in patients with good neurologic condition. The best functional outcomes are achieved in patients who have clots in the nondominant hemisphere but who do not have any baseline dementia. Given the underlying vasculopathy present throughout the brain, it should not be surprising that amyloid hemorrhage resection cavities carry a much higher recurrent hemorrhage risk than other surgical resection cavities.

Arteriovenous Malformations

AVMs are usually congenital. They consist of multiple arteriovenous communications that form a knot of feeding arteries and draining veins within brain tissue (Fig. 8-7). Because of the abnormal structure of the vessel walls and the direct communication between the feeding and draining vessels, clinical signs of rupture are common. The second most common presenting symptom is seizure. Bleeding is typically intraparenchymal rather than subarachnoid and is approximately 2% to 3% per year for typical AVMs. Hemorrhage usually occurs from the thinner walled venous portion of the malformation that still contains arterial pressure blood. AVMs with accentuated risks of hemorrhage include those with venous outflow obstruction and those with associated feeding artery aneurysms. Potentially curative treatment includes tightly focused and stereotactically delivered, single high-dose radiation (**stereotactic** radiosurgery), or microsurgical excision, and, rarely, endovascular embolization. Surgical morbidity and mortality for AVMs is related to size of the lesion, the eloquence of the brain involved, and the presence or absence of deep venous drainage to the vascular nidus. SR leads to myointimal cell proliferation on the

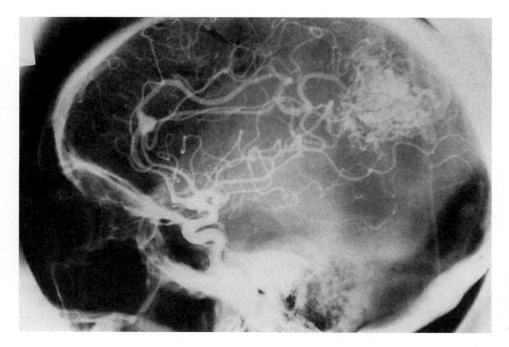

Figure 8-7 Lateral angiogram of a parietal arteriovenous malformation. An aneurysm is located proximally on an enlarged feeding vessel.

vascular channel walls, eventually leading to complete nidus occlusion in approximately 75% to 80% of cases over a period of 3 years. Endovascular embolization of AVMs is only rarely curative. It can, however, serve a temporizing protective role against initial rehemorrhage, as well as assist in optimizing the safety and efficacy of subsequent SR or microsurgical excision.

Aneurysmal Subarachnoid Hemorrhage

Unruptured berry (saccular) aneurysms tend to occur at vascular bifurcations and tend to project in the direction that the blood would have gone without the bifurcation present. Much rarer forms of cerebral aneurysm include fusiform aneurysms (often atherosclerosis-associated) and infectious aneurysms (mycotic aneurysms). Approximately 5% of people in the U.S. general population are thought to have berry aneurysms at any given time. They are named after the main branch occurring at their point of origin. Anterior circulation aneurysms are more common (85%) than posterior circulation aneurysms (15%), and, depending on the series reporting, either aCom A or pCom A aneurysms are most common (Fig. 8-8). Aneurysms are multiple in 20% of cases, with bilateral mirror aneurysms most commonly affecting the MCA, followed by the intracavernous ICA. The tendency for aneurysms can run in families, particularly for patients with multiple aneurysms. The annual rate of rupture for berry aneurysms greater than 9 mm diameter is estimated to be 2% to 3% per year, but is estimated to be 1% or less per year for aneurysms less than 1 cm in diameter.

Aneurysmal SAH is characterized by sudden onset of severe headache often associated with immediate loss of consciousness. In those with milder forms who do not lose consciousness, nausea, vomiting, stiff neck, photophobia, and drowsiness are common symptoms. Approximately 50% will have a history of a probable "sentinel bleed" marked by transient severe headache 1 to 2 weeks before their current SAH. The remaining patients presenting with normal level of consciousness may actually be presenting with their sentinel bleed. Examination may reveal meningismus, and funduscopic examination may reveal hemorrhages into the subhyaloid membrane. Approximately 35% of patients with aneurysmal SAH die before they reach a hospital or before they can be stabilized. Another 40% will die or remain functionally dependent from neurologic deficit as a result of rebleeding or ischemic vasospasm injury. Only 25% of patients will return to a functionally independent state after aneurysmal SAH. CT scanning is approximately 90% effective in detecting acute SAH, and sensitivity can be increased to approximately 95% to 98% by performing an LP in patients with a highly suggestive history but a negative or equivocal CT scan. CT angiogram can rapidly determine whether a cerebral aneurysm is present and guide subsequent treatment decisions. SAH is an extremely dangerous condition.

The initial risk of a ruptured aneurysm is the risk of rehemorrhage if the aneurysm is not sealed by either microsurgical clipping or endovascular coiling. Rehemorrhage is statistically maximal in the first 12 to 48 hours after initial hemorrhage. The mortality rate of a rehemorrhage is approximately 50%. The next risk after SAH is ischemic deficit from delayed vasospasm, which tends to begin 3 to 10 days after SAH and usually resolves by 2 weeks after SAH. The third risk is from the development of hydrocephalus from RBCs and subsequent CSF debris interfering with arachnoid villi CSF absorption. Clinical outcome after SAH and the subsequent risk of vasospasm is directly related to the patient's clinical condition on presentation (Hunt and Hess clinical grades 1–5) and the

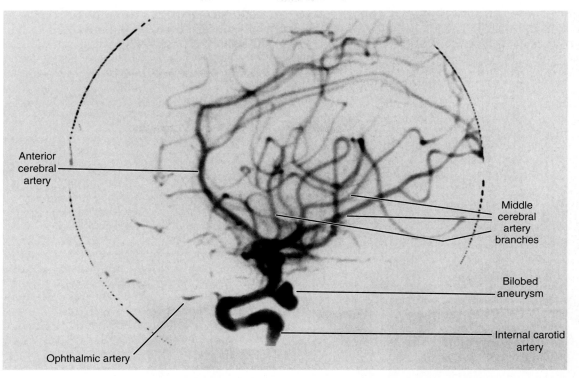

Anterior cerebral artery

Middle cerebral artery branches

Bilobed aneurysm

Internal carotid artery

Ophthalmic artery

Figure 8-8   Internal carotid artery with an aneurysm in the posterior communicating artery.

degree of blood present in the basal cisterns on CT scan (Fisher grades 0–3).

Patients diagnosed with SAH are admitted to the intensive care unit and are given phenytoin to prevent seizures and nimodipine (an oral calcium channel blocker) to help prevent vasospasm. An arterial line to monitor and strictly control blood pressure and a central line to monitor and optimize intravascular volume are usually needed. If hydrocephalus is present, consideration is given to placing a ventriculostomy without allowing rapid ventricular decompression. Until the aneurysm is protected by coiling or clipping, the patient is protected from anxiety, stress, or straining, by being placed in a quiet environment and given anxiolytics, stool softeners, and analgesics as needed. If intubated, the patient is premedicated before any endotracheal suctioning.

Initial clinical decision making usually centers on deciding whether to take the patient urgently to surgery or to have an angiogram performed. Angiography provides a better determination of anatomic detail and information as to the technical possibility of endovascular coiling. Because microvascular clipping is known to be both definitive and permanent, patients who are young, with uncomplicated anterior circulation aneurysms, and who are in good clinical condition (Hunt-Hess grades 1–3) are more often treated with microsurgical clipping. Patients who are elderly, have significant medical problems, have complex or posterior circulation aneurysms (PICA excepted), and who are in poor clinical condition (Hunt-Hess grades 4–5) currently tend to undergo endovascular coiling. In the fu-

ture, an increasing number of aneurysms are likely to be treated by endovascular means, thus avoiding craniotomy, if the early success rates prove to be durable over the long term.

Once the aneurysm is protected from rerupture, focus shifts to preventing and detecting vasospasm. Nimodipine is continued while daily transcranial Doppler cerebral artery velocities are monitored for upward trends that would indicate vasoconstriction. Intravascular volume is expanded to optimize cardiac preload and to optimize blood viscosity for small vessel rheology purposes through hemodilution down to a hematocrit of 30 to 32. If symptomatic vasospasm develops, the patient is treated with vasopressors to elevate systolic blood pressure to 160 mm Hg or greater. Vasospasm is best confirmed by cerebral angiography, which can also allow for endovascular treatment with either chemical (selective intra-arterial papaverine or a calcium channel blocker) or mechanical angioplasty with a soft balloon. Continued CSF drainage at this point can lower ICP and maximize CPP for a given MAP. Ultimately, approximately 20% of surviving patients will require a ventriculoperitoneal CSF shunt for persisting or delayed hydrocephalus. Delayed hydrocephalus usually presents 4 to 8 weeks after SAH and is characterized by loss of cognitive and consciousness recovery milestones.

Brain Tumors

Brain tumors are classified as either primary (arising from the brain, cranial nerves, and surrounding meninges) or secondary (metastasizing to the brain from a primary cancer elsewhere). Primary brain tumors can be further characterized by being either primary parenchymal tumors (either neuronal-glial or immune system in origin) or extraparenchymal. Pediatric primary brain tumors are also often considered as a separate category. Symptoms from brain tumors can arise from brain tissue destruction, brain tissue mass effect, or dysfunction resulting from compression by the brain tumor mass or associated vasogenic edema. The latter two causes are potentially reversible with surgical decompression of mass effect and treatment of vasogenic edema with steroids, respectively. Symptoms from brain tumors usually arise either from generalized phenomena such as increased ICP from tumor mass, vasogenic edema, hydrocephalus (e.g., headache, nausea, vomiting, papilledema, diplopia), or seizures (if the lesion is cortical and supratentorial). More specific symptoms relate to the area of the brain involved and commonly include motor weakness, sensory deficits or paresthesias, speech deficits, visual field cuts, ataxia, endocrine dysfunction, or deficits in other higher cortical functions. Seizures occur in 26% of cases of brain tumor, and a new-onset seizure in an adult should be considered to indicate a potential brain tumor until proven otherwise.

MRI is the test of choice for evaluating brain tumors. However, CT scanning and cerebral angiography can provide complementary information regarding presence of calcium; bone or skull erosion, destruction, or involvement; tumor vascularity; and the relationship of the mass to important cerebral blood vessels. These neuroimages indicate whether the tumor is intrinsic or extrinsic to the brain, show its location, and suggest its histology (Fig. 8-9). Stereotactic biopsy is often helpful to establish the cell type and confirm the diagnosis (Fig. 8-10).

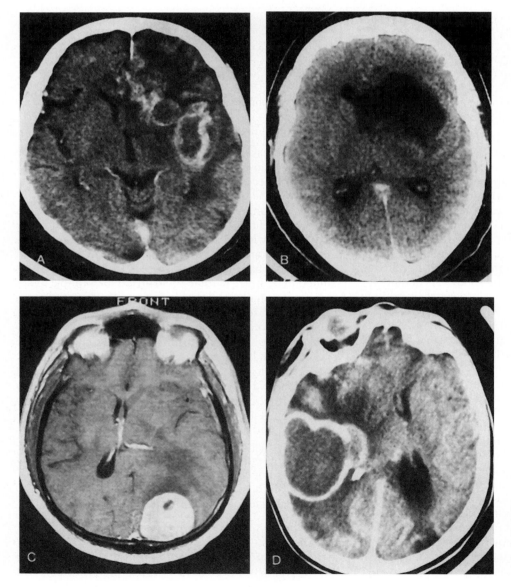

Figure 8-9 A, Enhanced computed tomography scans showing brain disorders. **A,** Glioblastomamultiforme. **B,** Low-grade astrocytoma. **C,** Metastatic melanoma. **D,** Brain abscess.

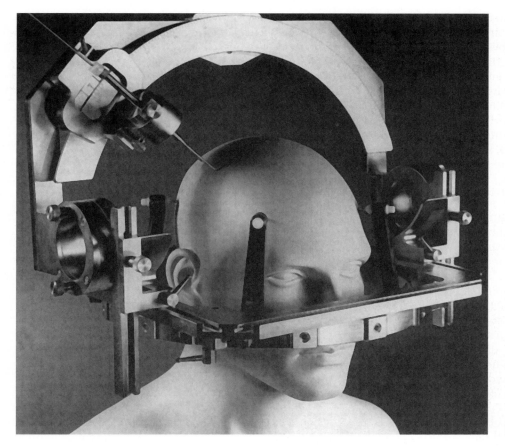

Figure 8-10   Stereotactic biopsy.

Secondary (Metastatic) Brain Tumors

Metastatic brain tumors are 4 times more common than primary brain tumors (Fig. 8-9C). They have an annual incidence of 36/100,000/yr. There are more than 100,000 new patients with metastatic brain tumor diagnosed each year in the United States. At the time of clinical diagnosis, approximately 37% to 50% of patients present with a single lesion and 50% to 63% have multiple tumors. Lung cancer is the most common CNS metastasis, closely followed by breast cancer in women. Melanoma is the most common histology to present with multiple lesions, and renal cell is the most likely histology to present with a single lesion. Most patients present with a brain metastasis within 6 months to 2 years of the diagnosis of their original primary tumor. Symptoms of the metastatic brain tumor lead to the initial discovery of cancer in 15% of cases. Approximately 43% to 60% of these patients will have an abnormal chest x-ray film, either from a primary lung tumor or from additional pulmonary metastases. In 1% to 5% of cases, the primary source of the metastasis is not found in initial work-up. Melanoma, choriocarcinoma, renal cell carcinoma, and thyroid carcinoma are the most common histologies to present with an intratumoral hemorrhage.

Untreated, a symptomatic patient with a single brain metastasis has a median life expectancy of 1 to 2 months, with an approximately 95% chance of dying from elevated ICP and herniation. Treatment of vasogenic edema with steroids only improves these figures to 2 months and 90%, respectively. Fractionated whole brain radiation therapy (WBRT) improves survival in a statistically significant manner to a median of 4 to 6 months. However, 50% of patients will still die a cerebral death, indicating a continued significant negative effect on quality of life (functional independence, ability for joy, and participation in relationships). Multiple prospective randomized controlled clinical trials have now demonstrated that improved local control through surgical resection of single brain metastases can improve median survival to 10 to 12 months and reduce the incidence of cerebral death to 25%. Compared with surgical resection, stereotactic radiosurgery appears to be able to achieve equivalent local control rates, median survival times, and cerebral death rates, although the two have yet to be compared in a randomized clinical trial (Fig. 8-10). Stereotactic radiosurgery with WBRT has been shown to provide improved survival compared to WBRT alone for single metastases in one randomized clinical trial, while it has been shown to provide improved local control for patients with up to four metastatic brain tumors in another randomized clinical trial.

WBRT is still necessary after surgical resection because local resection cavity recurrence rates increase from 10% with adjuvant WBRT to 40% when WBRT is withheld.

Stereotactic radiosurgery to eliminate the need for WBRT to prevent local recurrence is currently under study in clinical trials. In addition to improved median survival and better neurologic quality of life, the main advantage of improved local control through either surgical resection or stereotactic radiosurgery appears to be the unmasking of a subset of up to 20% of metastatic brain tumor patients with longer-term survival (2 to 3 years). With maximized CNS local control, the rate-limiting step for survival now shifts to extent of systemic disease and the responsiveness of the tumor histology to systemic therapy.

Primary Brain Tumors

Primary brain tumors have an annual incidence of 9.9/100,000/yr. Primary parenchymal brain tumors constitute 63.6% of the total and primary extraparenchymal tumors 36.4%. Primary parenchymal tumors are predominantly malignant tumors and include tumors of glial origin (~97%) and primary CNS lymphoma (PCNSL ~3%). Glial-origin tumors are truly benign in only 18% of cases. The remaining tumors consist of low-grade, intermediate-grade, and high-grade glial malignancies. All PCNSLs are malignant. On the other hand, only approximately 5% of primary extraparenchymal brain tumors are malignant. The majority are benign tumors and include meningiomas (65%), cranial nerve schwannomas (18%), pituitary tumors (16%), and craniopharyngiomas (2%).

Benign brain tumors are often best treated with surgical excision, which can be curative. If they are small enough and have an appropriate relationship to surrounding sensitive structures, many benign tumors can be treated with stereotactic radiosurgery. Fractionated radiotherapy is best avoided for patients with benign tumors and normal life expectancies, due to concerns for cognitive side effects. It is often reserved for recurrent tumors or for tumors too large or inauspicious for stereotactic radiosurgery. Malignant brain tumors can be treated with surgical resection or stereotactic radiosurgery to maximize local control. Surgical resection also provides histologic diagnosis and relief of symptomatic mass effect. Most malignant brain tumors can also be treated with varying combinations of fractionated radiotherapy and chemotherapy, with varying degrees of success. Long-term survival (>5 years) and cure are unfortunately rare for most malignant brain tumors.

Glial Tumors

Glia are the supporting cells in the CNS, and the overwhelming majority of primary parenchymal brain tumors are gliomas. Astrocytes are the structural scaffolding of the CNS neuropil. They serve as metabolic nurse cells for the neurons and help maintain extracellular ionic, neurotransmitter, and metabolic homeostasis. Oligodendrocytes manufacture myelin and provide electrical insulation for axons. Ependymal cells line the ventricular system. They are important in maintaining CSF barrier and have a role in CSF physiology and homeostasis. Both neurons and glia originally derived from a common multipotential stem cell that went on to differentiate into a glial-restricted pre-

cursor cell and a neuronal-restricted precursor cell. Ependymal cells diverged earliest from the glial-restricted precursor cell, leaving oligodendrocytes and astrocytes to develop from a bipotential progenitor cell. Primitive neuroectodermal tumors (PNETs), medulloblastomas in the posterior fossa and pineoblastomas in the pineal gland, are believed to arise from a multipotential neuronal-glial stem cell.

Gliomas include astrocytomas (most common), oligodendrogliomas, mixed oligo-astrocytomas, and ependymomas. All categories are classified by the World Health Organization (WHO) into numeric grades of malignancy based on histologic criteria: grades II to IV for astrocytoma and mixed oligo-astrocytoma and grades I to III for oligodendroglioma and ependymoma. It is not uncommon for low-grade gliomas to progress over time to a higher grade. Intermediate histologic grades are often referred to as anaplastic, and high-grade gliomas are termed malignant. A grade IV malignant astrocytoma is also known as a glioblastoma multiforme (GBM; Fig. 8-9A).

In general, prognosis for patients with gliomas is related to histologic grade of the tumor, functional clinical status (Karnofsky Performance Status [KPS]), and patient age (younger do better), in descending order of importance. GBM is one of the most malignant tumors of the brain. Median survival with surgery fractionated radiotherapy and chemotherapy is only 12 to 13 months, with only 12% alive at 2 years and 2% to 5% alive 5 years after diagnosis. Recently, clinical trials of concomitant temozolomide chemotherapy during radiotherapy and continuous temozolomide chemotherapy after radiotherapy has been completed have shown an improved median survival, as well as an increase in 2-year survival to 20%. Low-grade, anaplastic, and malignant oligodendrogliomas have now been shown to respond well to chemotherapy with either PCV (procarbazine, CCNU, and vincristine) or temozolomide. For malignant gliomas, molecular biomarkers are becoming increasingly important for estimating prognosis, as well as selecting therapy. Examples include loss of heterozygosity on chromosomes 1p and 19q, which predicts chemoresponsiveness of oligodendrogliomas, and methylguanine O'6'-methyltransferase promoter methylation, which predicts the accentuated responsiveness of anaplastic astrocytoma and GBM (WHO grades III and IV) to concomitant temozolomide and fractionated radiotherapy.

Unlike other malignancies in the body, gliomas rarely metastasize. They have a tendency to recur locally (95% recur within 2 cm of the original resection cavity), but also show a remarkable tendency for individual tumor cells to display impressive migratory and tissue invasion potential. Preferential pathways for invasion and migration include functional white matter connections of the area of the brain where the tumor developed, as well as along the basement membranes of blood vessels and the ependymal lining of the ventricles. It is this tendency toward diffuse normal functional tissue invasion that frustrates surgical attempts at more radical cure. CSF spread is most common with PNETs and ependymomas, but can rarely occur in other gliomas late in their clinical course.

Primary Central Nervous System Lymphoma

The incidence of PCNSL is rising, presumably due to the rising incidence of human immunodeficiency virus (HIV) infection in the world. In the United States, 50% of PCNSL is now acquired immunodeficiency syndrome (AIDS) associated. The majority of PCNSL is B cell in origin. When it is diagnosed, it is important to check the patient's fundi because up to 20% will have associated involvement of the eye. PCNSL is a nonsurgical disease that has an excellent and dramatic initial imaging response to either chemotherapy or fractionated radiotherapy. Unfortunately, this response is not durable over the long term. Surgery is usually limited to stereotactic needle biopsy. Currently, chemotherapy is usually tried first in an attempt to delay the potential congenitive side effects of radiotherapy, especially if intrathecal chemotherapy is used along with systemic chemotherapy. Intrathecal CSF therapy is indicated if CSF cytology is positive or if the ventricular lining or meninges are obviously involved on MRI scan.

Other Primary Brain Tumors

Pilocytic astrocytomas (WHO grade I astrocytoma), gangliogliomas, subependymal giant cell astrocytomas, central neurocytomas, and hemangioblastomas are examples of truly benign tumors that can be cured with surgical resection alone. Pilocytic astrocytomas can be associated with neurofibromatosis, type 1 (chromosome 17). Hemangioblastomas can be associated with von Hippel–Lindau syndrome. When this is the case, the tumors can be multiple, may involve the cerebellum or spinal cord, and may be associated with polycythemia from tumor secretion of erythropoietin and retinal hemangiomas. These patients may also suffer from atrial myxomas, retroperitoneal angiomyolipomas, and renal cell carcinomas. For these tumors, stereotactic radiosurgery is reserved for cases in locations too dangerous for safe resection and is best suited for solid rather than cystic tumors because of unpredictable cyst fluid dynamics after stereotactic radiosurgery.

Extraparenchymal Benign Tumors

Meningiomas are benign tumors that arise from arachnoid cap cells (Fig. 8-9E). They are multiple in about 10% of cases and can rarely be associated with genetic conditions such as neurofibromatosis type 2 (chromosome 22) or meningiomatosis. They can arise from either the dura of the convexity, the dura of the falx or tentorium, the dura of the skull base, or the arachnoid cap cells in the choroid plexus of the ventricles. They can directly involve adjacent bone (hyperostosis). Because they arise from the dura, meningiomas have an ECA blood supply via meningeal branches. Meningiomas are benign 92% of the time, anaplastic 6% of the time, and malignant 2% of the time. Benign meningiomas can be cured with surgical resection, but this requires resection of all the tumor, all the attached dura, and all the adjacent bone (Simpson grade 1 resec-

tion). Neuroimaging recurrence rates are 15% to 20% at 10 to 20 years for patients where Simpson grade 1 or 2 resection can be achieved. Recurrence rates are very high for Simpson grades 3 to 5 resections. Endovascular embolization preoperatively can assist with limiting surgical blood loss. Additional alternative therapies include stereotactic radiosurgery if the tumor is small enough and sufficiently distant from the optic nerve and chiasm and standard fractionated radiotherapy. Certain tumor locations and or structural involvements limit the ability to achieve a Simpson grade 1 or 2 resection, including cavernous sinus involvement, involvement of the posterior two thirds of the sagittal sinus, and involvement of the torcula or transverse sinus. In these cases, subtotal surgical resection followed by stereotactic radiosurgery for the residual tumor in the high-risk area is an alternative treatment strategy that maximizes preservation of neurologic and cranial nerve function. Fractionated radiotherapy is advisable in all cases of anaplastic and malignant meningioma, even after complete surgical resection. Chemotherapy with hydroxyurea has been utilized for patients with malignant meningioma with some degree of success in a subset of responsive patients.

Vestibular schwannomas are the most common cranial nerve schwannoma. Unilateral tumors are sporadic, while bilateral vestibular schwannomas are diagnostic for neurofibromatosis, type 2. These tumors arise from Schwann cells of the vestibular nerve at or inside the internal auditory canal (Fig. 8-11). The patient usually has a history of unilateral tinnitus with vertigo that disappears as the vestibular nerve is destroyed. As the tumor grows into the cranial cavity at the cerebellopontine angle, pressure on the auditory nerve eventually leads to deafness, which usually begins as preferential high-frequency hearing loss on the audiogram. The function of the adjacent, equally stretched facial nerve (motor) is preserved until very late in the course. Unilateral sensorineural hearing loss with impairment of taste on the same side is highly suggestive of vestibular schwannoma. As the tumor grows, it involves the fifth cranial nerve with facial numbness and eventual loss of the corneal reflex. Ultimately, cerebellar signs (staggering gait, veering toward the side of the lesion) and ninth and tenth cranial nerve deficits (i.e., hoarseness, dysphagia, aspiration) occur. Microsurgical treatment options include resection by way of a retrosigmoid, translabyrinthine, or middle cranial fossa approach. Hearing can only be spared by way of the retrosigmoid or middle cranial fossa approach, but the latter approach can only be used for very small tumors. Microsurgical cranial nerve preservation rates vary according to tumor size and the experience of the individual. Stereotactic radiosurgery is an alternative to microsurgical resection for tumors 33.5 cm or less in diameter. Ten-year neuroimaging control rates for current tumor doses are 95% for unilateral vestibular schwannomas. Cranial nerve preservation rates exceed those of microsurgery for all but the smallest intracanalicular tumors. Fractionated stereotactic radiotherapy has been tried in an attempt to further improve hearing preservation

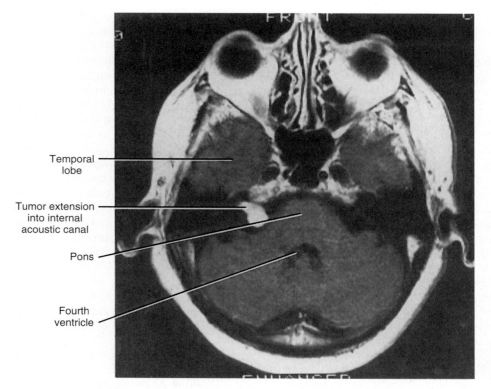

Temporal lobe

Tumor extension into internal acoustic canal

Pons

Fourth ventricle

Figure 8-11 Enhanced magnetic resonance imaging scan showing an acoustic neuroma.

rates, but current results do not exceed those achievable with gamma knife stereotactic radiosurgery, and the long-term durability of tumor control rates with fractionation for vestibular schwannomas is currently unknown.

Pituitary adenomas can be functional (hormone secreting) or nonsecretory. They are classified as either microadenomas (<1 cm diameter) or macroadenomas (≥1 cm diameter). Most secretory adenomas are diagnosed while they are still microadenomas because of the presence of hormone-related symptoms such as menstrual irregularities, galactorrhea, frontal sinus bossing, enlargement of hands and feet, and coarseness of facial features. Most non-secretory tumors are not diagnosed until they become macroadenomas and cause visual symptoms from downward pressure on the optic chiasm (bitemporal hemianopsia) or cranial nerve symptoms from invasion of the cavernous sinus (Fig. 8-12). Rarely, pituitary tumors present with sudden-onset headache, visual loss, and Addisonian crisis from sudden pituitary infarction or hemorrhage (pituitary apoplexy).

The most common functional tumor of the pituitary is prolactinoma, which causes amenorrhea-galactorrhea syndrome in women and impotence in men. Somatotrophic tumors secrete excess growth hormone and cause acromegaly. In addition to coarsened features, prognathism, and hand and foot growth, patients have hypertension, diabetes mellitus, and myopathy, including cardiomyopathy. Corticotrophic tumors secrete adrenocorticotropic hormone (ACTH) and cause Cushing's disease (see discussion of Cushing's disease and syndrome in Chapter 21

of Lawrence's *Essentials of General Surgery*, 4th ed.). In addition to truncal obesity, buffalo hump, striae, and easy bruising, these patients have hypertension, diabetes mellitus, and myopathy. These changes are caused by an excess of circulating cortisol because of an excess of circulating ACTH. Gonadotrophic tumors secrete follicle-stimulating hormone or luteinizing hormone. They are rare and cause sterility, loss of libido, and impotence.

Many secretory pituitary tumors can be treated medically (bromocriptine for prolactinoma, somatostatin for acromegaly, and ketoconazole for Cushing's disease) with both hormone reduction and some tumor shrinkage. Unfortunately, because these tumors require life-long therapy, some patients become intolerant of the drug and others are concerned with preserving fertility. In these settings, consideration should be given to either microsurgical or endoscopic trans-sphenoidal approach for tumor resection. Apparent complete removal of the microadenoma is accomplished in approximately 85% of cases. The recurrence rate is approximately 20% after 5 years. Hormonal cure is less common and only approaches 50% to 60% at 5 years.

For macroadenomas, surgical resection affords the opportunity to decompress the optic pathway, often leading to dramatic visual improvement, which can usually be accomplished transsphenoidally. Craniotomy is generally reserved for rare firm and adherent tumors and for extensions of the tumor lateral to the ICA or up into the root of the sylvian fissure. For pituitary adenomas, stereotactic radiosurgery is usually reserved for cavernous sinus residual dis-

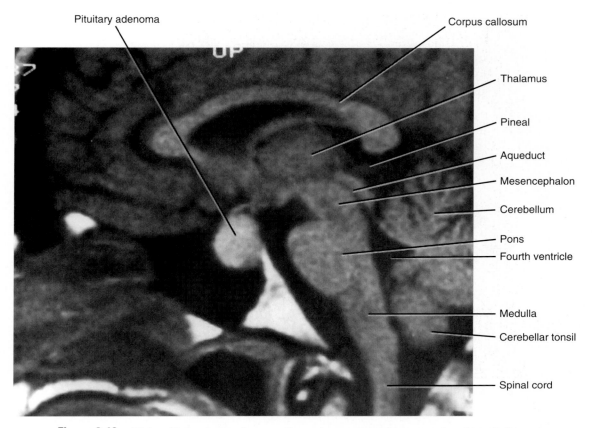

Figure 8-12   Midsagittal enhanced magnetic resonance imaging scan showing pituitary adenoma.

ease, recurrence, or cases in which the patient refuses open surgery and there is at least 2 mm of space separating the top of the tumor from the optic pathway. SR is extremely effective at controlling tumor growth and has, for the most part, replaced fractionated radiotherapy for recurrent or residual disease. It is less successful at normalizing hormonal secretory syndromes. Hormone normalization requires a higher stereotactic radiosurgery tumor dose and is successful only approximately 30% to 40% of the time by 3 years after therapy. The risk of hypopituitarism varies according to the ability to visualize and spare the normal gland and stalk during stereotactic radiosurgery.

Pediatric Brain Tumors

Brain tumors are the number one solid cancer in children (ahead of Wilms' tumor) and are second only to leukemia for leading malignancy overall. Brain tumors are much more common in the posterior fossa in children than they are in adults. Cerebellar tumors are much more common than brain stem gliomas. During the first 9 years, medulloblastoma is the most common tumor, but by age 9 through age 19, pilocytic astrocytoma is the most common (Figs. 8-13 and 8-14C). Pediatric cerebellar pilocytic astrocytomas are commonly cystic, with the neoplastic tissue

restricted to a mural nodule along the wall of the cyst. Ependymoma remains third at all age-groups, but is 2.5 times more common between ages before age 4 years than during later years (Fig. 8-14B). Other rare tumors that are more common in children include craniopharyngiomas, germ cell tumors, embryonal cell tumor, malignant teratomas, pineal tumors, choroid plexus tumors, and optic nerve and hypothalamic pilocytic astrocytomas (neurofibromatosis, type 1).

Infants and pretoddlers often present with irritability, fussiness, nausea, vomiting, and a full fontanelle (if open). Lethargy and cranial nerve palsies (usually VI and VII) tend to occur late. Toddlers and preadolescents tend to present with regression or delay in motor milestones, imbalance, dysmetria and incoordination, headache, nausea, and vomiting. Obstructive hydrocephalus is a significant risk and may need to be treated with ventriculostomy even before managing the primary or main tumor. Brain stem gliomas account for approximately 20% of pediatric posterior fossa tumors and may present with unilateral esotropia and ipsilateral facial weakness (Fig. 8-14A).

Medulloblastomas usually involve the roof of the fourth ventricle and arise in the midline in either the superior or inferior medullary velum. A gross total surgical resection often can be achieved without disrupting the floor of the

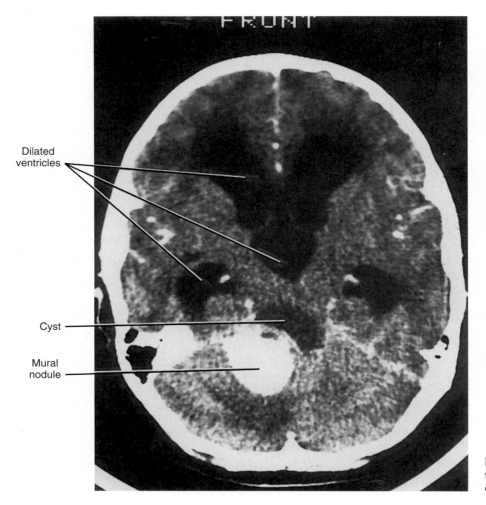

Dilated ventricles

Cyst

Mural nodule

Figure 8-13 Enhanced computed tomography scan showing a cerebellar astrocytoma.

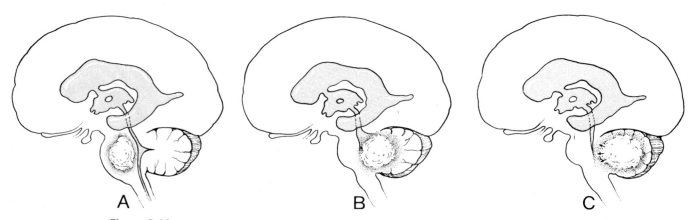

Figure 8-14 **A,** Brain stem tumor infiltrating up and down, displacing, but not occluding, the fourth ventricle (cranial nerve and long tract signs). **B,** Fourth ventricular tumor displacing the cerebellum and obliterating the fourth ventricle (hydrocephalus and cerebellar signs). **C,** Cerebellar tumor compressing and displacing the cerebellum and obliterating the fourth ventricle (hydrocephalus and cerebellar signs).

fourth ventricle (dorsal brain stem). Ependymomas can arise anywhere along the ependymal lining of the fourth ventricle, including the floor of the fourth ventricle and the foramina of Luschka. Complete surgical removal can be more problematic if removing the ependymal attachment requires disrupting the tissue of the dorsal brain stem. Near-total resection may be necessary to preserve important brain stem functions. Ependymomas also have an increased tendency to extend exophytically out of the foramina of Luschka into the cerebellopontine angle and ventral surface of the brain stem, where they wrap themselves around important lower cranial nerves and critical posterior circulation blood vessels. Very careful and meticulous dissection is required to remove them and preserve the surrounding structures under these circumstances. Both medulloblastoma and ependymoma patients benefit from staging by CSF sampling for cytology and spinal imaging for drop metastases (malignant cells that drop from above into the spinal fluid). Medulloblastoma patients also usually receive systemic staging with imaging and bone marrow biopsy. Both medulloblastoma patients and ependymoma patients benefit from fractionated radiotherapy. Controversy now exists as to whether full-dose craniospinal axis radiotherapy should be delivered routinely in these cases because of the tendency for CSF spread and drop metastases, or whether it should be reserved for high-risk patients. High-risk patients include those less than 3 years old, those with incomplete surgical tumor resection, and those with positive staging workup (CSF cytology or spinal MRI for drop metastases or positive systemic disease). Several chemotherapy regimens have proven beneficial for patients with medulloblastoma, but are less proven for those with ependymoma. Studies evaluating stereotactic radiosurgery as a boost for residual or recurrent disease are underway, and early results suggest promise, especially for ependymoma patients with small dorsal brain stem residual lesion and preserved neurologic function. For medulloblastoma treated with surgery, fractionated craniospinal radiotherapy, and chemotherapy, 5-year progression-free survival rates of 50% to 70% are now being achieved. Results are worse for high-risk patients. In very young patients (≤2 years), initial therapy is usually chemotherapy, with an attempt to delay radiotherapy until CNS myelination is complete (2–3 years old). Two-year progression-free survival in these high-risk patients is only 25% to 40%. For ependymoma, the 5-year survival rates with resection and radiotherapy, with or without chemotherapy, are about 50%. Once again, young age, residual disease, and evidence of tumor spread identify patients with worse prognosis.

For cerebellar pilocytic astrocytomas, surgical resection can be curative and is the treatment of choice. They more often arise in the cerebellar hemispheres in a paramedian location, but can involve the midline cerebellar structures. Brain stem gliomas have a uniformly poor prognosis, with survival rates of only about 18 months. Occasionally, they have a dorsally exophytic component that can be safely removed to decompress the brain stem and fourth ventricle. Pediatric diffuse pontine gliomas have such a characteristic imaging appearance that it is one of the rare tumors in which treatment can be initiated without tissue diagnosis. Ventriculoperitoneal shunting or endoscopic third ventriculostomy is often required for brain stem tumors and some cerebellar tumors.

Craniopharyngiomas arise in the sellar and suprasellar regions of the hypothalamic-pituitary axis from congenital ectodermal rests. They usually arise from, or are densely attached to, the pituitary stalk, and stalk preservation remains the greatest surgical challenge restricting complete resection and frustrating elimination of permanent DI as a sequela of surgery. Their histology often resembles that of the primitive tooth bud or skin. Like other epithelial structures, these tumors desquamate and secrete sebaceous substances and cholesterol that can collect in cysts. Rarely, this material is released into the subarachnoid space and causes sterile meningitis. These tumors can grow as a firm, solid mass that contains calcium, as a predominantly cystic mass with an extremely diaphanous and adherent cyst wall draped over and in between surrounding structures (cranial nerves, blood vessels, floor of these hypothalamus, and pituitary stalk), or even as a complex combination of the two. Although they are benign, they are difficult to remove completely and have a high recurrence rate. Syndromic hypothalamic damage and DI along with hypopituitarism are the dreaded complications of aggressive surgery; however, tumor cure is possible if the tumor can be delicately but completely removed on the first attempt. Aggressive resection of a recurrent tumor rarely leads to complete resection without significant collateral damage. Given these issues, additional multimodality therapies have evolved to assist with these complicated and individually unique circumstances. Tumor cyst growth and secretion can be controlled with P^{32} intracystic colloidal brachytherapy. Recurrent solid tumor components can be controlled with stereotactic radiosurgery. Fractionated radiotherapy has a role for cases that cannot be controlled with microsurgical or stereotactic surgical means.

Cerebral Infection

Cerebral infection is quite common worldwide as a cause of cerebral mass lesions. Whereas the most common intracranial mass lesion in the United States is tumor, in Mexico it is a parasitic infection known as cysticercosis and in India it is tuberculoma. Even in the United States, infectious bacterial meningitis is common in the pediatric age-group and among young people clustered together for the first time (e.g., schools, military barracks). Primary CNS viral infection is the rule rather than the exception in HIV-positive patients. Infections can be characterized by their organism of origin (e.g., bacterial, fungal, viral, parasitic, and prion). Although specific medical antimicrobial therapy is the mainstay of treatment, surgery occasionally plays a role in helping with confirming the correct diagnosis, as well as managing the complication that can arise from disease progression or evolution.

Meningitis, Tuberculosis and Subdural Empyema

Community-acquired, infectious bacterial meningitis most commonly arises from *Streptococcus pneumoniae* (pneumococcus), *Haemophilus influenzae*, *Neisseria meningitides*, and *Staphylococcus aureus*. The disease is most commonly seen in children, young adults newly collectively domiciled, and in the elderly. *H. influenzae* is the most common organism in young children, *N. meningitidis* and *S. pneumoniae* are the most common in adolescents and young adults, and *S. pneumoniae* is the most common in the elderly. Gram-negative bacilli such as *Escherichia coli* and *Klebsiella pneumoniae* should be considered in infants (<1 month of age). Acute suppurative meningitis can lead to altered level of consciousness, cerebral edema, seizures, central and cortical venous thrombosis, and hydrocephalus. It can lead, rarely, to subdural empyema.

Tuberculosis can manifest as cerebral mass lesions (tuberculoma or tuberculous abscess) or tuberculous meningitis. Tuberculous meningitis tends to be much more clinically indolent and insidious than pyogenic bacterial meningitis. It tends to affect the basal arachnoid cisterns with basal meningitis and can also lead to hydrocephalus.

If postmeningitic hydrocephalus is bacterial in origin, it is treated with external ventricular drainage until the infection is cleared, at which time a permanent ventriculoperitoneal shunt may be necessary if the hydrocephalus has not resolved. Hydrocephalus from tuberculous meningitis usually requires placement of a ventriculoperitoneal shunt even before the infection is cleared. Antituberculous agents are administered throughout the perioperative and postoperative period, and the infection can take 12 to 18 months to clear.

Subdural empyema is an emergent neurosurgical condition. These patients appear ill and febrile. They often have recurring or refractory seizures, despite antibiotics and anticonvulsants. CT scans and MR scans usually show an enhancing subdural fluid collection. MR is superior to CT for detecting subdural empyema because the volume of fluid collection can be subtle and MR can directly image in the coronal plane. Treatment is urgent surgical evacuation of the purulent matter and continued antibiotics. Evacuation can usually successfully be performed with irrigation between strategically placed burr holes, and conversion to craniotomy for fenestration of loculations is rarely necessary. Subdural empyema is a very serious clinical condition. Despite surgical intervention and aggressive medical therapy, mortality rates approach 21% to 35%. Seizures occur in the first few postoperative days in almost 50% of cases. The long-term, serious, disabling morbidity rate is reported to be approximately 20%.

Cerebral Abscess

Pyogenic brain abscesses evolve over approximately a 2-week period. At first, localized cerebritis occurs with the inoculation of bacteria into the brain. As polymorphonucleated white blood cells (WBCs) and lymphocytes invade, necrosis progresses centrifugally. Initially, the process is not walled off, and cerebral edema is maximal. Approximately 10 days later, a reticulin matrix develops and walls off the central zone of necrosis (pus) and inflammation. Two weeks or more after inoculation, a mature collagen wall forms around the pus. Intracranial abscesses are usually found in the cerebrum, but may also be found in the cerebellum. In approximately 80% of cases, the source of infection is identifiable. Previous surgery and penetrating head trauma account for approximately 10%. Another 20% are extensions from adjacent localized cranial infections (e.g., sinusitis, mastoiditis, dental infection). A further 20% have a cardiac source (e.g., valvular or congenital heart disease). In congenital heart disease, right-to-left shunts and pulmonary AVMs are common predisposing causes because they bypass the filter of the lungs. Hematogenous spread from infected loci elsewhere in the body accounts for 30%. Another 5% of cases (rapidly increasing in number) occur in patients who are immunocompromised because of organ transplants or AIDS.

The cause of infection depends on the source. Multiple organisms are common. Abscesses that arise after surgery or penetrating trauma are usually caused by *Staphylococcus aureus*, *Staphylococcus epidermidis*, or *Streptococcus*, although Gram-negative infections are increasing. Brain abscesses that arise from distant hematogenous sources, as well as from paranasal sinus, mastoid, or inner ear infections, are usually caused by anaerobic *Streptococci*, although *Bacteroides* or other species are often present as well. Many cerebral abscesses are polymicrobial (and should be assumed to be so) and treated with empiric broad-spectrum aerobic and anaerobic, as well as Gram-positive and Gram-negative, antibiotic coverage until disproven by aerobic and anaerobic cultures.

The classic symptoms of brain abscess are headache, fever, and focal neurologic deficits. However, this triad is found in fewer than 50% of patients. Headache is the most common symptom (70%–90%) and may be accompanied by nausea and vomiting. Fewer than 50% of patients have fever, which is usually low grade. There is usually little elevation of the sedimentation rate or peripheral WBC count. An abscess acts like any other cerebral mass lesion with surrounding vasogenic edema. Increased ICP can cause obtundation or confusion. Focal neurologic deficits depend on the location of the abscess. Seizures occur in approximately 30% of cases. Symptoms are those of a brain tumor, but evolve more rapidly; 75% of patients have symptoms for less than 2 weeks. Intraparenchymal abscesses tend to extend toward the ventricles. Intraventricular rupture, increased ICP, and local brain destruction are the major causes of disability and death.

Evaluation of the patient with headache and neurologic change begins with the realization that the suspected mass lesion could be a brain abscess or tumor. A history or finding of sinus, middle ear, lung, or other infection; recent head trauma; or cranial surgery is sought. Inquiry and examination should include the possibility of rheumatic and especially congenital heart disease, previous cardiac surgery, hemoptysis, immune compromise, or drug abuse. The presence of one or more of these factors suggests brain abscess rather than brain tumor. Fever should alert the examiner to the possibility of brain abscess, but its absence should never lead the examiner to dismiss the diagnosis.

Brain scans have helped to decrease the mortality rate from 30% to 40% to approximately 5% to 10%. CT or MRI scanning permits rapid diagnosis, localization, and identification of multiple abscesses. A uniform thin, enhancing wall surrounding a low-density core (Fig. 8-9D) suggests, but does not prove, the diagnosis. Lumbar puncture has little role in diagnosis or management because it decreases the pressure beneath a mass lesion and encourages transtentorial herniation. Further, the CSF is usually sterile, with few or no WBCs, unless the abscess is a secondary complication of bacterial meningitis (rare). In a significant number of patients, aggressive antibiotic therapy alone will resolve the infectious process in cerebritis, immature abscesses, and abscesses less than 1 cm in diameter. Trials of primary medical therapy should be carefully monitored by serial neurologic and neuroimaging examination to confirm evolution toward resolution. Surgical intervention is performed for patients with larger, mature lesions, and for patients with small lesions or immature abscesses that progress despite aggressive primary medical management.

Stereotactic aspiration (Fig. 8-10) under local anesthesia has evolved into the treatment of choice for brain abscess, particularly if the abscess is not readily accessible, is small, is associated with congenital heart disease that makes general anesthesia risky, or there are multiple lesions. Each lesion is punctured by a needle or catheter, and the contents are aspirated and sent for aerobic, anaerobic, fungal, and acid-fast bacilli cultures. Care is taken to aspirate slowly and gently and not to withdraw more than 50% of the preoperatively calculated volume of each lesion for fear of precipitating a hemorrhage from the collapsing wall, which contains fragile neovascularity. A drainage catheter is left in each abscess cavity and connected to gravity drainage to allow the abscess to spontaneously drain out any remaining pus over the next few days. The catheters are gradually withdrawn each day, over several days, once spontaneous drainage stops. Using this technique and culture-directed antibiotics, more than 90% of bacterial abscesses can be cured without disrupting the surrounding brain tissue. Open surgery is now usually reserved for cases of stereotactic failure, abscess recurrence, or those in which a skull-base defect with fistula is presumed to be the cause, thus requiring primary repair to prevent recurrence. Corticosteroids are usually reserved for patients who have significant and symptomatic mass effect and edema, because steroids will also suppress the patient's immune response.

Viral and Fungal Encephalitis

Viral encephalitis of the brain usually involves neurotrophic viruses. Currently, the most common encephalitis includes primary HIV CNS infection, primary CNS her-

petic encephalitis from herpes simplex virus (HSV-1), and rabies. Primary HIV infection is associated with AIDS dementia and a mild encephalopathy. Herpetic encephalitis is characterized by hemorrhagic bilateral temporal lobe involvement that can lead to dramatic limbic system and behavioral symptoms (Klüver-Bucy syndrome). More rarely, mumps, measles, polio, and coxsackie viruses and orthomyxovirus, papovavirus, ECHO virus, and arboviruses can cause encephalitis. In immunocompromised patients, Epstein-Barr virus can also be causative.

Fungal CNS infections include meningitis, encephalitis, and abscess formation. Commonly involved organisms include *Actinomyces, Aspergillus, Blastomyces, Candida, Coccidioides, Cryptococcus, Histoplasma, Mucormyces,* and *Nocardia* species. Most CNS fungal infections are associated with some form of immunosuppression (diabetes mellitus, chronic steroid use, systemic chemotherapy for cancer, systemic immunosuppression associated with organ transplant, or infectious immunosuppression from AIDS). Becausue aspergillosis is a primary infection of blood vessels, it is notorious for producing hemorrhagic encephalitis and areas of hemorrhagic infarction. Cryptococcal CNS infection is most often associated with AIDS as an opportunistic infection. Mucormycosis is a devastating, rapidly progressive, and usually fatal disease that often involves the CNS by way of direct extension from contiguous sinus disease in patients with diabetes mellitus and poorly controlled blood sugars. Nocardiosis is most common in organ transplant patients on systemic antirejection and immunosuppression agents.

When a correct diagnosis (for either category of condition) cannot be made with CSF and serum testing, a diagnostic biopsy can be performed. Although stereotactic needle biopsies may provide the diagnosis, the best chance of success often results from an open biopsy of an involved noneloquent area that includes meninges, cortex, and subcortical white matter for architectural histologic analysis. Treatment is appropriate diagnosis-directed antimicrobial therapy, and results are variable.

Parasitic Infection

Parasitic infections of the CNS include cysticercosis, toxoplasmosis, and echinococcosis. Cysticercosis is a very common infection in many parts of the world and results from infestation of the CNS with the larval form of the pork tapeworm (*Cysticercus*) acquired from eating poorly cooked, infested pork. Individual cysts are usually 3 to 18 mm in diameter and can be found anywhere in the CNS parenchyma, in an intraventricular location, or as clustered groups of multiple cysts in the subarachnoid basal cisterns. The cysts become symptomatic either when the larvae die and induce an inflammatory response in the surrounding brain or when they cause obstructive hydrocephalus (usually from an intraventricular cyst). Once the larvae die, the cysts usually calcify. Neurosurgical intervention is usually reserved for obstructive hydrocephalus, which can be treated by ventriculoperitoneal shunting or, more recently, with ventriculoscopic extraction of the obstructing cyst. CNS toxoplasmosis is usually associated with HIV-AIDS syndrome, and neurosurgical involvement is usually limited to distinguishing toxoplasmosis from PCNSL in a patient with AIDS by stereotactic needle biopsy. The larval form of *Echinococcus* leads to CNS hydatidosis. It is endemic in sheep-raising communities and can lead to symptomatic cysts in the brain, ventricles, or arachnoid cisterns. Because the cysts are usually larger and more fragile than cysticercosis cysts, when symptomatic they are usually removed with open surgery that relies on a minimal- or no-touch technique predominantly involving irrigation or background air insufflation to deliver the cyst without rupture.

Congenital Disorders

Infants, children, and even adults have congenital defects. Common cerebral defects include hydrocephalus, craniosynostosis, encephalocele, and Chiari malformations. These defects are also discussed in the chapter on Pediatric Surgery.

Hydrocephalus

Hydrocephalus is dilation of the ventricular system due to imbalance of CSF production and resorption leading to a relative excess of intracranial CSF. It is idiopathic and almost always is caused by obstruction of CSF flow rather than CSF overproduction. As such, most hydrocephalus is technically "obstructive" in nature. However, traditionally the terms communicating and obstructive have been utilized relative to the internal communications of the cerebral ventricles, and since this terminology is in common usage, it will be defined. The actual obstruction can occur at the site of arachnoid granulation CSF absorption or the site of fourth ventricular outflow, in which case all ventricles dilate symmetrically (communicating hydrocephalus). Communicating hydrocephalus can be congenital or can be acquired (intrauterine infection, prior meningitis, or SAH). It can also occur between the cerebral ventricles either at the foramen of Monroe, or more commonly, at the aqueduct of Sylvius, in which case only the upstream ventricles relative to normal CSF flow dilate (obstructive hydrocephalus). Obstructive hydrocephalus can be due to congenital narrowing and stiffening of the walls of the aqueduct of Sylvius (aqueductal stenosis), or it can be acquired as a result of intraventricular hemorrhage (usually associated with prematurity), or other obstructing intraventricular or periventricular compressive lesion (e.g., tumor, cyst, postinfectious loculation, or hematoma).

According to the Monroe-Kellie hypothesis, ICP increases due to increased CSF volume occupying the fixed, rigid, and enclosed, cranial space. Ventricular expansion occurs at the expense of normal brain tissue and therefore function is altered. Because the supratentorial periventricular tissues affected are predominantly white matter tract connections, the syndrome produced can resemble diffuse encephalopathy or a mild subcortical dementia. If the fontanelle is open it may become full and show reduced or absent pulsations. Serial occipital-frontal head circumference measurements may be large for age and weight and may cross standard growth curves over time. Because myelination is incomplete in very young patients, the cerebral aqueduct may physically distend and interfere with the crossing III nerve connections with one another in the tectum dorsal to the aqueduct. This can lead to loss of bilateral upgaze, or even to tonic conjugate downgaze (sunset or Collier's sign). If the skull is closed, as the ICP rises the child may become irritable, drowsy, or start to throw up. Unilateral or bilateral esotropia from cranial nerve VI dysfunction may develop. Papilledema may be present.

CT or MR scan confirms the diagnosis, and with an obstructive ventricular pattern, a contrast-enhanced MR study will rule out tumor as a cause of obstruction. Treatment for communicating hydrocephalus involves placement of a permanent ventricular shunt.

Although there have been successful systems that shunt the CSF to the heart, pleural space, ureter, and gall bladder, among other destinations, the modern system most used is the ventriculoperitoneal (VP) shunt. Hydrocephalus due to foramen of Monroe obstruction can be treated with endoscopic septostomy alone (if the other foramen of Monroe is patent), bilateral VP shunts (often distally connected into the same drainage catheter so that the function or fail symmetrically), or with an endoscopic septostomy followed by a unilateral VP shunt once the lateral ventricles communicate with one another (if the other foramen of Monroe is also obstructed). Hydrocephalus due to aqueduct or fourth ventricular outflow obstruction can be treated with a VP shunt or an endoscopic third ventriculostomy, communicating the third ventricle to the basal arachnoid cisterns through a hole created in the floor of the fourth ventricle just behind the mammillary bodies and in front of the midbrain. When supratentorial obstructive hydrocephalus is due to a separately trapped fourth ventricular cyst (Dandy-Walker syndrome), both supratentorial and fourth ventricular VP shunts are often utilized, once again, often with the two systems distally connected into the same drainage catheter so that the function or fail symmetrically.

Implantation of a foreign CSF diversion device always leads to the risk of subsequent shunt infection or system malfunction. Shunt infections usually occur due to skin organisms introduced at surgery (*S. aureus*, *S. epidermidis*, *Propionibacterium acnes*), and their risk is highest within 6 months of initial surgery. By a full year after implantation, infection from hematogenous spread of bacteria is just as likely as indolent perioperative contamination, and both risks have dropped to a low level. Shunt malfunction can be caused by shunt infection, proximal catheter obstruction with choroid plexus, shunt component disconnection, distal catheter obstruction, or normal growth leading to retraction of the distal catheter outside of the peritoneum due to inadequate catheter length. Suspected shunt malfunction is assessed with a series of plain x-rays (shunt series) to insure system integrity and catheter location, as well as a CT scan to check on ventricular size. Comparison with prior baseline ventricular size and shape on a CT scan obtained during normal shunt functioning is very useful. Shunt infections are assessed by sampling the CSF within the shunt system by means of a shunt tap. Occasionally, a shunt tap is also necessary to instill radionuclide tracer in equivocal cases of shunt malfunction in order to more directly visualize shunt function. Infected shunts are usually removed, and the patient is treated with external ventricular drainage while the infection is cleared and before a new shunt system is reinserted. Malfunctioning shunts are explored and repaired intraoperatively, taking care to assess CSF for potentially associated occult infection.

Craniosynostosis

Craniosynostosis is premature closure of one or more cranial sutures. Primary craniosynostosis may be sporadic or may occur as part of a congenital syndrome. With syndromic craniosynostosis, multiple sutures are usually involved, and more severe cosmetic deformities result. Normally, fibrous union of the sutures begins around 2 years of age and is completed by 8 years of age. When sutures close prematurely, continued brain growth causes compensatory growth of the skull at the remaining open sutures. Growth is halted in the direction perpendicular to the line of premature closure, and cosmetic deformities result.

When craniosynostosis involves the sagittal suture, the head is long and thin. When it involves the bilateral coronal sutures, it is short and wide anteriorly with retracted eyebrows. Premature closure of the midline forehead metopic suture results in a keel-shaped forehead. When it involves one coronal suture, the skull is asymmetrical, with flattening of the forehead and supraorbital ridge on the involved side and compensating contralateral frontal bossing. Corresponding changes occur posteriorly if one lambdoid suture is stenosed.

The appearance of the child usually prompts the parents to seek medical attention. Signs of increased ICP are usually only present in cases of multiple suture synostosis. If mental development is slow and all sutures are closed prematurely, and if there are no signs of increased ICP, then microcephaly, not primary craniosynostosis, is probably the correct diagnosis. The diagnosis is usually readily apparent on physical examination, plain skull x-rays, and bone window CT scans. Unless ICP is elevated, surgical intervention is for cosmetic and more normal psychosocial development purposes. Due to the potential blood loss from large scalp incisions and extensive bone work in infants, surgery is usually deferred until 2 to 6 months of age. At this age, the skull is still immature enough to expect the desired subsequent bone remodeling and new bone formation after surgical repair. The deformities are corrected with multiple osteotomies and bone plate remodel-

ing. If facial bone and/or orbital rim advancement is required, coordination with a plastic or craniofacial surgeon is often helpful.

Encephalocele

Encephaloceles are herniations of malformed brain through defects in the skull. They are usually covered with skin. Like myelomeningoceles, they probably arise when mesoderm somites do not properly form or close during development. Occipital and cerebellar encephaloceles are the most common and are readily apparent on examination. Nasofrontal encephaloceles may not be obvious externally, but they should be suspected if soft tissue swelling is found in the region of the medial canthus, in the nasal region, or even in the palate. Nasal encephaloceles are often associated with widening of the intraorbital distance as well as flattening or sinking of the upper nasal bridge. Encephaloceles can cause an apparent nasal polyp. Diagnosis is confirmed by CT (best for defining the bony defect) and MRI scanning (best for visualizing the contents of the meningeal extension. Treatment is surgical exploration to amputate and/or reduce the sac contents and repair the dura and osseus defect. For patients with cerebellum or brain stem contents in the sac, the outlook for satisfactory existence is limited. For occipital or suboccipital encephaloceles, care must be taken preoperatively to identify the course of the torcula, sagittal and transverse sinuses. Inadvertent occlusion of these structures during repair can lead to significant hydrocephalus due to venous outflow obstruction or even venous congestion or infarction of brain. For patients with nasofrontal encephaloceles, the prognosis is good if the hypothalamus has not herniated into the sac.

Chiari Malformations

Chiari malformations are congenital abnormalities of posterior fossa. Cerebellar development is characterized by extension of cerebellar tissue (the tonsils) through the foremen magnum to obstruct normal CSF flow, inhibit normal instantaneous equilibration of CSF pressures between the cranial and spinal CSF compartments, and place pressure on the dorsal medulla and upper spinal cord, which can become symptomatic. Disruption of CSF flow and pressure equilibration dynamics can lead to secondary spinal cord or brainstem syrinx formation, which can also be symptomatic.

Chiari I malformation is characterized by tonsillar displacement greater then 5 mm through the foramen magnum into the spinal canal. In severe cases, the end of the tonsils can be as low as the C2 or C3 level. It is associated with a reduced posterior fossa compartment volume, a low insertion of the torcula onto the skull, and a steepened tentorial angle rising up to the tentorial incisura. Syringomyelia is common with significant caudal displacement of the tonsils but rare in minor cases (Fig. 8-15). Chiari I malformations usually do not become symptomatic until adolescence or adulthood unless symptoms from an associ-

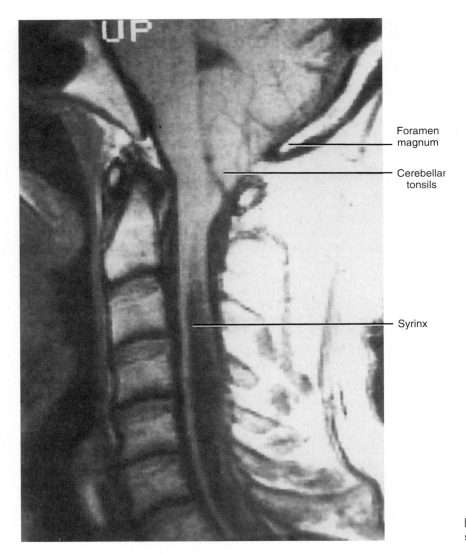

Figure 8-15 Magnetic resonance imaging scan showing a Chiari I malformation.

ated spinal cord syrinx (e.g., scoliosis) or tethered cord syndrome supervene during a growth spurt. Symptoms are broad and can include varying combinations of posterior occipital headaches radiating upwards (usually worse with Valsalva maneuvers), tinnitus, hearing loss, imbalance, oscillopsia from nystagmus, hiccups, nausea, dysphagia, hoarse voice, dysarthria, and bilateral hand numbness (presumably from dorsal pressure on the gracilis and cuneatus nuclei in the upper spinal cord at the top of the dorsal columns.

Chiari II (Arnold-Chiari) malformation is uniquely associated with myelomeningocele. In addition to reduction in posterior fossa volume, this syndrome is associated with intrinsic congenital migrational abnormalities of the brain stem including tectal beaking and actual physical kinking of the medulla. The brain is maldeveloped, with hypoplasia of the lower cranial nerve nuclei as well as cerebellar and cerebral microgyria and heterotopias common. Hydrocephalus occurs because the fourth ventricular outlet foramina are obstructed and because aqueductal stenosis

is common. Syringomyelia may occur as well. Both the tonsils and lower vermis of the cerebellum can descend down into the spinal canal and the caudal extent of descent can reach inferiorly as low as C3-5. The onset of symptoms from Chiari II malformation may occur in infancy, childhood, or even adult life. In infants, symptoms include opisthotonos (extensor posturing with arched spine), difficulty swallowing, regurgitation, stridor, and apnea. In children and adults, the manifestations are classified as brainstem (dysphagia, bulbar speech), cerebellar (nystagmus, oscillopsia), and upper motor neuron (hemiparesis, quadriparesis). In addition, syrinx, if present, can become symptomatic and cause lower motor neuron weakness in the upper extremities. The patient may also have a hanging sensory deficit over the shoulders that can extend to the arms and chest, sparing the lower body. With Chiari II malformations, urgent surgery is necessary to decompress the brain stem and reopen the foramen magnum CSF pathways as soon as the patient develops the first symptom, however slight. Multiple studies have now shown that once patients become symptomatic, syndrome progression can be rapid, and once function is lost, it is not likely to be recovered after subsequent decompression. Emphasis needs to be placed on preventing dysfunction in Chiari II patients, especially when they are infants and small children.

Surgery is performed to decompress the cerebellum, brain stem and upper spinal cord as well as restore foramen magnum CSF flow and fluid dynamics. This usually involves a limited decompressive suboccipital craniectomy as well as laminectomies to a level below the caudal extent of hindbrain herniation. The dura is usually opened in order to lyse thickened arachnoid adhesions at the cisterna magna and lateral medullary cisterns to ensure external CSF flow. Under the microscope, the tonsils can be separated in order to insure that the foramen of Magendie is open to the IV ventricle in order to reestablish internal CSF flow. With Chiari II malformations, a silastic tube can be used as a foramen of Magendie stent to ensure that communication with the subarachnoid space persists postoperatively. The dura is closed with a patch graft to insure adequate CSF communication between the posterior fossa and the spinal canal and to reduce the likelihood of recurrence. If syringomyelia is present, it is preferable to leave it alone and allow it to resolve spontaneously over the next 6 to 12 months (successful in the majority of cases). Syringosubarachnoid shunting or release of potential spinal cord tethering can be performed in a second stage, if syringomyelia does not adequately resolve once CSF flow and equilibration dynamics are reestablished across the foramen magnum.

Epilepsy

Epilepsy is a condition involving repeated seizures over time. Idiopathic epilepsy usually presents in childhood. New-onset seizure in an adult should prompt a thorough work-up to rule out cerebral mass lesion (e.g., tumor, AVM, or abscess) or drug or alcohol abuse. Epilepsy can be considered to be lesional (i.e., related to an image-defined mass lesion such as tumor, heterotopia, AVM, or abscess) or idiopathic. Idiopathic epilepsy is usually associated with primary neuronal focus that has developed a tendency towards electrical irritation and autonomous electrical activity. It can result from areas of prior brain injury where neurons become trapped in gliosis or scar (e.g., prior head injury, encephalitis, meningitis, brain surgery) or can be an area of stunted CNS development (e.g., mesial temporal sclerosis). Seizures can be simple partial, complex partial, partial with secondary generalization, or generalized (grand mal or petit-mal/absence). Most epilepsy is controllable with anticonvulsant therapy, and different medications work best for different types of seizures. Occasionally, multiple agents are required to control the disorder.

It is only when epilepsy becomes intractable and is significantly disabling to the patient that primary epilepsy surgery is considered. Intractability can be a slippery concept, but generally implies that adequate dose trials of at least three appropriate anticonvulsants for the particular seizure type have been tried, either singly or in combination, without success. Evaluation of a patient for potential epilepsy surgery involves standard diagnostic surface EEG and video-EEG monitoring to carefully confirm the type of seizure. MR neuroimaging is also used to assess anatomy and rule out structural lesions. Functional testing is used to localize speech function and hemispheric dominance. Formal neurocognitive testing is often performed as a baseline for postoperative comparison. If seizure focus localization cannot be adequately assured with standard EEG, then invasive three-dimensional monitoring with either subdural electrode grids, stereotactically implanted depth electrodes, or both may help confirm and define the precise point of seizure origin. The appropriateness of the patient for primary epilepsy surgery and the actual type of surgery attempted is usually decided by multidisciplinary epilepsy team consensus. Even if primary epilepsy surgery is not thought to be of help, some seizure control improvement can sometimes be obtained with surgical insertion of a vagal nerve stimulator.

Primary epilepsy surgeries include standard temporal lobectomy, selective amygdalohippocampectomy, cortical resections guided by intraoperative electrocorticography, partial corpus callosotomy, subcortical disconnections, and functional hemispherectomy. Patients may undergo only one surgery or may receive a series of incrementally more invasive procedures in an effort to do the minimum necessary to control the epilepsy. With carefully selected patients, a modern multidisciplinary epilepsy team can be expected to achieve epilepsy cure (no seizures, off all anticonvulsants) in up to 50% of patients. An additional group is either seizure-free or significantly controlled with continued anticonvulsant use. Overall, at least 70% to 80% of selected patients can expect significant benefit from the process. The effect on quality of life as well as subsequent cognitive function is very significant. Unfortunately, it is estimated that less than 20% of patients who are potential candidates for epilepsy surgery are currently referred to an epilepsy center for surgical evaluation.

Movement Disorders

Movement disorders are usually related to abnormalities localized to the corpus striatum, the thalamus, and the subthalamic and red nuclei. Surgically treatable conditions include hemifacial spasm (HFS), Parkinson's disease, other tremors of various types, dystonia, and athetosis.

HFS is a progressive disorder of the facial nerve and facial nerve nucleus that leads to unilateral rhythmic facial twitching of the facial musculature. It usually starts around the eye and then progresses over time to involve the lower face (in rare atypical situations the reverse is true). Eventually the spasms progress to involve the platysma and frontalis muscles. Tonus phenomenon occurs when the syndrome is severe. It consists of a titanic burst of repetitive muscle contractions without intervening relaxation that can grip the side of the face and hold it in a unilateral forced grimace smile while the eye is unable to open.

Medications do not work for HFS. Peripheral injections of botulinum toxins can temporarily mask the muscle twitches in mild cases, but it does not prevent syndrome progression. Furthermore, chronic repetitive injections are required, there is a risk of epiphora, and injections in the lower face can lead to unwelcome facial weakness. Posterior fossa cerebellopontine angle exploration with microvascular decompression (both arteries and veins) of the centrally myelinated portion of the facial nerve as it leaves the brainstem (root entry zone) leads to permanent cure of HFS in 80% of patients treated by an experienced surgeon.

With time, Parkinson's patients become refractory to pharmacologic agents and begin a progressive course of deterioration with worsened tremor, increased rigidity and bradykinesia, and changing on-off intervals. Stereotactic neurosurgical interventions can provide assistance when patients become refractory to medications. Stereotactic lesioning of select areas of the globus pallidus (pallidotomy) and thalamus (thalamotomy) can provide relief for both rigidity and tremor. More recently, efforts at selective thalamic stimulation after stereotactic insertion of stimulator electrodes have moved to the forefront for this condition. Stimulators have fewer complications, are reversible (they can be turned off), and are programmable in order to customize and titrate the desired response.

Dementia

Most causes of dementia are not surgically reversible. Normal pressure hydrocephalus (NPH) is an exception.

Normal Pressure Hydrocephalus

Normal pressure hydrocephalus is a clinical condition in which symmetric ventricular enlargement on CT or MR scan with normal ICP with diagnostic LP is associated with a triad of symptoms (gait disturbance, incontinence, and dementia) that improve or resolve with CSF diversion by VP shunting. They tend to occur in the order listed and tend to resolve in the same order. Once true dementia is present, the syndrome is advanced and complete resolution is rarely possible.

NPH must be distinguished from ex vacuo ventriculomegaly resulting from gradual brain loss (due to multiple ischemic insults, previous traumatic injuries, primary neurodegenerative disorder, or a combination of these three). This distinction is important because placing a VP shunt in an elderly patient with ex vacuo ventriculomegaly carries reported complication rates of between 20% to 50%, with subdural hygromas and hematomas being the most common. Attempts to diagnose those who truly have NPH (symptomatic, shunt-responsive ventriculomegaly) from those with ventriculomegaly from other causes have included high CSF volume LP "tap tests," radionuclide CSF cisternograms, and MR CSF flow studies. None of these studies has proven to have an acceptable positive and negative predictive value. The situation is compounded by a very high placebo effect and anticipational bias for patients and families (particularly with the LP tap test), as well as a high evaluator bias on the part of the neurosurgeon or the neurologist.

The key to understanding patient selection with NPH is realizing that the syndrome must be shunt-responsive. Therefore, the best test will either be a shunt or will accurately mimic a shunt. There are now two independent studies demonstrating that administering an ambulatory lumbar drainage test will correctly identify those patients who have a >90% chance of therapeutic response with placement of a permanent shunt. The test involves placing a lumbar drain and setting it to withdraw CSF at VP shunt rates while the patient is independently evaluated for gait by a physical therapist (with video gait analysis and balance master objective testing) as well as for cognitive function by a speech therapist (using validated testing instruments) on a daily basis for three days This test is currently the gold standard for assessing patients for NPH.

Although others have relied on empiric VP shunting, this practice is reported to have a high complication rate. Using a newer programmable shunt valve with the valve turned off at the time of insertion and then gradually turned on in an incremental manner over time, may help reduce the risk over acute overdrainage with subdural hygroma and subdural hematoma formation. However, this has yet to be proven empirically. This newer technology will not eliminate or lower the small risk of parenchymal or intraventricular hemorrhage associated with insertion, the risk of subsequent shunt and CSF infection, or the risk of bowel complications.

SPINE AND SPINAL CORD DISEASE

Anatomy and Physiology

The spine develops segmentally from each somite during fetal development. It consists of 7 cervical segments, 12 thoracic segments (each associated with a rib), 5 lumbar segments, and 5 sacral segments fused into one solid sacrum. It is composed of an anterior component that provides structural attachment for the axial skeleton and musculature, as well as the support necessary for upright ambulation. The posterior component serves a neural protective role. It consists of a spinal canal created by rings of bone extending posteriorly from each vertebral body (one pedicle and one lamina on either side) segmentally stacked upon one another (Fig. 8-16A,B). In between each segmental ring of bone is a neural foramen on each side through which passes the nerve root associated with each segment. Each vertebral segment can be considered a tripod with three joints. Anteriorly, the intravertebral disc serves as both a joint and an axial shock absorber. Posteriorly, paired facet joints on either side connect the pedicles and lamina above and below. The majority of cervical rotation occurs between C1 and C2 as well as between the occiput and C1. The majority of cervical flexion and extension occurs between C2 and T1. The majority of

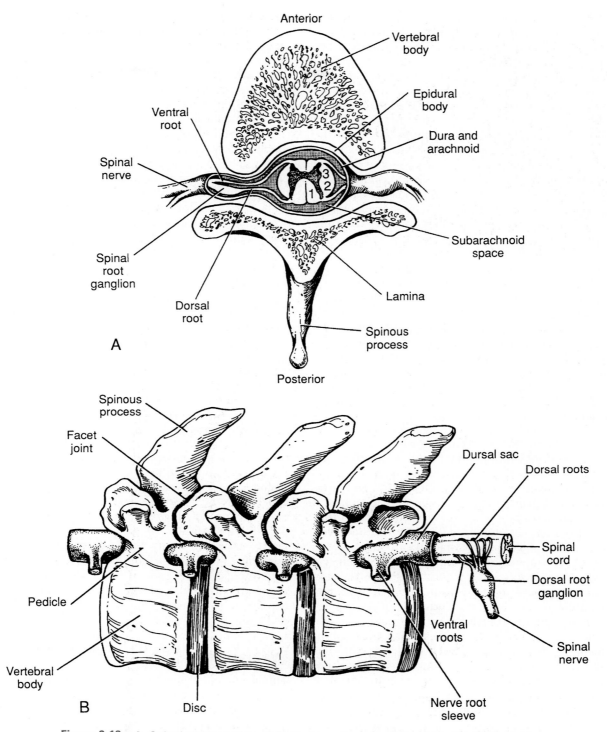

Figure 8-16   **A,** Spinal cross-section. *1,* Posterior column (position and vibration sense); *2,* posterolateral column (motor); *3,* anterolateral column (pain and temperature). **B,** Lateral view of the vertebral column and its contents.

thoracolumbar flexion occurs at T12–L2, while the majority of lumbar extension occurs at L4–S1. Both the cervical and lumbar segments have a natural lordosis, while the thoracic spine has a gentle kyphotic curve.

From a biomechanical stability standpoint, the spine can be considered to have three columns in the sagittal plane. The anterior column consists of the anterior longitudinal ligament and the anterior two thirds of the vertebral body and disc. The middle column consists of the posterior 1/3 of the vertebral body and disc as well as the posterior longitudinal ligament. The posterior column consists of the paired facet joints and the intraspinous ligament (extending between the spinous processes at each level). In general, a traumatic injury to the spine is considered to be unstable if it anatomically disrupts two of the three spinal columns.

The spinal cord continues down to the osseous L1–2 level, at which point it ends in a terminal fibrous filum that tethers it to the sacrum (filum terminale). From L2 down to S5, the lower spinal nerve roots continue downward within the dura of the spinal canal to the level of their foramen and exit as the cauda equina. The spinal cord extends from the foramen magnum to the lowest lumbar level in the newborn. As the child matures, the greater growth rate of the spinal canal causes relative ascent of the spinal cord within the canal. By adulthood, the tip of the cord reaches only as far as the top of L1–2. If the cord is tethered at its distal end during development, it is stretched as the child grows. Neurologic deficit can result.

Unlike the brain, the spinal cord has white matter tracts on its outer surface with the grey matter internally. Each cord segment is bilaterally symmetric and innervates a specific body segment (dermatome, sclerotome, and myotome) through its paired segmental nerves. The lemniscal sensory pathway (vibration and joint position sense) runs dorsally in the dorsal columns. The pyramidal tracts run laterally, and the spinothalamic tracts (pain and temperature sense) run anterolaterally on either side. Each segment relays the sensory information that it receives from its dorsal nerve roots up to the brain, through ascending reticular and lemniscal systems. Correspondingly, the segmental motor output through the ventral roots is brought under voluntary control by descending suprasegmental systems to the motor neurons of each cord segment. The level and vector direction of any compressive spinal cord lesion can be determined from the relative involvement of these three tracts as well as the dermatome and myotome level determined by examination.

With degenerative spine disease (disc degeneration and herniation as well as facet arthropathy), symptoms can result from either spinal canal stenosis, spinal foraminal stenosis, or a combination thereof. In the cervical and thoracic spine, **spinal stenosis** leads to symptoms of chronic partial spinal cord compression (myelopathy). In the lumbar spine, stenosis impinges upon the cauda equina and leads to a condition known as neurogenic claudication. With neurogenic claudication, back pain, radiating leg pain, and other cauda equina nerve root symptoms manifest with ambulation and are relieved by rest and flexing at the waist to increase the lumbar canal mid sagittal diameter. Foraminal stenosis, whether due to compression by anterior disc herniation, anterior vertebral body osteophyte, posterior facet joint osteophyte, or a combination of the three leads to pain, sensory loss, reflex change, and weakness signs and symptoms originating from the one nerve root affected (radiculopathy).

The blood supply to the spine comes from paired segmental arteries that accompany the nerve roots through each spinal foramen. The branch to the osseous segment penetrates the bone at the pedicle and then branches ventrally to supply the posterior three-fourths of the vertebral body as well as dorsally to supply the lamina, transverse process, and spinous process. This osseous vascular arrangement helps explain why metastatic tumors to the spine, which arrive as arterial emboli, tend to establish themselves initially within the pedicle of the spinal segment. Vertebral body or lamina involvement usually occurs by secondary extension. Blood supply to the spinal cord continues on to pierce the dura along with the nerve roots to supply the single anterior spinal artery (which runs in the ventral midline and supplies the anterior two-thirds of the spinal cord), as well as two smaller paired dorsal spinal arteries that run over each dorsal column and together supply the posterior medial one-third of the spinal cord. The spinal cord segmental arteries are not symmetric at each level. Generally, several dominant radicular arteries provide the majority of the blood flow. In the cervical cord the dominant contributors are the bilateral VA contributions to the anterior spinal artery, which come off after dural penetration and before they take off from the PICA. In the lower spinal cord the dominant radicular artery is called the artery of Adamkiewicz. It usually arises from the aorta on the left. It arises between T9–T12 in 75% of patients and between T9–L2 in 85% of patients. This artery is subject to injury with subsequent anterior spinal cord infarction during abdominal aortic aneurysm surgery. The vascular border zone between the major contributors to the anterior spinal artery (where the spinal cord is susceptible to ischemia in low flow states) is usually located at T4–5.

Evaluation

Spinal cord neurological evaluation includes both long tract and segmental assessments. Long tract evaluations include: (1) assessing the integrity of the pyramidal tracts and noting any upper motor neuron findings (increased tone, spasticity, hyperreflexia, and upper motor neuron pathological reflexes such as extensor plantar response or Hoffman's sign), (2) evaluating the upper and lower extremity distal joints for lemniscal pathway function (vibration — 128 Hz tuning fork and position sense), (3) evaluating the upper and lower extremity distal joints for spinothalamic function (pain-testing), and (4) presence of autonomic dysfunction (presence or absence of priapism, as well as bowel bladder and sexual function). Segmental examination includes assessing the muscle groups, patches of skin sensation, and reflexes associated with each significant appendicular nerve root.

The brachial and lumbar plexuses mix nerve roots into peripheral nerves so that muscles and reflexes have some overlap in impulse origin. To assist with segmental examination, there are a few rules for major nerve root contributions. The C5 nerve root is the only root supplying the rhomboid muscle and is the dominant root to the deltoid. It is the dominant root to the biceps reflex and supplies the skin on the upper outside of the shoulder (shoulder patch). The C6 nerve root is the dominant root to the brachioradialis muscle and reflex and supplies sensation to the first two fingers (six shooter). The C7 nerve root is the dominant root to the triceps muscle and reflex and supplies sensation to the middle finger (middle finger). The C8 nerve root is the dominant root supplying the intrinsic hand muscles (grip and finger abduction). It does not have a reliable reflex and provides sensation to the fifth finger (pinky). The L4 nerve root is the dominant root to the tibialis anterior (which dominates ankle dorsiflexion). It is the dominant root to the patellar reflex and supplies skin sensation on the medial calf down to the medial malleolus. The L5 nerve root is the dominant root to the extensor hallucis longus (great toe dorsiflexion). It does not have a reliable associated reflex and supplies skin sensation to the dorsal medial aspect of the foot (best tested in the first web space). The S1 nerve root is the dominant root supplying the gastrocnemius-soleus complex (controlling ankle plantar flexion). It is the dominant root to the Achilles reflex and supplies skin sensation to the ventral lateral aspect of the foot (best tested on the lateral aspect of the fifth toe).

Important clinical corollaries of these observations include noting that with the exception of C5, all C6–8 nerve roots extend below the elbow to the fingers for sensation. Therefore, with the exception of C5, arm pain should not be referred to as a "radicular pain" unless it extends down the arm to the fingers. Likewise, all L4–S1 verve roots extend below the knee to the calf or foot for sensation. Therefore, leg pain should not be referred to as "radicular pain" unless it extends below the knee. Likewise, a straight leg raise test is not considered positive for L4–S1 nerve root stretch unless the pain produced radiates below the knee.

Anterior Spinal Cord Syndrome

Anterior spinal cord syndrome leads to bilateral dysfunction of the spinothalamic pathways and pyramidal tracts with sparing of the lemniscal pathways. This leads to upper motor neuron findings and pin sensation reduction or loss bilaterally below the level of the lesion with sparing of joint vibration and position sense bilaterally. The level affected is determined by the segmental dermatome, myotome, and reflex examination. The severity of compression and/or depth of involvement is indicated by sparing versus dysfunction of the autonomic functions below the level of the lesion. Lesions that lead to variations of this syndrome

. include anterior spinal artery infarction, central disc herniation, ventral spondylotic myelopathy, spinal cord compression from a ventral meningioma, ventral compression from a spine tumor predominantly affecting the vertebral body, and ventral compression from an anterior canal burst fracture fragment.

Posterior Spinal Cord Syndrome

Posterior spinal cord syndrome leads to bilateral dysfunction of the lemniscal sensory pathways and pyramidal tracts with sparing of the spinothalamic pathways. This leads to upper motor neuron findings and vibration and joint position sense reduction or loss bilaterally below the level of the lesion with sparing of pin sharpness appreciation bilaterally. The level affected is determined by the segmental dermatome, myotome, and reflex examination. The severity of compression and/or depth of involvement is indicated by sparing versus dysfunction of the autonomic functions below the level of the lesion. Lesions that lead to variations of this syndrome include posterior spondylotic myelopathy, dorsal epidural hematoma or abscess, spinal cord compression from a dorsal meningioma, dorsal compression from tumor metastasis to Batson's plexus of epidural veins (e.g., lymphoma), or in-driven lamina fragment after spinal fracture.

Lateral Spinal Cord Syndrome

Also known as Brown-Séquard syndrome, lateral spinal cord syndrome leads to unilateral dysfunction of the lemniscal and spinothalamic sensory pathways as well as the ipsilateral pyramidal tract. This leads to ipsilateral upper motor neuron findings and vibration and joint position sense reduction or loss below the level of the lesion along with contralateral pin sensation reduction or loss below the level of the lesion. The level affected is determined by the segmental dermatome, myotome, and reflex examination. Careful pin examination may allow detection of a thin band of a suspended sensory level to pin testing at the specific level of the lesion in the spinal cord. The severity of compression and/or depth of involvement is indicated by sparing versus dysfunction of the autonomic functions below the level of the lesion. Lesions that lead to variations of this syndrome include lateral disc herniation, spinal cord compression from a lateral nerve root schwannoma, and compression from a spine tumor predominantly affecting the pedicle of the vertebra.

Central Spinal Cord Syndrome

Lesions in the center of the spinal cord (intramedullary tumors, syringomyelia) cause a loss of pain and temperature sensation at and just below the level of the lesion. An island of hypalgesia lies suspended between regions of normal sensation. This loss is caused by injury to second-order fibers that cross from the root entry zone to the contralateral anterior spinothalamic tract. As the lesion expands, the most medial aspects of the long fiber tracts are affected with spastic weakness, anesthesia, and dorsal column deficits that extend down from the level of the lesion.

Cauda Equina Versus Conus Medullaris Syndrome

Distinguishing between cauda equina and conus medullaris syndrome can be challenging. However, there are specific distinctions that can help. For example, cauda equina lesions are often associated with back or radicular pain, while conus lesions usually are not. Conus lesions are more likely to present suddenly with bilateral symptoms, while cauda equina lesions are more likely to present gradually and initially with unilateral symptoms. Both can lead to saddle sensory finding involving the sacral dermatomes bilaterally. However, cauda equina lesions are more likely to be asymmetric or unilateral, while conus lesions are more likely to exhibit sensory dissociation (sparing of the spinothalamic sensory pathway but not the lemniscal pathway, or visa versa). Cauda equina lesions are more likely to present with asymmetric motor loss, while conus lesions usually have symmetric motor loss. Autonomic findings are more common in conus lesions and tend to be present earlier than in cauda equina lesions. Common cauda equina syndrome lesions include large disc herniations, epidural hematoma or abscess, or intradural extramedullary tumor at the cauda equina level. Common lesions leading to conus medullaris syndrome include epidural hematoma or abscess, compressive epidural tumor, compressive canal bone fragment from a thoracolumbar burst fracture, and a myxopapillary ependymoma.

Neuroimaging

The same general comments and observations noted about CT and MR scanning in the cranial and cerebrovascular regions (and discussed in that section) apply to evaluation of the spine and spinal cord. MR is an excellent screening tool to assess the spine for canal mass, osseus spine tumor, disc herniation, spinal canal stenosis, and segmental foraminal stenosis. It is the imaging procedure of choice for assessing the spinal cord for diagnostic purposes, including, syrinx, tumor, or tethering, and for assessing the spine for infection or ligamentous injury. It is good at showing changes in vertebral body bone marrow and paraspinous soft tissue masses. CT scan is superior for assessing osseous fractures, facet joint alignment and integrity, and the presence of osteophytes, calcification of the posterior longitudinal ligament, or calcified spondylotic bars. CSF contrast myelography remains the best means of assessing nerve root sleeve CSF cutoff, confirming significant foraminal stenosis as well as assessing split spinal cord malformations. Spinal angiography remains the best means of detecting spinal AVMs or dural artery-venous fistulae. Each segmental spinal artery has to be individually and selectively sampled with the endovascular catheter in order to have a complete study. Plain spine films still have a role for the initial assessment of spine trauma and are a good screening tool for spine involvement with metastatic tumor. Bone scans are also an excellent screening tool for spine involvement with metastatic tumor, as well as spine infection and compression fractures.

Electrophysiology

Neurophysiology is an excellent means of sampling muscles in order to detect myotomal radicular denervation. Fibrillations and insertional irritability suggest acute denervation form the appropriate nerve root, while polyphasic action potentials suggest chronicity with reinnervation. Extremity EMG studies can be useful in assisting with nerve root localization for a suspected radiculopathy, but electrical findings take up to 6 weeks to appear after complete denervation.

Sensory-evoked potentials can be utilized to assess lemniscal pathway integrity and can be used intraoperatively to assess dorsal spinal cord function on a continuous basis. Motor-evoked potentials can only be performed with the patient under anesthesia and thus have their greatest use as an intraoperative monitor of the function of the lateral aspects of the spinal cord.

Spine Trauma

Spine trauma includes ligamentous injuries, spine fractures, fracture-dislocations, acute disc herniations, and incomplete and complete spinal cord injury.

Trauma Evaluation

Spinal cord injury patients should be assessed to determine whether their injury is complete or incomplete, according to the long tract and nerve root schemas outlined above (Table 8-4). Careful sacral examination is very important, since sacral sparing may be the only sign of an incomplete lesion and may go unnoticed if the sacral area is not carefully assessed. The presence or absence of priapism should be noted, and rectal tone, bulbocavernosus reflex, abdominal reflexes in all four quadrants, and the cremasteric reflexes should be carefully assessed. In addition to the neurological examination, examination of the spinal column includes palpation for deformity, tenderness, and spasm as well as tests of mobility. Tests of mobility are only performed once radiographs confirm no further injury would result from them. These tests include flexion, extension, rotation, and tilting of the neck and back.

Radiographs of the spine provide information about vertebral anomalies, displacement, destruction or remodeling, and disc space narrowing. Ninety percent of the diagnostic information gleaned from a simple A-P, lateral, and open-mouth trauma c-spine series is contained in the lateral view. It must have adequate technique and show the spine all the way down to the top of the T1 vertebral body. An additional swimmer's view is sometimes required to see this low. If no change is obvious, but the patient has significant symptoms or findings, or if some changes seem to merit further investigation, CT with coronal and sagittal

Table 8-4	**Potential Complications of Spinal Cord Lesions at or above Specific Levels**			
Level	**Innervation**	**Potential Risks**	**Treatment**	
S2–S5	Sphincters	Retention, incontinence (urinary tract infection)	Bladder catheterization	
L1–S2	Legs	Anesthesia and immobility (decubitus ulcers)	Careful, frequent positioning	
T1–12	Sympathetics	Temporary hypotension	Catecholamines	
	Chest cage	Respiration (pneumonia)	Respiratory care	
C5–T1	Upper extremities	Inability to perform self-care		
C3–C5	Diaphragms	Respiration (apnea, pneumonia)	Ventilatory assistance	

reconstructions or MRI scan is performed. An alternative study is myelography, with or without subsequent CT scan. Myelography requires lumbar puncture and may increase a neurologic deficit if the spinal canal is significantly compromised because of tumor or abscess. In these cases, no CSF is removed, and the amount of contrast material injected is small. Trauma myelography is now only rarely performed at most medical centers. If the patient has normal imaging studies and a normal examination but still has neck pain, dynamic flexion-extension views are obtained. If the patient cannot perform an adequate flexion-extension study due to muscle spasm, the cervical collar is left in place for 7 to 10 days. The patient is restudied once the spasms have decreased.

Stabilization

Patients are kept in a hard cervical collar until their cervical spine can be officially cleared, both clinically and radiographically. Clearing of a cervical spine requires a normal radiographic study (trauma series plain films or a fine-cut CT scan with axial and coronal reconstructions), a normal exam, and a pain-free patient with a normal mental status, or a patient with persisting pain but no abnormal motion on adequate dynamic films. Patients are kept on a long board until their thoracic and lumbar spines can be assessed with log rolling as well as screening A-P and lateral T-, and L-spine plain films.

Controversy currently exists as to whether incomplete spinal cord injury patients should be treated with either 24- or 48-hour high-dose methylprednisolone infusions. Both have been shown to lead to marginally statistically significant improvement of an extremely small magnitude compared with best supportive care without steroids in randomized clinical trials. However, the effect is very small in magnitude, barely reaches a significant level, and comes at the expense of a higher medical complication rate resulting from megadose steroid use. Currently, reasonable arguments can be made both for and against high-dose steroid use for trauma, and the determination is left to the responsible licensed staff physician whether or not to employ them. There is no proven role for high-dose steroids in patients with complete spinal cord injury or a currently asymptomatic adult patient (despite a history of transient extremity paresthesias that previously resolved) with a nor-

mal examination. Additional stabilization measures include bladder decompression with a self-retaining catheter, and maintaining oxygenation and systemic blood pressure. Systemic pressors such as dopamine are sometimes needed to maintain good spinal cord perfusion pressure in the face of sudden loss of systemic vascular tone from neurogenic shock.

Spinal Cord Injury Without Radiographic Abnormality

Spinal cord injury without radiographic abnormality (SCIWORA) is a special form of spinal cord injury that occurs in pediatric patients in the absence of osseus fracture due to the accentuated ligamentous laxity in children. In the absence of osseus abnormality on plain x-ray or CT scan, even in the face of a currently normal examination and asymptomatic state, a child (0 to 18 years) should be kept in a cervical collar if there has been a history of even transient neurological symptoms that could localize to the spinal cord. The patient should be evaluated by MR scan for ligamentous injury and probably evaluated by somatosensory evoked potentials to detect subclinical residual spinal cord dysfunction before risking assessment with dynamic flexion-extension views. SCIWORA patients are particularly prone to reinjuring their spinal cord with seemingly trivial movements or subsequent trauma. The second ictus is usually much more severe and may lead to permanent deficits. This syndrome is unique to the pediatric population.

Spine Fractures

Spinal fractures include specialized fractures of the C1–2 complex, fracture dislocations of the C3–7 cervical spine, thoracic compression fractures, thoracolumbar compression and burst fractures, and lumbosacral fracture-dislocations.

C1 (Jefferson) Fracture

A C1 Jefferson fracture is a fracture in two places of the atlas, usually due to axial load injury. The fracture is inferred from lateral spreading of the lateral masses on open-mouth c-spine views. It is directly visualized on axial CT scan views. Forty percent of Jefferson fractures are associated with C2 fractures. Jefferson fractures rarely present with neurological injury and usually heal with hard cervical collar immobilization for 3 months. After healing, the patient should be assessed with flexion-extension views to rule out C1–2 instability from anterior C1–2 ligamentous disruption.

C2 (Odontoid) Fracture

C2 odontoid fractures are transverse plane fractures through the stem of the axis that usually result from acute sudden extension as can occur when one falls forward like a tree trunk, with the forehead as the point of impact. Type II odontoid fractures occur right at the base of the odontoid peg. Type III fractures go down into the base of the body of C2, and type I fractures are avulsion fractures of the odontoid tip at the apical alar ligament insertion point. Type I and III lesions usually heal well with halo immobilization for 3 to 6 months. Type II odontoid fractures are more problematic. They have a high nonunion rate with halo immobilization due to tenuous vascular supply at this C1 and C2 somite fusion interface. Age plays an important role in determining the risk of nonunion. Generally, pa-

tients younger than age 40, who do not smoke and who have <4 mm fragment displacement, will likely heal with halo immobilization. For other patients, either halo immobilization or operative fusion can be employed. Surgical approaches for this lesion include anterior odontoid lag screw fixation (if the transverse check ligament is assessed to be intact), bilateral posterior transarticular screw fixation, or posterior C1–2 interlaminar fusion.

C2 (Hangman's) Fracture

C2 hangman's fracture (also known as C2 traumatic spondylolisthesis) is a bilateral pedicle fracture of C2, usually from acute hyperextension injury. Approximately 95% of these patients will be neurologically intact. The majority of these patients can be successfully treated with halo immobilization for 3 to 6 months. Rare cases with significant displacement and irreducible anterior angulation of the C2 on C3 may require operative fusion.

Subaxial C3–C7 Fractures

The majority of C3–7 fractures are traumatic fracture-dislocations (Fig. 8-17). Exceptions are the clay shoveler's

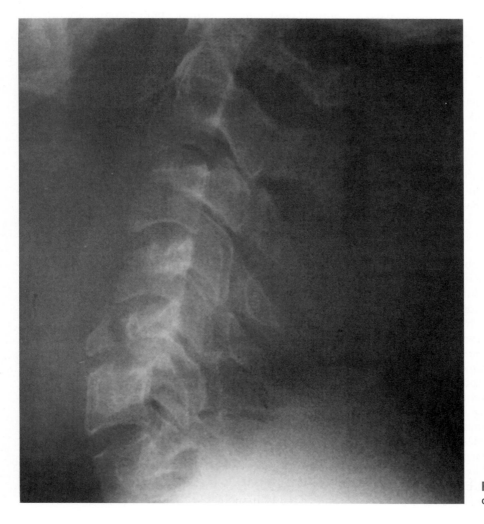

Figure 8-17 Fracture dislocation, C5 on C6.

fracture, which is a stable isolated spinous process fracture resulting from hyperextension that usually heals well with a cervical collar. Another fracture-dislocation is the anterior vertebral body corner tear-drop fracture, which also usually heals well with only collar immobilization.

Acute fracture dislocations usually result from hyperflexion injuries or hyperflexion injuries with axial loading. When an axial load is involved, there is usually an associated compression or burst fracture of the vertebral body, and there may be associated fracture of the lamina. The flexion component often leads to disruption of the intraspinous ligament posteriorly and can lead to either unilateral or bilateral jumped facets with anterior subluxation of the superior vertebral body in relation to the inferior vertebral body. Unilateral jumped facets can lead to a subluxation of up to a maximum of 25% vertebral body mid-sagittal width on lateral c-spine films. The A-P view is usually associated with misalignment of the spinous processes at this level due to the rotational component. Anterior subluxations greater than 25% of the vertebral body mid-sagittal width on lateral c-spine films should lead one to suspect bilateral facet dislocation.

To rule out ventral herniated disc or hematoma with C3–7 fracture-dislocations, an MR scan is useful before the fracture is reduced. If there is no burst or compression fracture component likely to warrant intraoperative reduction through anterior corpectomy and cervical plate fusion, then an attempt at closed reduction may be made. After placing Gardner-Wells tongs percutaneously to purchase the skull bilaterally above the ear canal, weighted in-line traction is gradually initiated along with muscle relaxants. It is customary to start with 5 to 10 lbs of traction and then proceed in 5-lb increments waiting a minimum of 20 to 30 minutes between each weight change and checking a lateral c-spine film prior to each new weight increment to assess for success of reduction or signs of overdistraction that might indicate ligamentous injury. Efforts continue until a maximum weight of 10 lbs per involved level is achieved, or until reduction is successful. Successful reduction gains should be held by halo immobilization for 3 to 6 months. Failure to achieve reduction usually leads to surgical exploration and intraoperative reduction and fusion. This can be done anteriorly with an anterior cervical discectomy with plate fixation after reduction or posteriorly with lateral mass plating fusion and/or intralaminar fusion sometimes supplemented by an intraspinous process dorsal tension band reconstitution, depending on the anatomy of the associated fractures. Facet fracture is a common reason for failure of closed reduction attempts. Very rarely, a C3–7 three-column spinal fracture is so unstable as to require a 360-degree fusion both posteriorly and anteriorly.

Vertebral Artery with Cervical Fractures

Fractures involving the transverse foramen C2–6 should raise the question of the status of the associated VA. Even cervical spine fracture not involving the transverse foramen can lead to VA occlusion or compromise due to traumatic dissection. While these injuries are rarely symptomatic due to the usual presence of a contralateral collateral VA, delayed embolization and posterior circulation stroke can occur. The VA should be examined for occlusion by means of CT angiogram, MR angiogram, or cerebral angiogram before considering a posterior lateral fusion with screws. Both C2-T1 lateral mass and C1–2 transarticular screw fixation run a small risk of VA injury. If the VA injured is the only remaining VA supplying the brainstem, then significant problems could result.

Thoracic Compression and Burst Fractures

Vertebral body compression fractures are the most common mid thoracic traumatic fractures. Due to the presence of the circumferential rib cage at T1–T10, these fractures usually heal well without surgery and only require an external thoracolumbar sacral orthosis (TLSO) to assist with pain control. Standing weight-bearing T-spine films should then be obtained. Surgical intervention should be considered for ≥50% loss of body height and/or ≥20 degrees of kyphotic angulation, which are risk factors for progressive kyphotic angulation. Burst fractures are very rare in the T1–10 thoracic spine, and operative indications include those for the compression fracture as well as ≥50% spinal canal mid sagittal canal compromise on axial CT scan.

Thoracolumbar Junction Compression and Burst Fractures

The thoracolumbar junction (T11-L2) is a point of maximum axial load as well as a pivot point for thoracolumbar flexion. As a result, it is particularly prone to compression and burst fracture resulting from axial load coupled with flexion. Compression fractures do not disrupt the posterior wall of the vertebral body, while burst fractures include the posterior wall and often lead to retropulsion of bone fragments into the spinal canal. Surgical intervention should be considered for ≥50% loss of body height and/or ≥20 degrees of kyphotic angulation, which are risk factors for progressive kyphotic angulation with either fracture type. An additional risk factor for progressive kyphotic angulation seen with burst fractures is ≥50% mid-sagittal spinal canal compromise on axial CT scan. In the absence of these indications, additional surgical exploration considerations include three-column spinal disruption and canal compromise in a patient with an incomplete spinal cord injury. Surgical fusion can be done from the front with corpectomy and short-segment anterior-lateral plate; from the back with short segment pedicle screw fixation with long moment arm chance screws utilized to maximize the chance of kyphotic correction, and anterior fragment reduction through ligamentotaxis (relying on the intactness of the posterior longitudinal ligament); from the back with long segment fixation (3 levels above and 3 levels below the injury); or from a combination of anterior and posterior approaches.

Thoracolumbar Junction Chance Fractures

More common before the shoulder harness and airbags were added to the traditional lap belt in automobiles, the

Chance fracture is the fracture that disobeys the 3-column stability rule. It results from thoracolumbar hyperflexion and extension, leading to an axial plane fracture that goes through the pedicles and facet joints as well as either the vertebral body or the disc space. Paradoxically, these fractures are usually stable and can usually be treated with a TLSO brace for pain control followed by early mobilization. Surgical fusion can be considered if there is a need to explore the spinal canal for bone or disc fragment in the presence of a partial spinal cord injury, if the patient wishes to have more rapid active mobilization as part of a posttraumatic rehabilitation program, or if doubt remains about the fracture stability based on anatomic concerns.

Lumbar-Sacral Fracture Dislocations

Lumbar-sacral fracture dislocations include traumatic L4–5 or L5–S1 spondylolisthesis and combinations of vertebral body compression and burst fractures. These levels are below the level of the conus medullaris and thus do not risk spinal cord injury. The need for surgical fusion versus conservative management in a TLSO or lumbar-sacral corset is based on the same three-column injury anatomic criteria and progressive kyphosis risk criteria listed above. In addition, traumatic anterolisthesis greater than 25% as well as lateral plane and rotational dislocations are given careful consideration. Surgical fusion can be performed posteriorly, anteriorly, or in a 360-degree combination.

Spinal Cord Injury Sequelae

Patients with spinal cord injuries are very susceptible to urinary reflux, urinary infection, decubitus ulcers of the skin, pneumonia, deep venous thrombosis, and pulmonary embolus. They are also at risk for septicemia from pyelonephritis, pneumonias, or infected decubitus. Autonomic dysreflexia can be a dangerous cardiovascular reflex response to overly rapid or aggressive bladder decompression.

Patients with spinal cord injury must begin mobilization soon after stabilization. A proper bowel regimen is critical, and both bowel training with daily suppositories and bladder training with intermittent catheterization begins as soon as spinal shock resolves. Compression stockings, sequential compression devices, and subcutaneous heparin are used as prophylaxis against deep venous thrombosis. Careful pulmonary toilet is maintained (usually with the assistance of a Roto-Rest bed in patients with high quadriplegia). Regular nursing positioning, skin care, and special antidecubitus beds are utilized. Physical therapists and occupational therapists begin working with the patient at the bedside, as soon as possible. Ultimately, early transfer to an in-patient spinal cord injury facility is ideal.

Degenerative Spine Disease

Degenerative diseases of the spine include disc herniation, spinal osteoarthritis and stenosis, and spondylolisthesis.

Disc Degeneration and Herniation

The intervertebral disc is composed of the nucleus pulposus and the surrounding annulus fibrosis. Degeneration of the disc occurs when the nucleus pulposus becomes desiccated because of age or recurrent trauma. This can be readily detected as a "black disc" on T2-weighted MR scan. In contrast, herniation of a disc occurs when the nucleus pulposus is extruded through a tear in the annulus. Extrusion usually occurs posterolaterally and often causes compression of a nerve root (radiculopathy). When it occurs centrally in the cervical or thoracic spinal canal, it can compress the spinal cord (myelopathy, anterior syndrome, lateral syndrome, or combination). Unlike disc herniation, disc degeneration is often asymptomatic.

Most symptomatic disc herniations occur in the lumbar or cervical regions. For the lumbar region, 95% occur at the L4–5 and L5–S1 levels (point of maximal lumbar lordosis), with L3–4 making up another 3% to 4%. Cervical disc herniation is also common, especially at the C5–6 and C6–7 levels (point of maximal cervical lordosis). C4–5 and C7–T1 can also be affected. Symptomatic thoracic discs are uncommon, but may cause paraplegia. Bulging of a disc posteriorly beneath the posterior longitudinal ligament is often asymptomatic. Greater protrusion, with herniation and extrusion beneath or through the posterior longitudinal ligament, is likely to cause radicular pain and even neurologic deficit (Fig. 8-18). Surgery for frank extrusion is more likely to relieve radicular pain than back or neck pain.

Symptoms of disc herniation almost always include pain, both in the spine and down one extremity. This pain is often exacerbated by straining, coughing, or sneezing, and by motion of the affected portion of the spine. Herniated discs and other cervical spine problems cause neck pain and often refer pain to the scapular region, arm, and hand. Lumbar disc herniations produce low back and leg pain that is usually worse on weight bearing. This leg pain is characteristically sciatic. It radiates down the posterior or lateral leg into the calf or even to the foot. Signs of disc herniation include radicular numbness and weakness within the innervation of a single nerve root as well as reflex loss (Table 8-5).

Herniation of an L4–5 disc usually compresses the L5 nerve root, although the L4 nerve root exits the spinal canal between the L4 and L5 vertebrae. Because the roots of the cauda equina leave the spinal foramina just above the corresponding disc, they escape compression by herniations of the disc. The root that begins to leave the dural sac at this level to exit the foramen below is at risk from the usual lumbar disc herniation.

The differential diagnosis of cervical disc disease (neck or arm pain) includes angina if the patient has left arm pain, cervical osteoarthritis and stenosis, upper limb nerve entrapment, tumor or infection within or adjacent to the spine, and shoulder and elbow disease. Corresponding considerations in the lumbar region include vascular claudication, hernia, gynecologic disease, abdominal aortic an-

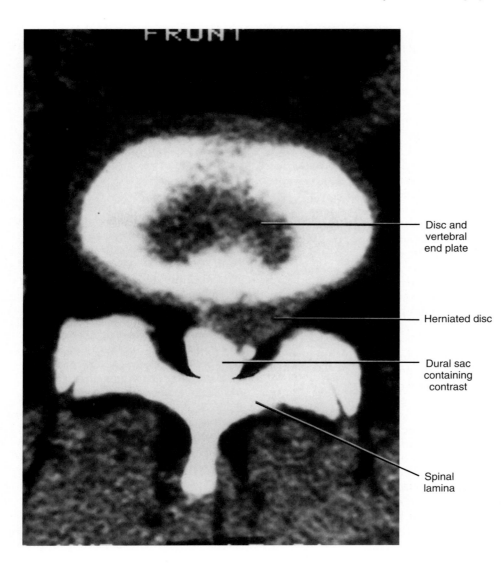

Disc and
vertebral
end plate

Herniated disc

Dural sac
containing
contrast

Spinal
lamina

Figure 8-18 Positive contrast computed tomography scan showing a herniated nucleus pulposus at L5-S1.

eurysm, spinal or retropelvic tumor or infection, lumbar osteoarthritis and stenosis, lower limb nerve entrapment, and hip and knee disease.

Initial treatment of most patients is conservative. The exception is patients who present with foot drop, bowel or bladder difficulties, or full-blown cauda equina syndrome or acute myelopathy. These patients should undergo urgent neuroimaging with consideration for early surgery if appropriate correlative abnormalities are identified. Initial conservative treatment consists of a short period of rest for the symptomatic spinal segment, analgesics, anti-inflammatory agents, and possibly muscle relaxants. In the cervi-

Table 8-5	Signs of Disk Herniation			
Level	**Root**	**Weakness**	**Reflex Loss**	**Numbness**
C4–5	C5	Deltoid	Biceps	Outer deltoid
C5–6	C6	Brachioradialis	Brachioradialis	Thumb, index
C6–7	C7	Triceps	Triceps	Middle
C7–T1	C8	Intrinsic hand	–	Pinky
L3–4	L4	Tibialis anterior	Patella	Medial calf
L4–5	L5	Extensor hallucis longus	–	Medial foot, 1st toe
L5–S1	S1	Gastrocnemius	Achilles	Lateral foot, left toe

cal region, treatment includes a collar to limit motion and may include traction. In the lumbar region, treatment consists of at least 24 to 48 hours of rest, followed by gradual increase of activity and progressive physical mobilization as tolerated. As improvement occurs, the patient may resume normal activities, but should avoid excessive lifting or bending. If progress is slow, physical therapy may be added to the regimen. Surgery is considered only if the patient shows no further progress over a period of weeks, if the condition worsens, or if there is marked weakness.

Disc herniation is suspected when examination and history localize the lesion to a specific nerve root. Diagnosis is confirmed by MR scan or myelo-CT scan. Back or neck pain with or without nonradicular arm or leg pain does not confirm that disc or foramen abnormalities seen on spine MR are the cause of the symptoms. Degenerative disc and spine abnormalities are seen in up to 70% of people in the United States over the age of 40 years. High confidence that the imaging abnormality of the source of the patient's symptoms requires clinical correlation to the correct affected nerve root.

Surgical treatment of disc herniation consists of microscopic or endoscopic excision. Percutaneous techniques are used, but their efficacy remains debatable and unproven. Standard techniques for lumbar or cervical discectomy include a posterior approach with limited removal of the adjacent lamina on the side of herniation, excision of the ligamentous flavum, gentle retraction of the nerve root, and removal of the underlying disc herniation. For cervical disc herniation, an anterior approach with or without spinal fusion with interposition bone graft and possible anterior cervical plate has become more common than posterior cervical discectomy. The disc is approached between the trachea and esophagus medially and at the carotid sheath laterally. The disc is excised through the anterior longitudinal ligament, back to and through the posterior longitudinal ligament. The herniated fragment is removed.

Good relief of radicular symptoms can be expected in >90% of patients with a clear radiculopathy that correlates with the lesion in question. Axial back and neck pain is less responsive with complete relief in only 60% to 70% of patients. Surgery is successful less often if these conditions are not met or if the patient has had a previous operation.

Foraminal Compression Syndrome

Even without frank disc herniation, radiculopathy can develop from foraminal or lateral recess stenosis due to a combination of three-dimensional factors. Disc bulge or herniation as well as endplate osteophyte can compress from the front, while posterior compression from facet joint arthropathy compounds the situation from behind. Due to the common absence of frank disc herniation and the poor resolution of MR for bony anatomy, the extent of nerve root compression can be underestimated with isolated MR scanning. For this setting plain CSF myelogra-phy with direct visualization of nerve root sleeve cut-off remains the most sensitive and specific test for confirming significant foraminal or lateral recess stenosis.

Treatment of this condition includes microscopic or endoscopic discectomy as described for disc herniation syndromes, but also critically depends upon decompressive microforaminotomy to deal with the facetal overgrowth and osteophyte compression. Results are equally effective so long as bony decompression is judicious and does not lead to spinal instability.

Cervical Stenosis

Cervical spinal canal stenosis leads to signs and symptoms of myelopathy. In cases of multilevel disc degeneration with chronic osteophyte formation, multiple segmental spondylotic "bars" can cause compression from a ventral vector. Degenerative thickening of the posterior ligamentum flavum often associated with ligamental folding and buckling with extension can lead to compression from a posterior vector. Ultimately, canal stenosis can be caused by a combination of ventral and dorsal factors. Patients are more susceptible to developing cervical stenosis with myelopathy if they are born with a congenitally tight cervical canal to start with, due to short pedicles bilaterally. Asians are particularly prone to a special stenotic syndrome known as ossification of the posterior longitudinal ligament (OPLL), which causes the PLL to ossify (usually with the ventral dural incorporation into the bone formed).

Treatment of myelopathy from cervical stenosis involves enlargement of the cervical canal. For ventral vector spondylotic bar lesions, this can be done anteriorly with multilevel anterior discectomy and fusions or with vertebrectomy and strut graft instrumentation. Good results can be achieved with actual improvement in myelopathy in the majority of patients for segments extending up to 3 disc and 2 vertebral body lengths. Longer segments have a tendency to forfeit cervical lordosis and carry a higher incidence of graft and instrumentation failure. For posterior vector compression, a multilevel decompressive laminectomy with or without lateral mass fusion to prevent loss of cervical lordosis and subsequent swan-neck deformity can be done. Alternatively, a decompressive multilevel laminoplasty that reconstructs the posterior spinal canal with a larger diameter can be performed. Posterior decompressive operations can more easily be performed for disease affecting more than 3 motion segments (C2 or 3 to C7 can be completed in the same sitting). Posterior decompressions usually stabilize the patient's clinical syndrome, but are less likely than anterior decompressions to actually reverse the process. Patients with OPLL are now more commonly treated with posterior decompressions due to the relatively high risk of disabling anterior dural tears and subsequent CSF leak seen with an anterior approaches to this difficult disease.

Preexisting cervical spinal stenosis can predispose patients to developing an acute central cord syndrome from sudden flexion-extension movements. If this occurs, the patient is immobilized in a hard cervical collar while the swelling of the spinal cord is allowed to resolve. Surgical decompression is performed in a delayed fashion to avoid the risk of further irritating an already damaged spinal cord.

Lumbar Stenosis

Lumbar stenosis develops from progressive encroachment of the spinal canal from the ventral aspect (disc degeneration, disc bulge, and reactive osteophyte formation) as well as the two posterior lateral directions (facetal hypertrophy and arthropathy). These three compass points of encroachment can collectively so indent the dural sac that it comes to appear as a tricornered hat in cross-sectional diameter. The points of maximal compression are at the inferior level of each lamina, with interval widening between the rings of constriction. On lateral CSF myelogram, the thecal sac can come to look like a string of sausage links.

As the lumbar stenosis progresses, it puts pressure on the nerve roots at the level of the cauda equina. At rest they may be asymptomatic, but with exertion such as walking, there is no room for the nerve roots to swell with increased blood flow necessary to meet their increased metabolic demands. This supply-demand mismatch leads to nerve root dysfunction and radicular symptoms (radiating radicular pain, numbness and tingling paresthesias, and myotomal weakness), which can affect multiple nerve roots bilaterally, and to lower back pain. These symptoms characteristically come on with walking and are relieved by rest, especially if the patient rests flexed at the waist (leaning over or sitting down) in such a way as to increase the mid-sagittal spinal canal diameter to provide the nerve roots with more room. With time and progression, the patient reports being able to walk shorter and shorter distances before having to stop to rest. This classic syndrome is called neurogenic claudication and must be distinguished from vascular claudication due to peripheral vascular disease (see Chapter 23 in Lawrence's *Essentials of General Surgery*, 4th ed).

Diagnosis is easily made on MR scan or CSF myelogram/CT scan. Treatment consists of posterior decompression of the involved segments. Although simple multilevel decompressive laminectomy was the treatment of choice for many years, and usually led to dramatic immediate improvement, unintentional disruption of the large degenerated facet joints on one or both sides often led to subsequent need for lumbar fusion in approximately 10% of cases. A newer approach involves bilateral multilevel inferior hemilaminotomies with resection of the segmental ligamentum flavum as well as bilateral undercutting medial facetectomies and foraminotomies at each affected level. With the superior lamina at each level as well as the intraspinous ligament preserved, it is hoped that this more involved procedure will lower the rates of secondary instability with multilevel wide decompressive laminectomy alone.

Spondylolysis and Spondylolisthesis

Forward slippage of one vertebral body on another (spondylolisthesis) most commonly occurs at the L4–5 or L5–S1 level. Bilateral defects (spondylolysis) across the spinal lamina diagonally, just below the pedicle, allow the most rostrolateral part of each lamina, with the attached pedicle and vertebral body, to separate and shift anteriorly. The spinal canal is sometimes compromised. These shifts are most common in children and adolescents, and tend to stabilize. Back pain and nerve root compression symptoms can occur in this younger age group. Adults, especially older adults, sometimes have spondylolisthesis without spondylolysis. In these patients, ligamentous laxity that accompanies osteoarthritic change permits slippage of adjacent vertebral bodies on one another to cause stenosis of the spinal canal. CT and MRI scans are extremely helpful in evaluating the patient and planning surgery. Operative stabilization and fusion may be necessary. Decompression is performed if there is neurologic deficit or radicular pain. The nerve root involved is usually one above that usually encountered for degenerative disc disease (L4 for L4–5, and L5 for L5–S1 spondylolisthesis).

Rheumatoid Arthritis and Congenital Atlantoaxial Dislocations

Rheumatoid arthritis compromises the spine, usually in the cervical region, and especially at the atlantoaxial (C1–2) level. Lesions at any cervical level may cause neural compression as a result of infiltration of vertebral bodies with collapse; ligamentous and disc degeneration with angulation and dislocation; or pannus (granulation tissue membrane) formation with mass effect. These changes, especially ligamentous laxity at the C1–2 level, cause chronic anterior dislocation of C1 on C2 and compress the spinal cord between the odontoid and the posterior arch of C1. Myelopathy can occur, but it progresses slowly, if at all. The resultant neurologic deficits are difficult to distinguish from more common neuropathies, motor degeneration, contractures, and arthritic deformities. Repeated evaluation, cervical collars, and surgical decompression, fixation, and fusion are important treatment considerations. Similar considerations govern congenital atlantoaxial (C1–2) dislocations, although symptoms are more episodic. Surgical stabilization is often performed, even if no neurologic deficit is detected.

Vascular Spine Disease

Vascular diseases of the spinal cord include AVMs, dural A-V fistulae, ischemic infarctions, and epidural hematomas. (See also Chapter 23 in Lawrence's *Essentials of General Surgery*, 4th ed.)

Spinal Cord AVM and Dural Arteriovenous Fistula

Spinal vascular malformations are uncommon, but are almost always AVMs, A-V dural fistulae, or cavernous malformations. Cavernous malformations occur within the cord, but AVMs may be located on the cord or within it. Dural A-V fistulae are always located adjacent to the spinal cord in intimate association with a segmental nerve root and its vascular pedicle. This relation to the cord defines the type and hazards of surgical treatment. Like tumors, lesions within the cord are more difficult to excise, and operation risks spinal paralysis to a far greater degree than operation on extramedullary AVMs. With dural A-V fistulae, the feeding arteries enter along the nerve root. Either surgical division of these feeders or, more recently, endovascular embolization of these feeders leads to cure. Vascular malformations of the cord often cause repeated attacks of spinal cord dysfunction or progressive spinal cord deficit. Spinal subarachnoid hemorrhage is uncommon.

Spinal Cord Stroke

Stroke can affect the spinal cord from embolic occlusion of the anterior spinal artery, or from border zone flow-related ischemia due to significant systemic hypotension or loss of a major segmental feeding artery such as the artery of Adamkiewicz. The cord is most susceptible to flow-related ischemia at the T4–5 level. The artery of Adamkiewicz is most susceptible to sacrifice during surgeries to repair abdominal aortic aneurysms, but can also be lost during left-sided retroperitoneal approaches to the thoracolumbar junction to repair and stabilize thoracolumbar compression or burst fracture. The syndrome is an anterior cord syndrome that spares the dorsal lemniscal pathways. Recent evidence suggests that lowering ICP by continuous perioperative lumbar drainage can lower the risk of anterior spinal artery infarction and reduce the severity of any subsequent stroke. It may be that this phenomenon works by optimizing spinal cord perfusion pressure by lowering ICP.

Epidural Hematoma

Spontaneous spinal epidural hematomas are associated with ruptured aneurysmal bone cysts involving the osseous spine, the rupture of dural A-V fistulae, and with iatrogenic coagulopathy. Iatrogenic epidural hematomas can be associated with LP, but are more commonly linked to placement of epidural catheters for pain control and/or lower extremity epidural anesthesia. In cases of abdominal aortic aneurysm repair performed under epidural anesthesia, neurosurgeons are often asked to distinguish catheter-related epidural hematoma from spinal cord infarction when the patient cannot move his or her legs postoperatively. The distinction is actually quite straightforward. Epidural hematomas lead to a posterior cord syndrome as opposed to the anterior syndrome seen with anterior spinal infarction. Even if the patient is intubated and sedated, somatosensory evoked potentials will indicate whether dorsal lemniscal function is preserved. An MR scan should be able to distinguish a dorsal hematoma from edema within the substance of the spinal cord. Epidural hematomas are treated with urgent correction of any coagulopathy that may be present. If they are small and asymptomatic,

they can be treated conservatively with observation. If they are symptomatic with cauda equina syndrome, conus medullaris syndrome, or any other cord compressive syndrome, they are surgically evacuated.

Spine Tumors

Spinal tumors are divided into three groups. These groups differ somewhat in age of presentation and prognosis. Extradural tumors arise from the osseous element of the spinal column (Figs. 8-19 and 8-20). Intradural extramedullary tumors arise from the dural sheath around the spinal cord or from the Schwann cell sheath around the spinal roots. Intramedullary tumors arise from the glial element of the spinal cord or from trapped ectodermal elements. Presenting symptoms of spinal tumors can be a variation of any of the spinal cord syndromes described above. Characteristically, they are also associated with back pain that is worse lying down, worse at night, and especially worse in the morning. A history of belt-like radiation of intercostal pain with Valsalva maneuver is also highly suggestive.

Secondary (Metastatic) Extradural Tumors

The most common spinal tumors in adults are extradural and are usually metastatic (Fig. 8-21). Metastases grow rapidly and usually cause symptoms of spinal cord compression that last from hours to a week. Most are carcinomas. Common primary lesions are located in the lung, breast, prostate, and kidneys. With the exception of lymphoma (which predominantly affects the dorsal and lateral epidural space), these tumors usually destroy bone. They compress the spinal cord either by growing in the epidural space or by causing collapse of the involved vertebrae. This collapse causes distortion, narrowing, and instability of the spinal column. Radiologic evaluation starts with plain spine films. Extradural (metastatic) tumors destroy bony elements. X-rays may show vertebral collapse that spares the disc spaces, but not the cortical end plates. Often there is loss of one or more pedicles (the winking owl sign — see Fig. 8-21A). If plain x-rays appear normal but strong suspicion persists, a nucleotide bone scan can be very sensitive to subtle early lesions. Both CT myelography and MR scanning are used to evaluate these patients. MR scanning avoids the danger of lumbar puncture and also visualizes the lesions, their effects on the spinal cord, and changes in the vertebrae. Gadolinium enhancement of MRI scan increases the definition of many spinal tumors. MRI scan is the most useful early step when a patient has spinal cord symptoms. It is especially urgent if the patient has a history of cancer.

As soon as spinal cord compression from metastatic tumor is suspected, the patient is treated with high-dose intravenous steroids. If the patient is in good clinical shape and the tumor is radiosensitive, then emergent radiotherapy is begun and the patient observed closely for neurological deterioration due to tumor swelling in reaction to the radia-

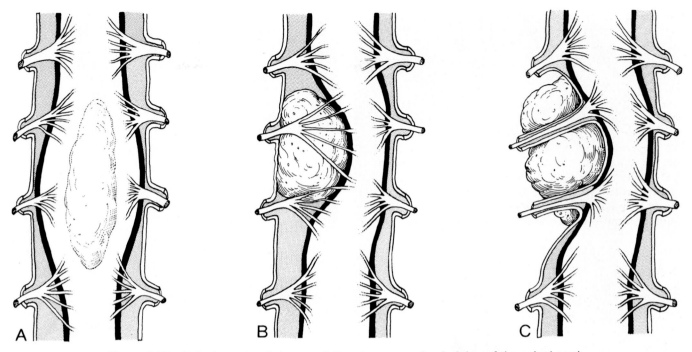

Figure 8-19 Spinal tumors. **A,** Intramedullary tumor causing bulging of the spinal cord. **B,** Extramedullary intradural tumor lying in the subarachnoid space, displacing and compressing the spinal cord, but not the dura. **C,** Extradural tumor lying in the epidural space, displacing the dural sac and spinal cord.

tion. In this setting, surgical decompression is reserved for evidence of neurological deterioration. If the tumor is radio-insensitive, the patient is already on the verge of losing ambulatory function. If the imaging suggests significant kyphotic or pending kyphotic deformity, then decompressive surgery with or without fusion is performed, followed by postoperative radiotherapy. The location of the compression dictates the type of operation performed. If the compression is from the back of the spinal canal or in the lateral gutters, laminectomy with tumor removal from the extradural space should suffice. Fusion is seldom necessary. If the compression is from the front because of vertebral collapse with angulation or because of tumor anterior to the cord, the operation is more difficult. Although a lateral posterior (costotransversectomy or lateral extracavitary) approach is advocated, the most common approach is anterior decompression with subsequent fusion (see Fig. 8-21C). Tumor surgery is most effective for patients who do not have complete loss of spinal cord function. The ability of the patient to walk prior to surgery is the single most important determinant of whether the patient will be ambulatory after surgery. The average survival after surgery for metastatic disease is generally 6 months.

Primary Spine Tumors

Primary spine tumors include both intradural extramedullary tumors and intradural intramedullary tumors

Intradural Extramedullary Spine Tumors

Intradural extramedullary tumors lie within the dural tube, but outside the confines of the spinal cord. In the cervical and thoracic spine, they lie adjacent to the spinal cord and the local nerve roots. They often distort and compress these structures and produce symptoms and signs of root or cord dysfunction. In the lumbar canal, they lie among the roots of the cauda equina and produce polyradicular symptoms and signs. These tumors are well circumscribed and do not extend over many segments. Since they are usually benign, the history is often long.

Neurofibromas are the most common intradural extramedullary tumors. They typically arise from a single dorsal sensory root. Multiple tumors are found in patients with neurofibromatosis. Neurofibromas can extend through an intervertebral foramen and grow out extradurally into the retropleural or retroperitoneal space. This dumbbell extension can become very large and may be the first portion of the tumor identified. For this reason, masses located near the spine require additional radiologic evaluation to determine whether they extend into the spinal canal.

Meningiomas are almost as common as neurofibromas and are based on the dura. They occur four times as often in women as in men. They are most common in the thoracic region and more commonly occur ventrally than dorsally.

The filum terminale within the cauda equina contains a continuation of the ependymal lining of the central

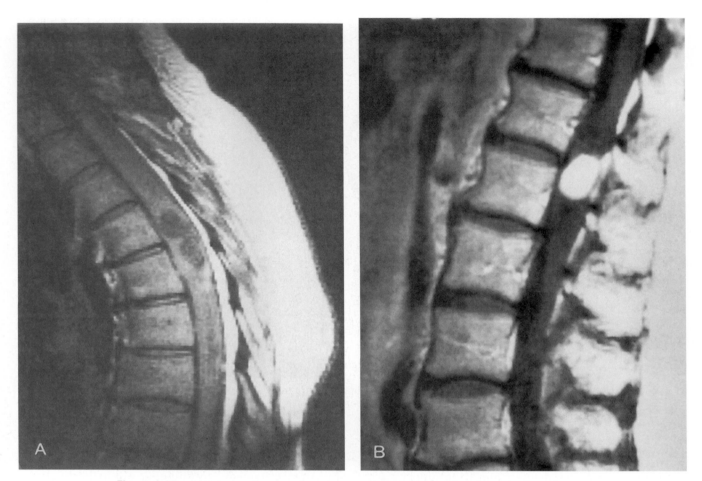

Figure 8-20   **A,** Enhanced magnetic resonance imaging scan showing spinal cord astrocytoma (intramedullary tumor). **B,** Enhanced magnetic resonance imaging scan showing spinal neurofibroma (extramedullary intradural tumor).

spinal canal. It is prone to develop a particularly benign form of ependymoma known as a myxopapillary ependymoma.

Contrast-enhanced MR is the imaging procedure of choice for seeing the type and extent of the tumor as well as its relationship to the spinal cord. CT scanning is better able to assess the surrounding bone changes resulting from the tumor. Neurofibromas may cause widening of a neural foramen on x-ray.

Intradural extramedullary tumors can be cured because they can usually be removed completely. Before the dura is opened, real-time ultrasound can be utilized to localize the tumor and ensure adequacy of rostral-caudal exposure. The operating microscope and microsurgical techniques, including the laser and ultrasonic aspirator, are used to remove the tumor. Laser is particularly effective and useful for dealing with lipomas. Neurologic function is monitored by repetitive testing of somatosensory and motor-evoked responses. Lower extremity and rectal EMG monitoring are useful for assisting with dissecting the cauda equina nerve roots free from a cauda equina schwannoma

or myxopapillary ependymoma. A recurrence rate of only 6% after 15 years is reported for meningioma. Similar or better results are expected for neurofibroma. Of these patients, 80% improve and 50% become completely normal.

Intradural Intramedullary Spine Tumors

Intramedullary tumors lie within the substance of the spinal cord. They are more common in children than in adults. Some are associated with a large cyst and may be confused with simple syrinx. Astrocytoma of the spinal cord is the most common intramedullary tumor of childhood (Fig. 8-20A). The biologic behavior of this tumor resembles that of low-grade cerebral astrocytoma, including the common presence of a cleavage plane between low-grade tumor and spinal cord. Malignant forms are rare. In some regions, the tumors blend with the spinal cord and limit the extent of surgical excision.

Ependymoma of the spinal cord is the most common intramedullary tumor in adults. These tumors arise from the ependyma of the central canal. They are usually well demarcated, and gross total excision is feasible.

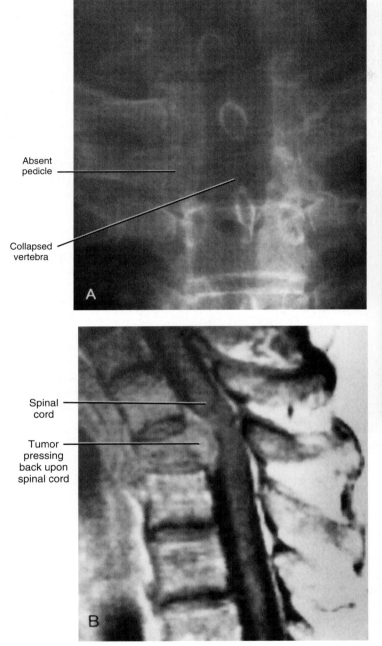

Absent
pedicle ——————

Collapsed
vertebra ——————

A

Spinal ——————
cord

Tumor ——————
pressing
back upon
spinal cord

B

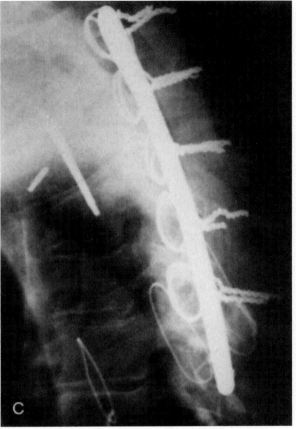

C

Figure 8-21 A, Metastatic tumor to the spine. **B,** Enhanced magnetic resonance imaging scan showing a metastatic spinal tumor. **C,** Lateral spine film after anterior decompression and fusion, with posterior stabilization and fusion, showing a metastatic spinal tumor.

Hemangioblastomas of the spinal cord account for fewer than 10% of intramedullary tumors. These tumors are sometimes cystic, are fairly well circumscribed, and do not extend over many segments. Total removal is possible in most cases, although bleeding can be a problem. Just as with cerebellar hemangioblastomas, these tumors are often associated with von Hippel-Lindau syndrome and are often multiple.

Dermoids, epidermoids, and lipomas are also found within the spinal cord or cauda equina, usually at or below the conus. A dermoid is often associated with a dermal sinus tract in the skin overlying the spine. This tract leads to the intraspinal tumor. Likewise, a lipoma that involves the conus or filum is usually in continuity with an overlying subcutaneous extension. The skin overlying this region may contain a hairy patch or cutaneous hemangioma.

Contrast-enhanced MR is the imaging procedure of choice for delineating the type and extent of the tumor as well as its relationship to the spinal cord. CT scanning allows assessment of the surrounding bone changes resulting from the tumor. Intramedullary lesions can enlarge the spinal canal and increase the interpedicular distance.

Intramedullary tumors are treated surgically in an attempt to remove the tumor and prevent further neurologic deterioration. Unlike intracranial ependymomas, ependymomas of the spinal cord can often be removed completely. The lack of a clear cleavage plane between an anaplastic or malignant astrocytoma and the spinal cord hinders attempts at complete removal. Only approximately 50% of spinal astrocytomas can be removed relatively completely. Microsurgical techniques greatly facilitate resection. Even if gross total resection is not possible, spinal cord internal decompression as well as spacious dural patch grafting can maximize additional functional time until deterioration restarts. Although most patients improve after surgery, spinal cord astrocytomas tend to recur, with increasing disability and even death. Radiation is an important adjunct in the management of chordoma. The role of radiotherapy the treatment of intramedullary tumors (e.g., incompletely removed intramedullary astrocytomas) is poorly defined to date, but it is probably helpful for residual ependymomas

Spine Infection

Spinal infections include discitis, osteomyelitis, and epidural abscess.

Osteomyelitis and Discitis

Discitis is far more common than osteomyelitis of the spine. It usually occurs in patients with diabetes, those who are immunocompromised, intravenous drug abusers, and patients with previous disc surgery. Infection is pyogenic (usually staphylococcal). Patients usually have severe back or neck pain and occasionally radicular pain. Local tenderness to both palpation and percussion is often present. Spinal cord or cauda equina compromise is rare. Within several months, spinal x-rays show dissolution of the vertebral end plates that define the disc space. Disc collapse and destruction follow. Ultimately, collapse and angulation of the adjacent vertebral bodies occur. MRI and CT scans show changes earlier than do x-rays. As with all types of spinal infection, the sedimentation rate is almost always elevated. Repeated studies provide a means to assess response to therapy. Fever and leukocytosis are uncommon because most cases are subacute or chronic and follow an indolent course.

Osteomyelitis can be bacterial, fungal, or tubercular in origin. Bacterial osteomyelitis often develops as contiguous spread of an adjacent discitis. The most common fungal osteomyelitis is due to coccidioidomycosis. Tuberculous osteomyelitis of the spine (Potts disease) is a chronic condition that usually begins beneath the two vertebral end plates that define a disc space and ultimately extends to involve both vertebral bodies. Unlike pyogenic osteomyelitis or discitis, in Potts disease the disc architecture and endplates remain relatively well preserved. Collapse of the vertebral bodies can lead to angulation of the spine and kyphotic deformity. Infection may spread to form an epidural abscess. Angulation, epidural abscess, and even disc prolapse can compress the spinal cord and lead to paralysis. Associated paraspinal abscess is common and has a telltale radiographic appearance

Discitis and osteomyelitis are treated with appropriate intravenous antibiotics for 6 to 8 weeks (which are best guided by culture results) and TLSO bracing to help control pain. Cultures can be obtained by CT-guided percutaneous needle biopsy, but can be sterile in up to 50% of postoperative discitis cases. Advanced osteomyelitis requires operative debridement and bone grafting. Tuberculous infection requires 12 to 18 months of multiple anti-TB agents. Coccidioidomycosis of the spine can be very difficult to clear, despite aggressive medical and surgical therapy

Epidural Abscess

Epidural abscess may be caused by hematogenous spread or direct extension from an abscess of the vertebral body, disc, or paraspinal tissues. These abscesses are usually pyogenic (mostly staphylococcal) and often occur in the thorax. Acute abscesses cause neck or back pain, fever, and spinal tenderness. Progression is similar to that of epidural tumors, with subsequent onset of radicular pain followed by spinal cord paralysis. Chronic abscesses progress more slowly and usually do not cause fever or leukocytosis. MRI scan is especially helpful in identifying the lesion. Treatment requires appropriate antibiotics and surgical drainage.

Congenital Spinal Lesions

Congenital spinal lesions include myelomeningocele and spina bifida, lipomeningocele, tethered spinal cord, split spinal cords, and sacral agenesis.

Spinal Dysraphism

Spina bifida encompasses a spectrum of dysraphic states that range from spina bifida occulta through meningocele and myelomeningocele

Spina Bifida and Myelomeningocele

Spina bifida is usually lumbar or lumbosacral. It occurs when there is inadequate closure of the neural tube, vertebral column, and overlying soft tissues. The most common, but least severe form is spina bifida occulta. It usually occurs without an underlying neural defect and presents as an incidental x-ray finding of an incomplete lamina (commonly at S2 or even L5). It is sometimes associated with an occult lipomeningocele (spinal lipoma) or intraspinal dermoid.

Meningocele is a more severe defect that does not cause neural malformation (approximately 1:500 births). Meningocele occurs when most of the elements dorsal to the spinal canal do not close. The dural sac protrudes through the vertebral defect to form a bulging sac beneath the skin. Although they are most common in the lumbosacral region, meningoceles can occur anywhere along the midline neuraxis, including the forehead and occiput. Neural elements are not present within the sac, except when they float up into it. Because the neural elements are not deformed, these children have no neurologic deficits. The incidence of myelomeningocele or meningocele has been steadily decreasing in the United States due to the regular use of large doses of folic acid in modern perinatal vitamins, as well as improved nutrition throughout our society. In order for supplemental folate to have beneficial effect, the mother should ideally be on folate supplements before she gets pregnant and for the first 8 to 12 weeks after conception.

When the malformation is more marked, neural tube closure is incomplete. A myelomeningocele forms, consisting of a protrusion of a central plaque of malformed neural elements posteriorly through a defect in the dura and vertebral lamina (Fig. 8-22). The neural elements are not usually covered by epidermis, and the myelomeningocele is considered open. The sac lies below the midthora-

cic region and is usually lumbar. Most children have hydrocephalus as well as significant deficits in sphincter and lower extremity functions. The sibling of a child who has myelomeningocele is at a twentyfold increased risk for having the condition.

Evaluation for myelomeningocele may begin in utero. Sampling of maternal blood for α-fetoprotein during the first trimester provides an adequate screen for the possible presence of an open myelomeningocele. If the result is positive, the diagnosis is confirmed with amniotic sampling for α-fetoprotein and ultrasound examination of the fetus in utero. Ultrasonography is also used to evaluate patients for neonatal hydrocephalus.

Meningoceles and myelomeningoceles are evident in the newborn. The examiner should record the site and dimensions of the lesion, whether it is open or closed, the level of any motor deficit, and the extent of reflex activity. The sensory level is often difficult to determine and depends on the infant's response to pain. The anal wink reflex and rectal tone are tested, and plain x-rays of the spine are

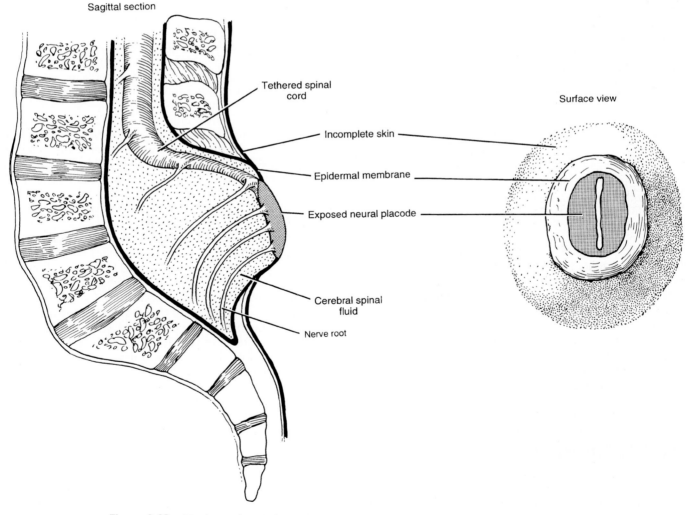

Figure 8-22   Myelomeningocele.

taken. If the lesion is a myelomeningocele, cranial CT scan or ultrasound is used to determine whether hydrocephalus is present and to visualize associated brain malformations. Early urologic consultation is obtained to evaluate bladder function. Orthopedic evaluation is necessary because dislocated hips and deformity of the lower extremities are often associated with myelomeningocele. High lesions are associated with scoliosis.

Surgery is required to repair meningoceles and myelomeningoceles. A meningocele is repaired according to the same principles as a hernia: the sac is dissected free, opened, divided, and closed level with the dura. The overlying soft tissue is closed in layers. Myelomeningoceles are usually repaired as soon after birth as feasible because early surgery is believed to avoid meningitis or ventriculitis if there is an open meningocele. Although this approach appears rational, it is debated because it places a significant strain on the parents, one of whom is recovering from childbirth and may not be in the same hospital as the newborn who is undergoing surgery. If CSF leakage is present, however, closure should not be delayed. Repair of a myelomeningocele requires dissection of the neural tissues from the surrounding cutaneous elements, with reconstruction of a dural tube about the neural tissue. A fascial layer may be mobilized to reinforce the closure. Skin closure often requires the development of cutaneous or myocutaneous flaps. Hydrocephalus may be present at the time of birth or develop after closure of the CSF defect. Whether to shunt at the time of defect closure or in a second stage is controversial, and the philosophy varies among surgeons.

Repeated follow-up is required to evaluate the many problems that occur in these patients. Expertise in a variety of fields is necessary: neurosurgery, urology, orthopedics, ophthalmology, developmental neurology, rehabilitation, and social services. This expertise can best be provided in a multidisciplinary clinic that focuses on the care of children with myelomeningocele. If leg function deteriorates or scoliosis progresses, MRI of the spinal cord to search for tethering or syrinx formation is warranted.

Tethered Spinal Cord

The normal spine grows more rapidly than the spinal cord. As a result, the tip of the spinal cord ascends from L5 at birth to L1 by adulthood. In myelomeningocele, the cord is tethered to the skin ectoderm. With growth, the spinal cord is stretched and distorted. Progressive scoliosis occurs, and a delayed neurologic deficit occurs above the static deficit. Tethering may also occur after repair because of scarring. Spinal cord tethering can lead to syrinx formation just as Chiari malformation can. Often, syrinxes do not spontaneously resorb unless both the Chiari malformation is decompressed and the tether released.

PERIPHERAL NERVE DISEASE

Anatomy and Physiology

Peripheral nerves are covered with an external connective tissue layer (epineurium). This sheath contains multiple nerve fascicles, and each is covered by its own connective tissue layer (perineurium). The fascicles branch and repeatedly interchange axons with one another over the length of the nerve. The fascicles contain motor axons from the spinal cord that end on effectors (muscles, blood vessels, glands, and other organs). They also contain sensory axons that conduct messages to the spinal cord from skin, joints, and other soft tissue receptors.

Each peripheral nerve is a simple extension of spinal nerve roots from a single segmental level (e.g., chest and abdomen) or the conjoined extension of roots from a number of adjacent levels (e.g., limbs). Limb nerves form as the ultimate extension of multiple recombinations of these nerve root contributions in the brachial and lumbosacral plexus. As a result of the simple segmental innervation of the trunk, myotomes and dermatomes are successively oriented in almost parallel fashion. Each receives the overlapping contribution of several spinal roots centered on that region.

The radicular and peripheral nerve distributions are similar. In the limbs, this simple radicular arrangement is oriented about a median axis. The progress of the dermatomes (and of the myotomes, to a much less recognizable extent) sequentially down one aspect of each extremity to the large digit, and up the other aspect from the smallest digit, is reflected in their innervation by successive overlapping spinal roots. In contrast to nerve roots, the peripheral nerves that innervate the limbs are composed of less orderly contributions from a variety of spinal roots. Consequently, lesions of the peripheral nerves that innervate the limbs usually produce neurologic deficits that are recognizably different from those caused by spinal root disease. Thus, the median nerve carries sensation from the palmar aspect of the radial 3.5 fingers of the hand and the adjacent palm. The corresponding dorsal aspects are largely the responsibility of the radial nerve. Sensation from the ulnar 1.5 fingers is transmitted by the ulnar nerve. In contrast, the sensory innervations of the sixth, seventh, and eighth cervical roots center, respectively, on all aspects of the thumb and the long and small fingers

Complete nerve transection leads to degeneration and loss of all axons beyond the point of transection (Wallerian degeneration). Reinnervation can occur by regeneration. For the first two weeks after transection, the proximal severed axons die back to the next viable Schwann cell at the first upstream node of Ranvier, where the cell membrane seals itself, while the distal axon degenerates leaving behind a hollow Schwann cell–lined tube. This time period also allows repair elements to reach the injury site form the cell body (which can be quite far away), utilizing axonal transport. Axonal sprouts from the proximal cut surface cross the gap and progress down the preserved Schwann cell sheaths of the transected axon. This outgrowth is provided by axoplasmic flow from the nerve cell bodies down the length of the regenerating axon. Axonal regrowth averages 1 to 2 mm/day. The time in days that EMG electrical evidence of reinnervation from a regenerating nerve can be expected can be estimated by measuring the distance from the injury to the mid portion of the muscle belly in question, dividing by 1.5, and then adding 14 days to account for the initial retraction and preparation period.

Peripheral Nerve Evaluation

The neurologic evaluation localizes the site of the lesion. Upper brachial plexus proximal nerve root avulsions should be suspected if ipsilateral diaphragm paralysis is present, and lower brachial plexus avulsions should be suspected if an ipsilateral Horner's syndrome is present. Tapping percussion over a portion of any nerve that contains unmyelinated axons produces a distal electrical sensation (**Tinel's sign**) within the regions of the skin that are normally supplied by the nerve. Sustained hyperflexion of the wrist for up to 60 seconds can lead to tingling sensory paresthesias in the distal median nerve distribution in patients with carpal tunnel median nerve entrapment neuropathy (**Phalen's sign**); generally the shorter the time until the onset of paresthesias, the more severe the compression syndrome. Electromyography is extremely useful for correct peripheral nerve and brachial and lumbar plexus lesion diagnosis, as well as detection of subclinical evidence of early nerve recovery. Nerve conduction studies are particularly useful in confirming the presence of a nerve entrapment syndrome as well as localizing the site of entrapment.

Evaluation of brachial plexus stretch injuries includes MRI scanning or myelography to identify pseudomeningoceles (posttraumatic outpouching of dura) that indicate root avulsion in the cervical spinal column. MR neurography is a newer technique that appears promising for assisting in the evaluation and confirmation of complex and elusive entrapment neuropathies such as thoracic outlet syndrome or piriformis syndrome.

Peripheral Nerve Trauma

Because injury causes architectural disruption of the proximal and distal nerve stumps at the point of transection, many new axons find their growth blocked or travel down paths that lead them to inappropriate terminals (e.g., motor instead of sensory). This problem is minimized when the transected nerve stumps are cleanly severed and accurately approximated. Open extremity injuries are explored surgically. If the wound is clean and the nerve transected sharply, then immediate direct repair by primary anastomosis or nerve grafting is done immediately. If the wound is contaminated and/or the transaction ragged or macerated, then the severed nerve ends are identified and tagged with a radioopaque marker to facilitate reexploration at a later date, after the extent of proximal regression is clear and the wound is no longer dirty. Nerves that are anatomically intact are left undisturbed in the short-term, even if they do not conduct intraoperative action potentials (lesion in continuity).

In crush or blunt nerve injury without transection, internal damage to the nerve can disrupt the axons and fascicular architecture, although the nerve remains in continuity. Some axons may cross the injury site and grow down the distal segment. Others do not and pile up blindly because fibroblasts have invaded the injured area. This fibrous tissue scar can prevent functional recovery. If natural recovery of the nerve has not progressed over a reasonable period of observation, the neuroma in continuity must be resected and the resulting nerve ends sutured together or grafted in order to permit adequate regeneration. Exploration can be delayed for 3 months (up to 6 months for more proximal plexus injuries) if regeneration is expected. However, delay to allow the chance of natural regeneration (which usually achieves an outcome superior to nerve grafting) must be weighed against the risk of atrophy or contracture of denervated muscle and changes in denervated skin receptors occur over time.

Minor injuries may disrupt only axons. Axons distal to the injury site degenerate, but the Schwann cell sheaths and fascicular architecture are preserved. Consequently, regenerating axons migrate down their original or adjacent channels and reinnervate the effectors and receptors that they originally supplied. Regeneration is possible without surgical intervention, and the prognosis for satisfactory spontaneous recovery is excellent. In even milder cases, axons may remain intact but fail to function (neuropraxia). A conduction block may be a component of nerve entrapment syndromes or posttraumatic epineural scarring. Minor nerve injuries may have a component of axonal disruption.

The etiology of the trauma indicates whether the injured nerve is likely to be in continuity. Penetrating trauma with a clean, sharp object is likely to cause transection and is amenable to repair. The outcome of injury caused by bullets and missiles is harder to predict. Missiles that travel close by nerves may produce damage without transection. These lesions in continuity may or may not recover satisfactorily. Closed injuries tend to produce neuromas in continuity. Stretch injuries of the peripheral nerves can produce irreparably long segments of intraneural scar. Traction on nerve roots of the brachial plexus often causes irreparable root avulsion

Peripheral Nerve Compression Syndromes

Nontraumatic nerve compression in the extremities is usually caused by further narrowing or compression of the normal passages through which the nerves travel. This compromise may occur spontaneously, but it is often promoted by conditions that affect the nerve or surrounding tissues. Entrapment syndromes are more common in patients with diabetes, connective tissue disease, myxedema, acromegaly, edema associated with menses or pregnancy, and scarring after focal trauma (e.g., Colles' fracture). Treatment of any underlying predisposing conditions, ergonomic adjustments to limit continued repetitive stress, and splinting of the effected area (if possible) are first-line therapies. If the problem is progressive despite these measures or is severe or disabling, surgical decompression of the nerve is indicated.

Common nerve compression syndromes include carpal tunnel syndrome, tardy ulnar palsy, and thoracic outlet syndrome. Lower extremity nerve entrapments are less common. These include entrapments of the lateral femoral cutaneous nerve to the anterolateral thigh by the inguinal ligament (meralgia paresthetica), the ilioinguinal nerve supplying the medial thigh, or the genitofemoral nerve supplying the uppermost medial thigh and scrotum.

Carpal Tunnel Syndrome

The most common nerve entrapment is carpal tunnel syndrome. This syndrome is caused by compression of the median nerve as it enters the hand beneath the carpal ligament. Symptoms include pain or paresthesia in the palmar aspect of the hand and fingers, especially at night or on awakening. Symptoms may extend above the wrist into the arm, but are not as pronounced as in the hand. Eventually, patients have numbness and difficulty with fine motor tasks. The diagnosis depends on the presence of these pain characteristics and the finding of Tinel's or Phalen's sign at the wrist (reproduction of symptoms after a minute of maintained wrist flexion). The diagnosis is supported by electrical studies that show slowed conduction in the median nerve at the wrist, although these studies are occasionally normal. Treatment is directed at any underlying pathology. Diuretics help in cases of edema. Splints and local steroid injections may provide relief, but it is often only temporary. Simple division of the carpal ligament is often necessary and can be done by means of an open procedure or endoscopically.

Ulnar Nerve Entrapment

Tardy ulnar palsy is largely caused by compression because of the anatomic relation of the nerve within the groove at the elbow. Patients with tardy ulnar palsy have numbness and weakness rather than pain. The condition is often far advanced by the time the patient is seen. Both physical signs and electrophysiologic abnormalities of muscle activity and nerve conduction are evident. Tinel's sign is elicited on tapping medially to the elbow. Sensory loss occurs in the ulnar distribution, and there is weakness and wasting of the interossei muscles. Surgical treatments include simple open decompression, or decompression with transposition of the ulnar nerve anteriorly to remove the pulley effect on the nerve posterior to the medial epicondyle. Often the former constitutes initial treatment, whereas the latter is reserved for recurrence.

The ulnar nerve can also become entrapped at the wrist in Guyon's canal. Much less common than Tardy ulnar palsy, this condition can be relieved with simple decompression at the wrist.

Thoracic Outlet Syndrome

Thoracic outlet syndrome, which causes nerve rather than vascular compression, shares some of the features of tardy ulnar palsy. It includes compression of the lower portion of the brachial plexus, which supplies the ulnar nerve. The compression occurs where the brachial plexus emerges into the axilla, through a narrow passage beneath the clavicle and between the anterior and middle scalene muscles, while resting on the first rib.

Abnormality of the anterior scalene is sometimes blamed for the symptoms, but it is not the only cause. Although a cervical rib may compromise the underside of the plexus and cause symptoms, asymptomatic cervical ribs are common. In patients with arm pain, symptoms should not be attributed to cervical ribs. Pain or neurologic deficit that occurs in the ulnar distribution, especially numbness that extends up the ulnar forearm, may be caused by any demonstrable cervical rib or especially prominent transverse process of C7. Surgical resection helps many of these patients. If no cervical rib is present, but the patient has pain and neurologic deficit in the ulnar distribution, with no other source of the problem identified, exploration with release of fibrous bands located where a cervical rib is usually located, release of the edge of the anterior scalene, or resection of the first rib is sometimes helpful.

The differential diagnoses of ulnar nerve entrapment and thoracic outlet syndrome include lesions of the lower cervical spine (e.g., cervical disc herniation). In addition, a tumor at the apex of the lung, usually metastatic from the pulmonary hilum, must be considered. These tumors produce Pancoast syndrome. They affect the lower brachial plexus and may mimic thoracic outlet syndrome. This type of tumor is suspected when arm pain is accompanied by a smaller pupil and ptosis of the ipsilateral eye (Horner's syndrome; an unusual finding in thoracic outlet syndrome). Diagnosis can be suggested from an apical lordotic chest x-ray. MR neurography is a newer neuroimaging technique that can demonstrate lower plexus nerve compression. However, the study is very technique-dependent and requires a very expert and experienced operator both for setting up the study and interpreting the results.

Peripheral Nerve Tumors

Tumors of the peripheral nerves are usually benign and cause swelling or pain. Neurilemomas (schwannomas) arise within the nerve (usually along a single fascicle) and displace the remaining nerve fiber fascicles around the tumor. With careful intraneural microdissection, they are often amenable to removal with preservation of the surrounding functional fascicles. Neurofibromas arise within a nerve, but grow between and around the nerve fibers. Any excision requires sacrifice of the nerve with or without subsequent nerve grafting. Schwannomas can be idiopathic or may be associated with neurocutaneous syndromes (especially with multiple neurofibromatosis, type 1, or schwannomatosis). Neurofibromas, whether single or associated with other neurofibromas or schwannomas, are often associated with neurofibromatosis type 1. If a nerve tumor expands rapidly, seems fixed to surrounding tissues, demonstrates loss of central contrast enhancement on MR imaging (necrosis), or becomes newly painful, malignancy is suspected. Most malignant degeneration of preexisting neurofibromas occurs in the setting of neurofibromatosis, type 1. With time, malignant tumors extend along the nerve and into surrounding tissues. These tumors can metastasize. Radical excision, with or without radiation therapy, is the treatment of choice.

PAIN

The best strategy for treating most pain involves determining and removing its cause. Unfortunately, this is not always possible. Some causes of pain cannot be removed. In addition there are situations and conditions where the upstream pain circuitry becomes either hypersensitive to even minor or trivial stimulation (e.g., dysesthesia, causalgia, reflex sympathetic dystrophy), or becomes autonomous at a CNS level with pain, occurring even in the absence of stimulus (e.g., anesthesia dolorosa or phantom limb pain). Cancer pain in terminally ill patients remains a major problem in our health system. While pain medications are the first line of defense for palliation in these situations, they do not always work (particularly for autonomous central pain), and patients can become refractory to relief even at supratherapeutic doses. Some chronic pain medications also come with unwanted end organ (liver or kidney) side effects, as well as physical and psychosocial dependence issues. When these situations are recognized, neurosurgeons can be of assistance. The best treatment for a given condition often varies with the specific requirements of the case and the surgeon's judgment. The issues can be complex and are not always straightforward or clearly defined. Attempting to treat a chronic pain syndrome form a purely organic or physical standpoint is not likely to work or lead to a durable response, unless the psychosocial issues intimately related to the syndrome are also addressed simultaneously.

Specifically Treatable Syndromes

There are specific pain syndromes, usually related to the cranial nerves, that have a long history of successful treatment with neurosurgical procedures. With these syndromes correct recognition and diagnosis of the syndrome and early referral to the neurosurgeon will often lead to the best outcome for affected patients.

Trigeminal Neuralgia
Trigeminal neuralgia is a facial pain syndrome that affects the distribution of the trigeminal nerve (cranial nerve V). It is usually unilateral, but in rare situations (2% to 4%) can be bilateral. It is characterized by sudden shock or sharp-stabbing episodes of pain radiating down one or more trigeminal divisions. Early in the syndrome the pain tends to last only seconds before ending just as abruptly as it started. Later in the syndrome painful shocks can

temporally group or cluster in a string of repetitive tetanic jolts that may make the pain seem like it lasts for a few minutes before it resolves. Early in the syndrome the patient experiences no pain or other trigeminal symptoms between episodes. The pain comes spontaneously in an unpredictable manner, but also can be triggered by trigeminal tactile stimulation (e.g., cold wind on the face, brushing teeth, washing face, putting on make-up, talking, or even chewing). Through operant conditioning, the patient soon learns which activities to avoid. Neurological examination is usually grossly normal, but very careful testing reveals subtle hypalgesia (10% to 20%) in the medial distribution of V2 or V3 in up to one third of patients. This incidence increases with chronicity of the syndrome and with surgical attempts at treatment. Spontaneous periods of remission lasting up to 6 months in length are common (up to 50% of patients), but recurrence is the rule, since the syndrome is slowly progressive in severity, frequency, and trigeminal nerve distribution. The pain of trigeminal neuralgia is so excruciating that patients will abruptly stop whatever they are doing and hold themselves immobile until it passes. Before the development of neurosurgical interventions, it was probably second only to cancer as the most common medical condition leading to patient suicide.

Differential diagnosis includes temporal-mandibular joint syndrome, postherpetic neuralgia, cluster headache, and deafferentation facial pain. Approximately 98% of cases are considered idiopathic in origin, with vascular cross-compression of the nerve affecting myelin insulation at the nerve root entry zone considered to be the likely cause. The remaining 2% of patients include patients with multiple sclerosis (~2% of multiple sclerosis patients will develop trigeminal neuralgia), brainstem lacunar infarctions in the trigeminal system, or cerebellopontine or Meckel's cave mass lesions (e.g., tumors, cysts, aneurysms or AVMs). MR scanning is useful to rule out these alternative causes. It does not, however, rule in or out vascular compression, given the size and multiplicity of vessels found to be involved at surgical exploration.

Initial therapy involves anticonvulsant medications to raise the threshold for electrical stimulation of the trigeminal system. Carbamazepine and oxcarbazepine have been proven to be the most effective agents in clinical trials and appear to be equivalent in terms of short-term efficacy. Oxcarbazepine is currently preferred due to a more favorable toxicity and side-effect profile, but lacks the long-term follow-up data available for carbamazepine. Approximately 95% of trigeminal neuralgia patients will respond to initial anticonvulsant therapy. Unfortunately, some are intolerant of side effects, some have idiosyncratic drug reactions, and some tend to gradually become refractory to increasing doses as the syndrome progresses. Approximately 56% of patients will fail carbamazepine therapy for one of these reasons over a period of 16 years. Despite these observations, it remains a sad truth that most trigeminal neuralgia patients will have undergone several dental procedures over a period of several years before the correct diagnosis is made, and the average trigeminal neuralgia patient has suffered with the syndrome for >5 years and has seen two to four neurologists before he or she is finally referred to a neurosurgeon.

In well-trained and experienced hands, microvascular decompression of the trigeminal nerve leads to initial cure (no pain, no medications) in approximately 80% of patients, and this success remains durable at 70% up to 20 years. Other important palliative treatment options include procedures that selectively and partially damage the ganglion or nerve root with either heat (percutaneous radiofrequency lesion), chemicals (percutaneous glycerol rhizotomy), mechanical crush (percutaneous balloon compression), or highly concentrated radiation (Gamma Knife stereotactic radiosurgery). The latter four procedures do not address the purported cause of the syndrome and are designed to treat the symptom. As palliative procedures they are all initially effective in about 65% to 80% of cases (pain-free with or without medications at 1 year). However, they each have an annual recurrence rate of approximately 6% to 10% per year, so that by 5 years after treatment this number drops to approximately 50%. The need for repeat palliative intervention is common. Currently, stereotactic radiosurgery appears to have the lowest rate of treatment-related numbness, and it avoids percutaneous needle placement from the cheek into the foramen ovale. Unfortunately, it is not immediately effective, with lesion maturation and therapeutic effect usually requiring 6 to 8 weeks (range, days to 6 months).

Glossopharyngeal Neuralgia

Glossopharyngeal neuralgia is much rarer then trigeminal neuralgia and affects the ninth and tenth cranial nerve distributions (back of the throat and, occasionally, inner ear). It otherwise has the same clinical characteristics, responds temporarily to the same medications, and likely has the same root entry zone vascular compressive cause. With glossopharyngeal neuralgia, the triggering events are swallowing, which can lead to dehydration and malnourishment due to swallowing aversion. While cranial nerve IX is one nerve, cranial nerve X has multiple fascicles in the cerebellopontine angle. This can make microvascular decompression technically much more challenging and may explain the slightly less successful results achieved. An alternative procedure is section of the ninth nerve root along with the upper 13-1/2 of the fascicles of cranial nerve X.

General Pain Syndrome Strategies

General strategies to improve chronic or incurable pain syndromes can target anywhere along the pain pathway from sensory nerve to sensory nerve root, to spinal cord, to brainstem, and to cortex. Some of the approaches involve lesioning, and others involve stimulation. Many peripheral nerve, nerve root, and spinal cord stimulation strategies are attempts to exploit the gate control theory of pain, first put forward by Melzak and Wall in 1965. They suggested a gating mechanism within the spinal cord that is closed in response to normal stimulation of the fast-conducting "touch" nerve fibers but that opens when the slow-conducting "pain" fibers transmit a high volume and intensity of sensory signals. The gate can be closed again if these signals are countered by renewed stimulation of the large fibers.

Nerve and Nerve Root Strategies

While nerve and nerve root injections with analgesics, steroids, or a combination of both can provide temporary relief for localized pain, the effects are not long lasting and require repeated injections. Transcutaneous electrical nerve stimulation (TENS), which targets and exploits the gate control theory of pain, can be subjectively helpful in some patients. Formal clinical studies with TENS units have shown only mild to modest improvement. Surgically implanted peripheral nerve stimulators have been tried based on a similar rationale with mixed results.

Cutting peripheral nerves leads to complete anesthesia in a given region, which can predispose the patient to unrecognized injury in the anesthetic area. It is also all-too-often complicated by the formation of a painful neuroma (ball of hypersensitive regenerating nerve endings trapped in a ball of scar tissue). Indeed, a posttraumatic neuroma can be a cause of chronic refractory pain syndromes. It can form at the ends of severed peripheral nerves or form within an anatomically intact and partially functional nerve that has suffered a stretch or crush injury, such as a neuroma incontinuity.

Surgical approaches to painful terminal neuromas include excision (risking recurrence), excision and burying the newly severed nerve ending within a muscle belly to protect it from easy stimulation, or excision followed by terminal end-to-end anastomoses of the terminal nerve fascicles to one another in order to inhibit axonal sprouting and new neuroma formation. Little can be done for neuromas in continuity associated with functional nerves short of external neurolysis to decompress epineurium to lower intraneuronal tissue pressure, or to risk loss of nerve function by resecting the neuroma and grafting the nerve.

Autonomic Nervous System Strategies

Causalgia and sympathetic dystrophy are peculiar burning pain syndromes that occur after partial injury of a major limb nerve. The pain is heightened by stress, is mediated through the autonomic nervous system, and usually begins some months after trauma. It may resolve spontaneously after a year or two. Sympathectomy or repeated local anesthetic injections into the sympathetic ganglion may be necessary.

Spinal Cord Strategies

Intrathecal narcotic administration directly into the CSF can provide a high degree of pain relief to pain sources in the abdomen, pelvis, and lower extremities with very little risk. Higher regions of the body are more risky to treat this way because the narcotic would have to ascend to levels that, if overshot, could affect respiratory function. Intrathecal morphine is remarkably effective at very low doses, and tolerance is not the problem that it is with chronic systemic administration of narcotics. Continuous dosing intrathecal morphine pumps have been one of the major advances in surgical pain management. It has all but replaced surgical lesioning procedures such as dorsal root rhizotomy, terminal cordectomy, anterior-lateral cordotomy, and anterior commissural myelotomy. A minipump that can be queried, programmed, and refilled percutaneously is implanted subcutaneously over the abdomen and is connected with a catheter that enters the dura in the lumbar spine.

The other spinal procedure that has proven to be effective and durable over time is stimulation of the lemniscal pathway (dorsal columns) by direct spinal cord stimulation using a subcutaneous programmable stimulator. Like the TENS unit, this procedure also targets and exploits the gate control theory of pain. However, direct dorsal column stimulation is much more effective than transcutaneous nerve stimulation. Dorsal column spinal cord stimulators can be set up with fine percutaneous multicontact leads that enter the epidural space in the lumbar spine and are subsequently positioned over each dorsal column up in the thoracic spine under fluoroscopic guidance. More definitive and permanent placement of larger contact leads in the form of an epidural strip of flat contact electrodes requires open thoracic laminectomy for placement.

Cranial Strategies
Most cranial lesioning strategies for controlling chronic or incurable pain have fallen out of favor over time (e.g., medullary tractotomy, thalamotomy, cingulotomy, and lobotomy). One exception appears to be pituitary ablation for intractable cancer pain. Using stereotactic radiosurgery, ablation can now be performed minimally invasively and nearly painlessly with no major surgical risks. The other exception is open radiofrequency trigeminal nucleus caudalis dorsal root entry zone (DREZ) lesioning of the posterior lateral medulla, which is still performed at select centers for anesthesia dolorosa (severe phantom limb-like, burning deafferentation pain associated with trigeminal distribution anesthesia).

Cranial stimulation strategies still have a role for chronic and refractory patients. They include stereotactically placing stimulator leads in the ventroposterior medial and lateral nuclei of the thalamus, as well as in the periaqueductal gray region of the midbrain. Motor cortex stimulation utilizing surgically placed surface contact electrodes on the frontal convexity are showing promise for treating patients with deafferentation facial pain, poststroke pain, phantom limb pain, and other intractable neuropathic pain syndromes.

SUGGESTED READINGS

DeMyer W. *Technique of the Neurologic Examination*. New York, NY: McGraw-Hill; 2004.

Guarantors of Brain. *Aids to the Examination of the Peripheral Nervous System*. Philadelphia, Pa: WB Saunders; 2000.

Nolte J. *The Human Brain: An Introduction to its Functional Anatomy*. St Louis, Mo.: CV Mosby; 1999.

Wilkins RH, Rengachary SS. *Neurosurgery*. New York, NY: McGraw-Hill; 1996.

Youmans JR. *Neurological Surgery*. Philadelphia, Pa: WB Saunders; 2004.

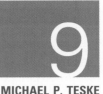

ALAN S. CRANDALL, JR. ■ IRVING RABER ■ MICHAEL P. TESKE
GEORGE L. WHITE, JR.

Ophthalmology: Diseases of the Eye

OBJECTIVES

Diseases of the Cornea

1 Describe the anatomy and function of the cornea and precorneal tear film.

2 Explain the use of the slitlamp to examine the cornea. Describe its value in determining the anatomic site of pathology within the cornea and anterior segment.

3 Describe the indications for corneal transplantation and the surgical procedures used.

4 Describe two surgical methods to correct aphakia.

5 Explain recurrent erosion syndrome.

6 Describe the evaluation and management of a corneal infiltrate.

7 Describe the various types of refractive surgery.

8 Define pterygia and describe their clinical management.

9 Identify three surgical methods to treat corneal surface disorders.

Diseases of the Anterior Chamber

1 Define glaucoma and its various categories.

2 Describe the pathophysiology of the different types of glaucoma and their presenting signs and symptoms.

3 Describe basic glaucoma treatment and the different therapies for the various kinds of glaucoma.

4 Discuss the indications for surgical rather than medical therapy for glaucoma.

Diseases of the Lens

1 Explain how the basic anatomy of the lens relates to the formation of the different types of cataract.

2 Explain how the anatomic location of the cataract determines its effect on visual function.

3 Describe the types of patient who would benefit most from cataract surgery.

4 Describe the various techniques of cataract surgery and the risks associated with them.

5 List the advantages and disadvantages of the various types of optical correction after cataract surgery.

Diseases of the Retina and Vitreous

1 Describe the signs and symptoms of retinal tears and detachments.

2 Discuss the principles and techniques of treatment of retinal tears and detachment.

3 List the major indications for vitreous surgery, as well as the goals and potential complications of this surgery.

4 Describe the management of penetrating eye injuries, with or without retained intraocular foreign bodies.

5 List the major indications for laser photocoagulation surgery involving the posterior segment of the eye. Describe the goals and potential complications of this surgery.

Diseases of the Nasolacrimal System, Eyelids, and Orbit

1 List the indications for nasolacrimal duct probing in infants.

2 Explain the differences between a dacryocystorhinostomy and a Jones tube procedure. Give the indications for each.

3 List the indications for tarsorrhaphy.

4 Describe the importance of ptosis as a finding on physical examination.

5 Describe and contrast the most common lesions that cause proptosis in children and adults.

6 List the indications for removal of an eye.

Diseases of the Extraocular Muscles

1 Describe the anatomy and function of the extraocular muscles.

2 Describe the innervation of the extraocular muscles. Explain how this innervation relates to strabismus.

3 Discuss how hyperopia, accommodation, and strabismus are related.

4 Describe single binocular vision, and explain how it relates to the treatment of congenital esotropia.

5 Describe the fundamentals, goals, and possible complications of strabismus surgery.

Ocular Disorders

1 List the common causes of red eye, especially those that threaten sight.

2 Discuss the significance of visual field defects, papillary disorders, hypertensive retinopathy, retinal vein occlusion and emboli, third and sixth nerve palsies, and diplopia.

Ophthalmology is the study of medical and surgical diseases of the eye. Intense study is required to understand the mechanism of action of the eye, its disease processes, and the methods to treat these disease processes. The eye is not an isolated organ; it interacts with the body and mind. There are no systemic diseases that do not have ocular effects. Some of the most common diseases (e.g., hypertension, diabetes) can have devastating effects on the eye. Blindness from diabetes (and trauma) is a major debilitating result that has extensive health care consequences. Such diseases as acquired immunodeficiency syndrome (AIDS) often have ocular involvement that requires surgery. However, the two most common ocular disease processes that affect health care in the United States are cataracts and glaucoma.

Everyone who lives long enough will eventually have **cataracts.** In a society in which people wish to remain active (e.g., driving, reading), cataract surgery is one of the most commonly performed surgeries. It requires tremendous health care expenditures every year. Fortunately, the high success rate of cataract surgery allows patients to return to normal activities.

Another common ocular disease is glaucoma, which affects up to 2% of the general population. It requires long-term treatment with medication or surgery. This disease also has a heavy impact on the public health care dollar because most patients with glaucoma are eligible for Medicare.

This chapter describes surgical diseases of the eye according to the subspecialties in ophthalmology: the cornea; the anterior chamber; the lens; the retina and vitreous; the nasolacrimal system, eyelids, and orbit; and the extraocular muscles. A short section at the end describes common ocular disorders. Figures 9-1 and 9-2 show the anatomy of the eye.

DISEASES OF THE CORNEA

Anatomy and Physiology

The cornea is a clear, avascular structure that provides structural integrity to the anterior segment of the eye. It is a major refractive component. Forming approximately one sixth of the surface of the eye, the cornea is similar in structure to neighboring sclera. Corneal collagen is more uniformly oriented, however, and the cornea itself is dehydrated. These two factors contribute to the maintenance of corneal clarity. The cornea and the overlying tear film provide two thirds of the refractive component of the eye. The lens accounts for the rest.

The precorneal tear film, which is crucial to the health of the eye, is produced by the lacrimal gland and specialized glands in the conjunctiva and eyelids. The tear film has three layers: (a) the superficial layer, produced by the meibomian glands, is oily and helps prevent evaporation; (b) the middle layer, produced by the lacrimal gland, is watery and comprises the bulk of tear film; and (c) the innermost layer, produced by goblet cells, is mucoid and contributes to even spreading of the tear film. Deficiencies in any of these layers can lead to optical disturbances and compromise the health of the eye.

The cornea has five layers. In anterior to posterior order, these are the epithelium, **Bowman's membrane,** the stroma, **Descemet's membrane,** and the endothelium. The epithelium is a nonkeratinized, stratified squamous cell layer that forms a smooth surface over the cornea. It can be damaged easily by minor trauma that causes cor-

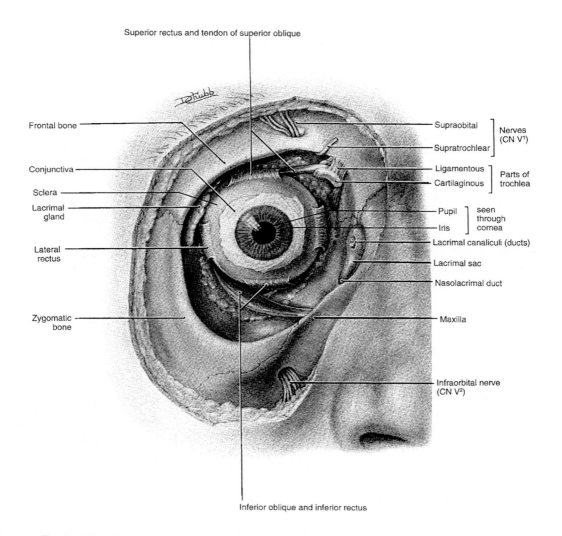

Superior rectus and tendon of superior oblique

Frontal bone

Conjunctiva

Sclera

Lacrimal gland

Lateral rectus

Zygomatic bone

Supraobital
Supratrochlear
} Nerves (CN V¹)

Ligamentous
Cartilaginous
} Parts of trochlea

Pupil
Iris
} seen through cornea

Lacrimal canaliculi (ducts)

Lacrimal sac

Nasolacrimal duct

Maxilla

Infraorbital nerve (CN V²)

Inferior oblique and inferior rectus

Figure 9-1   Orbital cavity, dissected from the front. *CN,* cranial nerve.

neal abrasions. If the epithelium basement membrane is damaged, adhesion of the epithelium is compromised and recurrent abrasions may result. Because the cornea is supplied by numerous nerve endings, these abrasions can be extremely painful. Supporting the epithelium is Bowman's membrane, which consists of randomly dispersed collagen that is firmly anchored into the corneal stroma. Although epithelium regenerates without scarring, Bowman's membrane does not. The next layer, stroma, accounts for 90% of normal corneal thickness. Its three main constituents (collagen-producing fibroblasts, collagen lamellae, and mucopolysaccharide ground substance) combine to produce a tough, elastic protective coat. Posterior to the corneal stroma is Descemet's membrane, the basement membrane for the fifth layer, endothelium. Corneal endothelium, derived from neuroectoderm, is a functionally complex monolayer of hexagonal cells that do not regenerate. The main function of this layer is to keep the

cornea in a partially dehydrated state and therefore to preserve its clarity. It accomplishes this function by maintaining a tight barrier between the corneal stroma and aqueous humor and by pumping water out of the corneal stroma. The cell density of this layer decreases with age. Although remaining cells enlarge to accommodate lower cell counts, corneal clarity is compromised when the endothelial cell count falls to 400 to 700 cells/mm². As the cell count falls, corneal stromal edema increases, followed by corneal epithelial edema. These developments lead to loss of vision and breakdown of the corneal epithelium.

The cornea metabolizes glucose primarily through glycolysis. It receives 90% of this substrate from aqueous humor. Oxygen is delivered to the corneal epithelium from the tear film and the environment. Corneal tissue posterior to and including the corneal stroma receives oxygen from the aqueous humor. Given its proximity to glucose-rich aqueous humor and oxygen-rich air, the cornea

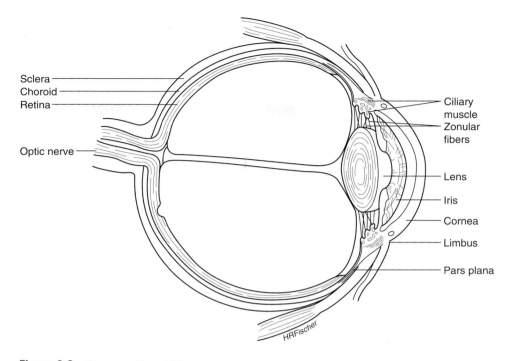

Figure 9-2 Cross-section of the eye.

functions well even though it is avascular. The tear film provides added immunologic protection in the form of enzymes and immunoglobulins.

Pathophysiology

The cornea can be damaged by trauma, infection, and metabolic imbalances. Additionally, the cornea can require treatment for structural defects or to replace diseased tissue.

Clinical Presentation and Evaluation

Examination of the cornea involves observation of the tissue and measurements of its curvature. The slitlamp is the most important instrument for evaluating the cornea because it allows creation of an optical cross section that permits direct visualization of any pathology. Examination is facilitated by the use of a topical anesthetic. By adjusting the light beam and the incident angle of observation, different areas within the cornea can be highlighted. Fluorescein stain is instilled to detect areas of corneal abrasion. In these areas, the cornea glows strongly under a cobalt blue light. Even a simple penlight can provide useful information, however. An irregular corneal surface can be detected by an irregular light reflex from any point source of light.

The curvature of the cornea, and therefore its refractive ability, is measured with a variety of instruments. The most common quantifiable method uses a **keratometer,** a device that measures the radius of curvature of the central cornea. These measurements are important in guiding refractive procedures and predicting appropriate intraocular lens (IOL) power. Newer, more expensive machines provide a topographic analysis of the corneal surface, much the same way that topographic maps represent the earth's surface. These are helpful for refractive procedures. The quality of the refracting surface of the cornea can be assessed with the keratometer and a keratoscope. A keratoscope projects a Placido's disc (concentric rings that show surface topography, analogous to elevation lines on topographic maps). These measurements are helpful in postoperative care, especially in suture removal.

The endothelial cell layer of the cornea is visualized and photographed with specular microscopy, a technique that uses an optical device that allows direct observation of the corneal endothelium. This technique provides information about the quality and quantity of the endothelial cells that are responsible for maintaining the relatively dehydrated state of the cornea, thus ensuring its clarity.

Treatment

Much corneal surgery arises from diseases that do not respond to nonsurgical treatment. Examples include **keratoconus** (corneal abnormality in which the cornea becomes misshapen into a conical shape) initially treated with a contact lens; infectious **keratitis** (inflammation of the cornea) treated with intensive fortified antibiotics; and herpes simplex keratitis treated with antivirals. Other cornea problems, such as **aphakic bullous keratopathy** (a breakdown in the cornea that leads to large defects in the epithelium) with diffuse corneal edema, are surgical diseases from the outset. This discussion involves only the diseases of the cornea that are treated primarily with corneal surgery. However, many medical interventions typically precede the necessary surgery.

Corneal surgery is performed for three main reasons: (a) to produce a clear visual pathway (e.g., cornea transplant for a corneal scar); (b) to maintain the integrity of the globe (e.g., lamellar cornea transplant for a perforation); and (c) to alter the inherent corneal structure to produce refractive or functional changes (e.g., radial keratotomy to reduce **myopia**). Much of the recent success with corneal surgery is the result of such technologic advances as the operating microscope, finer and better suture materials, improved instrumentation, and better tissue preservation.

For patients to have good vision after surgery, it is important to maintain a smooth corneal surface and clear corneal substance. Care is taken to approximate wounds carefully, without torque, to ensure that sutures are placed at equal depths within tissue, and to place an ideal tension on the suture. Various devices are used to help determine the correct tissue tension, although most surgeons find experience and practice the best aids.

Corneal Transplantation

Corneal transplantation is the most commonly performed tissue transplant in the United States (approximately 30,000 procedures/year). The success of this procedure has been facilitated by several factors (e.g., improved means of tissue preservation, the nationwide network of eye banks) that have increased the availability of corneal tissue. Because the cornea is avascular, aggressive immunosuppression therapy (required by most transplant patients) is not needed. Corneal transplantation involves replacing the full-thickness cornea (penetrating **keratoplasty;** Fig. 9-3)

or the partial-thickness cornea (lamellar keratoplasty; Fig. 9-4). The location of the corneal opacity determines the procedure. For full-thickness corneal lesions, only a full-thickness penetrating keratoplasty will suffice. For anteriorly placed corneal lesions, a lamellar keratoplasty can be performed. Often a full-thickness procedure is performed even though a partial-thickness procedure would do, because in most patients who undergo the partial-thickness procedure, scarring causes the development of a fine haze that interferes with vision (Fig. 9-5).

Indications

Corneal transplantation is used to treat pseudophakic and aphakic bullous keratopathy, keratoconus, corneal dystrophy, and infectious keratitis. Indications for penetrating keratoplasty (replacing full-thickness cornea) are listed in Table 9-1.

Pseudophakic bullous keratopathy, or permanent corneal clouding after IOL implant surgery, is the most common indication for corneal transplantation in the United States. All cataract surgery causes some loss of endothelial cells. In some patients, this loss brings the patient under the critical number of remaining cells required to maintain corneal clarity. Depending on the degree of endothelial damage, the cornea may become cloudy immediately after the surgery. More characteristically, this clouding occurs months to years after the surgery. Aphakic bullous keratopathy is corneal opacification after cataract surgery without an IOL implant.

IOL implants after cataract surgery became popular in the late 1970s. Early lens design led to a high incidence of corneal edema and problems (e.g., glaucoma, **hyphema** [blood in the anterior chamber of the eye]) that appeared years later. Sometimes these lenses can be replaced with better-designed implants before the cornea becomes permanently hazy. Once the cornea becomes opacified, visual

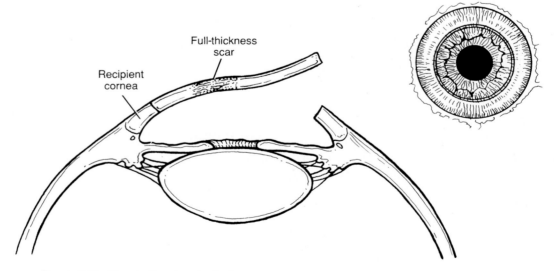

Figure 9-3 Penetrating keratoplasty.

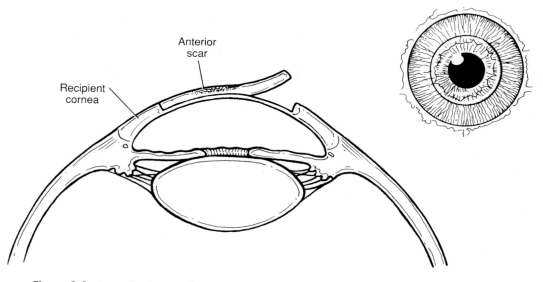

Figure 9-4   Lamellar keratoplasty.

rehabilitation requires a penetrating keratoplasty combined with IOL exchange. Although the incidence of pseudophakic bullous keratopathy is less than 1%, the sheer number of cataract surgeries performed in the United States annually makes this keratopathy the most common indication for corneal transplantation. As advances in cataract surgery produce less trauma to the eye, the incidence of pseudophakic bullous keratopathy is expected to decrease.

Patients with pseudophakic bullous keratopathy first notice diminution in vision as the cornea imbibes fluid. During the early stages of corneal edema, the patient has hazy, blurred vision that is worse on awakening and gradually clears. With the lids closed during sleep, fluid cannot evaporate from the corneal surface. After the eyes are open,

the imbibed fluid evaporates and the corneal haze decreases. Hypertonic saline drops and ointment promote corneal deturgescence, as does the use of a hair dryer on a low-heat setting held at arm's length and directed toward the eyes. As the cornea becomes more edematous, small blisters form in the corneal epithelium. These blisters tend to break down and cause severe ocular pain and irritation.

Penetrating keratoplasty alleviates discomfort from corneal epithelial breakdown and improves visual acuity. For patients who are poor candidates for corneal transplant, other procedures that can be tried include bandage contact lenses (extended-wear lenses that can remain in the eye), corneal surface scarification (with multiple fine-needle punctures or a diathermy probe), and conjunctival flaps. For a flap, a thin layer of healthy, intact conjunctiva is mobilized and pulled down over the corneal surface as a "hood" flap and sutured into place (Figs. 9-6 and 9-7). A conjunctival flap can also be used to treat corneal infections that are unresponsive to antimicrobial therapy. Applying the flap over the infected cornea apparently stimulates the body's immune system to eradicate infection. If

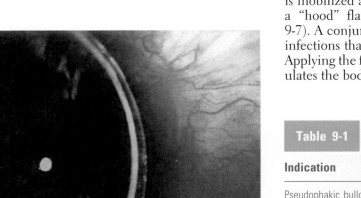

Figure 9-5   Slitlamp photo of lamellar keratoplasty. Residual opacification is seen in the host bed.

Table 9-1	Indications for Penetrating Keratoplasty
Indication	**Percent**
Pseudophakic bullous keratopathy	22.9
Fuch's dystrophy	16.3
Keratoconus	15.1
Aphakic bullous keratopathy	14.4
Regraft	10.1
Virus	4.4
Other	16.8
Total	100.0

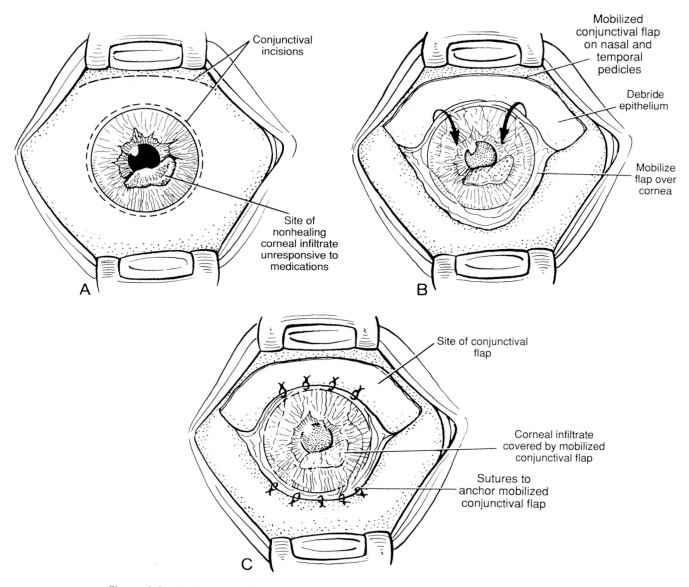

Figure 9-6   Conjunctival flap.

there is good visual potential, penetrating keratoplasty may be performed later, through the flap, after the inflamed corneal stroma becomes scarified.

Keratoconus is progressive dystrophy of the cornea in which the central cornea becomes thinner than normal, with a subsequent forward bulge. The bulge takes on a conoid shape that causes visual distortion and decreased visual acuity. It is usually bilateral, although one eye may be much more involved than the other. Most cases are sporadic, but 10% are hereditary. Keratoconus has a higher incidence in such systemic disorders as Down's syndrome, atopy (type I allergic reaction), and Marfan's syndrome. Eye rubbing may play a role in the development of keratoconus, and there is ongoing debate over whether contact lens wear may be a cause.

The disease tends to progress through adolescence and stabilize in young adulthood, although worsening may occur at any age. Most patients achieve excellent vision with rigid gas-permeable contact lenses. These lenses ameliorate associated irregular **astigmatism** (a refractive error in which the defect is not the same in all meridians). Surgery is indicated in patients who cannot use contact lenses because of steep or irregularly shaped corneas or in those who have central corneal scarring.

Penetrating keratoplasty is the procedure of choice for keratoconus, with a success rate of 80% to 90%. Some surgeons achieve good results with **epikeratophakia** (a procedure in which a graft is placed on the cornea) to flatten the corneas of patients who have small, central cones; have little scarring; and cannot tolerate contact lenses. This pro-

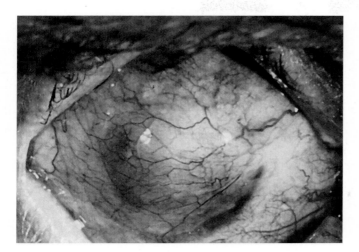

Figure 9-7   Well-healed conjunctival flap.

cedure uses a donor cornea that is frozen before being lathed commercially into a tissue contact lens. Epikeratophakia is advantageous because the globe does not have to be entered (reducing the risk of endophthalmitis). Immunologic rejection of the lens has never been reported. Visual results tend to be poorer than with penetrating keratoplasty, however. Occasionally, a patient's cornea has thinned to such a degree that penetrating keratoplasty is not possible: too little tissue is left on which to sew the donor graft. In these patients, lamellar keratoplasty is performed to "bulk up" the recipient cornea. After healing occurs, penetrating keratoplasty can be performed.

Some patients experience acute rupture of Descemet's membrane (if the membrane becomes thinned because of the keratoconus), with sudden inflow of aqueous humor into the corneal stroma. This condition, known as acute hydrops, is usually accompanied by acute pain and decreased vision. When the hydrops heals, the cornea often flattens. If the scarring does not involve the visual axis, patients who previously could not wear a rigid contact lens can now be fitted with one. However, most patients with acute hydrops ultimately need penetrating keratoplasty, which is best deferred until all of the corneal edema resolves.

Corneal dystrophies are inherited conditions that cause variable findings according to the anatomic layer affected. They are bilateral and largely autosomal dominant, with variable penetrance.

Superficial corneal dystrophies include map-dot-fingerprint dystrophy (Cogan's microcystic dystrophy). Abnormalities in the corneal epithelium cause changes in the epithelium basement membrane that manifest as fine map, dot, or fingerprint lines on slitlamp examination of the cornea. Patients with this condition may be asymptomatic, but spontaneous episodes of recurrent corneal erosion can occur. Conservative treatment includes topical lubricants, hypertonic saline drops or ointment, and bandage contact lenses. If these measures do not help the epithe-

lium adhere to its underlying basement membrane, paradoxically, debridement to the epithelium in the involved area may help achieve stability. Anterior stromal puncture is gaining acceptance. This procedure uses a fine needle to make small puncture marks just beyond Bowman's membrane, into the corneal stroma. These small scars allow the overlying epithelium to achieve better adhesion to its basement membrane. Even when the punctures are made within the visual axis, visual deficits are rare, although patients may complain of changes in the quality of their vision.

Many corneal stromal dystrophies occur, but the three classic ones are granular, lattice, and macular. Granular dystrophy is characterized by deposits of hyaline material into the corneal stroma. These deposits produce a "bread crumb" appearance, with intervening clear areas of cornea. This condition progresses slowly and leads to a gradual worsening of vision. Symptoms often do not start until midlife. Treatment with penetrating keratoplasty offers a good prognosis. Lattice dystrophy results from amyloid deposits within the corneal stroma. These deposits give the appearance of fine, refractile lines that form a web. This pattern is often best seen in retroillumination (slitlamp technique). Recurrent erosions are common and may lead to stromal haze and decreased vision. The treatment of choice is penetrating keratoplasty. Recurrences of lattice dystrophy in the corneal graft are common, but may take years to develop (Fig. 9-8). Macular dystrophy is usually more severe than granular or lattice dystrophy. Unlike the other types, macular dystrophy has an autosomal recessive inheritance pattern. Mucopolysaccharide deposits tend to spread diffusely through the corneal stroma, leading to decreased vision at an early age. These deposits reach the periphery, with no clear cornea between them. Penetrating keratoplasty is performed to improve vision.

Posterior dystrophies include Fuchs' endothelial dystrophy. This common autosomal dominant disorder is char-

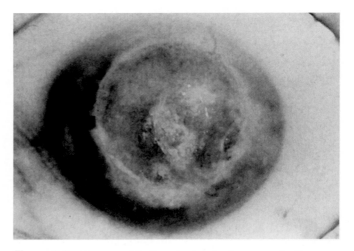

Figure 9-8   Recurrent lattice dystrophy in a penetrating keratoplasty.

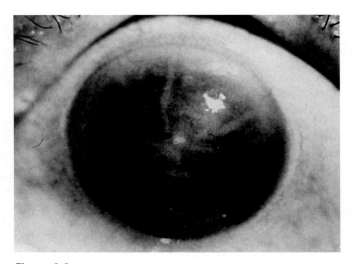

Figure 9-9   Corneal edema secondary to Fuchs' dystrophy.

acterized by the early development of endothelial dysfunction associated with decreased endothelial cell counts. This disorder is most commonly found in postmenopausal women. Slitlamp examination shows endothelial excrescences (**corneal guttae**), often associated with pigment. The amount of corneal edema depends on the severity of the disease (Fig. 9-9). As the disease progresses, epithelial breakdown may occur, eventually producing subepithelial scarring. Symptoms of blurred vision and irritation usually do not occur until the fifth or sixth decade. In the early stages, topical hypertonic saline may be used to dehydrate the cornea, and bandage contact lenses may be inserted to neutralize corneal astigmatism. In later stages, corneal transplantation is the only alternative to improve visual acuity.

Infectious keratitis is usually caused by bacteria, rarely by fungi or parasites. Infectious corneal infiltrates are associated with contact lenses, especially extended-wear soft contact lenses. Symptoms include pain, redness, purulent discharge, decreased vision, and **photophobia.** After appropriate cultures and smears are obtained by scraping the involved cornea under topical anesthesia, treatment is with broad-spectrum, fortified topical antibiotics. Fortified antibiotics are more concentrated than the usual ones and are specially formulated by a pharmacist. Typical antibiotics used are fortified vancomycin or gentamicin (50 mg/mL hourly), but these could change depending on patient sensitivities or the availability of new antibiotics. Most such "corneal ulcers" are successfully treated with medication. If a patient does not respond to initial treatment, cultures are repeated to look for more unusual organisms. Occasionally, corneal biopsy is needed to identify the microbial agent. For patients who do not respond to medical therapy, corneal transplantation is required to excise the infected tissue.

The corneal transplantation technique is modified slightly because of the presence of infectious organisms.

The size of the graft is determined by the size of the corneal infiltrate. If the corneal infiltrate is not totally excised, the residual organisms will reinfect the graft and possibly the inside of the eye. After the infected cornea is excised, the surgical tray is replaced with a new sterile tray of instruments. These instruments are used on the donor cornea to finish the surgery. The host corneal tissue button is sent not only to microbiology but also to pathology to check for organisms at the wound edge, just as one would look for evidence of tumor cells at the edge of a tumor resection. Fortified antibiotics are used topically after surgery, and the surgeon may use intraocular or intravenous antibiotics. Although preservation of a clear graft is desirable, the overriding concern is elimination of the infectious process. Consequently, topical steroids that suppress the immune system are used with caution, if at all.

The most common conditions that require cornea transplantation because of infection are fungal or amebic infectious keratitis and severe bacterial keratitis that has led to corneal perforation. If an infected cornea perforates, then cyanoacrylate tissue adhesive can be used to seal the perforation and allow the underlying tissue to heal after the acute infectious process is eradicated.

Sterile corneal ulceration may occur in association with such connective tissue disorders as rheumatoid arthritis, systemic lupus erythematosus, and Wegener's granulomatosis. The sterile infiltrates usually occur in the corneal periphery. They often respond to topical or anti-inflammatory therapy. If they perforate, cyanoacrylate tissue adhesive can be used. A bandage contact lens is placed over the cornea to protect against mechanical irritation from lid movement that can dislodge the adhesive. If successfully applied, the glue allows the corneal stroma to fill in beneath it. The glue usually spontaneously dislodges in a few months. Then the bandage contact lens is removed. The use of tissue adhesive is limited by the size of the corneal perforation. A perforation that is larger than 2 to 3 mm cannot be sealed with glue and requires a "patch" graft. This type of graft involves plugging the hole in the cornea with a piece of donor corneal tissue.

Technique

Donor Tissue. A cornea donor may be any deceased person who is younger than 75 years of age and has no transmissible disease or history of eye disease. Cornea tissue is refused from donors who test positive for human immunodeficiency virus, those who have had previous intraocular surgery, and those with hepatitis, rabies, sepsis, Jakob-Creutzfeldt disease, or glaucoma. The quality of donor tissue depends on the age of the donor, the time between death and tissue harvest, and the time spent in processing and preservation. Although younger donors and rapid harvest, processing, and preservation are preferred, many older donors can have excellent corneal quality as documented by endothelial cell counts. Both the eye bank and the surgeon assess the quality of the tissue. Tissue typing is not performed.

The donor cornea and a thin rim of surrounding sclera are preserved in solutions that contain nutritional, preservative, and antibiotic solutions. Although the risk of transplanting contaminated tissue is rare, cultures of the donor corneal rims are taken at the time of preservation and also at the time of surgery. Currently, donor tissue may be preserved for 5 to 7 days after death. Cryopreservation allows corneal preservation for many years, but is neither practical nor economical.

Full-Thickness Transplant. Corneal transplantation may be performed with an eyelid block and either local **retrobulbar** injection or general anesthesia. A lid speculum is placed in the conjunctival sac, avoiding pressure on the globe itself. Usually, a small stainless steel ring (Flieringa's ring) is sewn to the sclera to support the globe when the eye is open. Because the eye is an elastic structure, it tends to collapse when the cornea is removed, especially in children.

A corneal trephine (circular blade) of appropriate size is centered on the cornea, and a partial-thickness (80%) cut is made in the host. The donor cornea is prepared with a separate trephine. The endothelial side of the corneal button is up. To decrease the likelihood of postoperative complications and to simplify closure of the eye, this cut is approximately 0.5 mm larger in diameter than the host trephination. After the donor cornea is punched, it is placed on a protected Teflon block and covered by its preservative solution. Great care is taken to avoid trauma to the donor cornea that could cause endothelial cell loss and lead to graft failure.

After the donor cornea is prepared, the host eye is entered with a sharp blade. The host button is cut out with curved corneal scissors, and further intraocular surgery is performed as needed. Such surgery might include removal and replacement of an IOL, placement of a secondary IOL in a previously aphakic eye, removal of prolapsed vitreous humor from the anterior chamber of the eye, resection of scar tissue, or cataract extraction and primary IOL implant.

Once these other procedures are completed, the donor cornea is brought to the operative field and sewn into place. Various suturing methods are used, depending on the surgeon's preference (Figs. 9-10 and 9-11). The ultimate goal is to achieve a perfectly replaced cornea with no induced astigmatism. After the cornea is sewn to the recipient bed and the anterior chamber is reformed with balanced salt solution, the wound is inspected to make sure it is secure. The supporting ring is removed, antibiotics and steroids are administered if necessary, and a pressure patch with a shield is applied.

Postoperative management of penetrating keratoplasty includes topical steroids, topical antibiotics, and topical lubricants. If intraocular pressure is elevated, topical or systemic antiglaucoma medications are used. Because topical antibiotics are potentially toxic to the epithelium, they are gradually withdrawn over a period of several weeks.

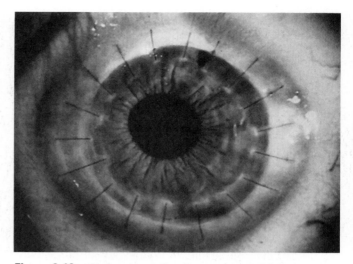

Figure 9-10 Clear penetrating keratoplasty with intact interrupted sutures.

Topical steroids are used for several months to reduce intraocular inflammation and prevent immunologic graft rejection.

Visual rehabilitation after penetrating keratoplasty takes much longer than that after other anterior segment surgical procedures. Avascular, clear corneal wounds heal much more slowly than limbal (vascular area between the cornea and the sclera) wounds. Complete visual recovery may take 1 year or longer. If patients obtain good visual acuity with a stable refraction and not too much astigmatism, sutures are best left in place. Removing them can cause large astigmatic errors. It is important to warn the patient about the potential for erosion and exposure of

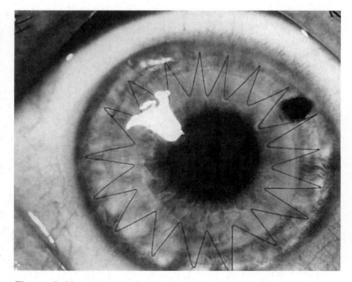

Figure 9-11 Clear penetrating keratoplasty with intact running sutures. A peripheral iridectomy (*hole in the iris to prevent glaucoma*) is seen at the 2 o'clock position.

disintegrating sutures, which can be a source of irritation and infection. All patients must be told to seek prompt ophthalmic evaluation if they experience pain, redness, irritation, or discharge that suggests suture exposure.

Intraoperative complications include damage to adjacent anterior segment structures (e.g., iris, lens). Bleeding from the iris or **anterior chamber angle** may occur during removal of a poorly designed or poorly positioned IOL. The most feared intraoperative complication is expulsive hemorrhage, the forceful expulsion of the intraocular contents after acute choroidal hemorrhage. This rare complication is more common in elderly patients, those with glaucoma, and those with previous eye surgery. The most important priority is closure of the eye. Secondary surgical intervention can be performed several days later, after the ocular status stabilizes.

Postoperative complications include rejection, endophthalmitis, persistent epithelial defects, infectious keratitis, elevated intraocular pressure, retinal detachment, and epithelial downgrowth. The incidence of rejection is approximately 10% to 20% for patients with a good prognosis (e.g., corneal scars, keratoconus, certain corneal dystrophies). Most rejection episodes occur 3 to 12 months after surgery. The incidence is higher in younger patients, presumably because of their more active immune systems. If caught early, rejection episodes can often be aborted by the intensive use of steroids, topically in the form of drops or ointment, subconjunctivally by injection, or orally. Patients who undergo penetrating keratoplasty are instructed to seek prompt ophthalmic evaluation at the first signs of rejection (e.g., conjunctival injection, pain, irritation, light sensitivity, decreased vision). In its early stages, rejection often is not noticed by patients, but it is observed during a routine follow-up visit. Permanently rejected corneas become cloudy. They may be retransplanted, although with each subsequent transplant, the chance of rejection increases.

The prognosis for corneal transplants depends primarily on the underlying disease. Favorable prognostic factors include the lack of preoperative inflammation, avascularity of the diseased cornea, normal intraocular pressure, and healthy ocular surface and adnexa. Poor indicators include active inflammation, surface disorders (e.g., dry eye syndrome, lid abnormalities, corneal vascularity, glaucoma, chemical burns). The results of penetrating keratoplasty in children are not as good as in adults because of such factors as associated congenital ocular abnormalities, difficulty with follow-up, and **amblyopia** (poor or decreased vision in an anatomically normal eye). Some disorders (e.g., certain corneal dystrophies, herpes simplex keratitis) tend to recur in corneal transplants. All of the stromal dystrophies recur in transplants, although it may take years for such recurrence to become apparent. The recurrence may differ from the characteristic appearance of the primary dystrophy.

The prognosis for a clear corneal transplant is fairly good, but in some cases, astigmatism and **anisometropia** (significant difference in refractive error between the eye that has had surgery and the one that has not) often preclude full visual rehabilitation. Contact lenses are helpful in neutralizing the astigmatism or anisometropia. Unfortunately, some patients cannot tolerate contact lenses (e.g., some elderly patients have difficulty handling or tolerating the lenses). Astigmatic keratorefractive surgery (discussed later) is sometimes required to correct excessive astigmatic or anisometropic refractive errors. Visual results after penetrating keratoplasty depend not only on the clarity and regularity of the transplanted corneal button, but also on the healthy function of the retina and optic nerve.

Partial-Thickness Transplant. Lamellar corneal transplant is useful for patients with anterior corneal disease (e.g., those who have scarring or inherited dystrophies). This procedure obviates the need to enter the eye, thereby virtually eliminating the risk of endophthalmitis. In addition, the recipient corneal endothelium is left intact, thereby eliminating the risk of immunologic endothelial rejection. The procedure also provides a patch graft in patients with acute corneal perforations that require immediate surgical closure.

The surgical procedure of lamellar keratoplasty is technically more demanding than that of penetrating keratoplasty. A corneal trephine is used to make a partial-thickness incision into the host cornea. Then a lamellar dissection is carried across the outlying trephination. The lamellar dissection is deep enough to remove the anterior stromal opacification while leaving a posterior bed of clear corneal stroma for the corneal donor. Donor tissue also requires precise lamellar dissection and is best performed from an intact donor globe.

The postoperative management is similar to that for penetrating keratoplasty, although fewer topical steroids are used. The healing of lamellar grafts tends to be quicker than that of penetrating keratoplasty. The major drawback of lamellar keratoplasty is the difficulty in achieving a smooth lamellar bed. Consequently, there is an increased potential for interface scarring that may restrict vision. However, in select patients with anterior corneal stromal opacification, lamellar transplant rather than penetrating keratoplasty is the treatment of choice.

Recently, new procedures have been developed to replace the damaged endothelial tissue without requiring a full corneal transplant. The technique is referred to as deep lamellar endothelial keratoplasty (DLEK). It involves surgically removing the diseased endothelium and replacing it with donor endothelium. This can be done through a small incision and does not require sutures. This procedure reduces astigmatism and other structural problems associated with a full-thickness corneal transplant.

Refractive Surgery

Refractive corneal surgery involves changing the refractive power of the eye by surgically modifying the shape of the cornea. A variety of procedures are used, but only the most common are discussed here.

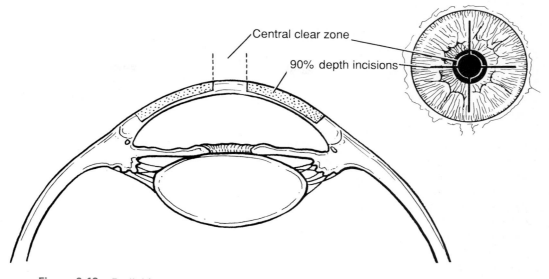

Central clear zone

90% depth incisions

Figure 9-12   Radial keratotomy.

Radial keratotomy, the most common refractive surgery performed, is used to correct myopia. Partial-thickness radial cuts are made in the cornea, sparing the visual axis (Figs. 9-12 and 9-13). This pattern of incisions tends to flatten the central cornea, thereby reducing the myopic refractive error. The procedure is usually performed under topical anesthesia. The amount of correction can be modified by varying the size of the spared central optical zone, the number of radial incisions, and the depth of the incisions. The predictability of radial keratotomy depends on the degree of myopia being treated. Patients with low to moderate myopia have an 80% to 90% chance of obtaining an uncorrected visual acuity of 20/40 or better. The chances of obtaining better visual acuity decrease with increasing myopia.

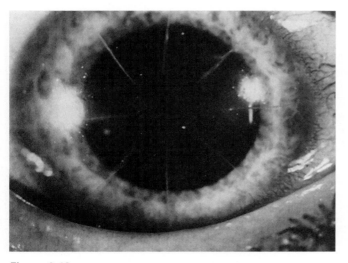

Figure 9-13   Eight-incision radial keratotomy.

Surgical complications are rare, although many patients note glare and fluctuating visual acuity in the early postoperative period. These problems tend to resolve with time. Repeat procedures are sometimes required. If the result still does not offer adequate uncorrected visual acuity, the patient must return to wearing spectacles or contact lenses. Questions have been raised about the stability of radial keratotomy. In some patients, the effect of surgery gradually increases over a period of several years. There is also concern that deep radial incisions may weaken the structural integrity of the cornea, increasing its susceptibility to traumatic rupture.

Other refractive procedures include corneal relaxing incisions, compression sutures, wedge resection, epikeratophakia (application of a donor cornea), and **keratomileusis** (grinding a new curvature on the cornea). Patients with congenital astigmatism or residual postoperative astigmatism usually can be managed with glasses or contact lenses. If astigmatism is excessive, surgical alternatives include relaxing incisions, compression sutures, and wedge resection. Relaxing incisions centered on the steep axis of the corneal astigmatism cause flattening of the cornea in that meridian, thereby reducing the amount of astigmatism. Corneal compression sutures and wedge resections are used to steepen a flat corneal meridian. Visual rehabilitation after wedge resection is much longer than with relaxing incisions. The effect of corneal compression sutures is variable and may not be permanent. The predictability of astigmatic surgery is less than ideal, but in patients with excessive postoperative astigmatism, there is nothing else to offer for visual rehabilitation.

Epikeratophakia and keratomileusis are examples of refractive procedures that use lamellar keratoplasty. Epikeratophakia is used primarily to correct **aphakia** in patients who cannot tolerate contact lenses and are not good candidates for a secondary IOL. The procedure involves suturing a commercially prepared lenticula of corneal tissue on top of the recipient cornea after the corneal epithelium is removed. Recovery is fast and the procedure is easily repeatable if necessary. Keratomileusis involves shaving off a thin anterior section of the cornea, freezing it, lathing it to the desired power and shape, thawing it, and resuturing it into its original site. This procedure is reserved for highly myopic patients whose vision cannot be corrected otherwise and who do not want to wear glasses or contact lenses. This procedure requires expensive equipment, the use of which can be difficult to master. Major drawbacks include poor predictability, irreversibility, and the potential for surgically induced irregular corneal astigmatism.

One of the most exciting developments in corneal surgery is the introduction of the Excimer laser, which vaporizes tissue with a high degree of precision. Although clinical trials are still technically underway, the laser is greatly in demand for sculpting the anterior cornea to produce refractive change. If the encouraging preliminary results hold up over the long term, this laser could revolutionize the practice of ophthalmology.

Pterygium Excision

A pterygium is a plaque-like extension of fibrovascular tissue onto the superficial cornea. Pterygia characteristically originate nasally from pinguecula (accumulation of connective tissue that thickens the conjunctiva) and grow onto the adjacent corneal surface. Their cause is unknown, but their incidence seems to correlate with exposure to ultraviolet light.

Pterygia are commonly restricted to the peripheral cornea, where they do not interfere with visual acuity. Some cause localized irritation that can be controlled with topical lubricants and vasoconstrictors. However, some pterygia extend toward the visual axis and cause corneal astigmatism and visual distortion. If a pterygium grows into the visual axis, it may interfere with visual acuity by causing opacification and obscuration of the central cornea. Surgical excision is recommended when vision begins to be distorted before the pterygium encroaches on the visual axis.

Surgery is usually performed under local anesthesia. The pterygium is dissected off the corneal surface with a fine lathe. Small cautery burns to the conjunctiva outlining the proposed graft site are helpful in delineating the proposed donor conjunctival site. After the initial incision into conjunctiva is made, retraction of the tissue makes these measurements difficult. The graft is carefully sewn into place over the pterygium excision site. Care is taken not to turn the donor tissue inside out.

Recurrence rates after primary pterygium removal vary from 10% to 50%, but tend to be lower in northern latitudes, where there is less exposure to ultraviolet light. The recurrence rate is diminished by the conjunctival transposition that covers the exposed bed of the excised pterygium. To decrease the chance of recurrence, beta irradiation or topical antimetabolites (Mitomycin C, thiotepa) are advocated.

A recurrent pterygium may become more extensive than the original one. Excessive scarring and involvement of underlying extraocular muscles can restrict ocular motility and cause double vision. Thus, pterygium surgery is best avoided unless it is absolutely necessary because of visual restriction, recurrent irritation, or cosmetic disfigurement. Before proceeding with surgery, the patient must be made aware of the potential for recurrence (Fig. 9-14).

Surface Disorders

Ocular surface disorders include dry eye syndrome, exposure keratopathy, and neurotrophic keratitis. Dry eye syndrome (**keratitis sicca**) is usually an isolated finding in menopausal women, but it can also occur as part of Sjögren's syndrome, ocular pemphigoid, or Stevens-Johnson syndrome. Exposure keratopathy occurs when the lids cannot cover the entire corneal surface on blinking or during sleep. It occurs in Bell's palsy and ocular trauma, where localized scarring of the lids prevents full corneal coverage. Neurotrophic keratitis is caused by dysfunction of the sensory nerve supply to the cornea (e.g., neurologic diseases that affect the first division of the trigeminal nerve).

All ocular surface disorders cause desiccation of the corneal epithelium and conjunctival squamous metaplasia and keratinizations. Patients often have ocular irritation and the sensation of a foreign body in the eye. Supplemental liquid tear substitutes and bland ointment may be all that is necessary to promote ocular comfort and maintain the integrity of the corneal epithelium. Occluding the puncta (shown in Fig. 9-33) with silicone plugs, cautery, or hyfrecation can also enhance ocular surface lubrication. In severe cases, however, permanent punctal occlusion may be necessary.

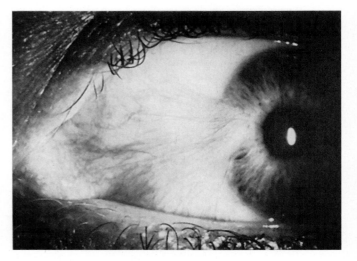

Figure 9-14   Recurrent pterygium.

Patients with severe dry eye syndrome, exposure kerato-pathy, or neurotrophic keratopathy are helped by tarsorrhaphy. The procedure involves sewing the edges of the superior and inferior lid margins together. Tarsorrhaphy is usually preceded by splitting the lid margin or excising a thin superficial layer of lid margin. The two opposing raw surfaces thus created remain permanently adjoined after the sutures are removed. Because this procedure is cosmetically disfiguring, it is reserved for patients with severe ocular surface disease and a potential for corneal ulceration and melting. After the cornea completely heals, the tarsorrhaphy can be separated by simple excision. However, the potential for recurrent epithelial breakdown remains.

A conjunctival flap is an alternative approach, but it is used only when the patient refuses a tarsorrhaphy or when the visual potential of the involved eye is poor.

Oculoplastic surgery is a third alternative to correct other eyelid deformities that cause corneal exposure. Conjunctival scarring disorders (e.g., ocular pemphigoid, Stevens-Johnson syndrome) are often resistant to all surgical and medical attempts to improve the ocular surface environment. In these cases, the only alternative is a keratoprosthesis in which a small telescope is sewn through the cornea, into the eye, and then brought out through a small opening in the eyelids that are otherwise sewn closed. Excellent results can be obtained for a few months to years, but the long-term prognosis is poor.

DISEASES OF THE ANTERIOR CHAMBER

Anatomy and Physiology

The anterior chamber is formed by the cornea, the angle (trabecular meshwork), the iris, and the lens of the eye. It is filled with aqueous humor, which is made by the ciliary body. Aqueous travels from the ciliary body through the pupil and leaves mainly through the trabecular meshwork and **Schlemm's canal.** The aqueous carries the nutrients for the cornea, lens, and trabecular meshwork. Intraocular pressure depends on the relation among aqueous production, aqueous outflow, and episcleral venous pressure.

Pathophysiology

An increase in ocular pressure that interferes with the normal functioning of the optic nerve head can lead to atrophy of the optic nerve, with progressive loss of the visual field. This disease is known as glaucoma. If untreated, it can lead to total, irreversible blindness.

Clinical Presentation and Evaluation

Patients with glaucoma have no symptoms. Detection depends on measurement of intraocular pressure with an applanation tonometer, an instrument used to determine ocular tension by application of a small, flat disc to the cornea. Normal intraocular pressure is 16 mm Hg (normal pressure is 10–22 mm Hg). Some patients have optic nerves that can withstand pressures greater than 22 mm Hg. Although these patients do not show optic nerve damage or visual field changes, they are considered ocular hypertensives or glaucoma suspects.

Prevention of lost vision depends on early detection and proper treatment with either medication or surgery. Glaucoma is commonly categorized according to the cause of the altered resistance to aqueous outflow as well as the clinical appearance of the anterior chamber angle. Glaucoma can be primary, secondary, or congenital.

Treatment

Primary Glaucoma

Primary glaucoma is classified as chronic open-angle, narrow-angle (or angle-closure), or mixed.

Chronic Open-Angle Glaucoma

Chronic open-angle glaucoma is the most common form of glaucoma; 2% of the general population older than 65 years old is at risk (Fig. 9-15). In chronic open-angle glaucoma, the trabecular meshwork appears anatomically normal, but its ability to remove aqueous fluid from the anterior chamber is diminished. This type of glaucoma is treated topically with such medications as timolol maleate, levobunolol, betaxolol, or pilocarpine as well as systemically with carbonic anhydrase inhibitors. If these medications do not reduce intraocular pressure to a safe level (i.e.,

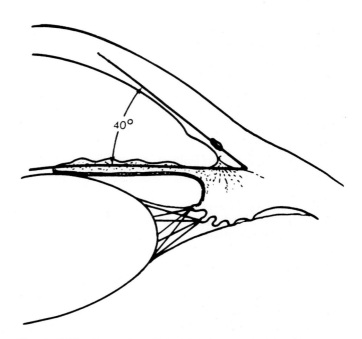

Figure 9-15 Typical configuration in open-angle glaucoma. The angle of the anterior chamber (*arrows*) is formed by the cornea and iris.

if further loss of vision is occurring at the current pressure) or if the patient cannot tolerate the medications, then laser trabeculoplasty may be attempted. Laser trabeculoplasty is performed under topical anesthesia. This procedure uses a special gonioscopic mirror to allow visualization of the anterior chamber (which cannot normally be seen because of the internal reflection caused by the anatomy and physiology of the anterior chamber). If a laser is used, approximately 75 spots are placed into the anterior trabecular meshwork in an area of 180 degrees. Usually, a 50-m, spot-sized, blue-green argon laser is used at 800 to 1,200 mW. The mechanism by which a laser trabeculoplasty effects change is not well understood, but the procedure reduces intraocular pressure by approximately 25% in 65% to 75% of patients. Although the procedure may relieve pressure for only months to a few years, it has few side effects and is sometimes used even before systemic medications.

If the patient is still losing vision, a surgical procedure may be required. In the United States, the most common surgical procedure is a trabeculectomy. This filtering procedure is effective in 75% to 90% of cases (Fig. 9-16). A trabeculectomy is usually performed under local anesthetic on an outpatient basis. After adequate anesthesia and preparation with a povidone-iodine solution, a lid speculum is inserted beneath the lids. The eye is rotated inferiorly, the superior rectus muscle is grasped with a forceps, and a 4-0 suture is passed under the muscle for traction. Peritomy is performed with blunt scissors. The conjunctiva is opened either near the cornea or 8 to 10 mm behind it. Cautery is used to obtain hemostasis, and the sclera is cleaned by scraping with a fine blade. With a very fine diamond knife, a half-scleral–thickness incision is made perpendicular to the limbus and extended approximately 3 to 4 mm behind it. A parallel incision is made approximately 4 mm away and is joined to the first one with an incision parallel to the limbus and 3 to 4 mm behind it (Fig. 9-16A). This area is dissected forward with a blunt blade. The flap is carried into clear cornea. The half-scleral–thickness flap may be triangular, rectangular, or even rhomboid. Studies show little difference in outcome because of the shape of the flap (Fig. 9-16B). A full-thickness piece of trabecular meshwork, approximately 1.5 to 2 mm, is removed (Fig. 9-16C, 9-16D, and 9-16E). A small iridectomy is performed to prevent closure of the opening by the iris (Fig. 9-16F). The flap is resutured with 10-0 sutures at the posterior edge of the incision. The conjunctiva and Tenon's capsule are resutured in place. At the time of trabeculectomy, antimetabolites (either 5-fluorouracil or mitomycin C) are often given to reduce the scarring that might lead to failure of the procedure. Even after trabeculectomy, patients may require additional medication to control pressure.

Narrow-Angle Glaucoma
Narrow-angle (angle-closure) glaucoma is caused by mechanical blockage of the angle by the iris (Fig. 9-17). Symptoms of acute-angle closure include halos around lights, headaches, nausea, and ocular pain. Signs are a steamy cornea, a partly dilated nonreactive pupil, a gonioscopically closed angle with high intraocular pressure, and red, injected eyes.

The blockage is usually easily broken by laser iridotomy (with either yttrium-aluminum-garnet [YAG] or argon laser), which creates a conduit for aqueous humor to flow from the posterior to the anterior chamber. This procedure deepens the anterior chamber and opens the angle by allowing the iris to fall back to its original position. After topical anesthesia, a special lens is used to focus the laser onto the iris surface. A **YAG laser** is then used to photodisrupt (or an argon laser to burn) the iris by producing a hole that breaks the pupillary block.

Occasionally, when the cornea is hazy and a laser cannot be used, surgical iridectomy is performed (Fig. 9-18). After adequate anesthesia, a 3- to 4-mm peritomy is performed, usually superiorly, to release the conjunctiva from its limbal attachments. The surgical limbus is identified, and the anterior chamber is entered with a knife. A forceps is used to grasp and retract the iris, and a small piece of iris is removed with scissors. The limbal incision is closed with a small 9-0 or 10-0 suture, and the peritomy is closed over that.

Medical treatment is used temporarily to lower pressure and relieve symptoms. This treatment is also used to clear the cornea to make laser iridotomy easier. The goal is to open the angle and reduce pressure. Usually the patient is given a β blocker to reduce aqueous production, oral or parenteral acetazolamide to further reduce aqueous production, oral glycerin to osmotically remove fluid from the eye, and pilocarpine drops to pull the iris from the cornea.

Mixed Chronic Open- and Narrow-Angle Glaucoma
In nearly 95% to 100% of patients with acute narrow-angle glaucoma, and with most nonchronic forms of glaucoma, either laser or surgical iridectomy is effective in preventing further attacks. Because a chronic, low-grade, narrow-angle attack may lead to damage of the trabecular meshwork, however, a patient may have mixed chronic open- and narrow-angle glaucoma that requires medication, even after iridectomy or iridotomy.

Secondary Glaucoma

Secondary glaucoma is characterized by associated ocular or systemic abnormalities that appear to account for the increased resistance to aqueous outflow. These glaucomas may be associated with intraocular tumors or hemorrhage; corneal endothelium, pigmentary, lens, or retinal disorders; ocular inflammation, trauma, or surgery; steroid ingestion; or elevated episcleral venous pressure.

Neovascular glaucoma is a secondary glaucoma in which new blood vessels form in the angle of the eye and on the iris. Histologically, connective tissue is also present. Neovascularization often starts at the pupillary margin. Eventually, vessels can cover the iris and progress into the angle. The fibrovascular membrane that is formed is con-

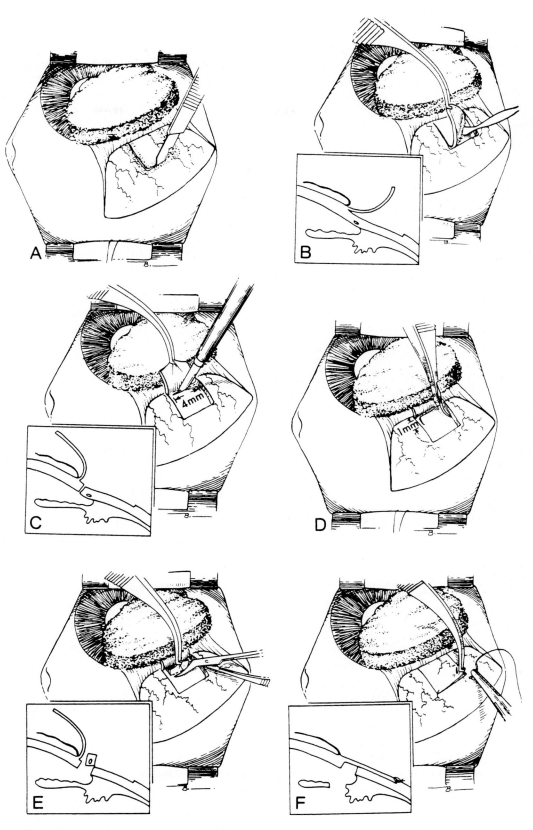

Figure 9-16 Basic technique for trabeculectomy. **A,** Margins of the scleral flap are outlined by partial-thickness incisions. **B,** Dissection of the scleral flap. **C,** The anterior chamber is entered with a knife just behind the hinge of the scleral flap. **D,** Completion of the anterior and lateral margins of a deep limbal incision with scissors. **E,** A flap of deep limbal tissue is excised by cutting along scleral spur. **F,** Approximation of the scleral flap.

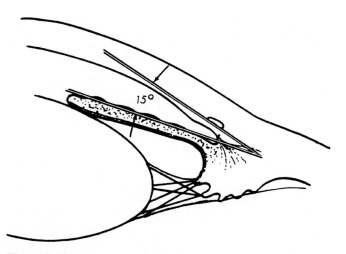

Figure 9-17 Narrow angle that typically precedes most forms of angle-closure glaucoma.

tracted, leading to **ectropion** uvea (i.e., the posterior pigment layer of the iris is pulled into the pupil and then onto the anterior surface) and also to anterior synechiae (i.e., the iris is pulled into the angle).

The cause of neovascular glaucoma is not fully understood. A common property of the many causes of **rubeosis iridis** (iris neovascularization) appears to be hypoxia, either anteriorly, or more commonly, posteriorly. Many believe that an angiogenesis factor is released and leads to the formation of new vessels. Some common causes of rubeosis iridis include diabetes mellitus, retinal vein occlusion, retinal artery occlusion, carotid artery disease, and intraocular surgery.

In general, the treatment for rubeosis is panretinal **photocoagulation** to reduce the stimulus for angiogenesis factors. Later stages may require surgery, including Setons (plastic one-way valves that drain externally). If these are unsuccessful, other therapies (e.g., destroying the ciliary body with a laser or alcohol injections) may be necessary to reduce the production of aqueous and lower the pressure.

Congenital Glaucoma

Congenital glaucoma is a rare, usually bilateral disease that affects approximately 1 in 20,000 live births. The exact mechanism that triggers this disease is not known, but the angle acts as if there were a membrane over the trabecular meshwork. The signs and symptoms of congenital glaucoma are photophobia, buphthalmos (large eye), large corneas, tearing, and corneal edema. Medications do not work well in affected infants, and surgery is required.

The principle of surgery for congenital glaucoma is to establish a pathway for aqueous to leave the anterior chamber and enter Schlemm's canal. The procedure can be done by goniotomy, in which a fine knife is passed across the anterior chamber to incise the trabecular meshwork (and usually into Schlemm's canal, the channel that collects aqueous from the trabecular meshwork) (Fig. 9-19).

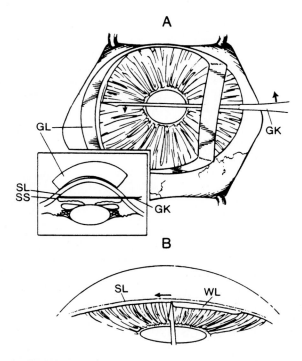

Figure 9-19 Goniotomy. **A,** With a surgical goniolens (*GL*) positioned on the cornea, a goniotomy knife (*GK*) is inserted through the peripheral cornea and passed across the anterior chamber to the angle in the opposite quadrant. **B,** Under direct gonioscopic visualization, angle tissue is excised between Schwalbe's line (*SL*) and the scleral spur (*SS*) for approximately one third of the circumference of the chamber angle. This excision creates a white line (*WL*) as the cut edge of tissue retracts from the incision. *Arrows* show the direction of knife movement during incision of the angle tissue.

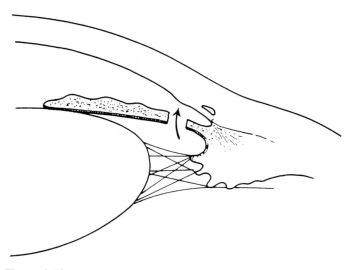

Figure 9-18 Mechanism of iridectomy. Communication between the anterior and posterior chambers (*arrow*) bypasses the pupillary block. The relatively higher pressure in the posterior chamber is relieved, and the peripheral iris falls away from the trabecular meshwork.

DISEASES OF THE LENS

Anatomy and Physiology

The lens is an avascular structure that grows throughout an individual's life. It has a dense nucleus that is surrounded by a softer cortex and is sequestered in a capsule. The lens epithelium produces new lens material that is analogous to the layers of an onion. The lens is responsible for the final bending of rays of light to focus them on the retina. The ciliary body (with the zonules) causes the lens to thicken to allow for close-up viewing (e.g., reading).

Pathophysiology

A cataract is any clouding of the lens of the eye. It may occur anywhere within the lens. The most common opacities occur within the nucleus, which naturally yellows and hardens with age. Opacities can occur in the anterior and posterior cortical areas, as well as in the posterior subcapsular area.

Etiology of Cataracts

Many factors are involved in the etiology of cataracts, including family history, general health, age, trauma, diabetes, steroid use, intraocular inflammation, and exposure to radiation. The lens is not only vulnerable to trauma, but because it is an avascular structure, it cannot rid itself easily of any metabolic injury.

A senile, or age-related, cataract is a yellowing of the lens because of natural by-products of the aging process. Density and coloration of the lens are extremely variable. In some early aging syndromes, the lens yellows at 30 to 35 years of age. Although almost all patients older than 65 years of age have some form of hardening or yellowing of the nucleus, some patients in their 80s and 90s have little lenticular change.

Blunt trauma, even without ocular perforation, may cause cataract formation, typically seen as a petal-form anterior cortical opacification in the central region of the lens (Fig. 9-20). It often appears in boxers who receive repeated blows to the head, but may be seen after a single blow. Another common cause is racquet sports, particularly racquetball and squash, in patients who do not wear protective eye gear. Recently, paint ball games and bungee cords have become common causes of blunt injuries.

Systemic and long-term topical steroid use can produce a posterior subcapsular cataract. Many believe that this phenomenon is dose-dependent, although the mechanism is not known. Another cause of these cataracts is intraocular inflammation, as seen in anterior and posterior uveitis syndromes (e.g., sarcoidosis, Reiter's syndrome, other human leukocyte antigen B27 subgroups). In patients with diabetes, swelling of the lens caused by high glucose levels can initiate a classic water cleft type of cataract. In uncontrolled diabetes, glucose enters the lens structure, where aldose reductase transforms it into sorbitol, which cannot

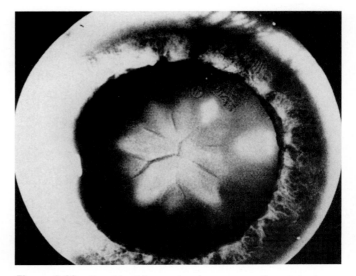

Figure 9-20 Petal-leaf formation in a traumatic cataract.

leave the lens. This process causes an osmotic gradient that results in swelling of the lens. Although the condition may be reversible, repeated offenses may lead to permanent lens changes.

Radiation exposure, usually greater than 400 rad, may also cause cataract formation. Radiation treatment for cancer around the head and neck is of particular concern. Some epidemiologic studies suggest that exposure to ultraviolet light over long periods (e.g., in farmers and fishermen) may also cause rapid cataract formation.

Clinical Presentation and Evaluation

Patients seek treatment because of reduced visual function. The subjective effect on the patient of such reduced visual function is the most important consideration in deciding whether to remove the cataract. Because a cataract does not harm the eye, indications for its removal are variable and require knowledge of the patient's capabilities, lifestyle, and desires. Although the success rate for cataract extraction is nearly 99%, a detailed discussion of its potential risks and benefits is needed before surgery is undertaken. Except in rare cases, the potential for good vision does not decrease by delaying surgery.

A senile cataract causes a myopic shift in refraction by increasing the refractive index of the lens, thus causing light to focus in front of the retina. This shift can allow the patient to read without glasses ("second sight"). The cataract also decreases night vision, increases glare at night, and because it absorbs blue light, leads to a dulling of colors ("browning effect"). Until it is well developed, however, a cataract does not usually affect reading and other close activities. In patients with poor distance vision (20/40 or less) who are nevertheless happy, surgery is not indicated.

In contrast to a nuclear cataract, which usually affects

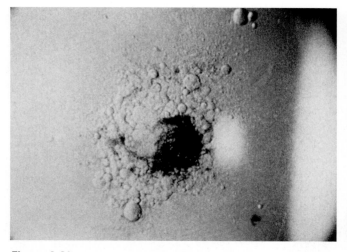

Figure 9-21   Light scattering from a posterior subcapsular cataract.

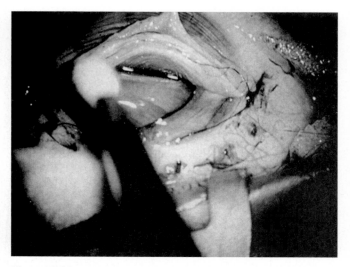

Figure 9-22   A freezing probe removing a cataract, including the capsule (intracapsular cataract extraction).

the elderly, a posterior subcapsular cataract often occurs in young patients, especially those who take steroids. This cataract diffracts light. Depending on its location (central or peripheral), it can cause severe disability in reading (Fig. 9-21). It can also cause extreme sensitivity to light and to glare from oncoming headlights. A patient may have 20/25, 20/30, or even better distance vision, but may be unable to read a newspaper. Individuals with excellent distance vision, but with occupations that require good close vision, may require early surgical intervention.

Treatment

Cataract Extraction Technique

Before the late 1970s, most cataract extractions were done by removing the entire lens, usually by cryosurgery. A probe reaching approximately −20°C was attached to the lens capsule, allowing complete removal of the lens and its capsule as a unit (intracapsular cataract extraction (Fig. 9-22). This technique had several drawbacks. It required a large incision that resulted in a slow healing process. In addition, the removal of the lens capsule structure and possible rupture of the anterior vitreous face led to a relatively high incidence of postoperative problems (e.g., retinal detachment, cystoid macular edema). In the late 1960s, the phacoemulsification technique invented by Charles Kelman renewed interest in extracapsular cataract extraction. This technique, in which a cataract is emulsified and aspirated with a high-frequency ultrasonic needle, leaves the posterior capsule intact for support. This support is good for the integrity of the eye and provides support for an implanted posterior chamber IOL.

The two techniques used for extracapsular cataract extraction are manual extraction and phacoemulsification. With the manual technique, the nucleus of the lens is removed whole. After the conjunctiva and Tenon's cap-

sule are dissected away from the surgical limbus, a 10.5- to 11-mm incision is made at the surgical limbus. The anterior capsule is opened (capsulotomy), and a central disc is removed. The nucleus is freed from its cortical attachments, usually by hydrodissection or with an intraocular instrument. The nucleus is then moved into the anterior chamber and removed with a lens loop (Fig. 9-23). Cortical material that remains within the capsule is removed by a unit that has an irrigation and aspiration port. In most cases, an IOL is implanted between the posterior and the remaining peripheral anterior capsule. The corneal wound is closed with 9-0, 10-0, or 11-0 suture material (usually nylon, although Mersilene is also used).

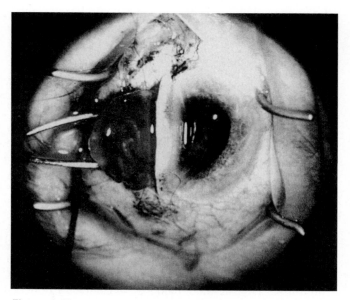

Figure 9-23   The nucleus is removed by extracapsular cataract extraction by a lens loop.

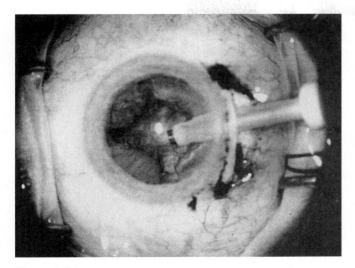

Figure 9-24 Phacoemulsification of the nucleus of a cataract.

With the phacoemulsification technique, ultrasound vibrates a titanium-tipped needle 27,000 to 54,000 cycles/sec to emulsify the nucleus, which is then aspirated through the tip of the needle (Fig. 9-24). The advantage of this technique is that it can be performed through a 1.9- to 3.2-mm incision. The incision is enlarged to accommodate an IOL (anywhere from 2.2 mm for a foldable silicone, acrylic, or hydrogel lens to 7.0 mm for a large optic lens). The smaller incision improves recovery time and minimizes postoperative astigmatic changes that occur with larger incisions. This technique also has disadvantages. Because it requires different skills than the manual technique, it can be difficult to learn, especially if no experienced surgeon is available to provide instruction and assistance. It also requires expensive equipment (up to $90,000/instrument), which necessitates a greater commitment to the instrumentation than does the manual technique. Nevertheless, there is a distinct trend toward the use of this procedure. In 1984, only 15% of cataract surgeons used phacoemulsification; today, nearly 96% use it.

Complications

Cataract surgery has several serious complications. First, choroidal hemorrhage occurs in approximately 1 of every 10,000 procedures, usually in elderly patients with arteriolar sclerosis. Choroidal hemorrhages usually lead to severe, if not total, loss of vision. The risk of choroidal hemorrhage approaches zero with phacoemulsification.

Endophthalmitis is an unusual, but potentially devastating event that often occurs 2 days to 2 weeks after surgery. Patients have ocular pain, eyelid swelling, and white blood cells that layer in the anterior chamber (**hypopyon**). The outcome depends on which microbe is involved and how quickly the condition is managed. Common microbes in early-onset endophthalmitis are *Staphylococcus aureus* and *Streptococcus epidermides*, and *Propionibacterium acnes* is

common in late onset. Management includes early diagnosis and treatment with antibiotics. A culture and Gram's stain from around the eye is taken. Anterior chamber and vitreous aspirates may also be needed. Intraocular broad-spectrum antibiotics are injected while awaiting culture results.

Retinal detachment may also occur after cataract extraction. The incidence of retinal detachment is approximately 5% in patients who undergo intracapsular cataract extraction. The incidence in uncomplicated extracapsular cataract surgery now approaches the spontaneous rate for that age-group (<1%).

Any surgical procedure causes the release of prostaglandins into the eye. Consequently, swelling may occur at the foveal region in the posterior segment. This swelling, known as **cystoid macular edema,** occurs temporarily in nearly all patients who undergo cataract extraction. After the blood–aqueous barrier stabilizes, the macular edema clears spontaneously. In 0.1% to 1% of patients, however, this edema may be a persistent and annoying problem that causes distortion of central vision. Treatment may include posterior injection of steroids or systemic treatment with nonsteroidal anti-inflammatory agents. Topical nonsteroidal anti-inflammatory drops are available both for prevention and treatment of cystoid macular edema.

Optical Correction after Surgery

Removal of the lens requires optical correction with glasses, contact lenses, or IOL implantation. Glasses can provide good optical correction, but only at large magnification compared with contact lenses (25% vs. 7%). The brain cannot fuse images seen by one eye as 25% disparate in size from those seen by the other eye. It is barely able to fuse images seen with a 7% disparity. Peripheral vision is better with contact lenses, but some patients have problems inserting and removing them. IOL implantation resolves the problems of both glasses and contact lenses (Fig. 9-25). Improvements in design and quality control since

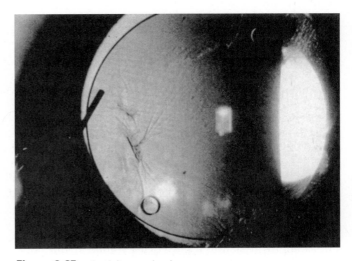

Figure 9-25 An intraocular lens.

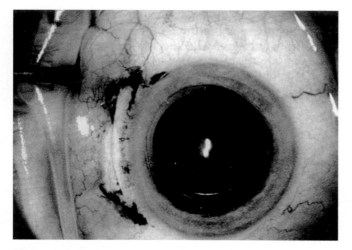

Figure 9-26 A well-positioned posterior chamber ("in-the-bag") intraocular lens.

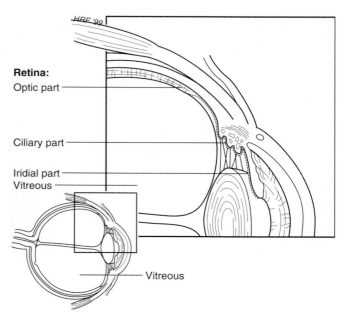

Figure 9-27 The retina and vitreous.

Harold Ridley launched the era of IOL implantation in 1947 in England have made IOLs the standard of care.

There are two major types. Anterior chamber lenses are placed on top of the iris, with footplates (haptics) resting in the anterior chamber angle. Posterior chamber lenses are placed within the remaining capsule, thus isolating the lens from the very sensitive tissues in the eye. Posterior ("in-the-bag") implantation is preferred (Fig. 9-26). After a few weeks, the lens becomes stable in the capsule, and dislocations are rare. However, because the capsule still contains live epithelial cells, 10% to 25% of patients experience a clouding of the posterior lens capsule after cataract surgery because the live cells can migrate behind the implant. This clouding (posterior capsule opacification) is also known as a secondary cataract because its symptoms resemble those of the primary cataract and can be treated with a YAG laser. The laser beam opens the capsule and immediately restores vision.

In pediatric patients, where the eye has not attained adult structure, IOLs are now the treatment of choice.

DISEASES OF THE RETINA AND VITREOUS

Anatomy and Physiology

The retina has three parts: optic, ciliary, and iridial (Fig. 9-27). The optic part receives the visual light rays and is further divided into pigmented and nervous parts. The ciliary and iridial parts of the retina are forward prolongations of the pigmented layer and a layer of supporting columnar or epithelial cells over the ciliary body and the posterior surface of the iris, respectively.

The vitreous is a connective tissue body made up of colloids (0.1%) and water (98%). It is transparent and occupies approximately four fifths of the volume of the globe. It provides a way for metabolites to move between the lens,

ciliary body, and retina. It also helps abort and redistribute energy applied to the globe. It is composed of collagen, hyaluronic acid, and proteins; albumin is the major protein.

Pathophysiology

The retina may break or detach. Retinal breaks can be either asymptomatic or acute. Asymptomatic retinal holes occur in approximately 6% of the population. Of this group, retinal detachment occurs in only 1 person in 10,000 each year. Acute symptomatic retinal tears (especially those associated with persistent vitreoretinal traction) are dangerous and carry a much higher risk of retinal detachment. The risk is increased in patients who have had previous cataract surgery, are highly myopic, have a family history of retinal detachment, or have had a retinal detachment in the other eye. Prophylactic treatment of these retinal breaks is indicated.

Full-thickness retinal defects (retinal breaks) may be small, atrophic holes or tears caused by vitreoretinal traction. Most retinal tears occur after a spontaneous or traumatic posterior vitreous detachment (PVD), in which the posterior attachments of the vitreous separate from the retina and the vitreous body collapses anteriorly. The vitreous is firmly attached over the vitreous base, a circumferential zone that straddles the **ora serrata** (the boundary between the retina and the pars plana) peripherally. Other areas of relatively firm vitreoretinal adhesions include retinal scars, areas of vitreoretinal degeneration (i.e., lattice degeneration), and major retinal blood vessels. The vitreoretinal traction caused by a PVD may cause tearing of the retina along any of these regions.

Most PVDs are spontaneous. Their prevalence increases with age (affecting 63% of persons older than 70 years of age) and after cataract surgery. A PVD may also occur after blunt or penetrating eye trauma.

Clinical Presentation and Evaluation

The symptoms of PVD and possible retinal tear include floating spots and flashing lights in the field of vision of one eye. The floaters are caused by shadows cast on the retina by vitreous opacities (e.g., condensed collagen fibers, glial tissue from the previous attachment of the posterior vitreous to the optic nerve [**Vogt's ring**], hemorrhage). Flashing lights are caused by physical stimulation of the retina by vitreous traction. Any patient who has new onset of flashing lights and floaters should undergo immediate fully dilated funduscopic examination to look for evidence of retinal tears or detachment. Of all patients who have new onset of PVD, approximately 10% have a retinal tear. Vitreous hemorrhage is an ominous sign. As many as 70% of patients with vitreous hemorrhage have a retinal tear, but fewer than 4% of patients without vitreous hemorrhage have a tear.

Treatment

Retinal Break Repair

The goal in prophylactic treatment of a retinal break is to prevent retinal detachment by creating a firm chorioreti-

nal scar that prevents liquid vitreous from leaking through the break into the subretinal space. The two most common methods used to achieve this scarring are cryotherapy and laser photocoagulation. Both methods are effective. The method used is dictated by the location of the tear, the presence of any subretinal fluid, and the preference of the surgeon. With both methods, the goal is to surround the break with confluent treatment to prevent subretinal fluid accumulation and retinal detachment. Cryotherapy is normally performed transconjunctivally. The freeze is allowed to penetrate the sclera, choroid, and retina. Visualization is performed with an indirect ophthalmoscope. The ice ball is allowed to thaw, the cryoprobe is moved slightly, and the process is repeated until the break is completely surrounded (Fig. 9-28). Laser photocoagulation is normally performed in conjunction with a fundus contact lens and either a slitlamp or an indirect ophthalmoscopic delivery system. Multiple 300- to 500-mm spots are placed until there are two or three rows of confluent surrounding treatment (Fig. 9-29). All patients are reexamined within 1 week to assess the adequacy of treatment. (Laser photocoagulation is discussed in greater detail later.)

Retinal Detachment Repair

Retinal detachments are usually the result of a retinal break. That is, they are **rhegmatogenous** (from the Greek *rhegma*, to break). They may also be tractional (e.g., severe

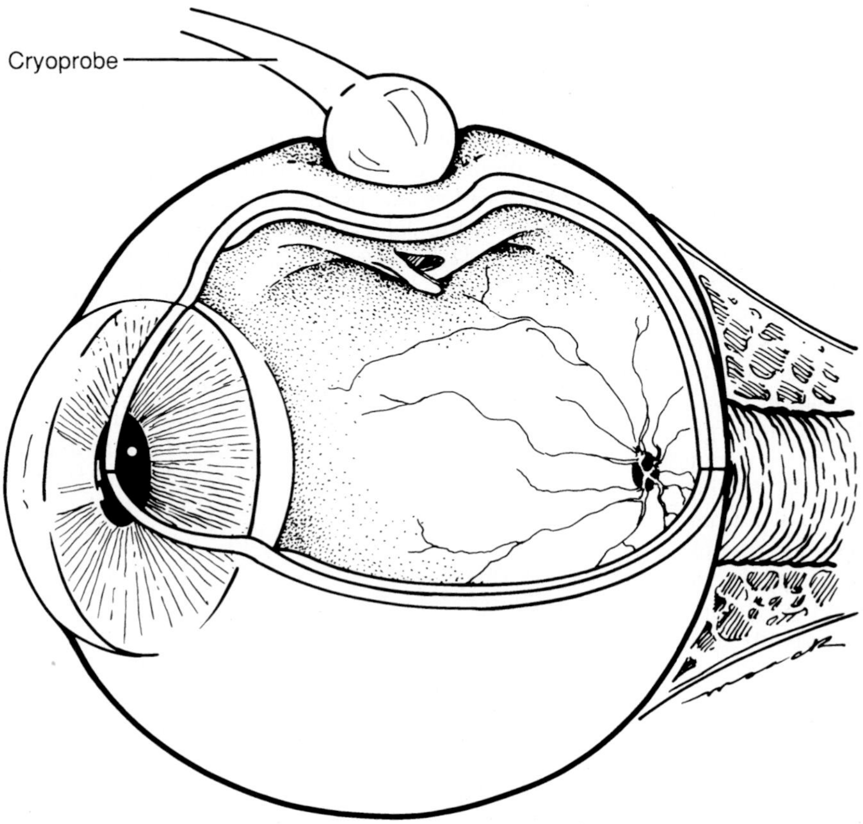

Figure 9-28 Cryotherapy treatment. Cryotherapy seals the retina

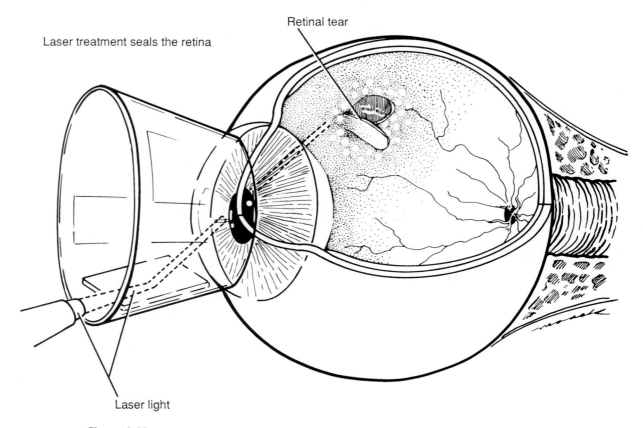

Laser treatment seals the retina

Retinal tear

Laser light

Figure 9-29   Laser treatment.

proliferative diabetic retinopathy) or exudative (e.g., some intraocular tumors, severe uveitis). This section discusses the surgical management of rhegmatogenous retinal detachments.

When subretinal fluid accumulates from an open retinal break, retinal detachment occurs (Fig. 9-30). Patients often have the same symptoms as in PVD (i.e., floaters, flashing lights), but may also have a "dark curtain" that obscures all or part of their vision. On examination, the detached retina usually has a corrugated appearance and often undulates with eye movement. To manage retinal detachment, a thorough preoperative examination to locate all retinal breaks is imperative. Regardless of the surgical technique used, the principles of retinal detachment surgery are to locate and close all retinal breaks. When these principles are followed, 90% to 95% of all retinal detachments can be anatomically reattached. The major reasons for failure are inability to locate and close all retinal breaks (early failure) and the development of proliferative vitreoretinopathy. Proliferative vitreoretinopathy is a fibrocellular response that causes membrane formation and contracture, and the reopening of retinal breaks or tractional retinal detachment.

The success of restoring good vision in retinal detachment repair depends on whether and for how long the macula is detached before surgery. If the retina is reat-

tached before macular detachment occurs, then the probability of retaining good central vision is excellent. If the macula is detached for longer than 1 week, only half of affected patients regain better than 20/70 vision.

The most widely accepted technique for retinal detachment repair is the **scleral buckle** procedure. Surgery is usually performed under a general anesthetic, but may also be performed with local retrobulbar anesthesia. Retinal breaks are located and treated with cryotherapy, as previously described. The breaks are closed by suturing either solid silicone or a silicone sponge to the sclera overlying the retinal breaks (Fig. 9-31). A buckling effect is created both to reoppose the break against the retinal pigment epithelium and to negate persistent vitreous traction. After the breaks are closed, the subretinal fluid is reabsorbed spontaneously, usually within 24 hours. Occasionally, the retinal breaks cannot be closed with the buckle alone. In these cases, the subretinal fluid is drained into the subretinal space with a small sclerotomy and micropuncture. This maneuver allows the retina to settle against the buckle and the breaks to close. The conjunctiva is carefully closed over the sclera and buckling elements. The procedure is done on an outpatient basis, but the patient is kept at minimal physical activity for at least 1 week.

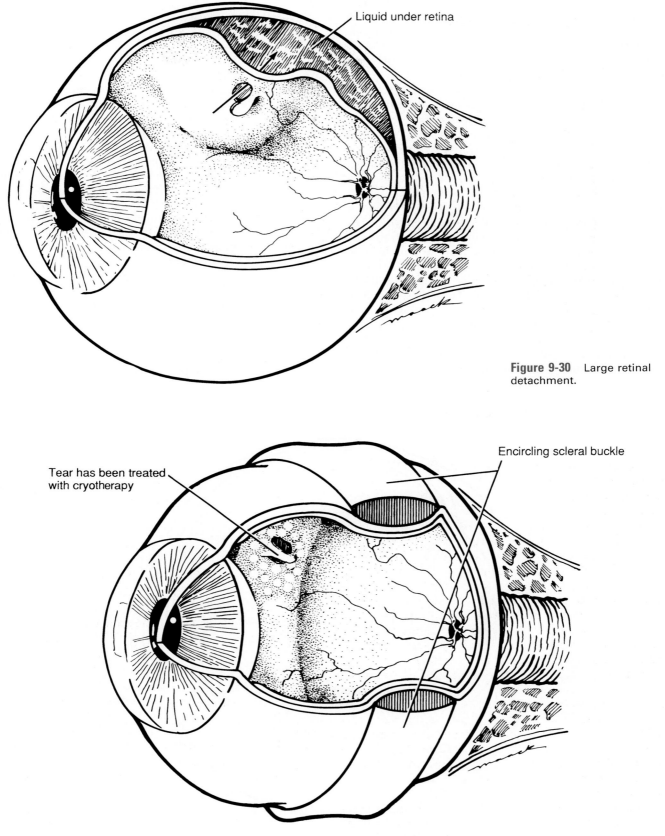

Liquid under retina

Figure 9-30   Large retinal detachment.

Tear has been treated with cryotherapy

Encircling scleral buckle

Figure 9-31   Scleral buckling surgery for retinal detachment.

Complications from scleral buckling surgery include subretinal or vitreous hemorrhage, intraocular infection, **strabismus** with associated double vision, glaucoma, cataract formation, and recurrent retinal detachment. The silicone buckling elements are left permanently in place unless signs of infection or extrusion occur.

Alternative techniques for retinal detachment repair include temporary scleral buckle and pneumatic retinopexy. With a temporary scleral buckle, an inflatable balloon is placed subconjunctivally over the retinal break. The break is then treated as previously described, with either laser photocoagulation or retinal cryopexy. The balloon is deflated and removed after an adequate chorioretinal scar forms (usually 1 week). This technique is particularly useful in small anteriorly located tears with little vitreous traction. In pneumatic retinopexy, sterile filtered air or expansile gas (C_3F_8, SF_6) is injected into the vitreous through the pars plana. The patient is positioned so that the bubble either creates an internal tamponade of the open break or breaks, allowing spontaneous resorption of the subretinal fluid. The breaks are treated with either cryotherapy or laser photocoagulation. The overall success rate with pneumatic retinopexy is somewhat less than that with scleral buckling surgery. However, because pneumatic retinopexy can be performed on an outpatient basis, thus avoiding the need for hospitalization and general anesthesia, it is an increasingly popular technique. The major complications are recurrent retinal detachment, cataract, glaucoma, and intraocular infection.

Vitreous Surgery

Most retinal breaks and resultant retinal detachments are the result of PVD. Most severe retinal problems that require surgery are directly related to the vitreous. This section discusses the principles behind vitreous surgery, the indications for it, and some of the specialized techniques used.

Vitreous surgery is performed in the hospital with an operating microscope. The patient is usually under general anesthesia. A multiport system is used. The entry sclerotomies to the vitreous cavity are performed through the pars plana (3–4 mm posterior to the corneal limbus). One port provides a constant infusion of a balanced salt solution to maintain normal intraocular pressure. The other two ports are "working" ports through which various instruments are passed: fiberoptic light, vitreous cutter, intraocular forceps, microscissors, or endolaser photocoagulation probes (Fig. 9-32).

The goals in vitreous surgery depend on specific indications, but include:

1 Removing opaque vitreous (e.g., vitreous hemorrhage)
2 Releasing vitreoretinal traction

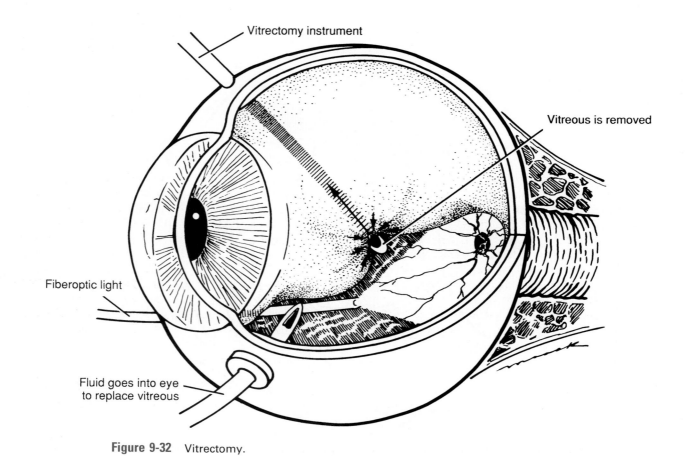

Figure 9-32   Vitrectomy.

3 Releasing or removing epiretinal membranes

4 Closing retinal breaks

5 Treating ischemic retina (i.e., endolaser photocoagulation)

6 Obtaining material for culture or cytologic examination

Indications for vitreous surgery include complex retinal detachments, proliferative diabetic retinopathy, trauma, and intraocular foreign bodies.

Some retinal detachments cannot be repaired by scleral buckling techniques alone. These include eyes with advanced proliferative vitreoretinopathy, retinal detachments with opaque media (e.g., vitreous hemorrhage), and eyes with large, complicated, retinal tears. Vitreous surgery in these eyes allows for improved visualization, release or removal of tractional membranes, and replacement of the vitreous with long-acting gas for prolonged internal tamponade. Even with these advanced techniques, however, the prognosis is poor.

Vitreous surgery in proliferative diabetic retinopathy produces visual improvement in approximately 75% of eyes with vitreous hemorrhage alone and approximately 60% of eyes with retinal detachments involving the macula. Patients with diabetes mellitus who have proliferative retinopathy are at risk for vitreous hemorrhage. In the absence of associated retinal detachment, it is usually recommended that vitreous surgery be deferred for several months to allow for possible spontaneous clearing. However, approximately 25% of vitreous hemorrhages do not clear, and vitrectomy is indicated for visual rehabilitation. Of surgically treated patients, 75% have visual improvement. In other diabetic patients, continued fibrovascular proliferation and contracture may cause either tractional or combined tractional and rhegmatogenous retinal detachment requiring vitreous surgery. Of patients with retinal detachments involving the macula who are treated with surgery, 60% have visual improvement.

The initial approach to any eye that is suspected of having a rupture, penetration, laceration, or retained intraocular foreign body (IOFB) is to protect the integrity of the globe by covering it with a protective shield and obtaining an immediate ophthalmologic consultation. Any significant trauma to the eye can lead to severe retinal problems that may necessitate vitreous surgery. In managing an eye with suspected trauma, the goal is to restore the integrity of the eye by achieving a watertight closure. Further surgery depends on specific indications, such as intraocular infection (endophthalmitis), a ruptured lens with an admixture of lens and vitreous, prolapse of vitreous through the wound, retinal detachment, and the type of IOFB that is present. A retained IOFB is suspected in an eye that has a projectile injury (e.g., from an explosion, from hammering metal on metal). The eye is examined carefully and evaluated radiologically. Most retained IOFBs should be removed as soon as possible after they are properly localized, especially those that are toxic to the eye (e.g., copper, iron). On rare occasions, small, inert IOFBs are left in the eye if they are not a threat to vision.

Penetrating eye injuries often have late complications related to intraocular cellular proliferation, membrane formation, and possible retinal detachment. Vitrectomy is indicated to remove the scaffolding on which these membranes proliferate. The timing of vitreous surgery after penetrating eye trauma is controversial. Some vitreoretinal surgeons advocate early intervention (within 1–3 days of injury). Others prefer to defer surgery for 7 to 10 days. The advantages of deferring surgery include decreasing the chances of significant intraoperative hemorrhage and allowing the vitreous to detach from the retina spontaneously to facilitate complete vitreous removal.

Blunt injuries to the globe can also cause scleral rupture. Signs of potential rupture include conjunctival **chemosis** (edema and swelling under the conjunctiva) and hemorrhage, a deep anterior chamber, low intraocular pressure, and severe vitreous hemorrhage. These signs indicate the need for immediate exploration and repair under general anesthesia.

Vitreous surgery is performed to manage endophthalmitis, to remove epiretinal membranes (macular pucker), to aid in the diagnosis of intraocular malignancies (large cell lymphoma), and to remove other causes of vitreous opacities (e.g., amyloidosis, inflammatory debris from chronic uveitis). Potential complications include retinal tears and detachment, hemorrhage, cataract (from touching the lens during surgery; all of the fluid used may stimulate growth), and glaucoma (from inflammation, hemorrhage, or gas bubbles). In patients with diabetes, the eyes are particularly susceptible to the development of iris neovascularization (rubeosis iridis), especially when vitreous surgery is combined with lens removal. Iris neovascularization may lead to neovascular glaucoma and possible loss of the eye.

Laser Photocoagulation Surgery

Laser photocoagulation treatment has become widely used over the past 20 years for a variety of ocular diseases. Most of these procedures are performed in an outpatient setting under topical or occasionally local retrobulbar anesthesia. The specific wavelength or type of laser used depends on the surgeon's preference, the specific entity being treated, and availability. In ophthalmology, argon blue-green, argon green, krypton red, and YAG are the most commonly used lasers. Most treatments are performed with a fundus contact lens with the patient seated comfortably at a slitlamp delivery system. (For further detail on the physical properties of the laser and the pathophysiologic effects of laser photocoagulation treatment, see Suggested Readings.)

Laser photocoagulation is used to treat retinal breaks, treat retinal ischemia, ablate choroidal or retinal neovascularization, create a chorioretinal adhesion or scar, and stimulate resorption of retinal or subretinal fluid. In the anterior segment of the eye, laser photocoagulation surgery is used to treat glaucoma and posterior lens capsule opacification after cataract surgery. In the posterior segment of the eye, the most common disease for which laser photocoagulation is used is proliferative diabetic retinopathy, the leading cause of blindness in the developed world. Untreated, many eyes progress to vitreous hemorrhage and fibrovascular proliferation with retinal detachment. Studies of diabetic retinopathy show that the risk of severe visual loss can be reduced with photocoagulation treatment. The mechanism by which this treatment causes regression of proliferative diabetic retinopathy is unknown. One theory is that treating or ablating the ischemic retina causes a decrease in the production of a "vasoproliferative factor," with subsequent regression of neovascularization. A similar response occurs when laser photocoagulation is used in other ophthalmic diseases that produce retinal ischemia and neovascularization (e.g., branch and central retinal vein occlusion, sickle cell retinopathy).

Laser photocoagulation is also used to treat macular edema in patients with diabetic retinopathy. Macular edema is the most common cause of visual loss in patients with diabetes. Leakage from macular capillaries or microaneurysms may result in either focal or diffuse areas of retinal thickening and edema. Lipid exudation may also be present. Studies show that treating the areas of macular edema that have either a focal or a grid pattern reduces or eliminates the edema in most cases. This treatment stabilizes and often improves central vision. This form of treatment is also beneficial for other retinal vascular disorders that cause macular edema (e.g., branch retinal vein occlusion).

Laser photocoagulation is also used to destroy the choroidal neovascularization that develops in a number of ocular disorders, including age-related macular degeneration, presumed ocular histoplasmosis syndrome, or any condition that disrupts the integrity of **Bruch's membrane.** This membrane separates the retina from the underlying choroid. Macular choroidal neovascularization may cause hemorrhaging in the subretinal, retinal, or vitreous spaces. A fibrous disciform scar may form and may cause permanent loss of central vision. The goal of laser photocoagulation treatment is to destroy the choroidal neovascularization before it involves the central macula (fovea). Because the laser treatment scar produces a permanent scotoma, choroidal neovascularization of the fovea is not usually treated.

The side effects and potential complications of laser photocoagulation are frequent, but rarely severe. They include loss of peripheral vision; decrease in night vision and dark adaptation; transient (and sometimes permanent) loss of central visual acuity; retinal holes; subretinal, retinal, or vitreous hemorrhage; recurrence of choroidal neovascularization; and accidental treatment of the fovea. Despite the potential hazards, however, laser photocoagulation is a valuable tool in the treatment of many eye diseases. It has clearly lowered the risk of severe visual loss in both diabetic retinopathy and age-related macular de-

generation, the two most common causes of blindness in the United States.

DISEASES OF THE NASOLACRIMAL SYSTEM, EYELIDS, AND ORBIT

Oculoplastic surgery is the interface between the specialties of ophthalmology and plastic surgery. The oculoplastic surgeon is concerned with conditions of the periocular bones and soft tissues that directly affect the health and functioning of the eyes. These include the nasolacrimal system, eyelids, and orbit. The oculoplastic surgeon is also concerned with removing the eye if necessary.

Anatomy and Physiology

The nasolacrimal system is the conduit for drainage of tears from the conjunctival sac to the inferior meatus of the nose (Fig. 9-33). The system has paired upper and lower eyelid puncta and canaliculi that run just below the mucocutaneous junction of the eyelids, beginning approximately 5 mm temporal to the angle of the medial **canthus.** The system converges into a short common canalicular segment that empties into the nasolacrimal sac. At this point, the flow of tears progresses down the nasolacrimal sac into the nasolacrimal duct, which opens into the inferior meatus. Located along this route are a series of valves that help to maintain unidirectional flow. Additionally, with each blink, the medial canthal region attachments of the orbicularis muscle create negative pressure within the lumen of the nasolacrimal sac. This pumping action actively draws tears into the system and thus ensures rapid turnover of the tear film.

Pathophysiology

A block at any point in the nasolacrimal system causes tearing or the symptomatic complaint of tearing. Of more

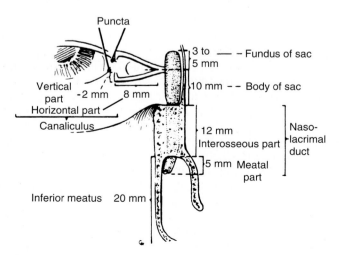

Figure 9-33   Lacrimal excretory system.

concern, blockage leads to the creation of a blind pouch in which infection and even abscess formation is common. The forms of blockage are variable, but in general, are considered either congenital or acquired.

In approximately 40% of normal infants, the opening of the nasolacrimal duct into the inferior meatus is occluded by a vestigial membrane at the time of birth. By 3 months of age, this membrane is patent in approximately 95% of infants.

Acquired lacrimal system obstructions, most commonly seen in adults, usually occur at the level of the nasolacrimal duct. Obstruction can result from trauma, infection, or tumor, but it is usually caused by idiopathic fibrosis from chronic inflammation. The second most common site of obstruction is at the level of the canalicular system. Trauma, topical eye medications, viral infections, and tumors cause most obstructions at this level.

Treatment

Congenital Obstruction

In the 5% of infants who do not have a patent vestigial nasolacrimal membrane, conservative measures (e.g., massaging the area overlying the nasolacrimal sac) are useful in attempting to open the nasolacrimal duct. If after 6 months of age the child still has epiphora, the nasolacrimal system is probed and the membrane physically opened. With the child placed under either mask or general anesthesia, a small metallic Bowman probe is introduced through either the upper or lower lid puncta. Once inside, the probe is gently passed through the canalicular system into the lumen of the nasolacrimal sac. After it contacts the medial wall of the nasolacrimal sac, the probe is rotated inferiorly 90 degrees and passed into the nasolacrimal duct, where it is gently advanced and the membrane ruptured. For most infants, this procedure is all that is required. If epiphora or infection recurs, however, the procedure may be repeated with a soft silicone stent to intubate the full length of the system. The stent is secured within the nose for approximately 6 weeks. After the stent is removed, the nasolacrimal duct remains patent in most children.

Acquired Obstruction

The management of acquired obstructions is almost entirely surgical. The adult drainage system is much more rigid than the child's and does not respond to probing or dilating maneuvers. These manipulations often lead to more scarring and stenosis. The two most common procedures involve the creation of an osteotomy through the lacrimal and maxillary bones. Through this site, vertical incisions are made in both the nasolacrimal sac and the nasal mucosa. These mucosal surfaces are united to create a mucosa-lined tract through which tears are conducted. If the nasolacrimal duct was the original site of obstruction, then this new tract bypasses the blockade. This procedure (dacryocystorhinostomy) is completed with the passage of a soft silicone stent through the intact canalicular system.

The stent is then brought out through the newly created mucosa-lined osteotomy site. The stent is secured inside the ala of the nose to ensure patency of the newly created tract during postoperative healing. The stent is removed after 3 to 6 months.

With a canalicular obstruction, a nasal osteotomy is created. Then the entire canalicular system is bypassed by inserting a Jones tube (a hollow glass tube 6–25 mm in length and 3–4 mm in diameter) through an incision in the caruncle and the underlying soft tissues into the osteotomy site. The conjunctival portion of the tube is fluted to facilitate the entry of tears into the lumen and to help position it properly deep within the medial canthus. The Jones tube remains in place and is removed only for yearly cleaning.

Eyelids

Anatomy and Physiology

Protection of the cornea and anterior segment of the eye depends on the correct position and functioning of the eyelids. Malposition of the eyelids can lead to many problems with the ocular surface, all of which can quickly lead to decreased vision or blindness. The importance of proper lid function cannot be overemphasized.

Clinical Presentation and Evaluation

Malposition of the eyelids can be attributed to **lagophthalmos, ptosis,** ectropion or **entropion,** and tumors. In the hospitalized patient, the most common eyelid malposition is lagophthalmos, an inability to close the eyelids completely that results in corneal exposure. Lagophthalmos is caused by eyelid retraction, proptosis, and seventh nerve palsies. It is usually seen in an intensive care setting, where the patient is typically comatose or obtunded. The resultant decrease in orbicularis tone allows the eyelids to open partially and the cornea to be exposed.

Another eyelid malposition is ptosis, a condition in which the upper eyelid margin droops, resulting in narrowing of the palpebral fissure. Ptosis may be congenital or acquired and may be either unilateral or bilateral. Congenital ptosis is usually the result of a poorly developed or nonfunctional levator muscle. Acquired ptosis is usually caused by disinsertion of the levator aponeurosis from its attachment to the rigid tarsus, the major supporting structure of the lid (Fig. 9-34). Acquired ptosis occurs most often with aging, but can occur after intraocular surgery, trauma, or protracted inflammatory conditions. Several other conditions can lead to acquired ptosis and must be considered when evaluating a patient. These include myasthenia gravis, myotonic dystrophy, and third nerve palsies. The fact that each of these conditions may be life threatening underscores the importance of recognizing ptosis during a general physical examination.

Ectropion and entropion are a turning outward or inward, respectively, of the eyelid margin. These conditions

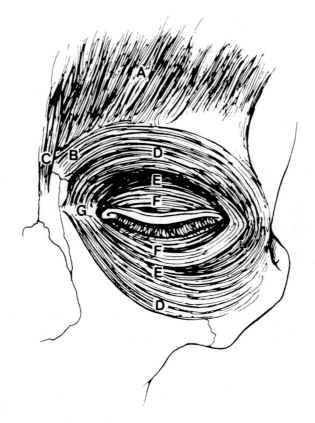

Figure 9-34 Musculature of the brow and eyelids. **A,** Frontalis muscle. **B,** Corrugator superciliaris muscle. **C,** Procerus muscle. **D,** Orbital orbicularis muscle. **E,** Preseptal orbicularis muscle. **F,** Pretarsal orbicularis muscle. **G,** Medial canthal tendon.

are related to an imbalance of forces between the outer surface (skin and orbicularis muscle) and the inner surface (eyelid retractors and conjunctival surface) of the eyelid. Age-related involutional changes and cicatrizing inflammatory conditions are the most common causes of these conditions, which can cause serious corneal exposure or marked corneal irritation from inward-turning eyelashes.

Eyelid tumors may cause almost any form of eyelid malposition. The most common tumors of the eyelids derive from skin. In order of relative frequency, they are basal cell carcinomas, squamous cell carcinomas, sebaceous gland carcinomas, and malignant melanomas. Basal cell carcinoma can only spread locally, but the other three can metastasize.

Treatment

The mainstay of therapy for lagophthalmos is topical ointment applied to the ocular surface at intervals varying from once a day to as often as every hour. If this treatment is insufficient, tarsorrhaphy, the surgical creation of permanent or temporary adhesions between the upper and lower eyelids, may be necessary. The entire lid margin, or only a portion of it, may be apposed. If full neurologic recovery

occurs, the entire tarsorrhaphy may be taken down. On the other hand, if a residual neurologic deficit (e.g., Bell's palsy) is present, a partial tarsorrhaphy may be left permanently to ensure adequate protection of the cornea.

Surgical correction of ptosis depends largely on the amount of levator muscle function that is present. In most cases, the preferred approach is to make a skin incision along the lid crease of the eyelid through which the levator aponeurosis is isolated. The aponeurosis is first resected an appropriate amount to correct the ptosis and then reattached to the tarsus. If levator function is very poor, the upper eyelid is connected to the overlying frontalis muscle by a sling made of alloplastic material or fascia lata harvested from the thigh.

Malpositions of ectropion and entropion are corrected surgically by tightening the lax structures and lysing adhesions. Skin grafts or mucous membrane spacer grafts are often required.

Surgical management of eyelid tumors requires resection of the tumor under frozen-section monitoring to ensure complete excision. The major portion of the eyelid often must be removed, followed by immediate eyelid reconstruction to ensure the safety of the eye. This process is complex and requires the combined use of myocutaneous tissue flaps, composite tissue grafts, and other plastic surgical techniques.

Orbital Disease

Because the orbit is one of the most complex areas of the body, pathologic processes involving the orbit are numerous and varied.

Clinical Presentation and Evaluation

The most common physical findings caused by orbital disease are proptosis and weakness of a particular cranial nerve or extraocular muscle. The symptoms of proptosis are related to exposure: tearing, corneal irritation, and pain. **Diplopia** is common because one eye usually protrudes. As in many areas of oculoplastics, the causes of orbital disease are differentiated between those found in children and those found in adults.

Children

The most common cause of proptosis in children is periocular infection, usually preseptal cellulitis or orbital cellulitis. It is important to differentiate between these two conditions because true orbital cellulitis is a medical emergency. Preseptal cellulitis is distinguished by eyelid swelling and erythema in the presence of a white, quiet eye with normal vision and ocular motility. The inflammatory process is limited to the periocular soft tissues and does not penetrate posterior to the orbital septum. It is usually caused by bacterial infection of an insect bite or a traumatic laceration.

In addition to periocular swelling and erythema, orbital cellulitis is associated with an inflamed ocular surface and decreased vision, extraocular motility disturbance, or both

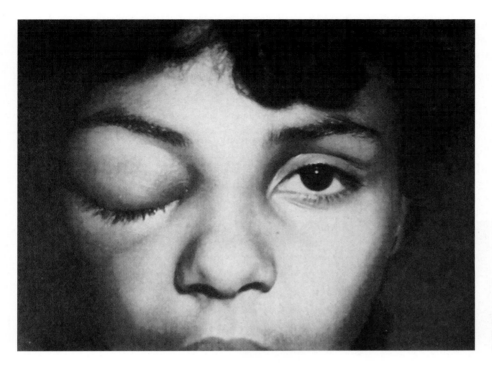

Figure 9-35 Clinical appearance of a patient with orbital cellulitis and subperiorbital abscess.

(Fig. 9-35). The infection is located posterior to the orbital septum and can spread to involve the eye, cranial nerves, and orbital vessels. The infection can also penetrate to the middle cranial fossa through the superior orbital fissure and can cause meningitis and brain abscess. Usually, the process is an extension of paranasal sinusitis that extends through the thin lamina papyracea of the medial wall of the orbit.

Other causes of proptosis in children include orbital pseudotumor, hemangioma, lymphangioma, dermoid cyst, neurofibroma, and various tumors, including optic nerve glioma, neuroblastoma, and rhabdomyosarcoma. The rapid development of unilateral proptosis in a child in the absence of inflammatory signs indicates rhabdomyosarcoma until proven otherwise. An emergency biopsy is needed to prove or disprove the diagnosis because the

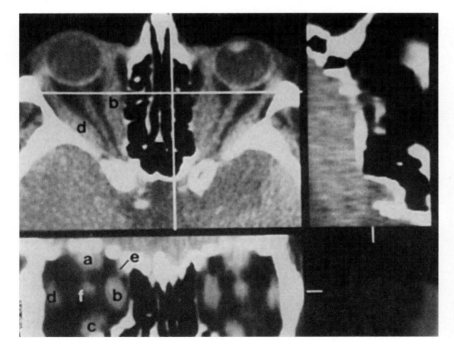

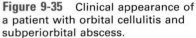

Figure 9-36 Orbital examination by computed tomography of a patient with thyroid ophthalmopathy. Greatly enlarged extraocular muscles and posterior compression of the optic nerve are shown. The direct scan was made in the axial plane at a mid-orbital level. Computer reconstructed coronal (*below*) and sagittal (*right*) sections provide multiplanar views of orbital structures. **a,** superior rectus muscle. **b,** medial rectus muscle. **c,** inferior rectus muscle. **d,** lateral rectus muscle. **e,** superior oblique muscle. **f,** optic nerve.

tumor can double in size in 24 hours. When limited to the orbit, up to 90% of cases of rhabdomyosarcoma are curable with a combination of chemotherapy and radiation therapy.

Adults

The most common cause of unilateral or bilateral proptosis in adults is Graves' ophthalmopathy (Fig. 9-36), followed by orbital pseudotumor, cavernous hemangioma, lymphangioma, and lymphoma (Fig. 9-37). Metastatic carcinoma, sphenoid meningioma, and lacrimal gland tumors are much less common.

Although neuroimaging studies (e.g., computed tomography, magnetic resonance imaging) aid immensely in the evaluation of orbital disease, in many cases, a correct diagnosis can be reached only with tissue biopsy.

Treatment

Children

Proper management of orbital cellulitis requires hospitalization for intravenous antibiotics. If vision is compromised, immediate surgical decompression and evacuation of the abscess should be performed.

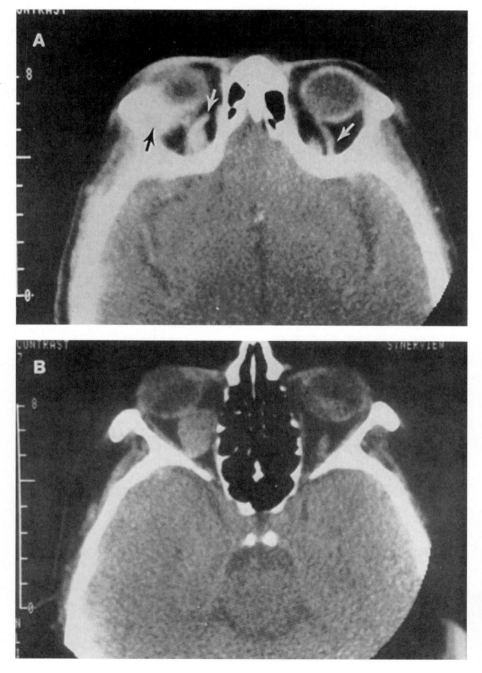

Figure 9-37   **A,** Computed axial tomography scan of a patient with lymphoma in the superolateral portion of the right orbit (*black arrow*). The superior ophthalmic veins are seen crossing the orbit from lateral to medial on both sides (*white arrows*). **B,** CT scan of a patient with a well-circumscribed cavernous hemangioma within the muscle cone of the right orbit.

Adults

The surgical approach to the orbit is based on whether the lesion is intraconal or extraconal (inside or outside the space bounded by the extraocular muscle cone). Intraconal lesions are usually approached with either a transcranial superior orbitotomy (which involves removal of the roof of the orbit) or a lateral orbitotomy, which requires removal of a portion of the zygomatic bone and the greater wing of the sphenoid. Both approaches provide excellent visualization of the intraconal structures, but the lateral approach is preferred because it avoids the morbidity associated with a craniotomy. The orbital apex is the only location within the orbit that requires a superior approach. A third approach for lesions located on the medial side of the optic nerve involves disinsertion of the medial rectus muscle followed by retraction of the globe laterally to visualize the intraconal space. This technique provides limited exposure and visualization.

Many techniques are used to approach lesions located outside the muscle cone. These lesions can usually be reached through well-camouflaged incisions placed within the lid crease or directly through the conjunctiva.

Removal of an Eye

The following are indications for removal of an eye:

1 A blind eye that is causing intractable pain and is unresponsive to conservative treatment
2 An irreparably traumatized eye that may incite sympathetic ophthalmia, an autoimmune condition that can cause blindness in the remaining eye
3 An untreatable intraocular malignancy
4 A blind eye that is cosmetically disfiguring and is not satisfactorily corrected with a cosmetic scleral prosthesis
5 Removal of a blind eye for diagnostic purposes if vision in the remaining eye is threatened

The two procedures used to remove an eye are enucleation and evisceration. Each has its own indications and limitations with which the oculoplastic surgeon must become familiar. For further information about the merits of each procedure, see Suggested Readings.

Enucleation involves removal of the entire eye. The rectus muscles are transected at their insertions, and the optic nerve is severed. The space previously occupied by the globe is taken up by an alloplastic implant (e.g., sphere). The extraocular muscles are attached to the implant. Consequently, its motility parallels the natural movement of the contralateral eye. The procedure is completed by closing the conjunctiva and related periocular soft tissues over the face of the implant.

Evisceration of an eye involves removing the entire contents of the eye through an incision in the scleral coat, leaving the extraocular muscles and the optic nerve attached to the sclera. An alloplastic implant is inserted into the scleral shell, and the wound is closed. The cornea is often excised as well because it has little inherent strength and may rupture and cause extrusion of the implant.

Six to eight weeks after enucleation or evisceration, the patient is fitted with an ocular prosthesis that is hand-painted to resemble the remaining normal eye.

DISEASES OF THE EXTRAOCULAR MUSCLES

Anatomy and Physiology

Structure and function are closely related in extraocular muscle activity. The four recti muscles insert on the globe either horizontally or vertically. Their primary action is as adductors or abductors (medial and lateral recti, respectively) or as elevators and depressors (superior and inferior recti, respectively) (Fig. 9-38). The orbit is pear-shaped, with its stem oriented posteriorly and medially. Therefore, the superior and inferior recti insert onto the globe at a slightly outward angle, affording these recti a secondary function of adduction. The inferior and superior oblique muscles insert obliquely on the globe. Their primary action is to extort and intort the eye, respectively (Figs. 9-39 and 9-40).

Because the superior division of the ocular motor nerve innervates the levator and superior rectus muscles, lid elevation is intimately associated with upgaze. The inferior division innervates the medial rectus, inferior rectus, and inferior oblique muscles. It also carries the parasympathetic fibers that are responsible for pupillary constriction.

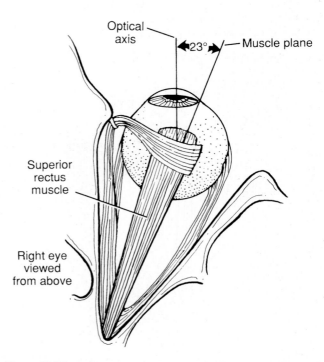

Figure 9-38   Muscle attachments and action.

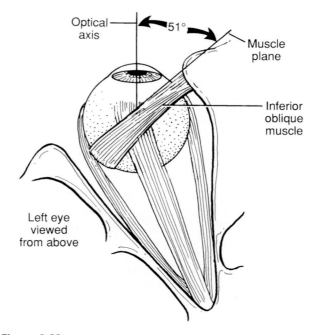

Figure 9-39   Muscle attachment and orbit orientation.

The trochlear nerve enervates the superior oblique muscle, and the abducens nerve innervates the lateral rectus muscle. All of the extraocular muscles have a basal level of tone that is manifest by **esotropia** caused by an unopposed medial rectus in sixth nerve palsy.

The blood supply to the extraocular muscles also supplies most of the anterior segment of the eye. Two anterior

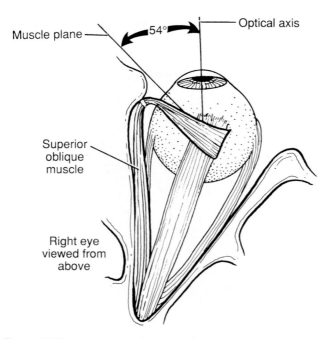

Figure 9-40   Primary action of the superior oblique muscle.

ciliary arteries course through every recti, except the lateral rectus, which has only one artery. Operating on more than two recti muscles at a time is not indicated because it could lead to anterior segment ischemia.

Pathophysiology

Strabismus, a misalignment of the eyes, is categorized as follows:

1 Esotropia, or inward turning
2 Exotropia, or outward turning
3 Hypertropia, or upward deviation
4 Hypotropia, or downward deviation

Pseudostrabismus refers to changes in the tissues surrounding the eye that simulate strabismus.

Congenital esotropia is usually apparent shortly after birth and is a leading indicator for strabismus surgery. Ideally, surgery is done at 6 months of age. Delay in correcting the condition denies the patient the prospect of using both eyes together. If the surgery is delayed past 10 months of age, there is less chance of obtaining some element of single binocular vision. Perceiving one image in the brain from the visual input of two eyes is the most rudimentary form of single binocular vision. Actual depth perception (stereopsis) is a higher order of binocular vision and is rarely attained with surgical correction of congenital esotropia. It is imperative that the general physician realize that treatment is surgical. The eyes do not have a tendency to realign spontaneously. Other situations (e.g., Duane's syndrome, congenital sixth nerve palsy) may simulate congenital esotropia, but these are beyond the scope of this discussion.

Esotropia can also be caused by excessive convergence. Because children tend to be hyperopic (light focuses behind the eye), the lens accommodates, or changes shape, to focus light on the retina (Fig. 9-41). Because **accommodation** is tied to convergence, hyperopic children must accommodate for clear distance vision. If this effort passes a critical level, it may lead to esotropia.

Exotropia, the tendency of the eye to deviate outward, increases with age. Often there is exotropia in the blind eye of elderly patients whose ability to fuse images previously kept the eyes aligned, preventing diplopia. In the case of one blind eye, obviously, there can be no diplopia; therefore, there is no incentive for spontaneous realignment (fusional convergence).

Hypertropic and hypotrophic deviations are less commonly seen as isolated entities, but often occur as part of the congenital esotropic complex.

Clinical Presentation and Evaluation

During the preoperative evaluation of the patient with strabismus, it is imperative to perform a full ophthalmologic examination, including a dilated fundus examination. Objective measurement of ametropia, which includes myopia

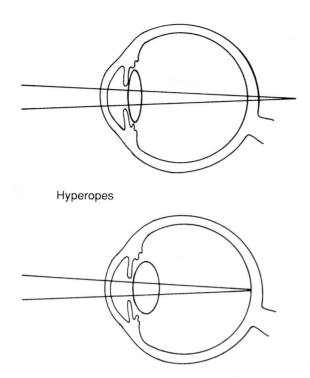

Figure 9-41   In hyperopia, the lens requires focusing, even at infinity.

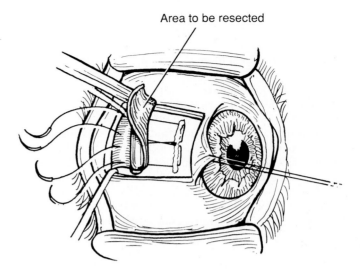

Figure 9-42   Resection of the lateral rectus muscle.

and **hyperopia,** and the degree of eye turn is indicated to rule out an accommodative component. If amblyopia is present, the better-seeing eye is occluded before surgery to force the amblyopic eye to be used. The earlier that occlusion therapy is initiated, the greater the likelihood of improved vision in the amblyopic eye.

Treatment

The goal of strabismus surgery in congenital esotropia is to attain some degree of single binocular vision. This goal requires that the eyes be aligned to within 10 prism diopters or 5 degrees of orthophoria (being straight). Of 106 patients with congenital esotropia, all of those who underwent surgical alignment by 6 months of age attained some degree of binocular vision. However, only 40% of those who underwent alignment after 24 months attained any degree of single binocular vision. Statistics on surgical treatment of exotropia vary widely. In new-onset exotropia, especially in an adult, surgical alignment is performed to treat diplopia. In long-standing exotropia, suppression may develop to alleviate the diplopia. In this case, success may be defined as adequate cosmesis.

Surgical correction of strabismus involves tightening or relaxing the extraocular muscles. In esotropia, the lateral rectus may be tightened or resected (Fig. 9-42) and the medial rectus relaxed or recessed (placed posterior to its original position; Fig. 9-43). This procedure results in more effective pulling by the lateral rectus and less effec-

tive pulling by the medial rectus, causing an outward turning of the esotropic eye.

Alternatively, both medial recti can be recessed. In some cases, the surgeon chooses this technique, understanding that it involves surgery on both eyes, whereas recession or resection surgery involves surgery on only one eye. In exotropia, surgical correction could involve resection of the medial rectus and recession of the lateral rectus in one eye, medial rectus resection in both eyes, or lateral rectus recession in both eyes. The approach depends on what is believed to be the underlying problem (e.g., a patient with poor ability to converge [convergence insuffi-

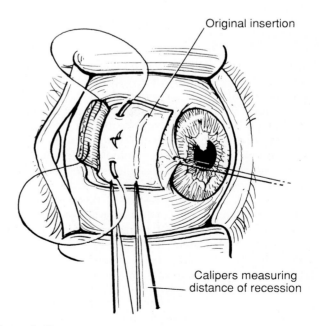

Figure 9-43   Recession of the medial rectus muscle.

ciency] might require bimedial resection). Superior and inferior rectus surgery is similar to horizontal rectus surgery, except that a small amount of muscle or tendon is resected or recessed to yield a greater effective change in alignment.

When muscle surgery is performed, the conjunctiva is opened to gain access to the extraocular muscles. A peritomy is often performed at the limbus, although some surgeons prefer to open the conjunctiva more posteriorly or directly over the muscle insertions. A 6-0 Vicryl traction suture may be used at the limbus to help pull the muscle that is being operated on into the surgeon's view. Once the muscle is visualized, it is isolated by slipping a muscle hook beneath it. Blunt dissection further isolates the muscle and frees it from intermuscular attachments.

In resection surgery, blunt dissection is more extensive than in recession surgery to expose the area of muscle to be resected. A caliper is used to measure the distance between the muscle insertion and the anticipated resection site where the muscle clamp is to be placed. Scissors are used to disinsert the muscle from the globe, leaving a small (<1 mm) stump. Two double 5-0 Vicryl sutures are placed, often with a mattress technique, to suture the remaining stump to the area of the muscle posterior to the clamp (Fig. 9-42). The excess muscle is excised and the muscle clamp removed.

In recession surgery, the muscle is isolated and hooked as in resection surgery. A 6-0 Vicryl suture is placed just posterior to the muscle insertion, and the muscle is disinserted from the globe with scissors. Because the muscle is placed more posteriorly on the globe, it is important to cut the muscle insertion flush with the globe, leaving as small a stump as possible. Calipers are used to mark the intended distance posterior to the original insertion. A partial-thickness Vicryl suture is placed in the sclera to suture the muscle in place (Fig. 9-43).

Complications

The greatest risk of complication in strabismus surgery is secondary to general anesthesia. In adults, local anesthesia is almost always preferred. In pediatric patients, general anesthesia is used. Malignant hyperthermia is a rare, but potentially fatal complication. Early signs include tachycardia or tachypnea with trismus or other muscular rigidity. Later signs include rapid increase in body temperature, metabolic acidosis, and cyanosis, followed by myocardial ischemia, hyperkalemia, and renal failure. If there is a family history of this condition, the patient should have a preoperative evaluation of serum creatine phosphokinase and pharmacologic testing of a muscle biopsy specimen.

Poor alignment is the most common complication of strabismus surgery. Excessive relaxation of the muscle in recession surgery leads to overcorrection. Insufficient relaxation leads to undercorrection. The same logic applies to muscle tightening in resection surgery. The level of alignment immediately after surgery is often transient, and

its instability may ultimately lead to a more or a less aligned permanent outcome. The use of adjustable sutures in the adult patient with strabismus has decreased the incidence of this complication. Another complication is loss of muscle arising from retraction of the muscle into the orbit after disinsertion. This problem can be avoided by always locking the muscle clamp and releasing it only after sutures are placed. Yet another complication is postoperative

Table 9-2	**Diagnosis of Common Eye Diseases**

Anatomy

All the muscles of the orbit are supplied by the oculomotor nerve *except* the lateral rectus (which is supplied by the abducent nerve) and the superior oblique (which is supplied by the trochlear nerve).

Lesions of the sympathetic nerve supply result in Horner's syndrome, which is a triad of constriction of pupil (miosis), slight ptosis (marked ptosis is caused by paralysis of the oculomotor nerve), and anhidrosis. A transient Horner's syndrome may occur in neuralgic migraine or in cluster headache. Presence of an apical lung tumor (Pancoast syndrome; lower brachial plexopathy and Horner's syndrome) should be ruled out.

The cornea is avascular and receives its nutrition from the aqueous humor.

History

Causes of painless loss of vision include:
Central retinal artery or vein occlusion
Giant cell arteritis
Ischemic optic neuropathy
Optic neuritis
Migraine (fortification spectra, scintillating scotoma)
Amaurosis fugax ("fleeting blindness" due to retinal emboli from ipsilateral carotid disease); significance: increased risk of retinal arterial occlusion or stroke; stuttering amaurosis may be precursor of permanent blindness
Neuritis and papillitis
Vitreous and retinal hemorrhages
Retinal detachment
Macular hole, cyst or hemorrhage
Macular edema
Macular degeneration
Malingering
Cataract
Acute (angle-closure) glaucoma

Examination

Common causes of absence of red reflex (on funduscopy) include:
Cataract
Vitreous hemorrhage
Retinal detachment

Sources: Berson FG, ed. *Basic Ophthalmology for Medical Students and Primary Care Residents,* 6th ed. San Francisco: American Academy of Ophthalmology; 1993.

eMedicine Clinical Knowledge Base. eMedicine.com, Inc. Available at http://www.emedicine.com/oph/contents.htm. Accessed May 1, 2006.

Lawrence PF, ed. *Essentials of General Surgery,* 4th ed. Philadelphia: Lippincott Williams & Wilkins; 2006.

University of Toronto, Faculty of Medicine, Department of Ophthalmology Webpage. Available at http://eyelearn.med.utoronto.ca/. Accessed May 1, 2006.

Table 9-3	Diseases of the Eye and Systemic Diseases with Ocular Manifestations

Diseases of the Eye and Adnexa

Pinguecula and pterygium

  Have histologically similar features (elastoid degeneration of the conjunctival substantia propria)

  Pinguecula (yellow, elevated nodule on either side of cornea; more common on the nasal side); rarely grows, no treatment is usually required

  Pterygium (triangular, plaque-like extension of fibrovascular tissue encroaching the conjunctiva onto the nasal side of cornea); if the pterygium continues growing and interferes with vision, excision is indicated

External and internal hordeolum and chalazion

  External hordeolum or stye: infection of the glands of the eyelids involving the glands of Zeis or Moll

  Internal hordeolum: infection of the Meibomian (tarsal) glands

  Chalazion: chronic granulomatous inflammation of Meibomian gland following internal hordeolum

Red eye

  Differential diagnosis of an "acute red eye" includes conjunctivitis, keratitis, uveitis (anterior, iritis; posterior uveitis can present with a "white eye"), episcleritis and scleritis, acute (angle-closure) glaucoma, and subconjunctival hemorrhage (due to trauma, coughing and straining, coagulation disorders, hypertension)

  If a "red eye" is associated with loss of vision, pain, opacities, irregular pupil, perilimbal erythema, increase in intraocular pressure, history of an eye disease, or is refractory to usual treatment, it signifies grave ocular pathology

Orbital cellulitis

  Especially in children, orbital cellulitis is an ocular emergency, because abscess formation and rapid increase in the orbital pressure may interfere with the blood supply to the eye and may compress the optic nerve. Immediate treatment with intravenous antibiotics is therefore indicated.

Cataract

  Cataract is the leading cause of curable blindness in the world, whereas age-related macular degeneration is the most common cause of blindness in the developed world. Vitamin A deficiency ("night blindness," Bitot's spots) is the most common cause of blindness in developing countries. The leading causes of "legal blindness" (partial, visual acuity of 20/200 or less), in the United States include glaucoma, diabetic retinopathy, and macular degeneration.

  Systemic diseases associated with cataract include diabetes mellitus, galactosemia, hypocalcemia, myotonic dystrophy, Down's syndrome, and atopic dermatitis. Corticosteroids and oxygen (retinopathy of prematurity) can also cause cataract.

Glaucoma

  Acute (angle-closure) glaucoma must be included in the differential diagnosis of abdominal discomfort and vomiting in elderly patients, because nausea and even abdominal pain may occur with this condition. Funduscopy should *always* be done if glaucoma is suspected.

Ocular burns

  Radiation burns

    Injuries to the corneal epithelium by ultraviolet rays (e.g., welding arc or flash burn, "snow blindness") classically manifest with symptoms 4 to 12 hours after injury

  Chemical burns

    Alkali burns of the eye are more serious because the agents tend to rapidly penetrate intraocularly and damage the tissue because of the devastating effect of saponifying lipid barriers. Acid burns, on the contrary, cause rapid damage but are usually less serious than alkali burns. The eye should be irrigated with water or saline solution (after instilling a topical anesthetic) for *at least* 20 minutes.

  Thermal burns

    Extensive edema in the eyelids and face after a thermal burn may interfere with the proper examination of the eye and may give a false impression of blindness until the swelling subsides

Ocular trauma

  An eyelid laceration can hide a perforated globe, which may, in turn, hide an intracranial injury

  In a case of laceration of the eyebrow, the eyebrow should *not* be shaved before repair because as much as 20% of the time the eyebrow may not grow back.

  All injuries involving the orbit (especially a blowout fracture of the floor of the orbit) should be assessed by *both* an ophthalmologist and an otolaryngologist because of the potential associated maxillofacial fractures

  One should *never* try to remove any foreign body in a case of penetrating or perforating ocular injury: the patient should be immediately referred to an ophthalmologist

Sympathetic ophthalmia

  Sympathetic ophthalmia is an autoimmune destruction of the normal eye following penetrating injury (causing blindness) of the other eye. In these cases, the blind eye should be removed within 2 weeks following injury to avoid this complication.

Intraocular tumors

  Malignant melanoma (of the uvea) is the most common primary intraocular tumor in adults (a blind painful eye may hide a melanoma), whereas retinoblastoma is the most frequent intraocular malignant tumor in children (with occasional spontaneous remission)

  All children with strabismus should have a funduscopy to exclude retinoblastoma

Cavernous sinus thrombosis

  Intracranial complications of acute or chronic infective sinusitis include cavernous sinus thrombosis, which is manifested by proptosis, swelling of the eyelids and conjunctiva, and ophthalmoplegia

(*continues*)

Table 9-3	*(continued)*

Systemic Diseases with Ocular Manifestations

Diabetes mellitus: retinopathy, macular edema or ischemia, vitreous hemorrhage
Hypertension: retinopathy, choroidopathy, and optic neuropathy
Sickle cell disease: vitreous and retinal hemorrhages, retinal detachment
HIV and acquired immunodeficiency syndrome (AIDS):
 Direct effect: retinal cotton wool spots and microaneurysms
 Opportunistic infections: viral (cytomegalovirus, herpes simplex, and varicella-zoster viruses); bacterial (staphylococcus, mycobacteria, syphilis); fungal
  (*Candida albicans, Cryptococcus neoformans*)
 Tumor: Kaposi's sarcoma
Thyroid disease: Grave's disease (toxic goiter)
Sarcoidosis uveitis
Rheumatoid arthritis: keratoconjunctivitis sicca, scleritis, and keratitis
Systemic lupus erythematosus: scleritis, corneal melt, retinal vasculitis, optic nerve infarction, Sjo;augren's syndrome
Giant cell arteritis: loss of vision (late)
Wegener's granulomatosis: keratoconjunctivitis sicca, scleritis, corneal melt, and orbital involvement
Multiple sclerosis: optic and retrobulbar neuritis, ocular motility disorders, visual field defects
Vascular emboli: transient visual loss, retinal artery occlusion
Systemic candidiasis: endophthalmitis, vitritis
Stevens-Johnson syndrome with associated ocular-mucous membrane syndrome: conjunctivitis, panophthalmitis, iritis

Sources: Berson FG, ed. *Basic Ophthalmology for Medical Students and Primary Care Residents,* 6th ed. San Francisco: American Academy of Ophthalmology; 1993.

eMedicine Clinical Knowledge Base. eMedicine.com, Inc. Available at http://www.emedicine.com/oph/contents.htm.

Lawrence PF, ed. *Essentials of General Surgery,* 4th ed. Philadelphia: Lippincott Williams & Wilkins; 2006.

University of Toronto, Faculty of Medicine, Department of Ophthalmology Webpage. Available at http://eyelearn.med.utoronto.ca/.

slippage of the sutured muscle, which is avoided by placing sutures deep into the muscle tendon and not into the outer muscular capsule.

To prevent changes in the size of the palpebral fissure in inferior rectus surgery, attachments are carefully dissected free. The inferior rectus is closely attached to the inferior oblique muscle and indirectly attached to the retractors of the lower lid. If the inferior rectus is recessed without separating its attachments to the eyelid retractors and orbital septum, the lid margins may be pulled inferiorly, opening the palpebral fissure and leading to fissure asymmetry.

Perforation of the globe can lead to another complication of recession surgery. If the globe is perforated as the muscle is disinserted and resutured more posteriorly to the sclera, the result is usually a benign chorioretinal scar. However, in some cases, perforation leads to endophthalmitis of the globe. Signs include pain, lid swelling, conjunctival injection, white blood cells layering in the anterior chamber (hypopyon), and fever. Endophthalmitis usually occurs within 2 to 5 days after surgery.

Finally, foreign body granulomas may appear at the incision site, as may conjunctival inclusion cysts. These and other sequelae that lead to elevated conjunctiva near the limbus may interfere with the ability of tears to reach the corneal surface, causing subsequent focal corneal dehydration and thinning (dellen). Excessive scarring or excessive muscle resection may also restrict ocular motility.

OCULAR DISORDERS

Common eye diseases and their diagnosis and description are listed in Tables 9-2 and 9-3. Adverse effects of drugs and indications of when to consult an ophthalmologist are listed in Table 9-4. Additional information on specific disorders is described below.

Red Eye

An acute red eye may be caused by a number of conditions, including conjunctivitis, corneal abrasion or ulceration, lid disorders, angle-closure glaucoma, and trauma. The most common cause is conjunctivitis. Conditions that threaten the loss of sight and therefore require immediate referral include corneal ulcer, acute iritis, angle-closure glaucoma, hyphema, and lacerated globe. Table 9-5 lists the causes of red eye, as well as diagnostic clues and recommended therapy.

Visual Field Defects

Visual field testing is an important part of the ophthalmic examination. The visual field is defined as the portion of space that is visible to the fixating eye. The defects found on visual field testing are useful in localizing the site of pathology. Confrontation visual fields are easy to perform and can yield a great amount of information. More formal forms of visual field testing include the use of a tangent

Table 9-4 — Adverse Effects of Drugs and When to Consult an Ophthalmologist

Adverse Ocular Effects of Systemic Drugs

Oxygen can cause retinopathy of prematurity

Chloramphenicol, streptomycin, ethambutol, and isoniazid can cause optic neuritis, whereas use of tetracycline may result in pseudotumor cerebri

Sulfonamides can cause Stevens-Johnson syndrome

Digitalis may cause disturbances of color vision, scotoma, and photopsia

Barbiturates can cause extraocular muscle palsies with diplopia, nystagmus, ptosis, or cortical blindness

Chlorpropamide can cause transient change in refractive error, diplopia, or Stevens-Johnson syndrome

Vitamin A can cause papilledema, retinal hemorrhage, loss of eyebrows and eyelashes, nystagmus, diplopia, and blurring of vision

Salicylates may result in nystagmus, retinal hemorrhage, and, rarely, cortical blindness

Repeated use of topical corticosteroids in the eye may result in herpes simplex (dendritic) keratitis, cataract formation, fungal infections, or open-angle glaucoma

When to Consult an Ophthalmologist

If the lacerations of the eyelid involve medial canthus, are deep or involve the tarsal plate, or are at the lid margin, the patient should be referred to an ophthalmologist. An ophthalmologist should also be consulted in cases of corneal ulcers, retinal detachment, iritis, glaucoma, retinal artery occlusion, endophthalmitis, orbital injury, and any foreign object penetration or perforation injury.

Sources: Berson FG, ed. *Basic Ophthalmology for Medical Students and Primary Care Residents,* 6th ed. San Francisco: American Academy of Ophthalmology; 1993.

eMedicine Clinical Knowledge Base. eMedicine.com, Inc. Available at http://www.emedicine.com/oph/contents.htm. Accessed May 1, 2006.

Lawrence PF, ed. *Essentials of General Surgery,* 4th ed. Philadelphia: Lippincott Williams & Wilkins; 2006.

University of Toronto, Faculty of Medicine, Department of Ophthalmology Webpage. Available at http://eyelearn.med.utoronto.ca/. Accessed May 1, 2006.

screen or computerized automated perimetry. These means are useful in following the progress of a disease and assessing the effect of treatment. Figure 9-44 shows examples of visual field defects.

Papillary Disorders

Disc edema is any swelling of the optic nerve with accumulation of abnormal fluid. Swelling that is associated with raised intracranial pressure is known as papilledema; swelling associated with inflammation is known as **papillitis.**

Papilledema is marked by loss of the central cup, indistinct disc margins, loss of spontaneous venous pulsations, and hyperemia of the disc tissue. There may also be disc hemorrhages, dilated veins, and exudates. Patients usually do not have any symptoms, although some have transient blurring of vision. Papillitis is marked by loss of vision, particularly central vision, and by an afferent pupillary defect. Visual field examinations are useful in distinguishing between the two. In papilledema, there is an enlarged

blind spot and constriction of the peripheral isopters. In papillitis, there is a central scotoma.

Ischemic optic neuropathy is a special form of disc edema that may be associated with cranial arteritis (giant cell). It causes sudden visual loss (usually an altitudinal field defect), with pale disc swelling and few hemorrhages. Systemic symptoms include weight loss, loss of appetite, pain on mastication, headache, and tenderness of the forehead over the temporal artery. Most patients also have an elevated sedimentation rate. Because these patients respond dramatically to steroids, it is important to make the correct diagnosis. Ischemic optic neuropathy can also be caused by atherosclerosis.

Hypertensive Retinopathy

Hypertension can cause vascular changes in the eye. These changes are of value both in diagnosing the hypertension and in gauging its severity. In the early stages, there may be focal narrowing of the arterioles (Fig. 9-45), beginning after the diastolic blood pressure is more than 120 mm Hg. Disc hemorrhage may occur early as well. Long-standing hypertension has a more generalized effect on the vessels. As the arterial wall thickens, the light reflex is altered. This condition may progress to give a copper wiring appearance to the eye (Fig. 9-46). Eventually, the eye may have a silver wiring appearance (Fig. 9-47) that signifies low blood flow and retinal ischemia. Arteriolar venous crossing changes also signify hypertensive changes that occur because the arteriole and the vein share a common adventitial sheath.

Retinal Vein Occlusion

Central retinal vein occlusion is a common problem, especially in the elderly. Vein occlusions are either nonischemic or ischemic. Ischemic vein occlusions have a worse visual prognosis and are often associated with neovascular glaucoma and retinal neovascularization, both of which may lead to blindness. The most common ocular cause of vein occlusion is glaucoma. The incidence of vein occlusion is also increased in patients with certain systemic diseases, including hypertension, diabetes mellitus (Fig. 9-48A,B), hyperviscosity syndromes, and collagen-vascular diseases, especially systemic lupus erythematosus.

Amaurosis Fugax

Amaurosis fugax is temporary loss of vision that is confined to one eye and lasts 5 to 10 minutes. Retinal emboli cause these transient ischemic attacks. There are three main types. A fibrin platelet embolus (Fisher plug) arises from the carotid bifurcation, from another great vessel, or from the heart, and represents platelet aggregates (Fig. 9-49). A calcific embolus arises from cardiac valves and appears as a solid plaque (Fig. 9-50). A cholesterol embolus (Hollenhorst's plaque) is formed from shed atheromatous plaques, usually from the carotid artery, and is composed of fibrin

Table 9-5	Red Eye: Causes, Diagnostic Clues, and Recommended Therapies		
Area	**Condition**	**Diagnostic Clues**	**Therapy**
Lid (vision fine)	Ectropion	Lid not against globe	Refer to surgery
	Entropion	Lashes against globe	Refer for surgery
	Chalazion	Not hot, minimal pain; slow evolution; lump in lid	Hot compresses; if no resolution, may excise
	Hordeolum externa	Acute onset, abscess on lid margin	Hot compresses followed by incision and drainage; topical antibiotics (gentamicin 0.3 mg/mL qid)
	Lid cellulitis (hordeolum interna)	Swollen, red, warm lid of acute onset; often follows a stye	Oral antibiotics (cephalexin 500 mg orally qid. or similar); follow closely; if getting worse, refer promptly
	Blepharitis	Red lid margin with scales and debris on lashes	Clean lid margins bid; intermittent topical antibiotic ointment (gentamicin or erythromycin bid); chronic condition, so refer for severe irritation or corneal complications only
	Trachoma	Tarsal plate scarring, superior corneal pannus	Tetracycline or erythromycin orally or topically; typical treatment tetracycline ointment bid $\times$ 4 wk, then first 5 days of each month $\times$ 3 mo
Conjunctiva (vision fine if discharge is removed)	Allergic conjunctivitis	Redness and swelling of conjunctiva with clear discharge; itching; chronic; seasonal	Topical astringents (naphazoline hydrochloride qid); cromolyn sodium qid in more severe cases; steroids on referral only
	Bacterial conjunctivitis	Conjunctival redness and swelling with purulent discharge; acute onset	Topical antibiotics (sulfacetamide or gentamicin qid); acute and severe, consider gonococcus; if Gram stain is suggestive, give penicillin G 100,000 units/mL 1 drop every 1 hr around the clock, with immediate ophthalmologic coverage
	Vernal conjunctivitis	Children with large bumps on upper tarsal plate; atopic children; photophobic	Cromolyn sodium qid; if unsuccessful, refer to ophthalmologist for steroid treatment
	Viral conjunctivitis	Conjunctival redness and swelling with a serous or seromucoid discharge; acute onset	Scrupulous hygiene (do not pass this around); topical antibiotics, as for bacterial conjunctivitis, if not sure; refer for any corneal complications
Cornea (vision often decreased)	Abrasion	Fluorescein stain shows epithelial defect; no corneal infiltrate; vision OK; marked pain	Antibiotic (e.g., gentamicin ointment) and tight pressure patch; monitor epithelial healing daily; refer for nonhealing or evidence of infiltrate; make sure there is no foreign body on the upper tarsal plate
	Corneal foreign body	Visible; irregularity in fluorescein staining; magnifier is used; painful	Remove foreign body with bevel of 25-gauge needle; remove all rust that is easily removable; patch and follow as for corneal abrasion
	Corneal ulcer	Epithelial defect with infiltrate; marked pain and photophobia	Emergency! Prompt referral; if any delay start gentamicin solution every 30 min around the clock
	Corneal herpes simplex	Irregular (dendritic) epithelial defect; not much pain	Acyclovir ointment 4 hr while awake; refer
	Pterygium	Advancing fleshy growth on cornea; usually nasal	Sunglasses; ocular lubricant qid; astringents (naphazoline hydrochloride qid); if advancing on cornea, refer for surgery
Iris	Iritis	Photophobia; perilimbal redness; vision may be decreased; pain variable, but usually more severe than casual examination would predict; irregular iris and deposits on back surface of cornea	Refer for appropriate workup and treatment
	Angle-closure glaucoma	Acute-onset pain, photophobia, and blurred vision; nausea common; cornea has "ground glass" appearance	Emergency! Prompt referral is critical; may start pilocarpine 2% drops every 10 min $\times$ 3 and acetazolamide 250 mg orally if delay is likely

qid, four times a day; bid, twice a day.

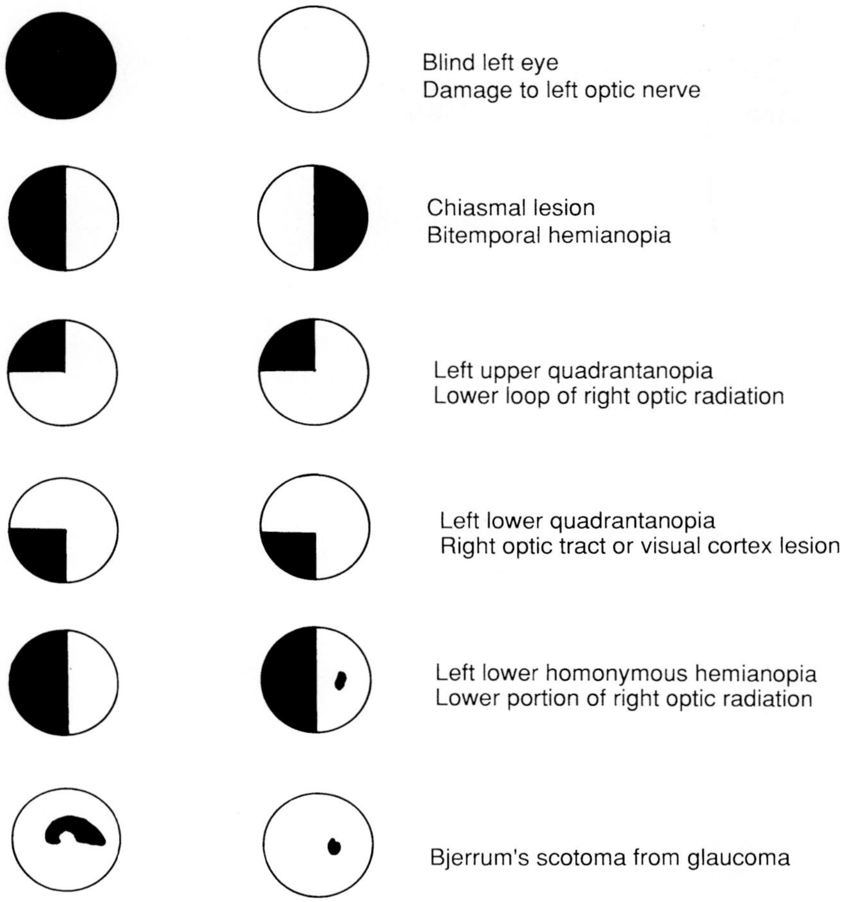

Blind left eye
Damage to left optic nerve

Chiasmal lesion
Bitemporal hemianopia

Left upper quadrantanopia
Lower loop of right optic radiation

Left lower quadrantanopia
Right optic tract or visual cortex lesion

Left lower homonymous hemianopia
Lower portion of right optic radiation

Bjerrum's scotoma from glaucoma

Figure 9-44   Example of visual field defects.

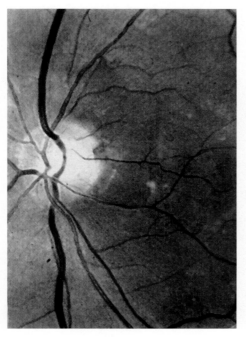

Figure 9-45   Arterial spasm in hypertension.

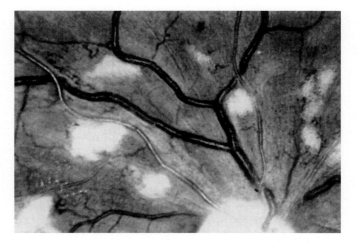

Figure 9-46   Copper wiring appearance in hypertensive retinopathy.

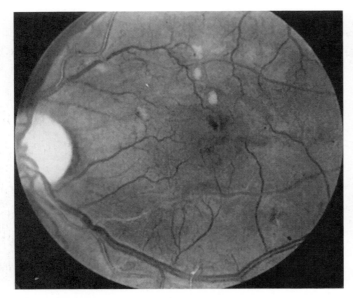

Figure 9-47 Silver wiring appearance in hypertensive retinopathy.

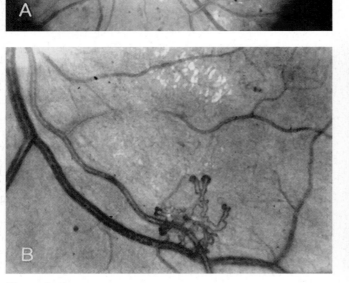

Figure 9-48 Diabetic neovascularization. **A,** Disc. **B,** Elsewhere.

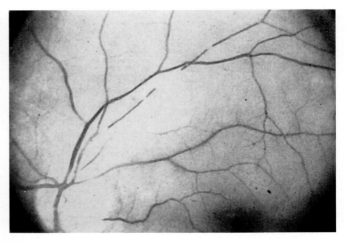

Figure 9-49 Fibrin embolus.

and cholesterol. Calcific plaques are dull, white, and chalky. Cholesterol plaques are bright orange or yellow and tend to glisten.

Third Nerve Palsy

The third nerve innervates the pupil, medial rectus, superior rectus, inferior rectus, levator of the lid, and inferior oblique. With total palsy, there is ptosis, the eye is deviated down and out, the pupil has no reaction, and accommodation is down. In an adult, third nerve palsy with pain is usually caused by compression from an aneurysm or ischemic disease (e.g., diabetes).

Sixth Nerve Palsy

Because of its long intracranial course, the sixth cranial nerve is susceptible to injury. This nerve may be damaged

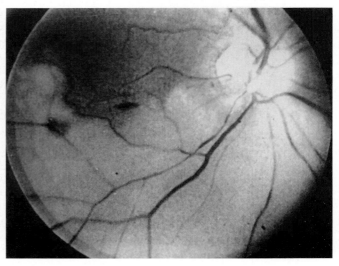

Figure 9-50 Calcific embolus.

by lesions in the orbit, cavernous sinus, or pontine region. Isolated sixth nerve palsies in adults may be caused by trauma, but usually result from vascular problems. These patients have horizontal diplopia.

Diplopia

Diplopia is double vision. A patient who has true double vision should return to single vision if either eye is occluded. "Monocular" diplopia can occur as a result of ocular causes (e.g., corneal disease, cataract formation) and should not be classified as diplopia. True diplopia requires that both eyes see (and have developed together since birth). Because different muscles and nerve pathways are involved, it is necessary to differentiate between horizontal diplopia and vertical diplopia. Each eye is examined separately and the individual muscles evaluated. For example, when the right lateral rectus muscle (innervated by the sixth cranial nerve) is evaluated, the patient is asked to move the eye to the right (laterally) in a horizontal plane. In this way, the muscle can be isolated.

SUGGESTED READINGS

Diseases of the Cornea

Kaufman HE, McDonald MB, Barron BA, Waltman SR, eds. *The Cornea*. New York: Churchill Livingstone; 1988.

Leibowitz H, ed. *Corneal Disorders: Clinical Diagnosis and Management*. Philadelphia: WB Saunders; 1984.

Smolin G, Thoft R, eds. *The Cornea: Scientific Foundations and Clinical Practice*. Boston: Little, Brown; 1987.

Diseases of the Anterior Chamber

Epstein DL. Trabeculectomy. In: Chandler PA, Grant WM, eds. *Glaucoma*, 3rd ed. Philadelphia: Lea & Febiger; 1986:204–218.

Kolker AE, Hetherington J Jr, eds. *Becker-Shaffer's Diagnoses and Therapy of the Glaucomas*, 5th ed. St. Louis: CV Mosby; 1983.

Ritch R, Shield MB, Krups T, eds. *The Glaucomas*. St. Louis: CV Mosby; 1989.

Diseases of the Lens

Clayman H. Intraocular lenses. In: Tasman W, Jaeger E, eds. *Duane's Clinical Ophthalmology*, Vol. 5. Philadelphia: JB Lippincott; 1989: 1–29.

Kelman C. Phacoemulsification and aspiration: The Kelman technique of cataract removal. In: Tasman W, Jaeger E, eds. *Duane's Clinical Ophthalmology*, Vol. 5. Philadelphia: JB Lippincott; 1989:1–13.

Weinstein G. Cataract surgery. In: Tasman W, Jaeger E, eds. *Duane's Clinical Ophthalmology*, Vol. 5. Philadelphia: JB Lippincott; 1989: 1–52.

Diseases of the Retina and Vitreous

Kini NM. Retina and vitreous. In: Pavan-Langston D, ed. *Manual of Ocular Diagnosis and Therapy*. Boston: Little, Brown; 1980: 133–155.

Kini NM. Vitreous. In: Vaughan D, Asbury T, eds. *General Ophthalmology*, 9th ed. Los Altos, Calif: Lange Medical; 1980:135–143.

Parker AJ, ed. *Manual of Retinal Surgery*. New York: Churchill Livingstone; 1989.

Diseases of the Nasolacrimal System, Eyelids, and Orbit

Smith BC, Della Rocca RC, Nesi FA, Lisman RD, eds. *Ophthalmic Plastic and Reconstructive Surgery*. St. Louis: CV Mosby; 1987.

Diseases of the Extraocular Muscles

Greenwald MJ. Amblyopia. In: Tasman W, ed. *Duane's Clinical Ophthalmology*, Vol. 1. Philadelphia: JB Lippincott; 1989.

Parks MM. Sensory tests and treatment of sensorial adaptations. In: Tasman W, ed. *Duane's Clinical Ophthalmology*, Vol. 1. Philadelphia: JB Lippincott; 1989.

Parks MM, Wheeler MB. Concomitant esodeviations. In: Tasman W, ed. *Duane's Clinical Ophthalmology*, Vol. 1. Philadelphia: JB Lippincott; 1989.

Reinecke RD. Muscle surgery. In: Tasman W, ed. *Duane's Clinical Ophthalmology*, Vol. 1. Philadelphia: JB Lippincott; 1989.

Von Noorden GK. *Atlas of Strabismus*. 4th ed. St. Louis: CV Mosby; 1983.

Ocular Disorders

Amaurosis Fugax Study Group. Amaurosis fugax (transient monocular blindness): A consensus statement. In: Bernstein EF, ed. *Amaurosis Fugax*. Heidelberg, Germany: Springer-Verlag; 1988.

Arruga J, Sanders M. Ophthalmologic findings in 70 patients with evidence of retinal embolism. *Ophthalmology* 1982;89:1336.

Hayuh SS. Hypertensive retinopathy: introduction. *Ophthalmologica* 1989;198:173.

Keith NM, Wagner HP, Barker NW. Some different types of essential hypertension, their course and prognosis. *Am J Med Sci* 1989;197: 332.

Glossary

accommodation process of ciliary muscle contraction that leads to an increase in the power of the lens of the eye.

Allen's test test performed on physical examination to determine the patency of the radial and ulnar arteries as they contribute to the circulation of the hand.

allograft graft between members of the same species.

amaurosis fugax temporary blindness; may be caused by transient ischemia from carotid artery insufficiency or centrifugal force.

amblyopia poor or decreased vision in an anatomically normal eye.

angina pectoris chest pain, heaviness, and pressure in a patient with cardiac ischemia.

anisometropia unequal refractive error between the two eyes.

annular pancreas ring of pancreas that encircles the duodenum; caused by failure of rotation of the dorsal pancreatic bud; often causes duodenal obstruction.

anterior chamber angle area of the eye where the iris meets the cornea; contains the trabecular meshwork where aqueous leaves the eye.

aphakia absence of the lens of the eye.

aphakic bullous keratopathy breakdown in the cornea that leads to bullae (large defects in the epithelium); related to damage to the endothelium from previous cataract surgery.

astigmatism refractive error in which the defect is not the same in all meridians; therefore, rays from a luminous point are not focused at a single point on the retina.

atresia congenital gap, stenosis, or intraluminal web in the esophagus or intestine; causes mechanical obstruction in the newborn.

augmentation mammaplasty surgery of the breast to increase its size.

axial pattern flap flap that is vascularized by a specific artery and vein; allows the length of the flap to significantly exceed its width.

Babinski response (Babinski sign) dorsiflexion of the great toe on painful stimulation of the sole.

Battle's sign ecchymosis overlying the mastoid process; associated with a basilar skull fracture.

bioprosthesis artificial heart valve that is composed, at least in part, by living tissue; chemically treated to prolong its viability.

Bjerrum's scotoma a wedge- or comet-shaped glaucoma defect.

blepharoplasty esthetic contouring of the eyelids.

blind spot (scotoma) nonseeing area within the visual field.

blow-out fracture isolated fracture of the orbital floor.

Bowman's membrane layer of the cornea just under the epithelium.

boxer's fracture fracture of the distal fourth or fifth metacarpal neck; usually caused by a blow to another object.

brain stem auditory evoked response (auditory brain stem response) test that measures the electroencephalographic responses to sound stimuli.

branchial cleft cyst cervical cyst that arises from developmental persistence of the ectodermal branchial grooves or endodermal pharyngeal pouches.

bronchoscope lighted instrument that is used to visualize the endobronchial anatomy; permits direct biopsy and sampling of abnormal findings.

Bruch's membrane innermost layer of the choroid, just under the retinal pigment epithelium.

canthus area formed by the junction of the upper and lower eyelids.

cardioplegia chemical paralysis of the heart in diastole; used to provide a quiet, bloodless field for surgery and to protect the myocardium during aortic cross-clamping, which precludes coronary blood flow.

cardiopulmonary bypass provision of substitute heart and lung function by a machine that transports and oxygenates blood extracorporeally.

cataract cloudiness in the crystalline lens of the eye.

cauda equina syndrome dull pain in the upper sacral region, with anesthesia or analgesia in the buttocks, genitalia, or thigh; accompanied by disturbed bowel and bladder function.

cervicofacial rhytidectomy a face-lift.

chemosis edema and swelling under the conjunctiva.

choanal atresia congenital absence of the posterior entrance into the nasopharynx from the nasal cavity.

cholesteatoma a skin-lined, keratin-producing cyst of the middle ear; probably caused by a diseased tympanic membrane.

cloaca a single perineal opening for the anus, vagina, and urethra; a rare, complex congenital anomaly.

Colles' fracture fracture of the lower end of the radius, with dorsal displacement of the distal fragment; sometimes called reversed Colles' fracture or Smith's fracture when volar displacement of the distal fragment occurs at the same site.

comminuted broken into several pieces; especially denoting a fractured bone.

compartment syndrome condition in which increased pressure in a confined anatomic space limits circulation and threatens tissue function and viability; the four leg compartments include anterior, deep posterior, lateral, and superficial posterior.

congenital diaphragmatic hernia congenital defect in a portion of the diaphragm; protrusion of intra-abdominal contents into the chest; the posterolateral Bochdalek hernia is much more common than the retrosternal hernia of Morgagni.

corneal guttae excrescences on Descemet's membrane.

coronary artery bypass grafting placement of a new conduit to circumvent coronary artery obstructions; may be autogenous (e.g., veins, arteries), a homograft, or synthetic.

coudé catheter urethral catheter with a curve along the tip; used in patients with prostate enlargement or a false passage (a straight catheter cannot be used in these patients because it cannot negotiate the upward curve of the posterior urethra); inserted with the curved tip directed upward; permits successful catheterization of the bladder.

cricothyrotomy surgical airway placed through the neck skin between the cricoid and thyroid cartilages, into the upper trachea or low subglottic space.

croup viral laryngotracheobronchitis; most commonly affects children 2 years of age or younger; usually affects the subglottic larynx, although it may extend the length of the trachea; over a period of several hours, a barking cough develops as the primary symptom; usually causes no fever or low-grade fever; physical examination shows an irritable infant with mild stridor and barking cough.

cryptorchidism failure of one or both testicles to descend to the normal scrotal position by the time of birth; if a testicle does not descend by the end of the first year, orchidopexy is performed to bring it down surgically; otherwise, spermatogenesis will not occur and the risk of subsequent malignancy is high.

cystoid macular edema swelling of the macular region, usually after surgery.

cystoscopy inspection of the interior of the bladder with a lighted tubular endoscope that allows visualization of the bladder and urethra.

decerebrate posturing extensor posturing (nonpurposeful and stereotyped) of the upper limbs, usually accompanied by extensor posturing of the lower limbs.

decorticate posturing flexor posturing (nonpurposeful and stereotyped) of the upper limbs, usually accompanied by extensor posturing of the lower limbs.

dental occlusion the manner in which the maxillary and mandibular teeth come into contact with each another.

depolarizing neuromuscular blocking agent drug that interrupts neuromuscular transmission by depolarizing the postsynaptic junction; causes transient muscle contraction; occupies the receptor to prevent further depolarization; an example is succinylcholine.

Descemet's membrane layer of cornea formed by the endothelium.

diaphysis shaft of a long bone, as distinguished from epiphysis (extremity) and apophysis (outgrowth).

diplopia double vision.

dislocation complete displacement of apposing joint surfaces.

drawer test in a knee examination, a test used to evaluate the integrity of the cruciate ligament; forward or backward sliding of the tibia indicates laxity or tear of the anterior (forward slide) or posterior (backward slide) cruciate ligaments.

Dupuytren's disease progressive palmar fasciitis and contraction.

ectropion outward rotation of the eyelid.

electronystagmography test that uses the predictable saccadic eye movements (nystagmus) that accompany various types of stimulation of the semicircular canals; periorbital electrodes are used to precisely sense and record nystagmus while the semicircular canals are stimulated with cooling, warming, and head rotation techniques.

enophthalmos posterior displacement of the globe in the orbit.

entropion inward rotation of the eyelid.

epidural hematoma blood clot that lies outside the dura (extradural), but inside the skull cavity or spinal canal.

epikeratophakia refractive corneal procedure in which a graft is placed on the patient's cornea; a living contact lens.

epiphysis part of a long bone developed from a center of ossification distinct from that of the shaft; separated at first from the shaft by a layer of cartilage.

epistaxis nasal bleeding.

esotropia misalignment of the eyes in which one eye deviates toward the other eye.

evoked otoacoustic emissions sounds that are emitted by the cochlea in response to acoustic stimulation; can be quantified to assess the hearing potential of a cochlea.

expressive (nonfluent) aphasia inability to say some or all words because of a problem with cerebral function rather than articulation; characterized by sparse speech.

external fixation method of fracture fixation that uses pins through the bone attached to an external frame.

extracorporeal membrane oxygenation type of prolonged cardiopulmonary bypass; gas exchange occurs in an external circuit that contains the patient's flowing blood; used mainly in infants with life-threatening respiratory failure.

extracorporeal shock wave lithotripsy method used to fragment urinary tract calculi (stones) with focused ultrasound energy.

fasciocutaneous flap reconstructive flap that provides thin and well-vascularized coverage from a named artery.

felon suppurative infection of the distal finger pulp.

free flap flap of skin, muscle, or bone that is transferred to a distant anatomic site with microvascular anastomosis of the blood vessels.

full-thickness skin graft graft of the full thickness of mucosa and submucosa or of skin and subcutaneous tissue, including epidermis, dermis, and a small portion of subcutaneous fat.

gamekeeper's thumb ulnar collateral ligament of the metacarpophalangeal joint of the thumb; vulnerable to the stress of thumb abduction.

ganglion cyst common benign tumor of the hand; originates from the joint spaces.

gastroschisis congenital defect of the abdominal wall to the side of the umbilical cord; the protruding viscera are not covered with a membrane, and they become chronically inflamed and edematous by the time of birth.

genu valgum knock-knee; tibia valga; deformity marked by abduction of the leg in relation to the thigh.

genu varum   bowleg; bandy leg; tibia vara; outward bowing of the leg.

greenstick fracture   bending of a bone, with incomplete fracture that involves only the convex side of the curve.

heart catheterization   injection of dye to enhance radiologic imaging; the dye outlines the coronary artery anatomy and shows ventricular and valvular function.

hemangioma   histologically benign vascular tumor; characterized initially by cellular proliferation, followed in many cases by involution; commonly located in the head and neck, but may be found anywhere; usually appears within the first few weeks after birth.

hemianopia   loss of vision in one-half of the visual field.

hemoptysis   expectoration of blood or bloody sputum.

Hirschsprung's disease   congenital absence of ganglion cells in the wall of the distal bowel (usually the rectosigmoid); leads to functional intestinal obstruction.

Hoffmann's response (Hoffmann's sign)   sudden flicking of the distal interphalangeal joint of the index, middle, or ring finger; causes flexion of one or more other fingers.

hydronephrosis   dilation of the collecting system and renal pelvis of the kidney; when seen on renal imaging studies, indicates possible ureteral or bladder outlet obstruction.

hyperopia   farsightedness; an eye that is "too short," or underpowered; corrected by adding power with "plus" lenses.

hypertrophic scar   raised, reddened scar that does not extend beyond the boundaries of the original scar.

hyphema   blood in the anterior chamber of the eye.

hypopyon   collection of pus (white cells) in the anterior chamber of the eye.

internal fixation   method of fracture fixation in which the hardware is completely contained within the body.

intra-aortic balloon pump   device that augments diastolic coronary blood flow and boosts cardiac output, thereby improving overall cardiac function; usually inserted through a femoral artery and placed just distal to the left subclavian artery.

intravenous pyelogram   imaging test used to evaluate the urinary tract; a preliminary abdominal film is obtained, contrast material is injected intravenously, and sequential films are obtained; as the dye is filtered and excreted, the films outline the urinary tract; this test also provides functional information (e.g., delay in excretion on one side suggests obstruction).

intussusception   telescoping, or invagination, of one part of the intestine into another; may cause intestinal obstruction and ischemia.

juvenile nasopharyngeal angiofibroma   highly vascular, benign tumor of adolescent boys; usually causes the classic symptoms of unilateral epistaxis and nasal obstruction.

Kanavel's signs   four signs used to diagnose tenosynovitis: fusiform swelling of the finger, finger held in a slightly flexed position, pain over the tendon sheath, and pain on passive extension of the finger.

keloid   exuberant scar tissue that mushrooms out and extends beyond the boundaries of the normal scar.

keratitis   inflammation of the cornea.

keratitis sicca   dry eye syndrome.

keratoacanthoma   rapidly growing, benign skin tumor.

keratoconus   corneal abnormality in which the cornea becomes misshapen into a conical shape; produces very distorted optics.

keratometer   device used to measure corneal curvature.

keratomileusis   lamellar keratoplasty in which the patient's cornea is lathed.

keratoplasty   corneal transplantation.

Ladd's bands   peritoneal attachments of an incompletely rotated cecum; may compress the underlying duodenum and cause obstruction.

lagophthalmos   inability to close the eyelids completely.

lateral humeral epicondylitis (tennis elbow)   overuse injury that originates in the extensor muscle of the wrist.

LeFort classification   system that classifies fractures of the maxilla based on their anatomic level.

Legg-Calve;aa-Perthes disease   epiphysial aseptic necrosis of the upper end of the femur.

limbus   vascular transition zone between the cornea and the sclera.

Luschka's joints   small synovial joints between adjacent lateral lips of the bodies of the lower cervical vertebrae.

lymphangioma   unencapsulated arcade of disorganized, thinly lined, fluid-filled spaces that often surround vital nerves and blood vessels; categorized according to the quality of the vascular structures as capillary, cavernous, or mixed.

Macintosh laryngoscope blade   gently curved instrument designed to expose the vocal cords for endotracheal intubation under direct vision when the tip is placed in the vallecula, between the epiglottis and the base of the tongue.

malignant otitis externa   osteomyelitis of the temporal bone; initiated by *Pseudomonas aeruginosa*; exposes the tympanic bone and moves into the other bones of the skull base.

mallet (baseball) finger   partial or complete avulsion of the long finger extensor from the base of the distal phalanx.

malrotation   failure of normal rotation of the intestinal tract during fetal development; the cecum is located in the right or left upper quadrant, and the duodenojejunal junction is located to the right of the midline; therefore, there is a predisposition to midgut volvulus or extrinsic duodenal compression by Ladd's bands.

mastopexy   aesthetic operation to lift the breast by removing excess skin; also known as dermal mastopexy.

mechanical (valvular) prosthesis   heart valve composed of manmade material.

Meckel's diverticulum   a blind-ending remnant of the vitelline sac that occurs in the distal ileum; may cause bleeding, obstruction, or inflammation.

meconium ileus   congenital obstruction of the distal ileum with sticky meconium; occurs in 15;pc of patients with cystic fibrosis.

metaphysis   growth zone between the epiphysis and diaphysis during development of a bone.

microtia   congenitally small or partially absent ears.

myocutaneous flap   reconstructive flap that consists of muscle and the overlying skin.

myopia   nearsightedness; an eye that is essentially too strong; rays of light are focused in the vitreous.

narrow-angle (angle-closure) glaucoma   glaucoma caused by anatomic proximity of the iris to the cornea; may be acute.

necrotizing enterocolitis   hemorrhagic necrosis of the intestine that usually occurs in premature neonates; the mucosa is initially affected, but the condition can progress to full-thickness necrosis and perforation; pneumatosis intestinalis (air in the wall of the bowel) is a pathognomonic finding on x-ray.

nevus   benign, usually pigmented skin lesion (e.g., mole).

obstructive sleep apnea   recurring periods of apnea during sleep; associated with respiratory efforts.

ora serrata   boundary between the retina and the pars plana.

organ of Corti   sensory organ found in the cochlea; transduces sound into a neural signal.

osteochondroma   solitary osteocartilaginous exostosis; benign cartilaginous neoplasm that consists of a pedicle of normal bone covered with a rim of proliferating cartilage.

osteoid osteoma   benign bone tumor that usually occurs in the femur and tibia.

osteomalacia   adult rickets; gradual softening and bending of the bones with pain of varying severity; softening is caused by inadequate bone mineralization, sometimes because of lack of vitamin D.

osteomeatal complex   region in the middle meatus of the lateral nasal wall; critical to appropriate sinus aeration; contains the anterior ethmoid sinuses, the ostia of the maxillary sinus, and the ostia of the frontal sinus.

osteoporosis   reduction in the quantity of bone or atrophy of skeletal tissue; occurs in postmenopausal women and elderly men.

otosclerosis   abnormality of the middle ear and occasionally the inner ear in which a small focus of spongy vascular bone involves all or part of the stapes footplate; causes fixation of the stapes footplate; results in conductive hearing loss.

Paget's disease   osteitis deformans; generalized skeletal disease, often familial, that affects older persons; bone resorption and formation are increased; leads to thickening and softening of bones.

papillitis   swelling of the optic disc caused by inflammation.

paronychia   infection of the perionychium (lateral nail fold).

percutaneous transluminal coronary angioplasty   percutaneous dilation to relieve coronary artery stenosis through an arterial catheter; relatively noninvasive and nonsurgical.

Phalen's sign   tingling in some or all of the radial 31\2 fingers when the wrist is flexed.

photocoagulation   laser-induced scarring.

photophobia   sensitivity to light.

plantar fasciitis (heel spur)   inflammation of the sole of the foot.

posterior fossa   the skull cavity below the tentorium.

postvoid residual   urine that is present in the bladder after voiding; can be assessed by catheterizing the bladder immediately after the patient voids and measuring the residual urine volume; a less invasive, but less accurate, test is to scan the bladder with a special ultrasound device.

prostate specific antigen   serine protease enzyme that is measured in the serum; an elevated level (>4.0) may indicate prostate cancer.

pseudophakic bullous keratopathy   permanent corneal clouding after implantation of an intraocular lens.

ptosis   drooping, often of the upper eyelid.

pulmonary artery catheter   catheter that is floated into a pulmonary artery; measures pressure, temperature, and oxygen tension to provide hemodynamic assessment.

pulmonary capillary wedge pressure   pressure measured in an end pulmonary artery; reflects left ventricular end-diastolic pressure; often used as a surrogate for volume status.

pulmonary function tests   series of measurements that assess the mechanics and physiology of breathing; used to stratify patients in terms of risk for pulmonary resection.

pulmonary resection   surgical removal of all or part of a lung to completely remove a targeted abnormality (e.g., abscess, cancer).

random-pattern skin flap   skin flap that does not contain a specific artery and vein; the length of the flap is limited to slightly greater than its width.

reduction mammaplasty   surgery of the breast to reduce its size.

reflux   usually refers to vesicoureteral reflux, a condition in which urine passes back up the ureter toward the kidney during voiding; normally, no urine should enter the ureters from the bladder at any time.

renal scan   nuclear medicine study in which a radioactive agent (with renal excretion) is administered intravenously; scanning shows renal function; in a Lasix renal scan, Lasix (furosemide) is given after tracer is injected; normally, the Lasix causes wash-out of the tracer; delayed clearance suggests obstruction.

retrobulbar   located behind the globe within the orbit.

retrograde urethrogram   study used to diagnose urethral strictures or injuries; contrast medium is injected through the urethral meatus, and a film is obtained during the injection.

rhegmatogenous   hole in the retina.

rhinitis medicamentosa   a drug-induced nasal inflammation; usually caused by abuse of decongestant nasal sprays; chronic use of the sprays causes rebound congestion sooner and sooner after each use; chronic vascular embarrassment eventually forces the abuser to spray more and more frequently to counteract this rebound congestion.

rhinoplasty   surgery to reshape and recontour the nose.

rubeosis iridis   neovascularization of the iris; an iris that has abnormal vessels that cause glaucoma when they fill the angle with vessels and cause scarring.

Salter-Harris classification   classification of epiphysial fractures into five groups (I to V), according to different prognoses regarding the effects of the injury on subsequent growth and deformity.

Schlemm's canal   channel that collects aqueous from the trabecular meshwork.

scleral buckle   surgical procedure to correct retinal detachment.

scoliosis   lateral curvature of the spine; may be flexible (correctable) or fixed (structural).

sialadenitis   inflammation of the salivary gland.

spinal stenosis   narrowing of the spinal canal with or without stenosis of the foramina.

split-thickness skin graft   a graft of portions of the skin (e.g., epidermis and part of the dermis, part of the mucosa and submucosa).

spondylolysis osteoarthritis; degeneration of the articulating part of a vertebra.

stereotactic three-dimensional localization, usually provided with a frame (to provide coordinates) and an imaging device (e.g., magnetic resonance imaging, computed tomography).

strabismus malalignment of the eyes.

stress fracture fatigue fracture that is usually caused by a sudden, strong, violent endogenous force.

stress test exercise or cardiac stimulation to provide cardiac ischemia that can be measured as to location and level of probable coronary artery obstruction.

subdural hematoma blood clot that lies outside the brain and arachnoid, but inside the dura within the skull cavity or spinal canal.

subluxation partial displacement of apposing joint surfaces.

supratentorial pertaining to the skull cavity above the tentorium.

syndactyly congenital webbing of the fingers.

syrinx (syringomyelia) a fluid-filled cavity that extends longitudinally within the center of the spinal cord; usually congenital.

talipes equinovarus (clubfoot) talipes equinus and talipes varus combined; the foot is plantar flexed, inverted, and adducted.

tenosynovitis infection of the tendon sheath, usually of the hand.

Thompson test test to determine whether the gastrocnemius soleus complex is intact; the examiner squeezes the calf muscle belly, and the foot responds with plantar flexion; lack of plantar flexion indicates a torn Achilles tendon.

thyroglossal duct cyst soft, painless, persistent midline neck mass seen in the first or second decade of life.

Tinel's sign tingling in all or part of the sensory distribution of a peripheral nerve elicited by tapping over a portion of the nerve (e.g., the median nerve at the wrist in cases of compression at that site).

tissue expansion use of an inflatable device buried beneath tissue to stretch the tissue for reconstructive purposes.

transurethral prostatectomy (transurethral resection of the prostate [TURP]) operation to treat benign prostate hypertrophy; a resectoscope is placed transurethrally, and a loop connected to a cautery is used to scoop out chips (fragments) of prostate.

transverse rectus abdominis myocutaneous (TRAM) flap method of breast reconstruction that uses the lower abdominal tissue to create the breast mound.

urinary flow rate (uroflow test) test used to evaluate the force of the urinary stream; the patient voids into a funnel-shaped container that is connected to a device that measures the urinary flow rate (volume/time); a low flow rate indicates obstruction or decreased bladder contractility.

urodynamics tests designed to evaluate bladder function; monitors and catheters are used to measure bladder pressure and flow rates; used to assess the ability of the bladder to store during filling and to empty during voiding.

VACTER association group of congenital anomalies that tend to occur together; named for their initial letters (i.e., vertebral, anorectal, cardiac, tracheal, esophageal, and radial or renal defects).

venous oxygen saturation percentage of filling of the available sites on the hemoglobin molecule by oxygen in the venous circulation.

vertigo hallucination of whirling motion when objective motion does not exist.

video-assisted thoracoscopic surgery endothoracic surgical intervention that uses telescope instrumentation to avoid open thoracotomy; can include biopsy, limited pulmonary resection, lymph node assessment, and pericardiocentesis; also called video-assisted thoracic surgery.

Vogt's ring benign, crescent-shaped white opacity at the limbus on the cornea.

wheal and flare typical cutaneous appearance of local histamine release; a central, white, raised fluid-filled wheal surrounded by an area of redness, with intense itching.

YAG laser laser that uses a neodymium-yttrium-aluminum-garnet light beam to coagulate and vaporize tissue; used to remove inflammatory or malignant tissue.

Z-plasty operation used to reorient a scar by lengthening it at the expense of width; the incisions resemble a Z.

Index

Page numbers followed by a *t* indicate a table, those followed by an *f* indicate a figure.